Transforming

Public Health Surveillance

Proactive Measures for Prevention, Detection, and Response

Transforming Public Health Surveillance

Proactive Measures for Prevention, Detection, and Response

EDITORS:

Scott JN McNabb, PhD, MS
Research Professor,
Emory University, Rollins School of Public Health
Managing Partner, Public Health Practice, LLC

J Mark Conde
Director IS and Associate Director EMPH/APHI,
Emory University, Rollins School of Public Health

Lisa Ferland, MPH
Senior Epidemiologist, Public Health Practice, LLC

William MacWright, MPH
Senior Technical Consultant, Public Health Practice, LLC

Ziad A Memish, MD
Senior Consultant Infectious Diseases,
Kingdom of Saudi Arabia, Ministry of Health
Professor, College of Medicine, Alfaisal University

Stacy Okutani, PhD
Principal Analyst, ANSER
Research Scholar, CISSM,
University of Maryland, College Park

Meeyoung M Park, MPH
Senior Public Health Program Associate,
Emory University, Rollins School of Public Health

Paige Ryland, MPH
Senior Epidemiologist, Public Health Practice, LLC

Affan T Shaikh, MPH
Senior Epidemiologist, Public Health Practice, LLC

Vivek Singh, MBBS, MPH
Associate Professor,
Public Health Foundation of India,
Indian Institute of Public Health - Hyderabad
Research Scholar, Department of Health, Ethics
and Society, CAPHRI School of Public Health
and Primary Care, Maastricht University

FOREWORDS BY:

David A Ross | James W Curran | FC Kasolo &
K Ofosu-Barko

ELSEVIER

ELSEVIER

Elsevier
7th Circle, Zahran Plaza, 7th Floor, PO Box 140825, Amman, 11814, Jordan

Transforming Public Health Surveillance: Proactive Measures for Prevention, Detection, and Response by Scott JN McNabb, J Mark Conde, Lisa Ferland, William MacWright, Ziad A Memish, Stacy Okutani, Meeyoung M Park, Paige Ryland, Affan T Shaikh, Vivek Singh

ISBN: 978-0-7020-6337-4
e-ISBN: 978-0-7020-6621-4

Printed in India

"If I have seen further than others, it is by standing upon the shoulders of giants."

– ***Sir Isaac Newton***

The authors and editors dedicate this work to ***Dr Steven Thacker****.* *At no time do we forget whose shoulders we stand upon.*

FOREWORD BY DAVID A ROSS

Early in the history of the United States, Thomas Jefferson noted that, "the health of the people is really the foundation upon which their happiness and all their power as a state depend." Creating the U.S. Public Health System was among the early of acts of a new Congress because they knew they must surveil the ports to protect against the importation of deadly diseases like syphilis, small pox, and tuberculosis.

In one form or another, mankind has always been collecting, analyzing, and responding to threats to health. One can imagine primitive man positioning lookouts to warn of threatening predators or passing along experience of what to eat and drink and what to avoid. The concept of gathering, distilling, and passing along information needed to help people adapt to their environment spans the arc of history. We mark the history of advances in surveillance with notable events like Edward Jenner observing the effects of cowpox on attenuating smallpox and John Snow making predictions based on the careful collection, analysis, and interpretation of data.

"Transforming Public Health Surveillance" advances this rich tradition of disease surveillance. This timely and needed text addresses the multiple challenges confronting health leaders as they respond to known and emerging health threats. Because people can travel to almost any corner of the earth within a few days, our world has become a new environment for monitoring, detecting, and responding to health threats. Increasingly, most people are within ready access of mobile communication devices that can inform their actions while also allowing them to inform others. Globalization and climate change are likely to have dramatic impacts on societies across the globe. Predictions about climate change tell us that we should expect significant displacement of populations due to extreme weather, rising seas, and desertification. Globalization has changed how and what we eat, thereby introducing complexity into foodborne disease surveillance. Technological innovation has transformed what people know, when they know it, and how they respond to health-related information.

Understanding our rapidly evolving ecology and social situation demands new approaches to and a keen awareness of the concepts underpinning health surveillance. Implementing surveillance systems in today's context presents challenges not previously faced. "Transforming Public Health Surveillance" presents contributions from leading experts who have years of experience confronting the unique ways in which surveillance systems are funded and governed, as well as expertise in conceptualizing, designing, and using surveillance data to protect the public's health.

Today's global health security environment demonstrates that effective health surveillance requires a conjunction of cross-sectoral political will, leadership, and economic self-interest supported by scientists knowledgeable in the concepts, models, and methods of making effective surveillance systems. The editors and authors of this text present expert and experienced guidance across the spectrum of challenges presented today.

Responding to emerging threats, like Ebola, challenges political and health leaders, threatens the social fabric of fragile economies, and emphasizes to health authorities the need for them to understand state-of-the-art surveillance system techniques and designs. "Transforming Public Health Surveillance" offers authoritative advice and examples covering the ways in which systems can be envisioned, the economics and evaluation of surveillance systems, workforce requirements, governance and geopolitical considerations, how multiple sectors can and must collaborate, and how informatics innovations will build an information ecology capable of producing more timely and accurate surveillance information.

Roman philosopher Marcus Tullius Cicero said, "let us not go over the old ground, let us rather prepare for what is to come." The editors of "Transforming Public Health Surveillance" have done just that. They have compiled an expert panel of contributing authors and have presented a timely text, aimed at preparing health and political leaders to prepare surveillance capabilities for what is to come. Today's health surveillance environment must accommodate point of care diagnostic technology as well as deal with locales that do not have electricity. Effective surveillance today must anticipate infectious and non-infectious causes of threats and must inform and, hopefully, support timely, targeted, and impactful interventions. This text provides the reference needed across continents to support improved surveillance capability.

David A Ross, ScD
Director, Public Health Informatics Institute and
CEO/President, The Task Force for Global Health

Public health has been defined as "what we, as a society, do collectively to assure the conditions in which people can be healthy."[1] In any jurisdiction, be it local, regional, or national, government has a major responsibility for the health of citizens and other residents and, hence, for public health. The core functions for public health agencies are assessment, policy development, and assurance.[2] All public health action should be based upon an accurate and timely assessment of the health conditions, current and potential threats, and risk factors of the population. The central activity of public health assessment is excellent surveillance. Timely surveillance is the conscience of public health and the guidepost for priority setting and public health action.

"Transforming Public Health Surveillance" provides essential information on the implementation of surveillance systems in a variety of situations in different countries with a wide array of health threats and varying capacity, emerging health threats know few geographic boundaries. Hence, the volume cogently addresses the international necessity for timeliness, consistency, and collaboration in conducting surveillance and rapidly communicating results. Authors from a dozen countries share lessons and address scientific, technical, and other implementation issues related to surveillance. The authors describe crucial contributions to be made for accurate surveillance for governments, academia, non-governmental organizations, and others and address how rapidly expanding biologic and communications technologies enhance surveillance capacity.

Over thirty years ago, clusters of fatal opportunistic infections and a rare cancer (Kaposi's sarcoma) were first noted in the United States.[3,4] The first step at the Centers for Disease Control and Prevention was to establish a case definition for active surveillance of the outbreak.[5] Other nations and the World Health Organization soon joined in the surveillance efforts. This surveillance approach rapidly identified the epidemiologic patterns for the condition soon to be named acquired immune deficiency syndrome, or AIDS. The epidemic was new and rapidly increasing. Populations affected and identified through surveillance suggested the cause was most likely an infectious agent transmitted through sexual contact or blood exposure. Thanks to excellent surveillance, even before the etiology was known, consensus recommendations for prevention of AIDS were published and promulgated by the US Public Health Service agencies.[6,7] Furthermore, this pattern assisted the focus of scientists who identified the human immunodeficiency virus (HIV) as the cause of AIDS within two years of the first reports.[8,9] HIV/AIDS and risk factor surveillance remain crucial throughout the world to prioritize scarce resources and evaluate prevention and care efforts for this global epidemic.

---

[1]The Future of Public Health; Committee for the Study of the Future of Public Health, Institute of Medicine, National Academy Press, p. 1, Washington, DC, 1988.

[2]Ibid, p. 7.

[3]CDC. Pneumocystis pneumonia – Los Angeles. *MMWR* 1981;30:1–3.

[4]CDC. Kaposi's sarcoma and Pneumocystis pneumonia among homosexual men – New York City and California. *MMWR* 1981;30:305–08.

[5]Curran JW, Jaffe HW. AIDS: the early years and CDC's response. *MMWR* 2011;60:64–9.

[6]CDC. Acquired immunodeficiency syndrome (AIDS) precautions for clinical and laboratory staffs. *MMWR* 1982;31:577–80.

[7]CDC. Prevention of acquired immune deficiency syndrome (AIDS): report of inter-agency recommendations. *MMWR* 1983;32:1–3.

[8]Barre-Sinoussi F, Chermann JHW, Rey F, et al. Isolation of a Flymphotropic retrovirus from a patient at risk for acquired immune deficiency syndrome (AIDS). *Science* 1983;220:868–71.

[9]Gallo RC, Salahuddin SZ, Popovic M, et al. Frequent detection and isolation of cytopathia retroviruses (HILV-III) from patients with AIDS and at risk for AIDS. *Science* 1984;224:500–03.

For all public health problems, accurate and timely surveillance is critical to identify threats, establish priorities, and identify the most effective response. Good public health surveillance is often expensive and therefore must select the highest priority topics and be conducted most efficiently. This timely volume addresses the issues necessary to establish and conduct effective surveillance to ensure the health of the public.

James W Curran MD, MPH
Dean, Rollins School of Public Health,
Emory University

FOREWORD BY FRANCIS CHISAKA KASOLO & KENNETH OFOSU-BARKO

We are at the dawn of a new era in public health surveillance (PHS), where widespread information and communication technologies (ICT) are utilized to increase our ability to detect, assess, report, and respond to public health threats and emergencies. The use of electronic systems for public health surveillance, e-Surveillance, is emerging as one of the most exciting and promising developments in public health.

Niccolo Machiavelli once said, "*in the beginning of the malady it is easy to cure but difficult to detect, but in the course of time, not having been either detected or treated in the beginning, it becomes easy to detect but difficult to cure*"[i]. He was only re-echoing what has been known for centuries.

The recent Ebola epidemic in West Africa speaks to this concept. The surveillance systems in the affected countries were incapable of detecting the presence of Ebola early, when it was small and easier to contain. As the outbreak grew and health professionals knew to suspect Ebola, it became easier to diagnose, but the situation became overwhelming and increasingly more difficult to contain.

The major reason leading to the delayed reports of the first Ebola cases was the inability of health workers and community members to transmit information to the national level for action in a timely and structured fashion. This can be partly attributed to the current methods of reporting, which largely depend on delivering hard copies of reports, investigation forms, and data.

The high number of deaths faced in the recent Ebola wake can be avoided. Take for example the lesser known and broadcasted Ebola outbreak that occurred in May 2011 in Uganda. A single case was detected in Nakisamata Village, Ngalonkalu Parish, Zirobwe sub-county, Luwero District in Uganda. The local community health worker who first detected the case was able to use the technology mTrac, a phone-based short messaging system (SMS) platform, to report the suspected case to the national level. This prompted an immediate investigation and allowed the body to be disposed of safely[ii]. These actions led to complete containment of the disease and a zero transmission rate. This success story demonstrates what we believe the transformation and strengthening of public health surveillance can achieve by ensuring the timely detection, investigation, and effective response to outbreaks.

Although some countries are using electronic systems for data collection and compilation, most African countries are still using paper based recording and reporting tools, especially at the peripheral and intermediate levels. This frequently leads to inadequate data management and suboptimal use of information for action. In addition, lack of policies for standardization of electronic tools makes it difficult to easily generate and share country and regional profiles of priority diseases, conditions, and events.

A thoughtfully planned e-Surveillance system would have offered more timely and structured detection, reporting, assessment, and response, at an earlier stage in the spread of the disease, when the number of cases were smaller and easier to contain. This is what makes e-Surveillance so vitally important, though not without its own difficulties.

In order for functional e-Surveillance to be realized in the African region and across the globe, a number of precursors are required including a well-trained workforce, international cooperation, regionally aligned and nationally enforced standards to ensure interoperability, and a complementary strategy. For this to be possible, political will and commitment from leaders (who understand the importance of an early disease warning system) for improved global security are vitally important.

In addition, e-Surveillance will require investment in the public health workforce. Current public health professionals will require in-service training on the standard operating procedures (SOPs) for use of e-Surveillance,

---

[i] Niccola Machiavelli; Rufus Goodwin, *The Prince, Dante University Press@2003.*

[ii] Shoemaker T, MacNeil A, Balinandi S, et al. Reemerging Sudan Ebola virus disease in Uganda, 2011. *Emerging Infectious Diseases* 2012;18(9):1480–83.

and e-Surveillance will need to be incorporated in current public health training programs. While public health professionals are at the very center of public health surveillance, the shift to e-Surveillance alters the necessary human resources to operate the changing systems. In addition to epidemiologists and the typical public health workforce, informaticians and ICT professionals must be trained and incorporated into the public health surveillance workflow. The addition of informaticians and ICT professionals in the public health surveillance workflow adds professionals with the necessary competencies to maintain, enhance, and manage the e-Surveillance system.

The recent Ebola epidemic clearly underscores the concept that a disease can, and will, move seamlessly across borders. To address this difficulty, partnerships across the public and private sectors are required. Of paramount importance is the understanding between countries that sharing surveillance data is crucial to halting the spread of disease. While policies are needed to ensure the sanctity of national sovereignty, sharing information must occur to make cross border surveillance easier and increase the index of suspicion.

To address weaknesses in the current surveillance systems, the WHO Regional Office for Africa in collaboration with other technical partners, such as the African Field Epidemiology Networks (AFENET), is developing an IDSR e-Surveillance policy and technical approach to be used by Member States to strengthen public health surveillance and response functions. It is envisioned that this will further facilitate the public health surveillance functions of prevention, detection, and response across borders in the region.

As this book discusses all of the ingredients necessary for functional e-Surveillance, it is being published at an opportune time and will provide a vision for what public health surveillance can and should do to meet the demands of today's world. The authors and editing team have provided content that spans from the historical contributions of public health surveillance to what innovations are possible in the future. The books' ideas are presented in six sections to highlight how governance, collaboration, informatics, and knowledge (data, analytics, and intelligence) are the necessary building blocks to propel the transformation of public health surveillance. These themes support the case that an enhanced workforce, strong international collaborations, and a complementary global strategy are key to enhanced prevention, prediction, detection, and response; which together work to meet the goal of strengthened global security.

Francis Chisaka Kasolo, MD, MSc, PHD, DTM&H (RCP)
Immediate Past Director, Disease Prevention and Control Cluster; WHO Regional Office for Africa, Brazzaville Congo

Kenneth Ofosu-Barko, MD, MPH
Executive Director, African Field Epidemiology Network, Kampala Uganda

PREFACE

Recent pandemics and the corresponding threats posed to global health security point out that strengthening public health surveillance is critical. *Transforming Public Health Surveillance* was conceived by a group of public health authorities working in the field of disease surveillance whose decades of combined experience enable them to see the current state of public health surveillance while envisioning how it is changing around the world in response to new challenges and opportunities. The way forward is not always clear and straightforward but several key issues have been identified as the necessary steps in ensuring that the path is smooth and successful.

As a reader, you will move through six sections: Current State of Public Health; Governance Unlocks Transformation; Collaboration Fuels Transformation; Informatics Enables Transformation; New Data, Analytics, and Intelligence (Knowledge) Enlightens Transformation; and Impacts of Transformed Public Health, taking you from a view of what is to the vision of what can be. As chapter authors present necessary considerations for this transformation, you will be convinced that public health surveillance must undergo this transformation successfully in order to sustain a safe and healthy world.

ACKNOWLEDGEMENTS

This work would not be possible without the contributions of a dedicated and engaged global team of passionate thought leaders in public health surveillance. We wish to acknowledge all those who have provided countless hours of administrative, editing, and research assistance in the completion of this work. Further, we would like to thank the institutions that have contributed the knowledge and experience necessary for understanding where we are going and how we can get there. Finally, we wish to offer a hearty and humble "thank you" to the editing, content, and marketing teams at Elsevier for their continued patience and steady guidance throughout the processes of conceptualizing, writing, and finalizing this project that we are very proud to present to you, the reader.

CONTRIBUTORS

Kaosar Afsana, MD, PhD, MPH
Director, Bangladesh Rural Advancement Committee (BRAC) Health Programme,
Professor, James P Grant School of Public Health, BRAC University, Bangladesh

Paul A Biedrzycki, MPH, MBA, CIH
Director, Division of Disease Control and Environmental Health
City of Milwaukee Health Department

Richard V Birtwhistle, MD
Departments of Family Medicine and Public Health Sciences, Queen's University
Canadian Primary Care Sentinel Surveillance Network

Leonard "Will" Chapman, MBA
Program Manager, Defense Threat Reduction Agency

JP Chretien, MD, PhD
Lead, Innovation & Evaluation Team, Armed Forces Health Surveillance Center

Stella Chungong, MD, MPH
National Surveillance System Strengthening and Monitoring for the International Health Regulations (IHR), World Health Organization, Geneva

Noelle M Cocoros, DSc, MPH
Epidemiologist, Department of Population Medicine, Harvard Medical School and Harvard Pilgrim Health Care Institute, Boston, MA

J Mark Conde
Director IS and Associate Director EMPH/APHI, Emory University, Rollins School of Public Health

Kara Contreary, PhD
Researcher, Mathematica Policy Research
Formerly Prevention Effectiveness Fellow, Centers for Disease Control & Prevention

Arthur J Davidson, MD
Denver Public Health, Denver Health, Denver, CO

Stephane de la Rocque, DVM, PhD
National Surveillance System Strengthening and Monitoring for the International Health Regulations (IHR), World Health Organization, Geneva

Alfred DeMaria, Jr, MD
Medical Director, Bureau of Infectious Disease
Senior Epidemiologist, Massachusetts Department of Public Health

Isabelle Devaux, PhD, MPH
European Centre for Disease Prevention and Control, Stockholm

Matthew D Dollacker
Managing Director, Inductive Health Informatics Atlanta, Georgia USA

Julia Dooher, PhD
Johns Hopkins University Applied Physics Laboratory
Formerly American Association for the Advancement of Science (AAAS) Science and Technology Policy Fellow, Department of Defense

Jeffrey Engel, MD
Executive Director, Council of State and Territorial Epidemiologists, Atlanta, GA

Ngozi Erondu, PhD
London School of Hygiene and Tropical Medicine

Julie E Fischer, PhD
Associate Research Professor, George Washington University

Betsy Foxman, PhD
Professor of Epidemiology, University of Michigan

Rajeev Gera, MBBS, MPH
Chief of Party, RMNCH+A/USAID, IP Global Private Limited
Formerly, Senior Advisor, Monitoring and Evaluation, Immunization Technical Support Unit, Public Health Foundation of India

Tracey Goldstein, PhD
Associate Director, One Health Institute, School of Veterinary Medicine, University of California, Davis

Gigi Kwik Gronvall, PhD
Senior Associate, University of Pittsburg Medical Center, Center for Health Security

Gillian Haney, MPH
Director, Office of Integrated Surveillance and Informatics Services, Bureau of Infectious Disease, Massachusetts Department of Public Health

Habib Hasan, MD
Associate Professor, Public Health Foundation of India, Indian Institute of Public Health - Delhi

David L Heymann, MD
Professor, Infectious Disease Epidemiology, London School of Hygiene and Tropical Medicine
Head and Senior Fellow, Chatham House Centre on Global Health Security (London)

Richard S Hopkins, MD, MSPH
Adjunct Professor, Department of Epidemiology, Colleges of Medicine and of Public Health and Health Professions, University of Florida

Edmund Howard
Research Assistant, Chatham House Centre on Global Health Security (London)

Edward L Ionides, PhD
Professor of Statistics, University of Michigan

Rebecca Katz, PhD, MPH, MPA
Associate Professor, Milken Institute School of Public Health, George Washington University

Hayat Khogali, MBBS, MSc, MD
Director National Epidemiology and Zoonotic Disease Program, Federal Ministry of Health, Republic of Sudan
Senior Medical Epidemiologist, Federal Ministry of Health, Republic of Sudan

Ann Marie Kimball, MD, MPH
Senior Consulting Fellow, Chatham House Royal Institute of Foreign Affairs
Global Health and Bioethics and Humanities, University of Washington

Michael Klompas, MD, MPH, FRCPC
Associate Professor, Department of Population Medicine, Harvard Medical School and Harvard Pilgrim Health Care Institute, Boston, MA

James S Koopman, MD, MPH
Professor, Department of Epidemiology University of Michigan

Thomas Krafft, MSc, Dr. rer. Nat.
Associate Professor, Department of Health, Ethics and Society, CAPHRI School of Public Health and Primary Care, Maastricht University the Netherlands

Ramesh Krishnamurthy, PhD, MPH, MS, MA
eHealth: Standardization and Interoperability, Health Systems and Innovation Cluster, World Health Organization

Anna S Kushnir, PhD
Gryphon Scientific LLC, Takoma Park, MD, USA

William MacWright, MPH
Senior Epidemiologist, Public Health Practice, LLC, Atlanta, GA,

Jonna AK Mazet, DVM, MPVM, PhD
Executive Director, One Health Institute, School of Veterinary Medicine, University of California Davis, California

Haley McDermott, MPH
Program Manager, Global Health & Internal Medicine, School of Medicine, University of California Davis

Scott JN McNabb, PhD, MS
Research Professor, Emory University, Rollins School of Public Health

Kieran Moore, MD, CCFP(EM), FCFP, MPH, DTM&H, FRCPC
Associate Medical Officer of Health, Kingtson, Frontenac and Lennox & Addington Public Health, Kingston Ontario
Program Director, Queen's Public Health and Preventive Medicine

Peter Nsubuga, MD, MPH
Medical Epidemiologist, Global Public Health Solutions

Jennifer B Nuzzo, DrPH, SM
Senior Associate, University of Pittsburg Medical Center, Center for Health Security

Meeyoung M Park, MPH
Senior Public Health Program Associate, Emory University, Rollins School of Public Health

Mahomed Said Patel, MBBCh, FRACP, FAFPHM
Associate Professor, Australian National University, Canberra, Australia

Christine Phillips, MBBS, BMedSc, MA, MPH, DipEd, FRACGP
Associate Professor, Australian National University, Canberra, Australia

Eva Pilot, MSc
Researcher, Department of Health, Ethics and Society, CAPHRI School of Public Health and Primary Care, Maastricht University, the Netherlands

Richard Platt, MD, MSc
Professor and Chair, Department of Population Medicine, Harvard Medical School and Harvard Pilgrim Health Care Institute, Boston, MA

Lauren Reeves, MPA
Senior Health Communication Specialist, Public Health Practice, LLC

Chesley L Richards, MD, MPH, FACP
Director, Office of Public Health Scientific Services, Centers for Disease Control and Prevention

Beth E Rivin, MD, MPH
Adjunct Research Associate Professor, Global Health and Bioethics and Humanities, University of Washington

Henry Rolka, MS
Formerly Division of Epidemiology, Analysis, and Library Services
Center for Surveillance, Epidemiology and Laboratory Services
Office of Public Health Scientific Services
Centers for Disease Control & Prevention

Kevin L Russell, MD, MTM&H, FIDSA
Country Director, Centers for Disease Control and Prevention, Bangladesh
Previous Director, Armed Forces Health Surveillance Center, US Department of Defense

Paige Ryland, MPH
Senior Epidemiologist, Public Health Practice, LLC

Bidyut K Sarkar, MD, PhD
Senior Research Scientist, Public Health Foundation of India (PHFI), India

Affan T Shaikh, MPH
Senior Epidemiologist, Public Health Practice, LLC

Prem Singh, MD
Associate Advisor, Evaluation, Immunization Technical Support Unit (ITSU), Public Health Foundation of India (PHFI) and Ministry of Health and Family Welfare (MOHFW), India

Vivek Singh, MBBS, MPH
Associate Professor, Public Health Foundation of India, Indian Institute of Public Health - Hyderabad
Research Scholar, Department of Health, Ethics and Society, CAPHRI School of Public Health and Primary Care, Maastricht University

Paula Soper, MS, MPH, PMP, DrPH
Senior Director, Public Health Informatics, Association of State and Territorial Health Officials (ASTHO)

Rajesh Sreedharan, MD, MPH
National Surveillance System Strengthening and Monitoring for the International Health Regulations (IHR), World Health Organization, Geneva

Arunkumar Srinivasan, PhD
Informatics Science Lead, National Center for Chronic Disease Prevention and Health Promotion, United States Centers for Disease Control and Prevention

Laura C Streichert, PhD, MPH
Executive Director, International Society for Disease Surveillance (ISDS)

Jennifer Ward, MS
Senior Analyst, SRA International

Ian Watson, MS, MA, MPH
Branch Chief for AFRICOM/CENTCOM, Cooperative Biological Engagement Program at Defense Threat Reduction Agency (DTRA)

Andy Weber, MS
Formerly Deputy Coordinator for Ebola Response, US Department of State
Formerly Assistant Secretary of Defense (ASD) for Nuclear, Chemical, and Biological Defense Programs (NCB), US Department of Defense, USA

Jun Xing, MD, MPPM
National Surveillance System Strengthening and Monitoring for the International Health Regulations (IHR), World Health Organization, Geneva

Sanjay Zodpey, MD, PhD
Director, Indian Institute of Public Health - Delhi
Vice President North, Public Health Foundation of India

CONTENTS

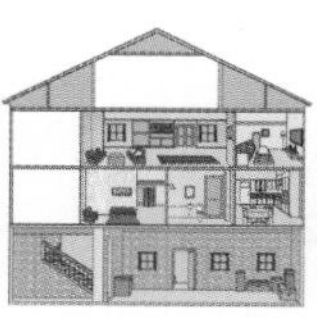

SECTION 4 Informatics Enables Transformation

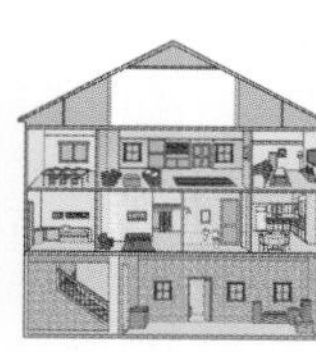

SECTION 5 New Data, Analytics, and Intelligence (Knowledge) Enlightens Transformation

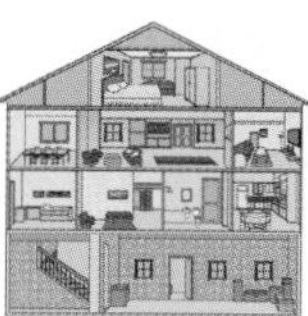

SECTION 6 Impacts of Transformed Public Health Surveillance

INTRODUCTION

The Next Generation of Public Health Surveillance

Scott JN McNabb, Leonard "Will" Chapman, Paige Ryland, William MacWright, Jennifer Ward, Hayat Khogali, Affan T Shaikh

There is nothing more difficult to take in hand, more perilous to conduct, or more uncertain in its success, than to take the lead in the introduction of a new order of things.

Niccolo Machiavelli, The Prince (1532)

KEY WORDS

Public health surveillance strengthening
Public health surveillance
e-Surveillance
One Health

THE PROMISE OF PUBLIC HEALTH SURVEILLANCE IN THE TWENTY-FIRST CENTURY

The world is different now. Public health—like other fields of health and medicine—must meet the challenges of our time and take advantage of emerging opportunities. **Public health surveillance** (**PHS**), the cornerstone science of public health,[1] must adapt. Our times do have historic uniqueness: extremely rapid human transportation and communication; frequent and large mass gatherings of people; broad climatic changes; and the growing immediacy of the interaction between animals and humans.

And while different, our times hold opportunities: information and communication technology (ICT) and tools; digital data standards; new data sources; and new analytic and visualization techniques. These promise to revolutionize our ability to prevent, detect, report, confirm, assess, communicate, and respond to emerging public health threats. In the coming era, public health data will be more comprehensive and precise, increasingly accessible, and more meaningful to decision-makers. One day it will be possible—with a few taps of a finger on a smartphone app—to collect and visualize public health data in real time to find epidemiologic information from anywhere in the world—public health information, when it is needed, where it is needed. This is a human right.

However, this vision must overcome gaps and impediments in four key areas that limit advances: governance, collaboration, informatics, and analytics. **Public health surveillance strengthening** (**PHSS**) means adopting thoughtful policies (e.g., reportable disease lists and frequencies, case definitions) based on global best practices. It involves harmonizing, synergizing, and integrating local, district, provincial, and national PHS workflow processes; standardizing reporting instruments; and training the workforce. It is the process of streamlining an antiquated workflow process; establishing global best practices in governance, policies, structures, and practices; building collaborations; and implementing standards to enhance the structure and platform that supports and bolsters the new opportunities to advance PHS in the twenty-first century. This includes the adoption of empowering ICT. But the tail does not wag the dog; meaning PHSS should precede the empowering of the renovated workflow processes by ICT, not be driven by it.

This book examines current models of PHS; analyzes the essential processes of PHSS; and explores how adapting or improving governance, collaboration, informatics, and analytics can enhance prevention, detection,

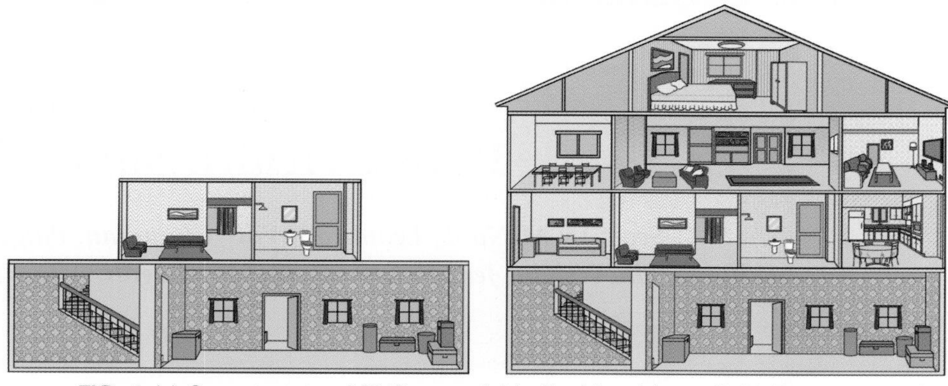

FIG. 1 (a) Current state of PHS as an "old, dilapidated house." (b) Future state of PHS as a "new, smart home."

and response. It describes how through respectful, mindful governance and mutually beneficial, multi-actor collaboration, the public health community can obtain the maximum benefit from modern advances in informatics and analytics.

Bringing together global thought leaders, policy makers, subject matter experts (SMEs), and practitioners who represent the disciplines required to transform PHS, this book visualizes and expresses (with applied intention) the transformation of PHS. And this transformation—using the metaphor of remodeling a dilapidated, old house—moves the field from its current state (imaged as an old, dilapidated house in Fig. 1a) to a future one (imaged as a remodeled, smart home in Fig. 1b). A vision now emerges where the PHS workforce implements the best techniques, uses the latest technologies, shares best practices, and networks locally, nationally, regionally, and globally. This book describes a road map of how to achieve this future state of a remodeled, smart home while pointing out the impediments, gaps, and milestones along the way.

Strengthening PHS is the key to prevent and reduce the impacts of global health security risks.[2] PHS offers the ability to predict and detect emerging heath threats. The ICT (i.e., standards for data coding, database structure, and data types, flow, and interchange methods) tools and analytic foundations necessary to achieve this future vision exist.[3] However, governance and collaboration are of varied effectiveness and need strengthening.[4]

Through the transformative processes of PHSS, the bricks are cemented, the roof is laid and the walls and interior doorways constructed into a new, smart home. PHS can be empowered by **electronic surveillance (e-Surveillance)** defined as the use of ICT to enable efficient and effective PHS workflow processes with functions designed to prevent, predict, detect, and respond.[1] And, just as the architect must follow local building codes and secure permits when remodeling a structure, there are key principles of PHSS and e-Surveillance that guide and govern its deployment (Fig. 2). Embracing innovation and mustering the political resolve to focus and financially invest in this transformation requires leadership and courage.

The scientific and technical transformation of PHS can only occur after up-to-date, mindful, transnational governance policies are adopted that meet current and future needs. This means expanding and building upon the existing International Health Regulations (IHR [2005]) framework.[5,6] This vision links nongovernmental organizations (NGOs) with government to strengthen PHS. The interventions proposed demonstrate the value, advantages, and potential of transforming PHS from an underfunded, siloed, and professionally neglected endeavor into an undertaking suited for the twenty-first century and beyond. And while not easy, it is necessary.

But I have promises to keep, and miles to go before I sleep, and miles to go before I sleep.[7]

Robert Frost, *Stopping by Woods on a Snowy Evening*

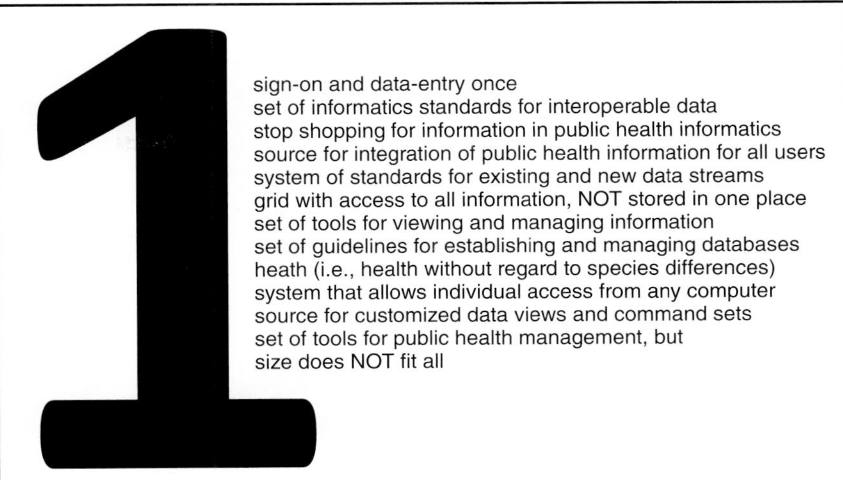

FIG. 2 Key principles of e-Surveillance.

SECTION 1—CURRENT STATE OF PUBLIC HEALTH SURVEILLANCE

The recent MERS-CoV and Ebola epidemics show that it is misguided to believe that hoarding of public health data, information, and messages (plus the technologies that support them) is advantageous to improve either a political or economic position; more so than ever, one nation's public health concerns impact all of us.[8]

This generation of public health leaders is poised to realize the full benefit that a remodeled and transformed PHS can provide to global health security; but a globally accepted, unified vision and concerted effort are missing.[9] As stated, transforming PHS to be effective and efficient for the twenty-first century could be analogous to the physical effort of renovating an old, dilapidated house (Fig. 1a) into a smart home; a home prepared to seamlessly integrate technology and the demands of modern life (Fig. 1b). In this metaphor of renovating an old house, we perceive the foundation of the house to be established and laid (Fig. 1a). The concrete footing (PHS purposes, objectives, and principles) and foundational bricks (PHS workflow processes) are aligned and in place. But the house is not equipped for the demands of the twenty-first century.

Transforming PHS first requires a comprehensive, insightful, and informed understanding of the current state (Section 1). Once surveyed (Chapter 3), the models of the systematic, ongoing collection of public health data to detect, report, confirm, analyze, communicate, and respond to emerging threats reveal an inefficient paradigm in need of reform ("restoration" using the metaphor). The use of various PHS models (i.e., indicator-based, event-based, predictive, participatory, and syndromic) (Chapter 3) depends on different circumstances faced by the PHS practitioner (i.e., routine time, seasonal occurrence of reportable conditions, outbreaks, or disaster/mass gathering). And the public health information—or situation awareness—needed by PHS practitioners to take action varies by circumstance (Fig. 3a–d).

While the purposes and objectives of PHS remain the same, different circumstances require new models, data, and methodologies. PHS models are stuck in a mire of siloed verticality (i.e., health outcome-specific funding and organizational structured systems) (Chapter 4). Based on *(i)* siloed funding streams (money and politics), *(ii)* narrow-minded and parochial public health attitudes and corporate culture (people), and *(iii)* outdated, administrative guidelines (policies), PHS now is neither efficient nor effective.

A recent report by the Council on Foreign Relations hinted at this by remarking, "Considering the merits and gaps of both horizontal and vertical healthcare approaches, [. . .] international health diplomacy should place greater emphasis on building horizontal, integrated healthcare systems to avoid similar pandemics like that of

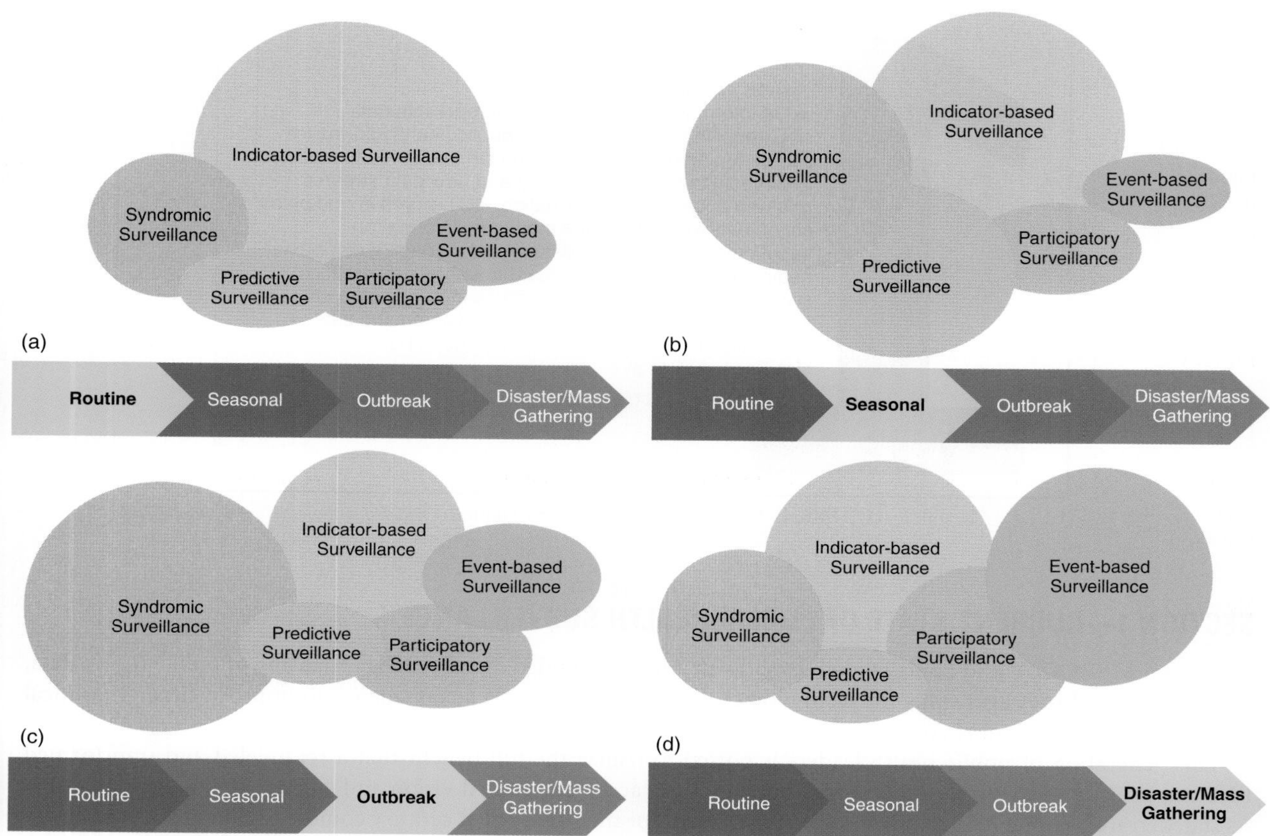

FIG. 3 Public health information useful to an epidemiologist during (a) routine times, by PHS model; (b) seasonal occurrences of reportable conditions, by PHS model; (c) outbreaks, by PHS model; (d) disaster or mass gathering, by PHS model.

Ebola."[10] Transforming existing legacy, siloed PHS (i.e., vertical systems that chase health outcome-specific data), into an integrated enterprise requires financial commitment and political will, which is driven by a clear, compelling vision and effective and efficient set of workflow processes. Success will require assertive efforts toward PHSS and e-Surveillance to "renovate the old, dilapidated house."

Another issue to consider is the role of reactive versus proactive PHS (Chapter 5). The drive to establish electronic health information systems (e-Health) creates new possibilities for PHS. In emerging proactive systems, triggered alerts can forecast future events. Innovative applications of these systems, including pharmacosurveillance, require collaboration among public and private partners. The internet and social media provide additional perspectives to population health and health system utilization. This new reality will lead to new legislative and policy frameworks to ensure proper collection of high-quality data from electronic health records (EHRs).

Monitoring measures the pulse of PHS and evaluation measures its functionality (effectiveness and efficiency). The U.S. Centers for Disease Control and Prevention (CDC) guidelines for evaluating PHS systems present an evaluation process that has been used for decades.[11-13] However, new PHS evaluation models (Chapters 6 and 7) are being developed that incorporate business concepts and the principles of health economics such as the workflow process analysis framework to determine gaps and impediments preventing efficient and effective PHS. These new models hold the promise of a more comprehensive evaluation linked to process, output, and outcome indicators. Evaluation plans should offer a clear and comprehensive understanding of the PHS system, complemented with contextual factors, costs, and potential areas for integration.

Health economics plays a significant role in determining the current state of PHS (Chapter 8). With new donors, stakeholders, and partners involved in global health, the expectations for measuring impact add emphasis to measuring outputs and outcomes and the return on investment, as opposed to just the process indicators. While there is no standard methodology for evaluating the benefit of a national PHS system, let alone a global one, researchers increasingly turn to calculating the benefits associated with number of cases and deaths averted. Linked to economics, workforce development is an important consideration that challenges efficient and effective PHS (Chapter 9). Public health professionals with epidemiologic training are few and far between, especially in underserved, underdeveloped countries. The rise of competency-based field epidemiology training programs (FETPs) gives countries opportunities to train the next generation of PHS professionals, but important gaps in competencies and capacity remain to be addressed.

FOUR KEY, HIGH-LEVEL, CONTEMPORARY MOVEMENTS

This book communicates how four key, high-level contemporary movements will empower and enable PHSS and e-Surveillance. They are governance (Section 2), collaboration (Section 3), informatics (Section 4), and analytics (Section 5). These movements map in a logic model showing inputs, outputs, and outcomes (Fig. 4).

Section 2—Governance Unlocks Transformation

Starting with the roof, the twentieth-century PHS model reinforces the idea that trade and commerce across national borders increase the risk of domestic plagues. This governance model fails in our fast-paced, globalized

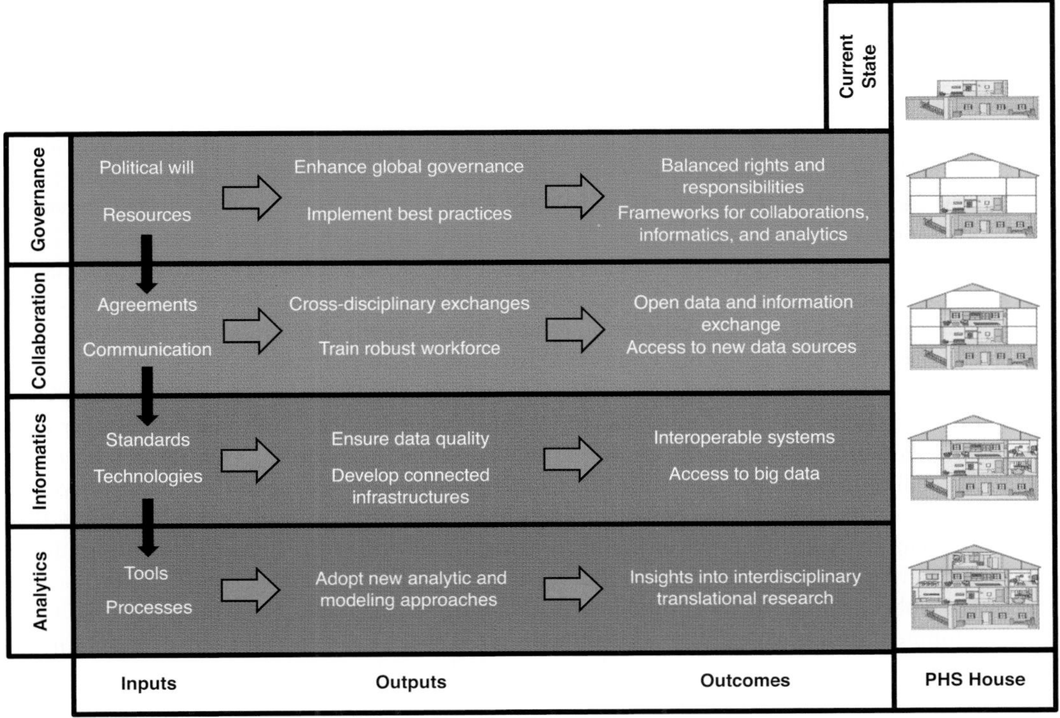

FIG. 4 Logic model of four movements to transform PHS.

twenty-first century world.[14,15] Current outdated governance models (e.g., policies, treaties, conventions) for global and domestic PHS must be updated to achieve an efficient and effective set of organized, integrated, and sequential workflow processes. The PHS "smart home" must be covered by the roof of transnational agreements aligned to twenty-first century realities (Fig. 5).

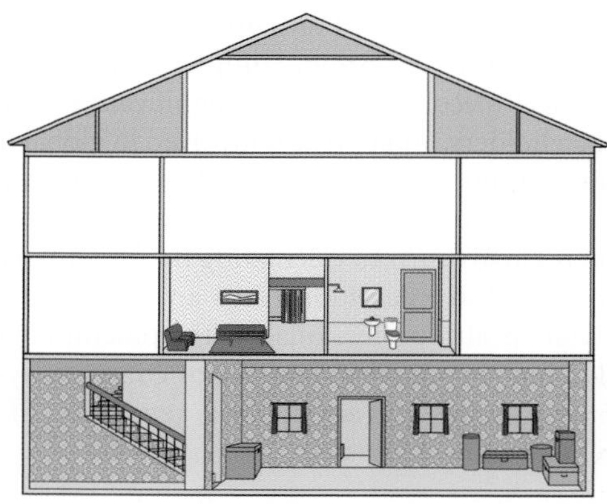

FIG. 5 Governance unlocks PHS transformation.

Today, PHS governance requires complete recognition of the mutual benefits and risks to global health and the economy; capacity investments; and transnational and national integration of public health information across public and private sectors. We should enhance the foundation built by the revised IHR (2005) to address the critical issues of our time including data stewardship; sovereignty of physical (e.g., patient specimens, isolates) and intellectual property; collaborative agreements for investigating public health events of international concern (PHEIC); and the democratizing power of the internet and social media.

Governance frameworks must be balanced by consideration of global PHS needs, while respecting national sovereign rights.[8] Governance models should embrace the adoption of new technologies in such a way as to maximize benefits and minimize risk. Adoption of novel applications of technology to support PHS could include smartphone apps, geographic information systems (GIS), and automated disease reporting algorithms and tools. We must be able to gather and analyze new data from nontraditional sources, and we must develop and adapt new technologies to improve data reporting and analyses. The technological revolution witnessed now will allow us to predict events, trigger more timely responses, and close the boundary between reacting to public health threats and preventing them.

Admittedly, there are concerns about openly sharing public health data, information, and messages.[16,17] However, it is important to realize that in the age of social media, information flows across borders just as freely as viruses. Legitimate concerns about privacy can be resolved through data stewardship agreements and informatics tools and techniques. These impediments must be overcome if our ultimate goal is to improve health and respond to imminent public health threats in a timely and effective manner. Only by working together, with transparent governance and mutual respect, can organizations and nations begin to build the trust necessary for our shared, global security.

To understand public health governance, we must understand the origin and development of the policies, standards, and best practices that shape PHS today (Chapter 10). The IHR (2005) have profoundly expanded the seminal efforts of the International Sanitary Conferences of the nineteenth and twentieth centuries. Section 2 explores the development and impact of global policies and practices to counteract the growing threat posed by emerging and re-emerging infectious diseases and endemic chronic conditions. This section examines the roots of PHS governance, a desire for standards and policies, and collaboration against mutual public health threats. The eventual formalization of the IHR (2005), a key and legally binding PHS document, is also discussed.

Adoption of these policies, standards, and best practices remains a vital issue, as the World Health Organization (WHO) is not a policing body and there are no sanctions for noncompliance.[18] National interests for global health security remain a significant motivating factor (Chapter 11). Public health security measures have increasingly become incorporated into national defense strategies. Global PHS and the sharing of its benefits provide a compelling case for better governance. Yet, global governance has been interpreted as being either a primary threat to the state or the individual; this focus determines the governance framework and language used to argue viewpoints (Chapter 12). This can be interpreted as either adopting a statist or globalist perspective. Often these perspectives use the language of global health security or human security to frame PHS issues, thus capturing health as a security, commodity, development of human right, or global public good issue. A smart governance model uses the appropriate mixture of perspectives for the situation and promotes holistic PHS to help balance goals and objectives and maximize benefits. This balanced approach is needed to transform the current state. Past successes such as the adoption of the Pandemic Influenza Preparedness Framework show it is possible (Chapter 13).

Section 3—Collaboration Fuels Transformation

Cutting passage ways in the internal walls of the old, dilapidated house to create collaborative space allows movement between rooms and opportunities to interact. This allows integration of different models of PHSS (Fig. 6). For example, the existing PHS silos in the USA are a huge problem[19], as they do not effectively or efficiently serve the community or patient.[19] Siloed, vertical PHS that (inefficiently) collects, analyzes, and interprets data about health outcome-specific events (e.g., HIV/AIDS and tuberculosis) should integrate funding structure. The U.S. model of funding vertical PHS systems is mirrored by the ineffective policies of some global NGOs that fund and drive outcome-specific program development in underserved, underresourced global settings.[20]

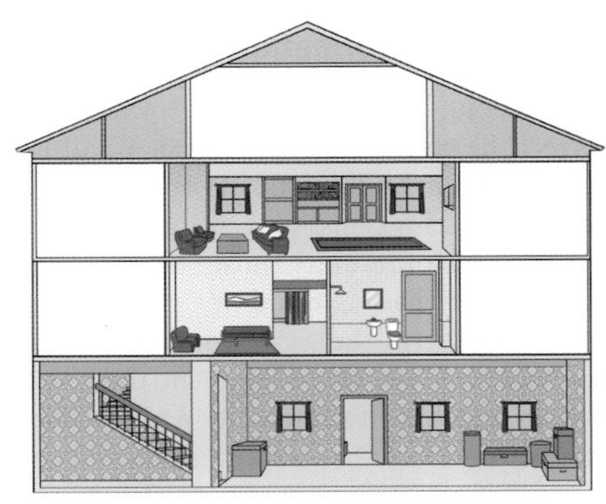

FIG. 6 Collaboration fuels PHS transformation.

Integration of PHS does not mean doing away with or negatively impacting the disease-specific outcome and prevention, treatment, and program-monitoring objectives critical to evaluate public health success. Rather, collaboration across programs, and disciplines, organizations, and nations would enhance our understanding of the complex interrelationships inherent to science, yet siloed by scientists.

An open door to a new partnership with technology can harness resources and technical expertise. Emerging diseases (e.g., pandemic influenza, MERS-CoV, Ebola) highlight the need for global cooperation that ensures health security. More specifically, the transparent exchange of data and knowledge creates synergy and the capacity to rapidly develop prevention and control measures against public health threats and encourage solutions to niche problems from a broader pool of ideas. These collaborative networks should include a range of sectors, including academic and private organizations.

A transformed PHS "smart home" means the door will be fully open to **One Health** (Chapter 14).[21] PHSS must include data, information, and messages about zoonotic diseases collected from veterinary medicine and laboratory.[1] For example, important initiatives are underway to monitor known threats such as highly pathogenic avian influenza.[22-27] Building on the recognition of this threat, it is important to expand the web of knowledge to include other animal diseases. Using technology to monitor, characterize, and report on animal diseases is a key aspect of transformed PHS. These efforts will leverage communities of interest to develop an awareness of emerging human health threats.

Additionally, we have yet to fully understand the contributions of multiple risk factors to the spread of disease. The effect of climate change and other human-driven ecological events and biological factors such as vectors' breeding patterns are understood but are not utilized effectively by PHS. For data from different disciplines to work in PHS, SMEs must understand PHS goals. The promise of collaboration supports predictive PHS—the ability to forecast disease trends based on past experiences using external and nontraditional data sources.

The military and NGOs have made significant contributions to global public health security. Although not readily perceived by the public, military PHS encompasses a range of areas (Chapters 15 and 16). PHS initiatives, best practices, and information overseen by the U.S. Department of Defense (DoD) are shared with other governmental institutions. NGOs have also increasingly become important actors in global health PHS; they serve as important advocates for PHS (Chapter 17) and globally, they contribute to building capacity, developing standards, and improving the public health workforce.

Among these actors, there is a need to improve communication, integrate public health programs, and actively engage the public in the process. Ultimately, partnerships strengthen and expedite the development and adoption of new technology and leverage resources to accomplish shared goals. For instance, public health and clinical medicine can both benefit from increased collaboration in PHS (Chapter 18). Community outreach is also essential to improve PHS (Chapter 19). We must recognize that different communities represent diverse economic, social, and political elements that need to be understood. Public health can benefit from reaching out to new and established communities to address routine and novel outbreaks.

Section 4—Informatics Enables Transformation

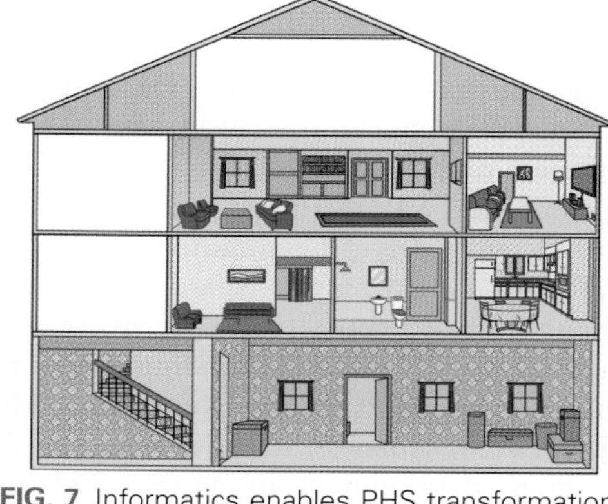

FIG. 7 Informatics enables PHS transformation.

Remodelling the "smart home" with electricity and water will correct the poor flow of territorial, unidirectional PHS data. Feedback of public health data, information, and messages to data providers (e.g., clinicians) and mutually beneficial collaboration with the medical community must be improved. Providers' PHS notification efforts have community value and providers should understand its benefit; the legal requirements for mandatory reporting are necessary but as we augment them with new sources of data that leverage new technologies and the democratizing force of the internet and Big Data analytics, we will see an inevitable convergence that will unlock a new era of PHS (Fig. 7).

PHS can be enabled by new technological advances (Section 4). There are key factors necessary to successfully enable PHS through informatics and ICT. Informatics promises to draw data from many sources enhancing trend and pattern recognition, creating actionable information for public health responses. The challenges to successfully leverage informatics and ICT include creating global information standards, finding creative ways to bring heterogeneous data together rapidly, and creating sustainable infrastructure investments.

Data interoperability is an increasingly important component of PHS. Interoperability will require diligence in implementing concepts such as data quality (Chapter 20). Interoperable systems extend beyond the tools used to accommodate data exchange. Once a partnership has been formed, thoughtful planning is required to harmonize the politics, policies, and protocols for data exchange.

Data can answer complex public health questions (Chapter 21). Knowing and understanding the behavior of data sources—volume, variety, velocity, and veracity—will help determine how to derive the appropriate information. We also must identify and understand the gaps that may challenge effective dissemination and implementation of innovative informatics solutions (Chapter 22). Emerging techniques for data visualization are another opportunity for transforming PHS (Chapter 23).

Section 5—New Data, Analytics, Intelligence (Knowledge) Enlightens Transformation

Fully wired, the PHS "smart home" (Fig. 8) receives a flow of new data from new sources (e.g., social, news media) and uses new analytic techniques to provide situation awareness and comprehensive public health intelligence. This information can be used to report timely, accurate, and predictive data, information, and messages for public health action (Section 5).

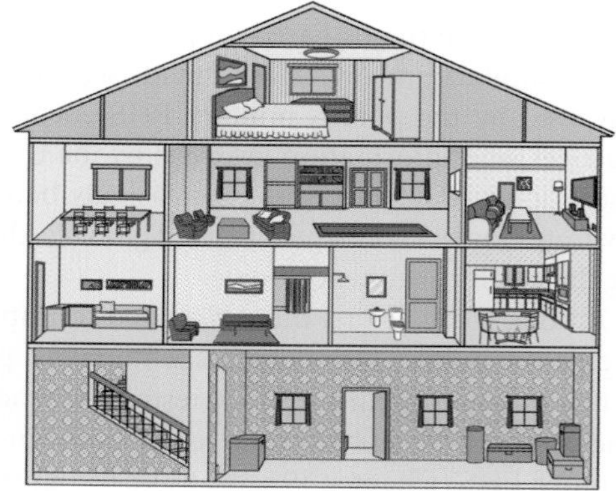

FIG. 8 New data, analytics, intelligence (knowledge) enlightens transformation.

The products of transformed PHS—new data, new analytics, and new intelligence—push through existing limitations of manual, paper-based data collection, aging data analysis methods, and siloed data systems (Section 6). However, moving forward it is important to find an appropriate balance between sensitivity and specificity, while maintaining timeliness in the face of public pressure with increasing access to unrestrained data flows from social media and other new media approaches. Appropriate integration and use of new data feeds can inform policy decisions and interventions, but it also brings new challenges. Development of sophisticated "Big Data" tools will change the way PHS is conducted that today's PHS practitioners are just starting to grasp.

Verifying and validating increasing amounts of public health data remain a challenge to public health—good surveillance requires good data (Chapter 24). With good data, modeling is, and will continue to be, increasingly important to inform disease control (Chapter 25). This requires awareness of how to use models properly.

New data sources are emerging with new technologies. For example, genomic data hold incredible promise for PHS (Chapter 26). However, with new data sources there is a gap that needs to be addressed. Genetic sequences could clarify complexities in disease patterns; but how can we gain the most useful PHS information? Frameworks for non-PHS experts present an ideal way forward as can be demonstrated for genetic system analysts aiming to use data for PHS. This added understanding could further refine the way we detect, assess, and respond to public health threats. New sources and types of data will inevitably lead to a variety of new approaches to analyzing public health data (Chapter 27). However, economic and logistical barriers to disseminating and adopting electronic information systems raise a number of important issues about the transferability of data, privacy, and security.

Establishing scientific exchanges and learning fora to share best practices are important for a fruitful and synergistic collaboration. With various organizational travel restrictions and limited resources and time, new ways of sharing scientific and public health innovations must be developed to spread best practices and novel ideas. Many organizations may be reluctant to reveal project shortcomings, for the fear of losing funding or support when, in fact, additional resources and support are needed to overcome these obstacles. Sharing novel and innovative ways of conducting PHS is paramount to increasing connectivity in the global community.

SECTION 6—IMPACTS OF TRANSFORMED PUBLIC HEALTH SURVEILLANCE

Once remodeled, the new PHS "smart home" can be linked to other public health actions as part of the greater "neighborhood." Ultimately, the transformation of PHS is incomplete without linking these advancements in governance, collaboration, informatics, and new data, analytics, and intelligence to public health action (Section 6). This link is made, for example, between PHS and the Millennium Development Goals. A key lesson from this linkage is that it is possible for nations to agree on aspirational goals for development, to collect and share data for monitoring progress and performance toward the goals, and attract global investments for these initiatives. However, the major barrier to collecting and using data for informing national decisions is weak and fragmented health systems.

Applying advances in public health actions for the Post-2015 Millennium Development Agenda offers an opportunity to address barriers (Chapter 29). Research and future innovations in key areas such as One Health, public health genomics, and new technologies such as Big Data, GIS, and social media will play an important role in the continuing transformation of PHS. Understanding and addressing the various challenges for leveraging PHS research and innovation such as interoperability, point-of-care diagnostics, workforce, and funding limitations will better enable and further enhance continued transformation (Chapter 30). And through its successful transformation, by utilizing balanced governance, multidisciplinary collaborations, cutting-edge informatics, and new data, analytics, and intelligence, PHS promises to facilitate sustainable and equitable health progress, addressing the disproportionate burden for the poor, undercounting and imprecision, and human right issues (Chapter 31).

WHAT YOU CAN LOOK FORWARD TO

As our world evolves with new challenges, so is our ability to overcome obstacles. ICT and tools; digital data standards and sources; and new analytic techniques will change our ability to report, assess, and respond to emerging and reemerging threats.

In this book, we utilize real threats presented as online case studies* (antimicrobial resistance, disaster/mass gathering, pandemic influenza, MERS-CoV, and polio) to demonstrate the transformational potential of PHS

*Available at http://booksite.elsevier.com/9780702063374/

from its current state to its future promise. Through respectful, mindful governance and mutually beneficial, multi-actor collaboration, the global public health community can effectively guide the transformation of PHS to fully realize advances in informatics, and new data, analytics, and intelligence to unlock the full impact of twenty-first century PHS.

KEY SUMMARY POINTS

- Public Health Surveillance (PHS) is the collection of health information for the purposes of monitoring, preventing or controlling the spread of disease in a population. It includes surveillance of infectious and chronic disease, adverse event monitoring, and syndromic surveillance.
- Public health knowledge should be readily available to the international public in a modern format.
- Public Health Surveillance Strengthening is at a tipping point where the latest innovations in public health science and business practices, including ICT, must be used to empower PHS.
- There is a need to reexamine and restructure PHS and funding streams so that inefficient vertical siloed health PHS programs are integrated into the larger PHS system.
- New collaborative networks are necessary to ensure global cooperation and transparent exchange of data to facilitate health security.
- PHS must adopt the One Health Concept, including data, information, and messages about diseases in animals with significance to human health and environmental factors and risks.

REFERENCES

1. Langmuir AD. The surveillance of communicable diseases of national importance. The New England Journal of Medicine 1963;268:182–92.
2. Brownson RC, Baker EA, Leet TL, Gillespie KN, True WR. Evidence-based public health. New York: Oxford University Press; 2010. p. 312.
3. Choi BC. The past, present, and future of public health surveillance. Scientifica 2012;2012:875253.
4. Mays GP, Scutchfield FD. Improving public health system performance through multiorganizational partnerships. Prev Chronic Dis 2010;7(6):A116.
5. Lindqvist J. Towards a healthy world–By co-operation or coercion? 2014.
6. Wilson K, Brownstein JS, Fidler DP. Strengthening the International Health Regulations: lessons from the H1N1 pandemic. Health Policy Plan 2010;25(6):505–9.
7. Robert F. "Stopping by Woods on a Snowy Evening" from The Poetry of Robert Frost, edited by Edward Connery Lathem. Copyright 1923, © 1969 by Henry Holt and Company, Inc., renewed 1951, by Robert Frost.
8. McNabb SJN, Shaikh AT, Nuzzo JB, Zumla AI, Heymann DL. Triumphs, trials, and tribulations of the global response to MERS coronavirus. Lancet Respir Med 2014;2(6):436–7.
9. Katz R, Rosenbaum S. Challenging custom: rethinking National Population Surveillance Policy in a global public health age. J Health Polit Policy Law 2010;35(6):1027–55.
10. Penfold E, Fourie P. Ebola and cultures of engagement: Chinese versus Western health diplomacy. In: Councils Co, editor. 2014.
11. Buehler JW, Hopkins RS, Overhage JM, Sosin DM, Tong V, Centers for Disease Control and Prevention. Framework for evaluating public health surveillance systems for early detection of outbreaks. MMRW Recomm Rep 2004;53(RR05):1–11.
12. German RR, Lee LM, Horan JM, Milstein RL, Pertowski CA, Waller MN. Updated guidelines for evaluating public health surveillance systems. MMRW Recomm Rep 2001;50(RR13):1–35.
13. Centers for Disease Control and Prevention. Guidelines for evaluating surveillance systems. MMRW Recomm Rep 1988;37(S-5):1–18.
14. Thacker SB. Historical development. In: Teutsch SM, Churchill RE, editors. Principles and practice of public health surveillance. (2nd ed.), New York: Oxford University Press; 2000. p. 1–15.
15. Fidler DP. From international sanitary conventions to global health security: the new International Health Regulations. Chinese J Int Law 2005;4(2):325–92.
16. Diamond CC, Mostashari F, Shirky C. Collecting and sharing data for population health: a new paradigm. Health Aff 2009;28(2):454–66.
17. Verity C, Manning D, Nicoll A. Consent, confidentiality, and the threat to public health surveillance. Commentary: don't waive consent lightly—involve the public. BMJ 2002;324(7347):1210–13.
18. World Health Organization. Severe acute respiratory syndrome - press briefing, <http://www.who.int/csr/sars/press2003_04_01/en/>; 2003.
19. Thacker SB, Stroup DF. Future directions for comprehensive public health surveillance and health information systems in the United States. Am J Epidemiol 1994;140(5):383–97.
20. McNabb SJN, Chungong S, Ryan M, Wuhib T, Nsubuga P, Alemu W, et al. Conceptual framework of public health surveillance and action and its application in health sector reform. BMC Public Health 2002;2:2.
21. Scotch M, Odofin L, Rabinowitz P. Linkages between animal and human health sentinel data. BMC Vet Res 2009;5:15.
22. Breed AC, Harris K, Hesterberg U, Gould G, Londt BZ, Brown IH, et al. Surveillance for avian influenza in wild birds in the European Union in 2007. Avian Dis 2010;54(Suppl. 1):399–404.
23. Escorcia M, Attene-Ramos MS, Estrada MJ, Nava GM. Improving global influenza surveillance: trends of A(H5N1) virus in Africa and Asia. BMC Res Notes 2012;5:62.
24. Hesterberg U, Harris K, Stroud D, Guberti V, Busani L, Pittman M, et al. Avian influenza surveillance in wild birds in the European Union in 2006. Influenza Other Respir Viruses 2009;3(1):1–14.
25. Kang HM, Jeong OM, Kim MC, Kwon JS, Paek MR, Choi JG, et al. Surveillance of avian influenza virus in wild bird fecal samples from South Korea, 2003-2008. J Wildl Dis 2010;46(3):878–88.
26. Mariner JC, Jones BA, Hendrickx S, El Masry I, Jobre Y, Jost CC. Experiences in participatory surveillance and community-based reporting systems for H5N1 highly pathogenic avian influenza: a case study approach. Ecohealth 2014;11:22–35.
27. Slavec B, Krapez U, Racnik AJ, Hari A, Wernig JM, Dovc A, et al. Surveillance of influenza A viruses in wild birds in Slovenia from 2006 to 2010. Avian Dis 2012;56(Suppl. 4):999–1005.

1

SECTION

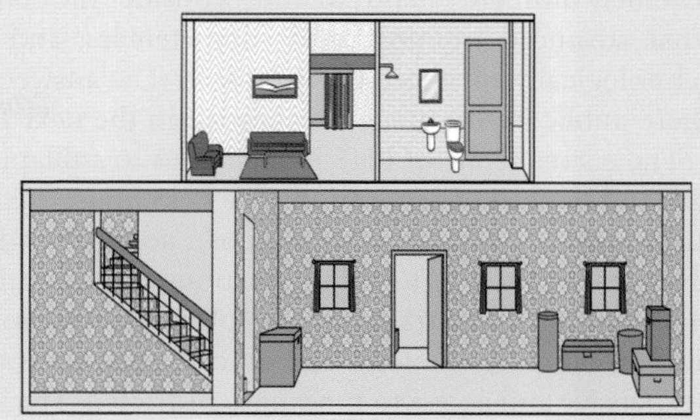

Current State of Public Health Surveillance

Lisa Ferland, Scott JN McNabb

Section Outline

The systematic collection of data is essential for ongoing analysis and interpretation by public health practitioners to detect, report, and respond to conditions and events of public health importance. As technological advances are incorporated into routine public health practice, practitioners must adapt to new situations related to travel, technology, disasters, population growth, and migration that affect how public health conducts public health surveillance (PHS). New methodologies, solutions, and adaptations to modern PHS address these new dynamics in the ongoing effort to maintain the public's health.

Current PHS takes various forms and follows different models, but all focus on collecting, analyzing, and interpreting data for public health action. PHS systems related to disease eradication or funded by single funding streams are often constructed in a vertical, siloed nature and transforming PHS systems into an integrated enterprise is often difficult, costly, and politically challenging. Collectively, we must move toward systems that can adjust to public health threats while remaining sensitive to the core objectives of PHS.

PHS systems must be frequently monitored and evaluated to continue to meet population's health needs. Requirements for any PHS system must also be balanced with the costs associated with detection and response. What is the cost if public health fails to properly manage an outbreak? Unfortunately, the difficulty to justify investments in technology is due to the nature of PHS—costs are only seen when the systems fail. Quantifying the true cost of good public health practice is extremely difficult. Finally, we must consider the demands of these systems in relation to the public health workforce. What advanced training, new competencies, and experiences will they need in order to execute PHS in this technologically advanced environment? The answers to these questions remain paramount to our understanding of where public health practice is headed in the next 10 years and beyond.

The current state of PHS is analogous to a dilapidated house that while built has a faulty foundation, is in disrepair, and in need of renovation. The PHS house has a poorly designed floor plan including single rooms that do not interconnect (program vertical silos); some that do connect at all with one another. The house contains some advanced technology to help operations run smoothly, but is occupied with people who are not equipped to utilize all of the functions; training takes place mainly on-site. These people (i.e., the workforce) need additional training in informatics, technology, and other special skills to move practice forward. The budget for the house renovation is expensive and access to funding is restricted. The builders struggle to adequately justify all costs before the funders can approve the renovation budget.

LEARNING OBJECTIVES

- Explain why PHS must adapt to overcome new challenges presented and how these challenges also present new opportunities.
- Explain the process of PHSS.
- Describe the evolution of public health surveillance systems in the USA and the challenges.
- Identify the vision for PHS that lays on the horizon.
- Define the roles of CDC and CSTE in PHS.
- Describe CDC's future vision and strategic plan for PHS.
- Describe the different types and approaches used for conducting public health surveillance.
- Understand the benefits and limitations to public health data from differing types of surveillance systems.
- Communicate the advantages and disadvantages of differing types of surveillance systems.
- Describe the differences between vertical and integrated surveillance systems.
- Explain the challenges involved with implementing vertical and integrated surveillance systems.
- Describe the differences between proactive and reactive surveillance.
- Articulate how Electronic Health Records enable proactive surveillance.
- Describe the importance of Big Data, internet, and social media for upcoming proactive surveillance structures and systems.
- Explain the most commonly used methods for evaluation of surveillance as well as the newly introduced models.
- Describe the Work Process Analysis evaluation framework.
- Articulate the elements of surveillance evaluation unaccounted for within the CDC's guidelines and the need for a new approach for evaluation.
- Explain the relationship between health and wealth.
- Describe the need and challenges of determining ROI, cost utility, cost-effectiveness, and cost–benefit analysis.
- Describe the need for workforce development and capacity strengthening in epidemiology and its impact on public health surveillance.

CHAPTER

1

Past Contributions

Henry Rolka, Kara Contreary

If we dwell on the past, we rob the present. But if we ignore the past, we may rob the future.

Taoist saying

KEY WORDS

Surveillance system
Data management
Data analysis
Notifiable disease (or priority disease)

We define public health surveillance as the systematic collection of health information for the purposes of monitoring, preventing, or controlling the spread of disease in a population. The type of information collected and used can vary from confirmed cases of disease to individual symptoms, from indicators like body mass index (BMI) to purchase of over-the-counter medicines. The practice of surveillance has changed significantly over time but remains an invaluable tool that public health practitioners can use to prevent illness and promote health in populations. This chapter will provide a brief overview of several types of public health surveillance and how selected surveillance efforts respond to internal and external challenges. It will attempt to illustrate the challenges inherent in designing and sustaining surveillance programs and make recommendations for incorporating lessons learned into future efforts.

Public health officials are tasked with the difficult job of improving and protecting the health of the population. The decisions they face have evolved and expanded over time, from electing to shut off access to contaminated well water to electing to participate in large international outbreak control responses. The point of surveillance is to support sound decision-making. It is important to keep this in mind at all levels of surveillance practice. Alexander D. Langmuir,[1] who founded the Epidemic Intelligence Service Program, said, "Good surveillance does not necessarily ensure the making of right decisions, but it reduces the chance of wrong ones." During times of very rapidly evolving knowledge and technology, it can be easy to become distracted by new tools that seem to enable revolutionary changes in surveillance practice. However, in order to avoid dead ends, false starts, and missteps, it is necessary to frequently remind ourselves of why we put time, effort, and resources into public health surveillance. Before each unit of investment, no matter how small, it is necessary to answer the question, "How will this step help support sound decision-making?"

While there have been a number of remarkable health issues that highlight the necessary transformation of public health surveillance, this book has chosen seven case studies (pandemic influenza, antimicrobial resistance, diabetes, exposomes, MERS-CoV, nuclear disaster, and polio) to highlight the important role surveillance plays in achieving better health outcomes for all. These case studies can be found at http://booksite.elsevier.com/9780702063374/ and are referenced throughout the following chapters to help illustrate how current PHS efforts need to be renovated.

TYPES OF PUBLIC HEALTH SURVEILLANCE

The issue of surveillance is not new, with the early focus of public health surveillance being infectious diseases. As far back as the mid-fourteenth century in the Republic of Venice, three keepers were designated to detect and keep away ships with passengers infected with Black Death (pneumonic plague). This was perhaps the first official public health measure in the prevention of disease spread. Varying surveillance measures were put in place in subsequent centuries in Europe and the Americas.

Basic local surveillance in the western hemisphere appeared in Rhode Island in 1741 with an act requiring tavern owners to report contagious disease among patrons[2,3] and in New York City in 1796 when physicians were required to report infectious disease cases.[4] At the US national level, surveillance began in 1878 with the US Marine Hospital Service (the forerunner of the modern Public Health Service) collecting data on foreign occurrences of diseases such as cholera, smallpox, plague, and yellow fever from US consuls overseas, which were used to establish quarantines aimed at preventing the spread of those diseases to the USA. Publicly reporting the results of these surveillance efforts began in 1879, and by 1928, all states, the District of Columbia, Hawaii, and Puerto Rico were reporting to the Surgeon General on 29 "notifiable" diseases. A **notifiable disease** is one for which regular, frequent, and timely information regarding individual cases is considered necessary for the prevention and control of the disease.[5]

The role of international disease spread in furthering public health surveillance can also be seen in Europe. In 1829 a cholera epidemic prompted European leaders to review the factors that contributed to the spread of disease. Variation in quarantine measures by country was implicated in the epidemic, prompting a series of international sanitary conferences starting in 1851 to agree upon quarantine measures against cholera, plague, and yellow fever.[6] A number of conventions came out of these meetings, which were consolidated into a single International Sanitary Convention in 1903. These cooperative efforts were echoed across the Atlantic, where the republics of the Americas established the International Sanitary Bureau in 1902.[7]

Over time, as the chronic disease burden increased in western countries, new surveillance systems were created in response to the shifting health profile of the population. A **surveillance system** is the ongoing systematic collection and analysis of data. The data may lead to actions taken to prevent and control an infectious disease.[8] In the USA, in addition to tracking infectious diseases, the Centers for Disease Control and Prevention (CDC) currently houses 16 major surveillance systems covering chronic diseases.[9] These systems collect data on health-risk behaviors, preventive care practices, and the burden of chronic diseases.

In addition to infectious and chronic diseases, adverse reactions to drugs, vaccines, and other products are tracked through surveillance programs (Fig. 1-1). The US Food and Drug Administration (FDA) Adverse Event Reporting System (FAERS) is a database that contains information about adverse events and medication errors reported to the FDA. It supports the FDA's postmarketing safety surveillance program for drugs and therapeutic products. The closely related Vaccine Adverse Event Reporting System (VAERS) is a national vaccine safety surveillance program cosponsored by the CDC and FDA. It collects information about signs and symptoms that occur after administration of vaccines licensed for use in the USA.

A final and increasingly important type of surveillance involves vigilance for the signs of deliberate infection. The heightened awareness of the potential for bioweapons use during the first decade of the new millennium affected priorities in public health surveillance. During the years following the terrorist attacks on the USA on September 11, 2001 (9/11), there was a heightened emphasis on leading edge indicators of human disease.[10–12] This new emphasis led to accelerated development and deployment of *syndromic surveillance* (or *biosurveillance*), which uses prediagnostic signs and symptoms (e.g., rash and fever) instead of confirmed disease case reports. These early indicators were used to attempt more timely inference into population events that posed a public health threat.[13]

Syndromic surveillance introduced an array of novel data sources into the practice of surveillance. Sources range from very early indicators such as increased sales of orange juice in a business or academic cafeteria (a proxy for cold/flu symptoms), over-the-counter medicine sales, nurse call-line volumes, and social network word usage to the gold standard—but often time-delayed—laboratory confirmation of disease. These various data sources are

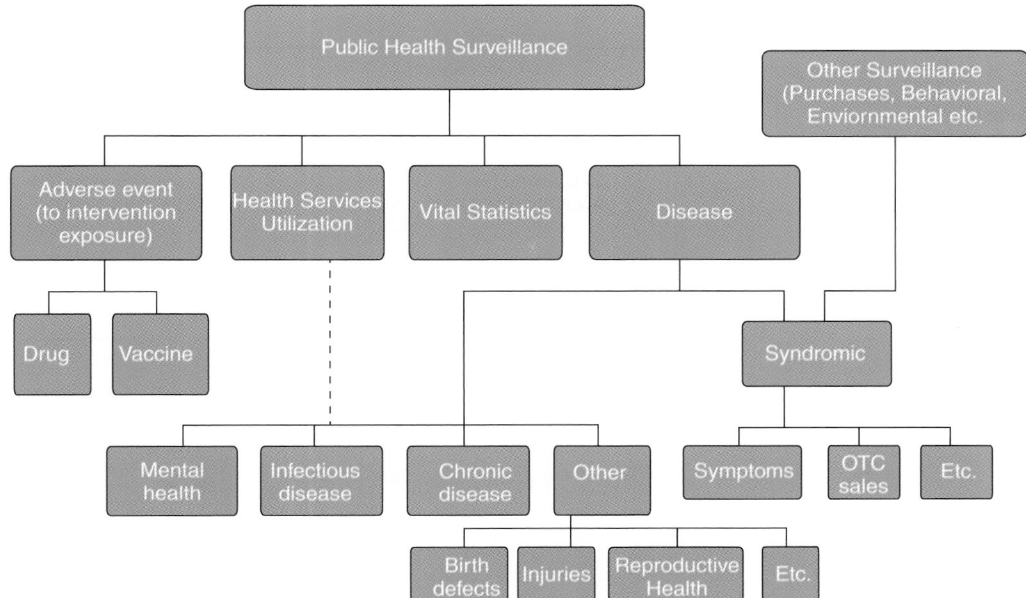

FIG. 1-1 Landscape of public health surveillance activities.

generated differently; they capture different stages of the disease cycle and may be more or less specific to the disease of interest in the population.[14,15] Subject matter professionals from several fields are needed to cover the knowledge base necessary to make use of syndromic surveillance. The difficulty faced in covering this knowledge base, along with other issues, has not allowed syndromic surveillance to progress as far as early enthusiasts had imagined it would.[16,17] A discussion of influences hampering development of syndromic surveillance can be found later in this chapter.

EVOLUTION OF SURVEILLANCE SYSTEMS

Over the long history of public health surveillance (Fig. 1-2), numerous factors have affected and will continue to influence the development of surveillance systems.[18] These factors may be considered in three groups, which are neither comprehensive nor mutually exclusive but useful for practical considerations. The first group is responses to uncontrolled external events or perceived threats. Examples include (a) the public health experience with human immunodeficiency virus/acquired immunodeficiency syndrome (HIV/AIDS), (b) the growing perception of a bioterrorism threat in the early twenty-first century, and (c) disease outbreaks like the continuing global influenza epidemic and the yearly viral characterization, vaccine production, and cyclic immunization program. The second group of factors affecting the development of surveillance systems is deliberate efforts to shape how surveillance is conducted. Examples include (a) the movement from paper-based to electronic recording, (b) the automation of data processing, and (c) system interoperability efforts. The final group of factors is legislative or regulatory decisions by governments to address public health issues. Examples of this group include (a) vaccine recommendations and (b) the International Health Regulations (IHR) reporting obligations established by World Health Organization (WHO) in 2007.[19]

As an example of the first group, uncontrolled external events, consider the consequences of the AIDS epidemic. The first report of AIDS in the medical literature was in June of 1981.[20] In 1982, researchers presented evidence that AIDS was caused by an infectious agent and soon most researchers were in agreement that it was transmitted through sexual and blood contact.[21] With the spread of HIV all over the world, starting in Africa in the late 1970s and

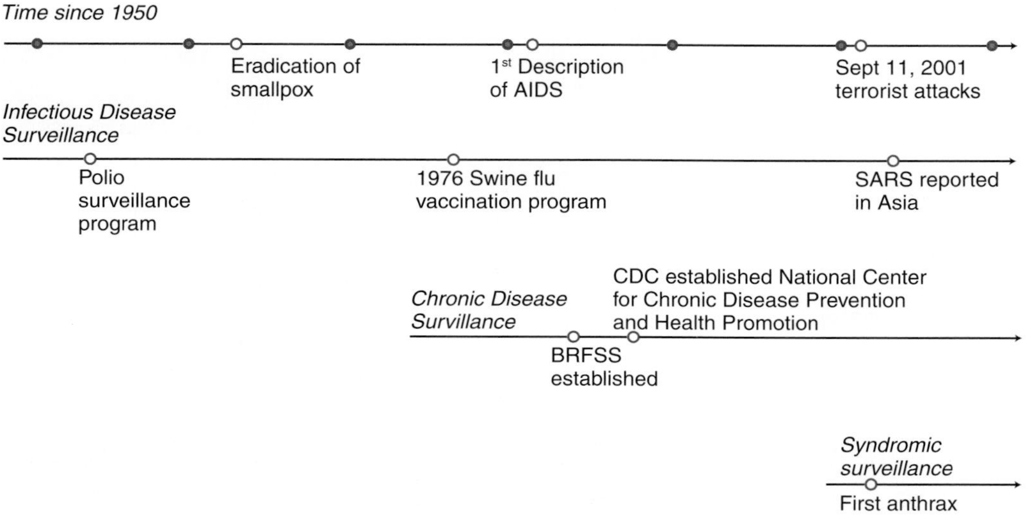

FIG. 1-2 Timeline of selected public health surveillance efforts in the USA.

spreading to Western Europe and the Americas by the early 1980s, eventually reaching Asia and Eastern Europe by the early 1990s, surveillance has been a priority in global public health for the past 3 decades. Until the early twenty-first century, coordinated surveillance was hampered by the use of multiple case definitions around the world. Not until 2006 did the WHO publish a set of standardized case definitions for HIV and AIDS specifically for surveillance purposes. With standard definitions, it became possible not only to monitor the spread and progress of the disease, but also to evaluate interventions and prevention programs against a common rubric.

A major initiative that demonstrates the second type of factor, deliberate efforts to shape surveillance, is a 1998 integration project at the CDC that established the framework for the National Electronic Disease Surveillance System (NEDSS). The purpose of NEDSS was to tie together many of the currently separate systems used for public health surveillance by implementing uniform data standards, communication networks, and policy-level agreements regarding data access, sharing, and reduction of data collection burden.[22] This would avoid duplicating efforts and, in the long term (it was hoped), lead to an integrated system that would gather more timely health data from numerous sources, making it easier to monitor the health of communities and detect emerging public health problems from infectious disease or terrorist activity.[23] Unfortunately, not all the goals of the integration project were realized. The following section offers more information about NEDSS.

The third group of factors, legislative decisions to address public health issues, includes, for example, government sponsorship of health interventions that affect surveillance. Specifically, consider the hosting of vaccination programs, including both population-wide vaccination efforts and more targeted programs like ring vaccination. The USA, Germany, and Great Britain have had laws regarding routine vaccination since the 1800s, when smallpox vaccination was adopted as a public health measure.[24] When smallpox became less prevalent, ring vaccination (in which surveillance is used to track down individuals who could have been exposed to an infected person and vaccinating them) was used to limit the spread from isolated cases. Together, these techniques enabled the elimination of smallpox.[25]

IHR, established by the WHO and formally adopted by the 22nd World Health Assembly in 1969, provide a good example of international regulatory measures taken to promote public health. For over 40 years, the IHR have been the primary legally binding global agreement addressing the risks of the international spread of infectious disease. The IHR evolved from the international sanitary conferences of the last half of the nineteenth century and the public health institutions founded in the first half of the twentieth century.[26] These international agreements and institutions established and coordinated related functions including limited notification obligations and surveillance for certain infectious diseases.

Today, under the IHR, countries have a legal obligation to conduct surveillance for infectious diseases and to share information about outbreaks with the international community. The IHR codify the measures that countries must take to limit the international spread of disease while ensuring minimum interference with trade and travel.

CRUCIAL CHALLENGES

The field of public health is constantly changing in response to new challenges and new opportunities. As the discipline progresses, each new development provides a learning opportunity for future generations of public health practitioners. This is equally true about public health surveillance, especially as it strives to incorporate advances in information-sharing technology into existing methods and practices. In this section, we discuss some of the crucial challenges of public health surveillance. At times, we draw on past successes and failures, documenting lessons learned and, we hope, giving surveillance practitioners of the future a perspective that will help prevent repetition of past mistakes. The examples are not intended to be comprehensive but to provide examples. In particular, we will discuss NEDSS and BioSense, each of which has contributed greatly to our understanding of the interaction between the technological and human components of surveillance activities. The purpose of this narrative is not to specifically criticize the programs used as examples or the people or organizations who worked on them. It is designed to point out easily overlooked planning and implementation factors associated with success and to enable insight into ways to avoid potential pitfalls using previous surveillance system development experiences. A number of factors can potentially impede surveillance efforts, and many of them are outside the control of developers. Annual government budget cycles, and the inherent uncertainty involved in funding large-scale, long-term projects, can make smooth development difficult. The fact that development efforts will need to contend with these impediments makes it all the more important to get it right on factors that *are* under developer control.

One of the most prominent challenges for governments involved in planning surveillance activities concerns the amount and nature of data to collect and store. Surveillance is, by its nature, a somewhat intrusive enterprise in that it is essential to collect information about individuals' health statuses, their symptoms, and their behaviors in order to maintain a health and disease awareness of a population. Such data collection by governments may make some individuals uneasy. There is also an attendant risk of unintended personal identification that requires balance with the utility of the collected, stored, or otherwise accessed data.[17,27] There is thus a balance to be struck between respecting individual privacy and accommodating the considerable data needs of public health surveillance efforts.

Moving forward, as technology enables the collection and processing of ever-larger data sets, with increased potential for cross-indexing data sources, the tension between effective surveillance and personal privacy will only increase. One way to address this issue has been to suggest that data should only be collected if they are currently part of a planned analysis. This results in collection of the "minimum currently necessary" set of information. However, as new threats emerge (or new surveillance techniques are developed), information that was not anticipated to be useful might turn out to be important (e.g., over-the-counter purchases, environmental exposure records). Collecting more than the minimum currently necessary data expands future surveillance capacity by providing time series data on variables that may be of interest to future public health efforts. Investment in future capacity must therefore be balanced against present and future threats to individual privacy. The depth of this responsibility can be reviewed in connection with a historical perspective of the interface between human rights and governmental statistical policy.[28]

We turn now to more operational challenges. In order to focus the discussion, we will deal mainly with the difficulty inherent in maintaining user involvement during the development and deployment of new highly technical surveillance efforts. All surveillance is (and should be) done in order that the end users might apply the information collected to improve decision-making. These end users should be kept in mind and should have input at all stages of program development, in order to ensure that the final product provides the intended public health benefit. The need for surveillance to link to larger public health efforts has been recognized since 1850.[29] Furthermore, the need for user involvement in highly technological undertakings has been recognized at least since the mid-1990s,[30,31] but despite program officials being aware of this precept, some recent large-scale surveillance efforts have struggled to build systems that work optimally for the intended end users.[17,23,32] As a case study, consider the Surveillance System Integration Project that spawned NEDSS.

This is not meant to be a comprehensive end-to-end review of all that has worked or not worked in surveillance program efforts. It is simply to point out a few ideas in example cases from an earlier historical perspective on known efforts, namely, NEDSS and BioSense. Thus, the purpose is that new programs can consider these experiences for learning and building on past success.

NEDSS and the Challenge of Surveillance Integration

As of the time of NEDSS's conception, the program in place for tracking diseases of particular interest to public health officials was the National Notifiable Disease Surveillance System (NNDSS). Under NNDSS, weekly case counts of notifiable diseases were collected by state health departments and published in the CDC's *MMWR*. This program has been in place since the 1960s, but by the 1990s, US public health leaders recognized the potential benefits of interoperable surveillance to facilitate efficient collection, analysis, and use of the data, as well as sharing of necessary computer software. The hope was that eventually the integrated electronic information system would gather real-time health data from multiple sources, including state and local health departments, public and private laboratories, managed care and health maintenance organizations, medical examiners, hospitals, and emergency departments. It would monitor the health of communities, perform ongoing trend analysis, detect emerging public health problems, and provide information for setting public health policy.

In order to facilitate rapid and seamless sharing of electronic data, the system was to be designed in collaboration between CDC and its traditional partners in public health (e.g., state public health departments), as well as with new partners such as health maintenance organizations, private laboratories, and other nonhealth state and federal agencies. The developers wished to satisfy the requirements of stakeholders across various levels of public health administration, across a wide geographic range, and across multiple stakeholder perspectives. In a deliberate attempt to create a system that would satisfy requirements across these broad categories (and thereby be sustainable in the long term), the NEDSS developers adopted a decision-by-consensus model of development. Specifications, components, and implementation procedures were developed, discussed, planned, and implemented through exhaustive group vetting.

The forerunner of NEDSS for transmitting data, called the National Electronic Telecommunications System for Surveillance (NETSS) was scheduled to be phased out as states gradually adopted NEDSS, which made use of updated and more efficient technology and standards.[33] The transition process was begun in the late 1990s and certainly many technical data standard and message transmission accomplishments were achieved, but, as of June 2012, only 19 of the 50 states and Washington, DC, were using the NEDSS Base System.[34] Numerous states were, however, using other NEDSS-compatible transmission solutions. It is debatable and would be a speculation to assert a clear reason for implementation shortfalls. It is important to keep in mind that unanticipated challenges are to be expected when diverse users of a system are involved in a system plan and implementation. Identifying users, engaging with them, and maintaining the partnership are all necessary for striking the correct balance.

It is not enough, however, to strike the right balance between progress and stakeholder involvement. As an example of a surveillance project that was initiated a few years after NEDSS and encountered additional challenges, let us look at the BioSense program.[35,36]

BioSense and the Challenge of Analytic Data Management

Traditionally, public health surveillance in the USA starts with health care practitioners reporting disease cases to local public health agencies. The local agencies then report to state public health agencies or health departments, who in turn voluntarily report to the CDC. In 2003, this multistage approach became newly seen as insufficient for new population health threats, particularly for highly infectious agents such as those associated with bioterrorism.[37] The elevated concern over bioterror attacks inspired nontraditional approaches to public health surveillance in order to obtain new types and sources of relevant data, substantially speed up information flow, increase completeness and accuracy, and improve national coverage.

BioSense was initially designed to collect very timely electronic data.[23,38] It was to include electronic data generated in the course of individuals' interactions with health care providers and other health-related services. This would expedite initial detection and quantification of public health threats. A number of newly expanded surveillance activities would provide data from hospital emergency rooms, ambulatory care clinics, health plans, claims clearinghouses, clinical testing laboratories, retail pharmacies, and nurse call lines. Consideration of other early detection sources included emergency medical service dispatches, school and work absenteeism, and others.

At the federal level, BioSense was part of a larger initiative to detect and defend against a bioterror threat.[13] As such, the federal mandate for quick implementation was particularly urgent, and developers could not use the same consensus-based strategy they had with NEDSS. Thus, an operational system of unprecedented scope was put in place and made usable within a year. However, vetting the details of the system with most of the user stakeholders was planned for after implementation and initiated in April 2004.[35]

Program managers recognized that in order for BioSense to be sustainable, it could not be *just* a specialized anti-bioterror system. The system and the data would have to be relevant for decision support in practical, everyday public health practice, and not just for the rare instance of a deliberate exposure event. Public health programs would have to use BioSense data for routine public health efforts. Obstacles to engaging users at this point included a lack of technical capabilities such as analytic data management.[17,32,38] **Data management** is an administrative process by which the required data are acquired, validated, stored, protected, and processed, and by which its accessibility, reliability, and timeliness is ensured to satisfy the needs of the data users.[39] One of the biggest issues was likely the volume, variety, and frequency of data updates, which was novel to CDC at the time.

At the time of BioSense's initial implementation, civilian and military health data from the Department of Defense, Veteran's Affairs data, the National Retail Data Monitor and laboratory test order data were included. A few states had developed functional syndromic surveillance functions (e.g., PA) but most had not. They lacked the resources to build the technical and analytic infrastructures for using real-time patient encounter data for population surveillance. Moreover, it was not reasonable to expect each state and local health department to work independently on such development. At that point, the federal government assumed the role of coordinating procedures and best practices across states.[40]

BioSense continued to grow in 2005–2006, recruiting civilian hospitals into the program so that emergency room patient encounter data would be transmitted into the system. Data from hospitals all over the country were being loaded into the BioSense database multiple times each hour, and often did not share a common format. This massively increased the complexity of the system, which necessarily increased the requirements for analyzing the new data. Unfortunately, while there were sufficient resources allocated to acquiring, loading, and storing the data, the federal resources allocated to the analytic component could not keep pace.[17]

The lesson here is that in any surveillance program, the capacity to analyze data generated from surveillance activity is not a luxury—it is a necessity. Evidence comes from data that have been drawn from the surveillance system and analyzed to provide information of value. Without human resources conducting the analytic functions, the data cannot be brought to bear to help make better public health decisions. Speaking metaphorically, analytic capacity is the keystone of the bridge that connects health events on the ground to public health decision-making.

Surveillance's Unique Demands on Human Resources

As data sources and systems have grown in size and complexity, so have methods for studying and addressing public health problems (e.g., interconnectedness of behavioral, environmental and nutritional factors with chronic diseases such as diabetes, obesity, and stroke). In order to make sound judgments about data requirements for a specific purpose, professionals with broad experience and deep knowledge about data are needed. In general, as more integrated systems develop in complexity the epidemiologist must be joined by various other types of personnel in order to be successful with surveillance. More specifically, however, it is critically essential to have skilled data managers who can comfortably manage the transition from transactional data, generated on the ground and stored in a relational database structure, to analytical data sets in the flat file structure that statisticians and epidemiologists require (Fig. 1-3). This process involves rather unique skill sets that have grown in demand with the increase in the volume and complexity of data. The term "analytic data management" is not a standardized term but in this context describes the work process necessary for preparing analytic data files from raw data. Other steps such as stripping out identifying information to protect individual confidentiality may be included in this process. This staffing component—getting individuals with these skills into the surveillance project development stream—will be the lynchpin for connecting across the information space from data generation and storage to subject matter inquiry and decision support (Fig. 1-4).[41]

Recruiting, acquiring, and maintaining these skill sets can be problematic for several reasons. It is not often recognized as an exciting part of the surveillance or research landscape, and indeed it is not often chosen or even available as a career path. Analytic data managers are rarely glorified in public health or in general. The work can be tedious and very empirical in that the knowledge of a data source is based on close, repetitious, and redundant scrutiny of data details and very organized documentation.[38] When executives deciding on resource allocations lack experience in this type of work, it is easily overlooked or underestimated in scope.[42] Epidemiologists, statisticians, social scientists, engineers, and others may learn to carry out this function for one or more projects in the course of obtaining their academic credentials, but they usually have other career goals and therefore are generally not

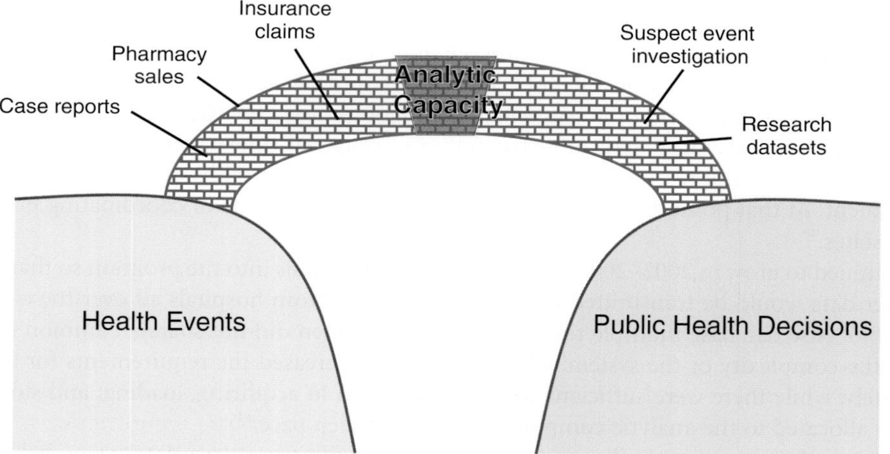

FIG. 1-3 Public health surveillance is the bridge between on-the-ground health events and good public health decision-making. The data are the bricks that form the bridge, but analytic capacity is the keystone that holds the bridge up. Without it, it is not possible to bridge the gap.

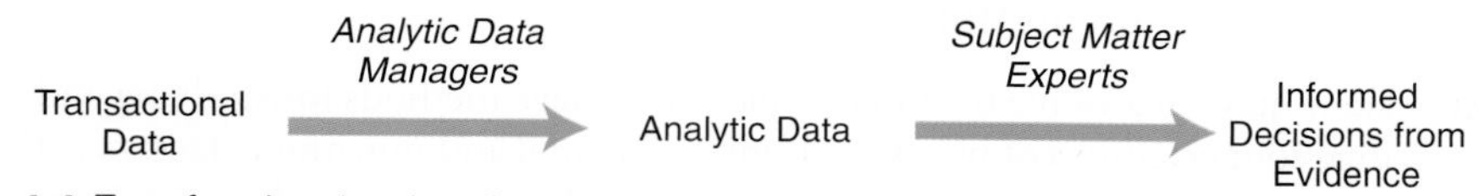
Transactional Data
Analytic Data Managers
Analytic Data
Subject Matter Experts
Informed Decisions from Evidence

FIG. 1-4 Transforming data into formats useful for public health decision-making requires skilled analytic data managers.

attracted to such work as a profession. Failure to adequately plan and staff this function can contribute to poor decision-making or invalid scientific findings, and can hamper operations of complex surveillance systems.[38]

This creates a specialized human resource management requirement for accomplishing the task of analytic data management in a sustainable manner. This is a serious management challenge in order to carry out the overall purpose of conducting surveillance in the public health setting and has become problematic to implement as data sources have grown and become more complex.

Summary

Although NEDSS and BioSense were funded and initiated separately, they are related. They both involve public health stakeholder objectives and analysis of public health data to support decisions that fulfill those objectives. **Data analysis** is the process of systematically applying statistical and/or logical techniques to describe and illustrate, condense and recap, and evaluate data.[43] We point out the shortcomings of the programs not to criticize but to emphasize the complexity of modern surveillance systems and their development. BioSense, in particular, was initiated with very little in the way of precursor. In the absence of information, the only way to generate information is to take an action and observe the results. Viewed in that context, both NEDSS and BioSense are remarkable accomplishments in that they successfully mobilized the many and various resources necessary to achieve national-level real-time surveillance, and made significant strides in that direction. Now, with the NEDSS and BioSense experiences in hand, it is the responsibility of new public health surveillance efforts to study and consider what went right, what went wrong, and how to proceed efficiently, learning from the efforts that came before.

WHAT IS ON THE HORIZON IN PUBLIC HEALTH SURVEILLANCE?

With accessible data and the human resource requirements for understanding and analyzing those data, modern surveillance can achieve its stated goals. A number of new data sources are entering mainstream use and presenting opportunities the early practitioners of public health surveillance could never have imagined. Electronic health records (EHRs) promise efficiencies to providers, hospitals, insurers, and the government, and are enabling more automated case identification to support traditional surveillance.[44–47] Administrative billing records, although not as complete with respect to individual health events as EHRs, are also becoming more widely used.[48] Such sources will likely be more and more utilized for their value in syndromic surveillance[49] as well as in health utilization assessments and population health metrics.

It is important to note that the methods for using data from administrative records or other "spontaneously" generated data are substantially different from those for using data acquired from controlled experiments or designed surveys. When data are collected for designed experiments and surveys, care is taken to ensure that the population of interest is accurately represented by the sample data. When data are simply acquired through administrative processes without a target population in mind, drawing inference from the resulting data requires different statistical methods.[38] In public health this is an ongoing methods development challenge for epidemiologists, statisticians, economists, policy analysts, and others.

Another benefit of using new data sources for surveillance is that the methodological innovation required for EHRs and billing data will open up the possibility of assimilating even less orthodox data sources and approaches to surveillance. Social networks, search word volume analyses (such as Google Flu Trends), and over-the-counter purchases present rich new possibilities in public health surveillance, but only if the information they provide can be parsed in a way that is useful for decision-making. Ensuring that analytic methods keep pace with expanding data sources will be a continuing challenge for public health surveillance.

Other opportunities come not from technological innovations per se but from the changing nature of life in a globalizing world. With people more internationally mobile than ever before, public health practitioners in different countries must accept the reality that public health events do not respect boundaries. National and local public health authorities will come under increasing pressure to cooperate with an international system that aims to address global public health risks.[19] Furthermore, in recognition of the relationship between human health and the health of nonhuman populations (e.g., avian flu H5N1 and swine flu H1N1), the ties between human and animal health are being considered in more depth. This is one of the primary goals of the One Health Initiative (see Chapter 14), which aims to expand worldwide collaboration in health care for humans, animals, and the environment.[50]

The horizon holds great promise for new knowledge from innovative public health professionals, methods, and tools as long as we maintain focus on collecting the best-quality information and putting it to use to improve public health decision-making.

KEY SUMMARY POINTS

- The purpose of public health surveillance is to support sound decision-making in order to prevent or control the spread of disease in a population.
- It is important to learn from past surveillance efforts to avoid repeating mistakes and capitalize on the successes.
- Proper governance and implementation strategies are of the upmost importance to ensure a proper balance between stakeholder engagement and forward momentum.
- There is a lack of skilled analytic data managers in public health workforce and the need for this workforce is often underestimated when establishing and carrying out a surveillance system
- Public health surveillance is continuing to grow and evolve. New data sources and analytic techniques are constantly being developed (e.g., EHRs, surveillance of over-the-counter purchases).
- As the world becomes more connected, greater international collaboration will be necessary to prevent the spread of diseases across borders.

DISCUSSION QUESTIONS

1. How have uncontrolled events affected surveillance of nosocomial infections?
2. How might developing countries benefit from the experience of the developed world in combating diabetes?
3. What are some ways to resolve the tension between respecting individual privacy and ensuring adequate collection of data for public health surveillance?
4. When funding is limited, which types of surveillance should be prioritized? Why?
5. What are some of the challenges in incorporating nontraditional surveillance data into traditional surveillance programs?

Disclaimer

Materials appearing in this book prepared by individuals as part of their official duties as US government employees are not covered by copyright, and any views expressed therein do not necessarily represent the views of the US government. Such individuals' participation in this Work is not meant to serve as an official endorsement of any statement to the extent that such statement may conflict with any official position of the US government.

REFERENCES

1. Langmuir AD. The surveillance of communicable diseases of national importance. New Engl J Med 1963;268:182–92.
2. Hinman A. Surveillance of communicable diseases. Presented at the 100th annual meeting of the American Public Health Association. Atlantic City, NJ; November 15, 1972.
3. Thacker SB, Qualters JR, Lee LM. Public health surveillance in the United States: evolution and challenges. MMWR Surveill Summ 2012;61(Suppl):3–9.
4. Baumgartner L. One hundred years of health: New York City, 1866–1966. Bull N Y Acad Med 1969;45(6):555–86.
5. Adams DA, Gallagher KM, Jajosky RA, Kriseman J, Sharp P, Anderson WJ, et al. Summary of notifiable diseases – United States, 2011. MMWR Morb Mortal Wkly Rep 2013;60(53):1–117.
6. Howard-Jones N. The scientific background of the International Sanitary Conferences, 1851-1938. 5. The ninth conference: Paris, 1894. WHO Chronicle 1974;28(10):455–70.
7. WHO. Origin and development of health cooperation, <http://www.who.int/global_health_histories/background/en/>; September 25, 2015.
8. Centers for Disease Control and Prevention. About antimicrobial resistance, <http://www.cdc.gov/drugresistance/about.html/>; September 25, 2015.

9. Centers for Disease Control and Prevention. Chronic disease prevention and health promotion: statistics and tracking, <http://www.cdc.gov/chronicdisease/stats/index.htm/>; 2013.
10. Buckeridge DL. Outbreak detection through automated surveillance: a review of the determinants of detection. J Biomed Inform 2007;40(4):370–9.
11. Buckeridge DL, Switzer P, Owens D, Siegrist D, Pavlin J, Musen M. An evaluation model for syndromic surveillance: assessing the performance of a temporal algorithm. MMWR Morb Mortal Wkly Rep 2005;54(Suppl):109–15.
12. Siegrist D, Pavlin J. Bio-ALIRT biosurveillance detection algorithm evaluation. MMWR Morb Mortal Wkly Rep 2004;53(Suppl):152–8.
13. Rolka H, O'Connor JC. Real-time public health biosurveillance: systems and policy considerations. In: Zeng D, Chen H, Castillo-Chavez C, Lober B, Thurmond M, editors. Infectious disease informatics and biosurveillance: research, systems, and case studies. New York: Springer; 2011. p. 8.
14. Fricker Jr RD. Some methodological issues in biosurveillance. Stat Med 2011;30(5):403–15.
15. Rolka H, Bracy D, Russell C, Fram D, Ball R. Using simulation to assess the sensitivity and specificity of a signal detection tool for multidimensional public health surveillance data. Stat Med 2005;24(4):551–62.
16. Reingold A. If syndromic surveillance is the answer, what is the question? Biosecur Bioterror 2003;1(2):77–81.
17. Eban K. Biosense or biononsense. The Scientist, <http://www.the-scientist.com/?articles.view/articleNo/24864/title/Biosense-or-Biononsense/2007/>; 2007.
18. Mayer K, Pizer H, editors. HIV prevention: a comprehensive approach. Amsterdam: Elsevier, Academic Press; 2009.
19. [WHO. International Health Regulations, <http://www.who.int/topics/international_health_regulations/en/>; September 25, 2015.
20. Centers for Disease Control. Pneumocystis pneumonia — Los Angeles. MMWR Morb Mortal Wkly Rep 1981;30(21):250–52.
21. Gallo RC, Salahuddin SZ, Popovic M, Shearer GM, Kaplan M, Haynes BF, et al. Frequent detection and isolation of cytopathic retroviruses (HTLV-III) from patients with AIDS and at risk for AIDS. Science 1984;224(4648):500–503.
22. Morris G, Snider D, Katz M. Integrating public health information and surveillance systems. J Public Health Manag Pract. 1996;2(4):24–7.
23. Pezzino G. A guide to the implementation of NEDSS in state public health agencies. Council of State and Territorial Epidemiologists; Atlanta, GA. 2001.
24. The College of Physicians of Philadelphia. Government regulation. The history of vaccines, <http://www.historyofvaccines.org/content/articles/government-regulation/>; January 22, 2014. Last updated: July 31, 2014.
25. Strassburg MA. The global eradication of smallpox. Am J Infect Control 1982;10(2):53–9.
26. Eylenbosch W, Noah Ne. Surveillance in health and disease, Vol 9. Oxford: Oxford University Press; 1988.
27. Duncan G, Keller-McNulty S, Stokes S. Disclosure risk vs. data utility: the R-U confidentiality map. Research Triangle Park, NC: National Institute of Statistical Sciences; 2001.
28. Seltzer W. Population statistics, the holocaust, and the Nuremberg Trials. Popul Dev Rev 1998;24(3):511–52.
29. Choi BC. The past, present, and future of public health surveillance. Scientifica 2012;2012:75253.
30. The Standish Group International Inc. The chaos report, <http://www.csus.edu/indiv/v/velianitis/161/ChaosReport.pdf/>; 1995.
31. The Standish Group International Inc. Chaos Manifesto 2013: think big, act small, <http://versionone.com/assets/img/files/ChaosManifesto2013.pdf/>; 2013.
32. Barlas S. CDC's biosense network identifying possible bioterrorism, but skeptics abound. Emergency Medicine News 2007;29(9):17.
33. McNabb SJN, Jajosky RA, Fagan R, Danos S. Evolution of integrated surveillance in the United States. Program briefing, <http://www.google.com/url?sa=t&rct=j&q=&esrc=s&frm=1&source=web&cd=6&cad=rja&uact=8&ved=0CEQQFjAF&url=http%3A%2F%2Fwww2.cdc.gov%2Fncphi%2Fdisss%2Fseminars%2Fdocs%2FNETSS-to-NEDSS_Briefing.ppt&ei=n_iZU-HzJcu3sATezYHYBQ&usg=AFQjCNENcFo0z6EBH1jRAThTvUWXFDGYEw/>; February 15, 2008.
34. Council of State and Territorial Epidemiologists. Review of and recommendations for the National Notifiable Disease Surveillance System: a state and local health department perspective. April 2013. Atlanta, GA.
35. Bradley CA, Rolka H, Walker D, Loonsk J. BioSense: implementation of a National Early Event Detection and Situational Awareness System. MMWR Morb Mortal Wkly Rep 2005;54(Suppl):11–19.
36. Loonsk JW. BioSense—a national initiative for early detection and quantification of public health emergencies. MMWR Morb Mortal Wkly Rep 2004;53(Suppl):53–5.
37. Homeland Security Presidential Directive 21: Public Health and Medical Preparedness, <http://fas.org/irp/offdocs/nspd/hspd-21.htm> Published on: October 18, 2007.
38. Fricker R. Introduction to statistical methods for biosurveillance. Cambridge: Cambridge University Press; 2013.
39. Data management. <http://www.businessdictionary.com/definition/data-management.html/>; 2015.
40. Loonsk JW. The Public Health Information Network (PHIN) Preparedness Initiative. J Am Med Inform Assoc. 2006;13(1):1–4. <http://www.ncbi.nlm.nih.gov/pmc/articles/PMC1380188/>; September 25, 2015.
41. Rolka H, Walker DW, English R, Katzoff MJ, Scogin G, Xeunaus E. Analytical challenges for emerging public health surveillance. MMWR Surveill Summ 2012;61(Suppl):35–40.
42. Davenport T, Harris J. Competing on analytics: the new science of winning. Cambridge, MA: Harvard Business School Press; 2007.
43. Faculty Development and Instructional Design Center, Northern Illinois University, DeKalb, Illinois. 2005. <https://ori.hhs.gov/education/products/n_illinois_u/datamanagement/datopic.html>; September 25, 2015.
44. Klompas M, McVetta J, Lazarus R, Eggleston E, Haney G, Kruskal BA, et al. Integrating clinical practice and public health surveillance using electronic medical record systems. Am J Public Health 2012;102(Suppl. 3):S325–32.
45. Klompas M, Eggleston E, McVetta J, Lazarus R, Li L, Platt R. Automated detection and classification of type 1 versus type 2 diabetes using electronic health record data. Diabetes Care 2013;36(4):914–21.
46. Allen-Dicker J, Klompas M. Comparison of electronic laboratory reports, administrative claims, and electronic health record data for acute viral hepatitis surveillance. J Public Health Manag Pract 2012;18(3):209–14.
47. Calderwood MS, Platt R, Hou X, Malenfant J, Haney G, Kruskal B, et al. Real-time surveillance for tuberculosis using electronic health record data from an ambulatory practice in eastern Massachusetts. Public Health Rep 2010;125(6):843–50.
48. Hales CM, Harpaz R, Joesoef MR, Bialek SR. Examination of links between herpes zoster incidence and childhood varicella vaccination. Ann Intern Med 2013;159(11):739–45.
49. Singer M, Clair S. Syndemics and public health: reconceptualizing disease in bio-social context. Med Anthropol Q 2003;17(4):423–41.
50. One Health Initiative, <http://www.onehealthinitiative.com/about.php>; September 25, 2015.

CHAPTER

2

CDC Perspectives and Strategy on Emerging Public Health Surveillance Issues and Opportunities

Chesley L Richards

Not everything that can be counted counts, and not everything that counts can be counted.

Albert Einstein

KEY WORDS

CDC Surveillance Strategy
Health information technology policy
Informatics
Electronic laboratory reporting
MMWR
HITECH
NNDSS
Health Information Innovation Consortium
BioSense
National Vital Statistics System
CDC

INTRODUCTION

Public health surveillance is the cornerstone of public health practice and can be defined as the " . . . systematic, ongoing collection, management, analysis, and interpretation of data followed by the dissemination of these data to public health programs to stimulate public health action . . . ."[1] More succinctly, public health surveillance produces data for action to improve or protect health. In the USA, public health surveillance is at a crossroads.[2-5] With decreasing public financing for public health in many jurisdictions and emerging health information technologies that offer tremendous opportunities for rapid and flexible data collection, evolution of the methods, systems, and workforce needs for public health surveillance is underway. High-quality public health surveillance can rapidly detect and monitor diseases and injuries, assess the impact of interventions, and assist in the management of and recovery from large-scale public health incidents. Today's media and communications environment pressures public health scientists, researchers, and frontline practitioners to provide information, on an almost instantaneous basis, that is responsive to public and policy maker concerns about specific geographies and populations. Actions informed by surveillance data take many forms, such as policy changes, new program interventions, public communication, and investments in research. Local, state, and federal public health professionals, government leaders, public health partners, and the public depend on high-quality, timely, and actionable public health surveillance data.

Public Health Surveillance in the USA

In the USA, public health surveillance occurs as a partnership between state, territorial, local, and tribal (STLT) jurisdictions and the federal government. The statutory responsibility for disease reporting is at the state and local level, and, through voluntary reporting, surveillance data are provided to the federal government at the **Centers for Disease Control and Prevention (CDC)**. The US CDC "is one of the major operating components of the US

Department of Health and Human Services and is recognized as the nation's premiere health promotion, prevention, and preparedness agencies. CDC focuses in five strategic areas: supporting state and local health departments, improving global health, implementing measures to decrease leading causes of death, strengthening surveillance and epidemiology, and reforming health policies."[6]

Surveillance at the national level can be used to drive or assess national public health policy (e.g., surveillance for vaccine preventable diseases informs immunization policies and programs), to identify the national scope and trajectory of emerging infections (e.g., H1N1 influenza, West Nile Virus, MERS), or to monitor changes in common diseases (e.g., sexually transmitted diseases, cancer). At the local level, surveillance data informs local public health action and is served by national and state data to provide context and comparison. While beyond the scope of this chapter, several thorough reviews on public health surveillance in the USA have been published.[2-5] Taken together, these reviews paint a picture of public health surveillance in the USA that identifies challenges and opportunities. First, a series of fundamental challenges exist, including insufficient funding and technical expertise in many STLT health agencies, differing information standards and requirements among jurisdictions, concerns about confidentiality protection and data sharing, lack of access to data in health care systems, insufficient linkages to nonhealth social determinant data, and insufficient analytic approaches, tools, and workforce. Many of these challenges are addressed in other chapters in this textbook. These challenges are substantial, but they also highlight exciting opportunities to more fully integrate, analyze, and visualize a broad array of data toward more robust information to support public health action.

CDC'S ROLE AND ACTIVITIES

CDC plays important roles for public health surveillance issues, including coordination, support, and technical expertise. CDC works with the Council of State and Territorial Epidemiologists (CSTE) to establish reportable conditions for the USA.[7] Data on these conditions are collected by state and local health agencies per their statutory powers and then voluntarily shared with CDC to create a national awareness of reportable conditions through weekly reportable conditions tables published in the ***Morbidity and Mortality Weekly Report*** *which is a publication series prepared by CDC, and an annual summary report.*[8,9] Other data shared with CDC are collected as part of a broad array of federally funded programs and projects. Consequently, these many programs and projects have generally relied on purpose-built systems or tools that are not necessarily aligned across the agency. This distributed approach, while in many cases effective in producing actionable public health data, can create challenges for efficiency, common standards, and repurposing of existing systems for new or emerging surveillance issues.

CDC'S VISION AND STRATEGIC APPROACH

The vision for surveillance activities supported or operated by CDC is to be able to get the right public health data and information into the right hands at the right time. Building off of earlier work to outline a strategic framework to address challenges with public health surveillance in the USA, CDC launched a surveillance strategy in February 2014 to drive agency activities, investments, and priorities for public health surveillance.[4,10] The **CDC Surveillance Strategy** is the US CDC's strategy that guides efforts to make essential surveillance systems more adaptable to the rapidly changing technology landscape, more versatile in meeting demands for expanding knowledge about evolving threats to health, and more able to meet the demands for timely and population-specific and geographically specific surveillance information.[10] The strategy will also facilitate work to consolidate systems, eliminate unnecessary redundancies in reporting, and reduce reporting burden.[10] This strategy laid out three overriding goals and a series of specific activities to improve surveillance, which are as follows:

- To enhance the accountability, resource use, workforce, and innovation for surveillance by establishing a Surveillance Leadership Board, a surveillance workforce plan, and an innovation consortium.[10]
- To accelerate the utilization of emerging tools and approaches to improve the availability, quality, and timeliness of surveillance data by establishing enhanced health information technology (HIT) policy engagement, HIT vendor forums, and informatics innovation projects.[10]

- To demonstrate early success through four crosscutting surveillance system initiatives to improve surveillance by addressing data availability, system usability, redundancies, and incorporation of new information technologies.

While specific to CDC, the goals and activities described are in alignment with the National Strategy for Biosurveillance and are also intended to provide guidance and improved support to the needs of STLT health agencies in the USA with whom CDC works.[11]

CDC SURVEILLANCE STRATEGY GOALS

In outlining the strategy, CDC aims to rapidly improve its surveillance activities and investments while also laying the groundwork for long-lasting system evolution. The goals and activities address fundamental gaps identified through external peer review, stakeholder consultations, and internal assessments.

Goal 1. Surveillance Decision-making and Structure

The first goal of the surveillance strategy is aimed at enhancing the accountability, resource use, workforce, and innovation for surveillance at CDC and in support of STLT agencies. This goal creates a structural framework to advance strategic surveillance investments and activities at CDC by creating a leadership board, a surveillance/informatics workforce plan, and an innovation consortium. The leadership board will make recommendations to the CDC Director and senior leaders regarding key strategic decisions on surveillance (e.g., harmonizing systems, common funding language and approaches, and use of information standards). The workforce plan will be critical in supporting future implementation of surveillance and data tools and platforms at both CDC and in STLT agencies. The innovation consortium will connect currently disparate innovation activities to a forum for sharing successes, learning from failures, and ensuring that informatics innovations are connected to the current national IT standards and policy directions.

CDC Surveillance Leadership Board

In 2014, CDC established a Surveillance Leadership Board comprising key senior leaders in the agency. The board was charged with reviewing, guiding, and overseeing the evolution of CDC surveillance systems in accordance with principles established in the strategy document. The board is chaired by the CDC Deputy Director for Public Health Scientific Services and is composed of members appointed from CDC operating divisions responsible for aspects of disease, injury, and condition surveillance. Through the board, CDC aims to enhance its accountability to policy makers and public health programs that should benefit from a robust surveillance information infrastructure. The board is focusing on agency policies and programs to optimize resource investments devoted to the emerging surveillance systems infrastructure. This will be accomplished by assuring coordination among partners and transparency in decision-making, harmonizing CDC's efforts to work with HIT standards development organizations and work toward streamlining requests for public health reporting functionality in commercial electronic health record systems, monitoring progress in new system implementation, facilitating the use of best practices for surveillance, and ensuring that CDC is making progress toward achieving its broad strategic goals.

Workforce Plan

CDC will develop a federal and STLT workforce training and support plan that integrates CDC's strategy for improving surveillance systems and technological considerations practitioners will face with CDC workforce investments. While the plan will focus on the resources CDC has to promote the surveillance and informatics workforce, it will be informed by collaboration with an array of partners also interested in these workforce issues.[12] The aim is for this plan to support improved preparation of surveillance practitioners to assess new data sources, interface with technologies used by clinical health care providers, and evaluate commercial, governmental, and open source surveillance system products. The plan will address both the short-term training needs of new and current public health practitioners and the longer term future training and ongoing support for the surveillance workforce.

CDC Health Information Innovation Consortium

CDC has created a **CDC Health Information Innovation Consortium** to foster and promote creative solutions to surveillance challenges implemented through innovative projects in CDC programs and STLT agencies. This consortium identifies and accelerates emerging tools and approaches to improve the availability, quality, and timeliness of surveillance data while also connecting these efforts to the other activities of the surveillance strategy.[10]

Goal 2. Emerging Information Tools and Approaches

The second goal of the surveillance strategy aims to accelerate the utilization of emerging tools and approaches to improve the availability, quality, and timeliness of surveillance data.

Emerging HIT improvements offer tremendous potential to improve the timeliness, quality, quantity, and efficiency of public health data, enabling decision-makers to take action while more effectively linking public health agencies and systems with clinical systems and health care professionals. The **Health Information Technology for Economic and Clinical Health Act** (HITECH) and the associated Meaningful Use requirements allow clinicians, health care providers, and public health systems to benefit from greater electronic connectivity, public health reporting, and population health monitoring.[10] HITECH is an act that was enacted as part of the American Recovery and Reinvestment Act of 2009 and was signed into law on February 17, 2009, to promote the adoption and meaningful use of health information technology.[13] However, with these tremendous opportunities come formidable challenges for public health agencies, particularly regarding the informatics workforce, tools, and resources to effectively connect with the health care community.[14]

The utilization and incorporation of emerging HIT tools and approaches by CDC and public health can be improved through more effective policy, vendor engagement, and leveraging of emerging information technologies.[10] In addition to the innovation consortium described above, CDC is working with STLT agencies to improve policy and vendor engagement and to provide support for innovation projects.

HIT Policy Engagement

The HITECH act and other health information technology policies have brought about an environment in which public health data activities are increasingly impacted by broader HIT policies as set by the Office of the National Information Technology Coordinator (ONC) and other federal information technology regulators. The Federal Health Information Technology Strategic Plan, 2011–2015,[15] and the HIT Policy Committee are the foundations for ONC's work. Through collaboration with ONC, CDC has increased its involvement and participation in the HIT policy committee and actively participated in crafting of the Federal HIT Strategic Plan for 2015–2020. To complement these policy engagements, CDC is collaborating on a series of projects with ONC to further STLT health agencies' capacity to implement HIT strategies.

Strategic HIT Vendor Engagement

CDC is developing a forum to systematically engage vendors regarding informatics technologies and tools that can advance surveillance practice and systems. Vendor engagement provides opportunities for CDC programs and STLT agencies to more consistently communicate key functionality and application needs to an array of information technology and electronic health record vendors.

Support for Innovative Informatics Projects

We define **informatics** as the science concerned with gathering, manipulating, storing, retrieving, and classifying recorded information.[16] Beginning in 2014, CDC is providing seed funding and technical support for small project awards generated through the aforementioned Health Information Innovation Consortium to advance specific innovations in areas of interest such as data collection, transport, storage, analysis, visualization, and availability. These projects will (1) advance innovation on a specific interest area; (2) if successful, provide insights or tools that can be generalized to other surveillance systems or activities; and (3) improve effectiveness or efficiency of existing surveillance systems by leveraging emerging information technologies. Projects may be related to electronic health records, or they may include innovations using mobile technologies and social media as potentially important new tools for public health surveillance.[17,18]

Goal 3. Crosscutting Agency Initiatives

Finally, CDC initiated four crosscutting agency initiatives in 2014 to improve surveillance by addressing data availability, system usability, redundancies, and incorporation of new information technologies in major systems or activities. These initiatives are aimed at improving existing platforms or tools that have wide applicability and can benefit both STLT agencies and multiple programs at CDC. By focusing on these systems or tools, CDC is creating higher performing broad platforms that can increasingly be used for other surveillance needs or activities. In coming years, additional initiatives may be added to make similar progress on other crosscutting platforms in the agency.

Initiative 1. National Notifiable Diseases Surveillance System Modernization Initiative

The **National Notifiable Diseases Surveillance System (NNDSS)** is the USA's public system for monitoring the occurrence and spread of the diseases and conditions that STLT agencies have agreed to report voluntarily to CDC. Currently, there are over 70 reportable diseases and conditions. This complex system is supported and used by numerous stakeholders and is expected to provide accurate, timely, and sufficient information for surveillance and response on notifiable conditions.[19] The National Electronic Disease Surveillance System (NEDSS) facilitates the electronic transfer of public health surveillance data from the health care system to public health departments and is a major conduit for exchanging information that supports NNDSS. NEDSS provides standards, IT infrastructure, and incentives for rapid electronic NNDSS reporting. However, some states have not fully implemented NEDSS and submit data utilizing the legacy National Electronic Telecommunications System for Surveillance (NETSS) format from 1990. Evolution in technology, data and exchange standards offer more robust and timely opportunities for data reporting, analysis, and visualization, but may also face challenges in implementation. Consequently, CDC is reexamining and enhancing the infrastructure supporting public health surveillance for notifiable diseases and conditions.

The NNDSS Modernization Initiative seeks to enhance surveillance capabilities in response to stakeholders' concerns and needs for more comprehensive, timely, and higher quality data. It will also provide a robust infrastructure based on interoperable, standardized data and exchange mechanisms.[10] The specific performance objective for this initiative is to have 90% of data reported through NNDSS using standard HL7 messages, enabling the retirement of the NETSS legacy system. By retiring NETSS, NNDSS will have improved timeliness, standardization, and data usability by CDC programs and STLT agencies.

Initiative 2. BioSense Enhancement Initiative

Syndromic surveillance can offer potentially important contributions to public health surveillance, especially for situational awareness of emerging public health threats.[20,21] At CDC, the **BioSense program**, established in 2003 after 9/11 and the subsequent anthrax attacks, is a syndromic surveillance system that provides data necessary for public health officials to monitor and respond to possible disease or hazardous conditions.[10] It is an electronic health information system with standardized tools and procedures for rapidly collecting, sharing, and evaluating information about emergency department visits and other health-related data from health care sources and clinical care facilities.[10,22] Findings from a recent investment internal review of BioSense highlighted the promise and potential that this surveillance system holds for public health, particularly around increasing use of electronic health records, strengthening our partnership with the health care sector, extending surveillance practices and methods, and reducing costs.[10] The BioSense Enhancement Initiative will build on the successes of the past, fix areas that need improvement, and enhance both the national view of syndromic surveillance data and the ability for STLT agencies to analyze, compare, and ultimately take action on their local data.[10] The performance goal is to establish, by mid-2015, enhanced public health situational awareness utilizing electronic health record data and active CDC and STLT analyses that support public health decisions and programs at the local, state, and national levels.

Initiative 3. Accelerating Electronic Laboratory Reporting

Electronic laboratory reporting, the electronic transmission from laboratories to public health of laboratory reports, which identify reportable conditions, of results to public health agencies can improve public health surveillance for reportable diseases and conditions by making reporting more timely and complete.[10,23] At the end of July 2013, approximately 62% of 20 million laboratory reports were being received electronically, compared with 54% in 2012.[10,24] Strong relationships between clinical laboratories, laboratory information management system vendors, and public health agencies are necessary for this continued improvement. The performance metric for this initiative is to have at least 80% of laboratory reports to public health agencies (at CDC or states) received as electronic laboratory reports. As electronic reporting of laboratory data becomes more universal, it will be important to properly assess the impact on public health practitioners regarding both volume and quality of the data so as not to create undue, unplanned burdens.[25,26]

Initiative 4. Mortality Surveillance-Related Initiatives with the National Vital Statistics System

National Vital Statistics System (**NVSS**) is "the oldest and most successful example of intergovernmental data sharing in US Public Health and the shared relationships, standards, and procedures form the mechanism by which NCHS collects and disseminates the Nation's official vital statistics. These data are provided through contracts between NCHS and vital registration systems operated in the various jurisdictions legally responsible for the registration of vital events—births, deaths, marriages, divorces, and fetal deaths."[27] Making over the NVSS into a system capable of supporting near real-time public health surveillance has been needed for a long time. Electronic death certificates, for example, can be used to conduct mortality surveillance for health conditions such as influenza.[28] While much progress has been made, substantial focus is needed to fully realize NVSS's potential as a public health surveillance tool.[28] By 2016, 80% of death reports occurring in at least 25 states will be reported electronically.

EXPECTED OUTCOMES AND FUTURE DIRECTIONS

Over the next 3–5 years, the CDC Surveillance Strategy will increasingly guide both program and agency-wide surveillance activities. By establishing a framework within which to make coordinated and strategic investments in surveillance programs and infrastructure, the agency aims to use its resources efficiently and with high value to STLT health agencies. By reducing the number of stand-alone systems and increasing the use of highly functional, multi-program platforms, CDC seeks to increase functionality and decrease duplication and redundant burden on STLT agencies. And, by leveraging emerging technologies in a more coordinated fashion across the agency and with STLT agencies, CDC aims to accelerate movement toward a digital infrastructure that can provide data and information to those who need it when they need it and in a form that allows them to act. The CDC Surveillance Strategy is not a static document but a leadership framework to achieve these goals.

JOB FUNCTIONS

Jobs focused on surveillance strategy implementation will require broad epidemiologic, public health, informatics, and leadership skills. Key competencies for implementing the CDC Surveillance Strategy relate to emerging skills needed at both national and STLT agencies. In addition to competencies in applied epidemiology, informatics, and public health,[29] training and experience in strategy and innovation, public health leadership, and program management is desirable to maximize the opportunities for implementation of key elements of the surveillance strategy.

KEY SUMMARY POINTS

- Public health surveillance is evolving, given the challenges of decreasing public financing and emerging health information technologies.
- High-quality public health surveillance can rapidly detect and monitor disease and injuries, assess the impact of interventions, and assist in the management of and recovery from large-scale public health incidents.
- Public health surveillance occurs as a partnership between STLT jurisdictions and the federal government. The statutory responsibility for disease reporting is at the state and local levels, and surveillance data are provided through voluntary reporting to CDC.
- CDC's vision for surveillance is to be able to get the right public health data and information into the right hands at the right time. CDC launched a surveillance strategy to drive activities, investments, and priorities for public health surveillance.
- The strategy's goals are (i) to enhance the accountability, resource use, workforce, and innovation for surveillance at CDC and in support of STLT agencies; (ii) to accelerate the utilization of emerging tools and approaches to improve the availability, quality, and timeliness of surveillance data; and (iii) to improve existing platforms or tools that have wide applicability and can benefit both STLT agencies and multiple programs at CDC.

DISCUSSION QUESTIONS

1. What are some of the challenges public health surveillance is facing?
2. Give examples of CDC's role in public health surveillance activities.
3. How are workforce issues and challenges addressed throughout the CDC Surveillance Strategy presented in this chapter?
4. How are data from electronic health records and other clinical sources used throughout the strategy?
5. How do the strategy's initiatives, plans, and approaches seek to benefit both CDC and STLT agencies? Why is this important?

REFERENCES

1. Thacker SB, Qualters JR, Lee LM. Centers for Disease Control and Prevention. Public health surveillance in the United States: evolution and challenges. MMWR Surveill Summ 2012;61(Suppl):3–9.
2. Mirza N, Reynolds T, Coletta M, Suda K, Soyiri I, Markle A, et al. Steps to a sustainable public health surveillance enterprise a commentary from the international society for disease surveillance. Online J Public Health Inform 2013;5(2):210.
3. Smith PF, Hadler JL, Stanbury M, Rolfs RT, Hopkins RS. "Blueprint version 2.0": updating public health surveillance for the 21st century. J Public Health Manag Pract 2013;19(3):231–9.
4. Buehler JW. CDC's vision for public health surveillance in the 21st century. Introduction. MMWR Surveill Summ 2012;61(Suppl):1–2.
5. NORC. Assessing the status and prospects of state and local health department information technology infrastructure. Chicago: University of Chicago; 2013.
6. About CDC 24-7. Our History - Our Story: U.S. Centers for Disease Control and Prevention, <http://www.cdc.gov/about/history/index.html/>; October 1, 2015..
7. CSTE. CSTE List of Nationally Notifiable Conditions 2012, <http://c.ymcdn.com/sites/www.cste.org/resource/resmgr/PDFs/CSTENotifiableConditionListA.pdf/>; May 10, 2014.
8. Adams DA, Gallagher KM, Jajosky RA, Kriseman J, Sharp P, Anderson WJ, et al. Summary of notifiable diseases - United States, 2011. MMWR Morb Mortal Wkly Rep 2013;60(53):1–117.
9. Morbidity and Mortality Weekly Report (MMWR). U.S. Centers for Disease Control and Prevention, <http://www.cdc.gov/mmwr/about.html/>; 2015.
10. Prevention US CfDCa. Surveillance strategy; 2014.
11. National Strategy for Biosurveillance. Washington, DC: The White House; 2012. <https://www.whitehouse.gov/sites/default/files/National_Strategy_for_Biosurveillance_July_2012.pdf>; October 1, 2015.
12. Drehobl PA, Roush SW, Stover BH, Koo D. Public health surveillance workforce of the future. MMWR Surveill Summ 2012;61(Suppl):25–9.
13. Health Information Privacy HITECH Act enforcement interim final rule: U.S. department of health and human services, <http://www.hhs.gov/>; 2013. [updated July 26, 2013; cited 2015].
14. Lenert L, Sundwall DN. Public health surveillance and meaningful use regulations: a crisis of opportunity. Am J Public Health 2012;102(3):e1–7.
15. Office of the National Information Technology Coordinator. Department of Health and Human Services. Federal Health Information Technology Strategic Plan 2015-2020. <https://www.healthit.gov/sites/default/files/9-5-federalhealthitstratplanfinal_0.pdf>; October 1, 2015.
16. National Program of Cancer Registries (NPCR) Informatics. U.S. Centers for Disease Control and Prevention, <http://www.cdc.gov/cancer/npcr/informatics/>; 2015.
17. Eggleston EM, Weitzman ER. Innovative uses of electronic health records and social media for public health surveillance. Curr Diab Rep 2014;14(3):468.
18. Hartley DM. Using social media and internet data for public health surveillance: the importance of talking. Milbank Q 2014;92(1):34–9.
19. National Notifiable Disease Surveillance System (NNDSS): U.S. Centers for Disease Control and Prevention, <http://wwwn.cdc.gov/nndss/>; 2015 [updated May 6, 2015].
20. Fan S, Blair C, Brown A, Gabos S, Honish L, Hughes T, et al. A multifunction public health surveillance system and the lessons learned in its development: the Alberta real time syndromic surveillance net. Can J Public Health 2010;101(6):454–8.
21. Wilson EL, Egger JR, Konty KJ, Paladini M, Weiss D, Nguyen TQ. Description of a school nurse visit syndromic surveillance system and comparison to emergency department visits, New York City. Am J Public Health 2014;104(1):e50–6.

22. BioSense Program BioSense. U.S. Centers for Disease Control and Prevention, <http://www.cdc.gov/biosense/>; 2015.
23. Meaningful Use Electronic Laboratory Reporting (ELR). U.S. Centers for Disease Control and Prevention, <http://www.cdc.gov/ehrmeaningfuluse/elr.html/>; 2015.
24. Progress in increasing electronic reporting of laboratory results to public health agencies—United States, 2013. MMWR Morb Mortal Wkly Rep 2013;62(38):797–999.
25. Dixon BE, Gibson PJ, Grannis SJ. Estimating increased electronic laboratory reporting volumes for meaningful use: implications for the public health workforce. Online J Public Health Inform 2014;5(3):225.
26. Dixon BE, Siegel JA, Oemig TV, Grannis SJ. Electronic health information quality challenges and interventions to improve public health surveillance data and practice. Public Health Rep 2013;128(6):546–53.
27. National Vital Statistics System. U.S. Centers for Disease Control and Prevention, <http://www.cdc.gov/nchs/nvss.htm>; 2015.
28. Bancroft EA, Lee S. Use of electronic death certificates for influenza death surveillance. Emerg Infect Dis 2014;20(1):78–82.
29. Prevention USCfDCa. Workforce Development Resources: Competencies, <http://www.cdc.gov/ophss/csels/dsepd/resources.html/>; May 30, 2014.

CHAPTER

3

Models of Public Health Surveillance

Meeyoung M Park, Lauren Reeves

You must be in tune with the times and prepared to break with tradition.

James Agee

KEY WORDS

Passive surveillance
Sentinel surveillance
One Health Approach
Community-based surveillance
Digital surveillance
Syndromic surveillance
Event-based surveillance
Population-based surveillance
Indicator-based surveillance
Predictive surveillance
Participatory surveillance
Laboratory surveillance
Genetic surveillance

OVERVIEW AND EVOLUTION OF PUBLIC HEALTH SURVEILLANCE

Economic globalization has advanced with innovations in communication and transport technologies. The resulting increase in the intersection of humans, livestock, and agriculture results in increased volume of disease carrying vectors and imported infectious diseases around the world through international trade. For this reason, we must be especially cognizant of dynamic disease transmission models that weigh variables beyond traditional public health surveillance, to collectively consider risk factors across human, animal, and environmental spectra (i.e., One Health, see Chapter 14) to identify and address individual-level and community public health issues. Recent disease outbreaks, such as the massive Ebola outbreak originating in Guinea in December 2013, demonstrate the necessity of public awareness as well as multinational and multisectoral collaboration for effective surveillance and response.[2]

We define new eras of public health surveillance (PHS) by changes in the underlying paradigm, analytic approach, and preventive approach.[3] For instance, just as advances in clinical care practices and technologies enabled the population to combat and resist infectious diseases, an increasing focus on chronic conditions in the late twentieth century resulted in analytic approaches and preventive measures for chronic disease epidemiology.[3,4] Surveillance continues to undergo paradigm shifts as its methods and tools evolve.[5,6] In the twenty-first century, epidemiologists have adopted technologies that enhance diagnostic capabilities, expand scope of data collection, improve timeliness and data quality, and support sophisticated analyses and modeling to address global One Health priorities.

This chapter will introduce and describe different modes and models of surveillance to provide a foundation for the rest of the book, highlighting new technologies that are key contributors to novel methods. These surveillance modes and models will be referred to and discussed throughout the remaining chapters. Understanding these systems is an important aspect of understanding PHS and its practice.

PUBLIC HEALTH SURVEILLANCE OBJECTIVES

Information derived from analysis of surveillance data are used to estimate the scope, severity, and characteristics of a public health issue.[7] This information informs public health actions and measures the impact and efficacy of interventions, both of which help facilitate planning for future health threats.[8] To do so, surveillance data are monitored to identify changes in disease occurrence and are characterized by person, place, and time, the minimum case data required for basic surveillance.[8–11] Enhanced surveillance includes more detailed variables increasingly accessible with more sophisticated techniques, integrated data, specialized software, and tools for analysis discussed elsewhere in this book.[9] (See Chapters 18, 21, 23, and 25–27.) Data analysis helps epidemiologists identify disease trends.[11] PHS also helps to detect outbreaks and cases for epidemiologic research and to develop hypotheses for study.[8,12,13] Comprehensive surveillance involves not only monitoring the disease, condition, or event but also evaluating risk factors and prevention services.[8]

The specific surveillance objectives of an individual public health program depend on the information needs and intended use of data of relevant stakeholders.[11] Data analysis and results help public health practitioners prioritize different activities and interventions; analyses designed to evaluate programs subsequently inform resource allocation, whereby limited funds are distributed to effective or promising programs.[8,14] In general, surveillance systems should be established to detect and characterize diseases, conditions, or events of public health concern in order to implement prevention and control programs. As such, health information systems (e.g., vital events registries or electronic medical records) do not strictly constitute surveillance systems; however, these databases may be an important data source and therefore part of the broader surveillance network.[8]

MODES OF PUBLIC HEALTH SURVEILLANCE

The modes of surveillance described in this section refer to broad, overarching approaches to surveillance. One or more modes of surveillance may be incorporated into the design of a surveillance system model (described in the next section), depending on the surveillance objectives and nature of the condition, disease, or event.

Passive Surveillance

Definition

Passive surveillance is a type of surveillance that relies on regular reporting of disease data by all institutions that attend to patients (or test specimens) and are part of a reporting network. In passive surveillance there is no active search for cases; rather, it involves voluntary submission of reports generated at the local level.[15] In passive surveillance, health care workers and laboratorians at peripheral levels collect and report data on conditions or events using standard case definitions. Workers at health facilities and laboratories also collect, transfer, and test specimens for laboratory diagnosis and case confirmation.[16] Data from these tests and diagnoses are generated and sent to public health departments at a specified frequency depending on the urgency or importance related to the condition under surveillance.[15,16] Successful passive surveillance is dependent on the ability of health care workers to accurately identify and report cases in a timely fashion, and requires medical and laboratory workers to be well trained and laboratories to have adequate supplies and equipment.[16]

While passive surveillance requires fewer resources on the part of the public health department, the data collected may be skewed or incomplete due to reliance on reporters. Many cases are undiagnosed because of a lack of disease awareness by health care workers, nonspecificity of symptoms, mild presentation of symptoms, or shortage of laboratory resources to perform diagnostics.[16–18] Health care providers who are undertrained or unmotivated further hinder case detection and reporting.[16] The population within the catchment area may also have poor access to health care, exacerbating issues with underdiagnosis, incomplete surveillance data, delayed response, and diluted health impacts, especially in under-resourced countries.[8,16,19] Examples of passive surveillance include the Vaccine Adverse Events Reporting System, monitoring patient safety in the USA, and most of the health-care-associated infection surveillance systems.[20,21] Passive surveillance is most useful for routine monitoring of well-characterized, endemic conditions with specific case definitions and case classification criteria.

Sentinel Surveillance

Sentinel surveillance is a type of surveillance that relies on data from selected reporters (e.g., hospitals) with a 1) high probability of seeing cases of the target disease, 2) adequate laboratory facilities, 3) and qualified staff. "Sentinel surveillance is used when high-quality data are needed about a particular disease that cannot be obtained through a passive system."[22] Sentinel surveillance provides more robust and comprehensive data than passive surveillance systems.[16,22] Data may be sent more frequently and for additional diseases beyond what is routinely reported in a passive surveillance system.[16] Reports may include various types of laboratory diagnostic results, such as genetic typing, serotyping, and antibiotic resistance.[23–25] Sentinel surveillance is conducted by a selection of voluntary reporters within a closed network, in contrast to a passive system that receives data from all reporters within a catchment area.[22] Reporters in the network should have access to high-quality diagnostics, adequately trained medical personnel, and a sufficiently large population served with access to public health and health care services.[22] This method of data collection is not useful for surveillance of rare diseases, as data are gathered within a restricted network for a subset of the population and are thereby not representative of the general population.[16,22]

Sentinel surveillance is usually conducted for a particular reason, such as the surveillance for a specific subpopulation or condition. For example, conducting routine, passive surveillance for malaria has been inadequate due to poorly defined indicators, incomplete data, and inconsistent report frequency; therefore, sentinel surveillance for malaria was launched in Oromia Regional State, Ethiopia. This surveillance system was composed of 10 sentinel sites to fill information gaps and improve public health response.[26] This mode of surveillance is also effective to monitor trends in antibiotic resistance; however, it is not well suited to determine the efficacy of interventions within defined populations.[23]

Population-Based Surveillance

Population-based surveillance is a type of surveillance that "involves identifying all new cases of the disease under surveillance in a defined population" using community-based cohort studies and active surveillance of households to determine attack rates and disease burden.[18,23] Population-based surveillance is the counterpart to sentinel surveillance and it complements routine surveillance.[23] The granularity of the data allows for data analysis involving comorbidities or high-risk groups and development of disease transmission models.[18] In addition, the World Health Organization (WHO) has recommended using population-based surveillance to measure the efficacy of new vaccines, as it is very useful for determining a vaccine's overall effect on the population.[23] As data collection for this type of surveillance requires field visits to collect representative samples, population-based surveillance is more resource and labor intensive than passive and sentinel surveillance.[23]

An example of population-based surveillance involved the study of trivalent inactivated influenza vaccine effectiveness in pregnant women. This case–control study was conducted over two influenza seasons in two metropolitan areas within a health care network and the laboratory-confirmed results affirmed the efficacy of the vaccine intervention.[27] Population-based surveillance may also be conducted to characterize rates and risks for morbidity and mortality in target populations.[28,29]

Active Surveillance

Active surveillance is a type of surveillance that dynamically seeks data from participants in the surveillance system on a regular basis.[30] It involves the proactive collection of data from health facilities through interviews with health care providers and direct review of medical records to identify suspect and confirmed cases.[31] Public health professionals systematically visit health care facilities to identify infected persons and investigate potential cases using clinical data and laboratory test results.[31] (See Chapter 5 for discussion on active and passive surveillance.) This method of surveillance is intensive, sensitive, and expensive. It is particularly effective during the final stages of a disease eradication process. An example is the active virological surveillance using genomic sequencing to identify and track isolates of poliovirus and pinpoint gaps in surveillance, established in 2012 by WHO.[31,32] (See Chapters 25, 30, and 31 for a discussion of the role of polio surveillance in disease eradication efforts.)

Laboratory-Based Surveillance

Laboratory-based surveillance uses laboratory data to detect trends and outbreaks, estimate burden of illness, and allows for subtyping of pathogens, which is critical for linking illness to vehicles and reservoirs.[33] Laboratory-based surveillance is critical for confirming outbreak detection and management and public health program evaluation. Laboratory data provide details on pathogen classification and subtyping (e.g., *Vibrio cholerae* O1) and other information, such as antimicrobial susceptibility, in order to confirm diagnoses, refine case classifications, identify new pathogens, and otherwise characterize etiologic agents. Analysis of these data can help investigators conduct contact tracing to map the transmission of disease, identify potential interventions, and provide intelligence for post-outbreak surveillance. At other times, laboratory surveillance supports trend monitoring, measures the efficacy of interventions, and provides data to gauge achievement of surveillance objectives, such as reducing nosocomial infections.[34]

To support laboratory surveillance, staff must be trained in proper biosafety and biosecurity procedures and on all proper laboratory standard operating procedures. Laboratories must also have resources to procure essential equipment, reagents, and supplies to conduct diagnostic tests. In addition, sample collection requires specific protocols not only to protect handlers during transport but also to ensure samples are not contaminated.[35]

Laboratories serve as a cornerstone of PHS; without laboratory surveillance capacity, many case reports remain unconfirmed and surveillance data are incomplete. Most infectious disease case classification criteria include laboratory result criteria. Even some noninfectious conditions and events include data from laboratory testing (e.g., carbon monoxide poisoning) in confirmation of cases.[36]

Genetic Surveillance

Genetic surveillance is a specialized branch of laboratory-based surveillance focusing on molecular subtyping to identify pathogens and genetic markers for heritable diseases or increased susceptibility to risk factors.[37–40] Laboratory criteria for case classification in case definitions increasingly include genetic pathogen typing for infectious disease and food-borne illnesses.[41–43] Genetic markers identify strains of pathogens and are used to characterize antimicrobial resistant genotypes.[43] (See chapter 26 for a detailed discussion of genetic pathogen surveillance.) Analysis of genetic pathogen surveillance data may facilitate earlier detection of outbreaks through investigation of genetic divergence in chains of transmission. Genetic surveillance also informs disease transmission models, which incorporate factors such as pathogen virulence and behavior, spatial-temporal distribution among host population, antigenic shift, and antimicrobial resistance.[44]

Typing using molecular tools such as multiplex real-time polymerase chain reaction (PCR) and sequence-based detection alleviates burdens on reference laboratories that conduct serotyping to identify subtypes, as there are many more laboratories able to execute genetic surveillance protocols.[37,45,46] Whole genome sequencing techniques permit scientists to discover and study novel genetic variations in humans and pathogens that impact risk of disease.[47,48] In addition to laboratory equipment and reagents, genetic surveillance requires access to a database of molecular typing data and specialized protocols and tools to capture, process, and analyze these inherently large data sets.

Genetic surveillance is not commonly conducted for routine surveillance of infectious diseases, though some programs exist, such as PulseNet in the USA.[42,44] The cost of equipment, reagents, and analytic tools; access to laboratory training and appropriate protocols; and ability to analyze genetic data are each barriers to establishing routine genetic surveillance programs in many countries.[44]

Community-Based Surveillance

Community-based surveillance is a type of surveillance that uses community volunteers or leaders to actively participate in discovery and reporting of cases. This type of surveillance puts public health and health officials in direct contact with suspected, probable, and confirmed cases of disease and allows for rapid, if not immediate, medical response and quarantine. This is the most effective type of surveillance to monitor diseases nearing eradication.[49] Community volunteers and leaders participate in the active discovery and reporting of cases.[49]

Data from community-based surveillance can complement data gathered through other approaches from health facilities, providing vital information during outbreaks for targeted interventions.[50] Community-based surveillance can also inform detailed needs assessments, capturing baseline data, and delineating public health issues.[51]

Digital Surveillance

Digital surveillance entails data collection via web-based protocols and is increasingly critical in improving the timeliness of surveillance and response.[52] For decades, public health data have been transferred over the internet for passive and sentinel surveillance networks. The US Centers for Disease Control and Prevention (CDC) launched the National Electronic Telecommunications System for Surveillance (NETSS) in 1990, facilitating the electronic transfer of notifiable disease data.[53] The National Electronic Disease Surveillance System (NEDSS) project was initiated in 2001 as CDC's next-generation solution for integrated electronic PHS data exchange, using industry health information technology (IT) vocabulary (e.g., ICD-9, SNOMED, LOINC) and messaging standards (e.g., HL7) to enable interoperability.[54]

Several technologies now in development will enable automated near real-time public health reporting and further reduce the resource burden in detecting and confirming cases. Screening algorithms have been developed, which can automatically detect cases of tuberculosis and hepatitis B in electronic medical records with very high sensitivity and positive predictive value.[55,56] With the development of the Reportable Conditions Knowledge Management System (RCKMS) by the Council of State and Territorial Epidemiologists (CSTE) and the US CDC, reporting requirements for state reportable and notifiable diseases will be machine readable, further reducing the burden for reporting entities to identify and report cases.[57] The RCKMS also would support automated laboratory reporting, which will lead to faster case confirmation.[57]

Social Media Use in Public Health

Public health researchers have explored nontraditional, internet-based sources in the Web 2.0 environment, such as Facebook, Twitter, and other social media sites, for early event detection signals to augment formal channels of public health information.[58,59] While not helpful data collection tools, social media sources provide a conduit for public health organizations to quickly and almost effortlessly contact millions of people within their surveillance network, in many ways simplifying the means to effectively communicate risk (although as we have seen with other media frenzies during sensationalized public health events, this is a double-edged sword).[59] An effect of enabling peer-to-peer communications are community-driven participatory surveillance (described under Models of Surveillance) groups in which patient groups have initiated and shared surveillance data within their networks.[60] Sites such as PatientsLikeMe connect individuals, many with rare, chronic conditions, to supportive peer groups representing over 2000 conditions.[60] The pioneering founders of PatientsLikeMe have provided paid access to Genentech, a biotechnology company, for access to their database and users for research, marking a precedent for partnerships between health-centric social media and industry.[61] However, until more research can validate the use of social media sources for structured surveillance, the subjectivity of personal health data from social media make it challenging to incorporate these data into official surveillance systems.[62] Natural language processing, crowdsourcing, and artificial intelligence are some of the sophisticated methods and tools used to conduct research using social media data.[58,63–65] These methods, among others, have been used to conduct digital surveillance for conditions such as influenza and diabetes, as well as other topics such as prescription and illicit drug use, patient safety, health care quality, and mental and behavioral health.[66,67]

MODELS OF SURVEILLANCE

The following models of surveillance describe generic strategies for conducting surveillance that may employ one or more modes of surveillance discussed above. Public health organizations should plan and implement their surveillance systems based on best practices that leverage the inherent strengths of a given model of surveillance. Likewise, different models of surveillance have differing weaknesses, but public health organizations can sidestep these shortcomings with reasonable foresight. Key objectives of surveillance systems are to achieve early outbreak and cluster detection, to plan prevention and control programs, and to evaluate interventions and policy decisions; it can be more efficient to deploy a combination of surveillance models, as results are complementary, bolstering downstream outcomes for preparedness and response.

Indicator-Based Surveillance

Characteristics of Indicator-Based Surveillance

Indicator-based surveillance (IBS) involves the routine reporting of diseases, conditions, and events through notifiable disease surveillance systems, including sentinel surveillance channels and laboratory-based surveillance.[68] Most IBS data are collected through passive surveillance. Public health agencies collect IBS data for a predefined list of diseases or conditions using standardized definitions.[9] In many national systems, IBS data are collected according to regulatory requirements or guidelines.

IBS is best used for routine monitoring of disease trends and has high sensitivity for detection of outbreaks, in which case many diseases, conditions, and events have a predefined threshold for investigation and/or response.[68] For zoonotic disease surveillance, integration with veterinary data increases the strength of the system.[9] Due to the lag between data capture, reporting, and laboratory confirmation, IBS is less efficient at early response to emerging health threats versus other models of surveillance described below; however, outbreak response should be designed into the system.[9,68]

Data for IBS are typically gathered from health care settings, though other individuals or institutions may be defined as a reporting entity (e.g., laboratory, hospital) based on the characteristics of the catchment area.[68] The reporting hierarchy of these entities is clearly defined within a closed system.[68] In a robust, fully comprehensive system, many data sources are incorporated into the IBS system. Non-health-care sources of IBS data include poison centers, behavioral surveillance, environmental surveillance, veterinary surveillance, food/water supply safety, vital records, and drug postlicensing monitoring. Surveillance of emerging risks is monitored through data gathered via morbidity surveillance, health care activity reports, and prescription monitoring. Finally, laboratory surveillance is very important for case classification, especially as many notifiable or priority diseases have laboratory confirmation criteria.[9]

Surveillance data vary by disease, but at a minimum, data typically include variables for demographics, health outcome, basis of diagnosis, risk factors, and clinical management data.[69] Data reporting for specific diseases and syndromes are aggregated, and zero reporting is used to clarify against null answers.[68] Data may be categorized by demographic factors or other variables; cases may be conditionally notifiable, limiting requested reports by age (e.g., <5 years old), antimicrobial resistance, or maternal status, for instance, when children and pregnant women were especially tracked during the 2009 H1N1 influenza pandemic due to their heightened susceptibility to serious illness and mortality.[68,70–74]

Data formats are structured and predefined, captured in forms used to send data at specified intervals for subsequent collation and regular analysis by surveillance teams.[9,68] Standardized reporting forms improve data quality and overall surveillance system performance, utilizing standardized data field formats and vocabulary and defining the core (minimum) data set to structure the data for more accurate analysis. For example, the "date of diagnosis" could be entered into an unstructured data field in several different formats (e.g., 4/6/2014, April 6, 2014, 2014/4/6). Standardizing this field simplifies data analysis, especially for large data sets, facilitating more rapid characterization of trends and detection of anomalies for earlier response.

International Health Regulations (2005) Surveillance and Nationally Notifiable Conditions

WHO International Health Regulations (IHR [2005]) identifies three categories of diseases or events that may constitute a public health event of international concern (PHEIC). The first category includes four diseases that are immediately notifiable to WHO: smallpox, wild-type polio, novel influenza, and severe acute respiratory syndrome (SARS). Another subset of diseases and disease groups (e.g., cholera and other diseases of national or regional concern) will always be considered for international notification based on a decision algorithm of the IHR (2005). The final categorization includes "diseases or events that may constitute a PHEIC" and is a catchall category important for international notification of emerging diseases not listed elsewhere.[75] In addition to IHR (2005)-specified diseases for international alert, there are other diseases considered high priority for surveillance, including HIV/AIDS, bovine spongiform encephalopathy (mad cow disease), weaponized anthrax, syphilis, drug-resistant tuberculosis, and West Nile Virus.[76]

The specific list of diseases, conditions, and events under surveillance varies from country to country and, in some cases, between subnational jurisdictions within the same country based on local public health priorities. While WHO urges member states to include smallpox, wild-type polio, novel influenza, and SARS on their national priority disease list for surveillance, priority conditions and their reporting requirements (e.g., frequency, reporting method) are ultimately the discretion of a country's Ministry of Health.[75] For example, the US CDC publishes an annual list of "notifiable" conditions, case definitions, and reporting requirements, which is determined by the states and CSTE.[77] This list also indicates the timeliness of report case notification to CDC by a state. Notification of cases by US states to CDC is voluntary, while reporting within state boundaries is mandated and required by state governments. Each notifiable condition has a national case definition (also developed by CSTE) to aid case notification.

It is common to see weekly or monthly cycles designated for reporting notifiable diseases, but some diseases require daily or immediate reporting for rapid response.[68] Conditions that may be related to bioterrorism, such as anthrax or plague, must be reported immediately. Pertussis, while important to report promptly, does not have as stringent timeliness requirements. In comparison, the impetus to report chronic diseases is not as urgent and may only require quarterly or annual reporting. Reporters are generally required to submit reports of notifiable diseases through an IBS.

Limitations of Indicator-Based Surveillance Systems

A notable disadvantage of IBS is the delay between case identification and the report of aggregated data to public health, with further delays in reporting if laboratory diagnoses are required for case confirmation.[68] Delays in surveillance are experienced in food-borne disease outbreaks, for example, because of the time lag between the onset of the illness, doctor visit and specimen collection and laboratory confirmation. Reporting delays in communicable disease outbreaks can lead to delays in outbreak investigation and, ultimately, disease control. Electronic and automated data transmission and processing using machine-readable reporting requirements (as provided by RCKMS) and reporting algorithms can reduce burden and improve timeliness.

Another limitation of IBS is its relative rigidity. A period of preparation and transition is needed for a public health system to develop standardized case definitions and then to create and deploy data collection tools for newly reportable conditions. The gradual conversion to integrated data in interoperable electronic information systems for IBS introduces additional complexity, such as common data elements between medical, laboratory, veterinary, and public health sectors (in a One Health environment) and also between disease-specific programs, need to be harmonized.

Event-Based Surveillance

Characteristics of Event-Based Surveillance

Event-based surveillance (EBS) is the "organized rapid capture of information about events that are a risk to public health, and is complementary to IBS, particularly during the course of an outbreak."[68] As the name suggests, EBS frequently occurs around specific events or incidents from or during which categorized symptoms occur. EBS is distinct from IBS in that community groups, schools, religious institutions, the media, and other organizations are encouraged to report unusual events. Because of this distinction, case definitions are not always required, although they can be used for EBS.[67]

Events are captured in structured definitions. Definitions are intentionally broad, more sensitive than with IBS, and delineate geospatial and temporal parameters. They can be symptom-based, such as clusters of deaths at a location or site (e.g., health care facility, school, and community organization) during a certain period of time or clusters of disease of unknown etiology during a certain period of time. Definitions can also be unusual events, including those that cause particular concern or fear and those that could harm or negatively impact the population's health.[68]

EBS is designed to detect rare or new events not included in IBS, such as events in populations without access to health care.[68] Data are captured on events related to disease incidence (e.g., disease clusters, unusual disease patterns, and unexpected deaths); events related to potential human exposure (e.g., animal deaths, food or water contamination, and environmental hazards); and informal reports through formal surveillance channels or the media.[68] The data collection process for EBS is usually active, although funding is often limited, requiring data sources to be prioritized according to their sensitivity and sustainability.[68,78] Data sensitivity is based on confirmed public health events that have been detected, assessed, and responded to.[68]

Internationally, EBS is supported among many organizations that use a variety of data mining algorithms, news aggregators, distribution lists, and visualization tools.[9] According to IHR (2005) self-assessments from 2012, responding countries have relatively high levels of capacity for EBS and IBS (74% and 87%, respectively), and nearly all (91%) have identified EBS information sources.[78] Domestic data sources include health care workers, local media, and community focal points.[9,68]

Mass Gatherings

EBS has provided an excellent complementary epidemic intelligence to national surveillance systems during mass gatherings, such as the Hajj or the Olympics.[79,80] An evaluation of an EBS system conducted during the 2012 London Olympic and Paralympic Games found reports to be timely and data to be sensitive, complete, and stable. Overall, the EBS system was judged to be "efficient, fast, and responsive" with nominal effort expended by staff.[80]

The Hajj is an annual pilgrimage of over 2 million Muslim men and women who travel to Mecca from over 100 countries.[81] During the 2009 Hajj, surveillance applications deployed mobile devices that strengthened public health preparedness in the midst of the H1N1 influenza A virus pandemic.[79,82] Recent public health threats, such as the Middle East respiratory syndrome coronavirus (MERS-Cov) and Ebola virus in West Africa, pique concerns and punctuate the need for EBS support during mass gatherings.[83]

Limitations of Event-Based Surveillance

In EBS, reporters are often the media and health care workers, both of whom tend to provide credible, timely, and directly sourced information. It is important to note, however, that media EBS reports may be biased from their perceptions of the newsworthiness of an event and not its public health importance. Media reports may not be as reliable or effective in countries with heavily censored media. Health care workers already participate in a reporting network, so existing communication channels can be leveraged for EBS without significant burden. However, reports from health care facilities may be representative of those seeking care and not the population at large. More investment is needed to assess, confirm, and respond to reports from the general community. For example, reporting infrastructures such as hotlines or hubs at community centers can be established. This type of infrastructure would require advertisement to the community and volunteer or leader recruitment and training. Direct community outreach tends to yield high sensitivity for individuals who self-report ailments or unusual events, but low specificity.[68]

A disadvantage of EBS is that it requires designated public health staff to collect data and, when possible, to facilitate event confirmation and assessment. EBS reports are sometimes undefined, and the data are often unstructured and not standardized. At a minimum, public health staff should record a unique identifier, location, date and reporter contact information, date and time of event, event description, and actions taken to date. Public health professionals review and escalate reported events to trigger responses as appropriate.[68]

Syndromic Surveillance

Characteristics of Syndromic Surveillance

In 2001, anthrax bioterrorist attacks prompted the implementation of syndromic surveillance (SS) systems across the USA and since then, an increasing number of jurisdictions have implemented such programs.[84–88] SS has shifted from its original purpose for terrorism preparedness; it can be used to determine the severity of an outbreak and monitor disease trends, especially as longitudinal data become available and definitions are refined.[86] Data from SS systems are often used by public health programs to complement IBS data during the course of an outbreak. **Syndromic surveillance** uses existing health data in real time to provide immediate analysis and feedback to those charged with investigation and follow-up of potential outbreaks.[89] SS has been used for early detection of outbreaks, to follow the size, spread, and tempo of outbreaks, to monitor disease trends, and to provide reassurance that an outbreak has not occurred.[89]

For infectious diseases, SS focuses on the early symptom period before clinical or laboratory confirmation of diagnosis by using clinical and alternative data sources.[86] Early detection and warning supports timely and effective prevention and response, more so than IBS, which detects outbreaks much later.[90] Buehler et al. characterize SS systems as those that conduct ongoing (versus time-limited or "drop-in") surveillance for human health-related events or outcomes and early event detection or situational awareness in near real time to support IBS.[88]

Use of SS systems and data is more prevalent than in the early stages of SS, including the use of CDC's BioSense program by CDC and state and local jurisdictions. In the USA, capacity to conduct SS is now included in Meaningful Use requirements.[90,91] SS was reported to be most useful for monitoring influenza, as it can detect the onset of influenza before laboratory confirmation.[88]

Most SS systems rely on automated data collection from health-related events in existing electronic databases.[88] Using preexisting data sources to collect syndromic data reduces cost and burden.[86] Certain systems collect alternative data, such as school/work absenteeism and veterinary data, in addition to more common types of data like clinical data.[86] ICD-9 codes used in emergency department (ED) and outpatient settings are commonly used to classify syndromes.[86] Health-related events include health care services (e.g., ED visits or hotline calls) or health-related behaviors (e.g., over-the-counter medication purchases or absenteeism).[88] SS also monitors disease outbreaks, seasonal illnesses, health consequences of natural or other disasters, and noninfectious conditions.[88,92]

The methods for SS vary by planned duration and the method of gathering data.[86] Collection and reporting of SS data can leverage existing communication channels, similar to EBS leveraging existing relationships with health care workers.[86] Data from SS are used for epidemiologic analysis and electronic collection of near real-time patient data that allows for timely assessments of population health. Results of SS data analysis are displayed with web-based applications, often mapping data to geospatial markers and aggregate counts with associated case data.[88,93] Among other analytic methods, the SaTScan™ approach has been used to analyze data from contiguous zip codes and with a given range of dates to consider day-to-day or day and time variables based on historic data.[87,93,94] SS data can lead to public health action and is useful for event detection, situation awareness, and response.[90] SS data can trigger action based on a threshold number of early symptomatic cases. Diagnostic confirmation is a "paramount step in investigating alerts," given the high sensitivity and low specificity of certain syndrome categories.[86]

SS is used for early outbreaks or cluster detection before confirmed diagnosis (through IBS) to mobilize a more rapid response. That being said, response based on SS data depends on the size and spread of the outbreak, data accuracy and availability, syndrome definitions used, threshold alert criteria, and the medical community's ability to detect and report unusual cases.[86] SS is very useful for situational awareness of ongoing outbreaks and provides affordable, sensitive, and rapid geocoding.[87,88] In addition, SS can provide more timely and more granular geospatial details than data from sentinel networks, and the data are useful for detecting variation in mortality patterns.[88]

Veterinary Surveillance

Options for sustainable, routine collection of animal health data are limited, given the nature of veterinary disease surveillance. A study published in 2014 described implementation of an SS system at veterinary diagnostic laboratories that have proven to be a timely and dependable source of veterinary surveillance data.[95] This systematic, automated influx of electronic animal health data provides the public health sector the opportunity to leverage animal sentinels for early outbreak detection using a One Health approach.[96] Lessons learned from laboratory-based veterinary SS include the need for classification system of cases to syndromes, the development of a baseline profile to facilitate aberration detection, "the identification of temporal effects," a pilot assessment of detection algorithms, and real-time monitoring of surveillance data.[97] In Europe, a 2013 report identified 27 veterinary SS systems in 12 separate European countries, providing a glimpse of burgeoning interest in SS in the veterinary sector. As evidenced by recent reports, SS continues to be a useful beacon for imminent and unexpected health events threatening human and animal health populations.[96,98]

Limitations of Syndromic Surveillance

A challenge with SS is that alternative data sources have low specificity for syndromes of interest. It is still a technical challenge to easily isolate a signal that corresponds to a particular outbreak, cluster, or event.[86] SS is also less useful for small outbreaks versus other surveillance methods.[88]

Behavioral Risk Factor Surveillance

Characteristics of Behavioral Risk Factor Surveillance

Behavioral risk factor surveillance is the tracking of health-related risk behaviors, chronic conditions, and use of preventative services.[99] The USA conducts an annual survey using random-digit dialing (using both landlines and cell phones) survey methodology in all 50 states, District of Columbia and three US territories. Behavioral risk factor surveillance systems (BRFSS) collects data on issues such as vaccine shortages and influenza-like illness (ILI) that can help federal, state, and local public health agencies plan for potential pandemics.[99]

The World Alliance for Risk Factor Surveillance is a global working group that supports the development of BRFSS and methodologies to monitor and evaluate disease prevention and health promotion policies.[100] This group serves as a collaboration space for researchers, behavioral risk factor practitioners, and countries that are developing behavioral risk factor surveillance.

BRFSS are ongoing and flexible, as items can be modified or added to address new emerging health issues or risk factors. This also allows for seasonal variation and the ability to identify trends in behavior. The task of collecting behavioral risk factor data is arduous and requires a trained public health professional to call and solicit respondents using a random sampling methodology.[101] Comparisons within and across geographic regions can easily be done with a standardized questionnaire that is deployed nationwide.

Limitations of Behavioral Risk Factor Surveillance

The questionnaires used for behavioral risk factor surveillance must be revised annually to reflect changing public health policies and address emerging issues. All data are self-reported so there may be bias in the results and though they are anonymous, they cannot be validated at the individual level.[101] Collecting behavioral risk factor data can be a time-consuming task, with the USA collecting 400,000 interviews/year,[99] Italy's behavioral risk factor system collecting 60,000 interviews in 2007 and 2008,[101] and the analysis of these data is complex to address survey design. Factors that must be considered are not limited to unequal probability of selection, clustering of observations, stratification, and nonresponse.[102] Telephone surveys used to be an excellent approach to collecting data as it allowed for anonymity, quality control as the questions are asked in the same manner by trained professionals, and easy accessibility to respondents as most households had landline phones. Currently, one of the biggest challenges for telephone surveys is that 41% of US households no longer have a landline telephone.[103] People at or below poverty levels are less likely to maintain a landline, with 56% of Americans in or near poverty levels having a wireless-only/cell phone household.[103] In 2004, Africa became the first continent to have more cellular users than landline holders. Africans have the world's lowest rate of landline use at just 2.8% of Africans having a regular telephone.[104]

To address the growing issue of not being able to reach the entire population due to the increasing mobile phone use, public health professionals will need to seek out ways to incorporate mobile phone users, SMS-survey options, and internet-based surveys to reach the masses.

Predictive Surveillance

Characteristics of Predictive Surveillance

Predictive surveillance can provide advanced awareness of emerging infectious disease threats, much beyond what is possible with EBS or SS.[105] It utilizes state-of-the-art computer models and algorithms to simulate interrelated and, at times, interdependent pathogen, vector (arthropod), and host (animal and human) behaviors and to forecast disease outbreaks.[106] That being said, the basic premise of the model is to predict the presence or absence of pathogen in geographic area, not the behavior of pathogen.[105] Data components include environmental, vector, animal, and human elements.[105,107]

Predictive surveillance may use regional or localized climatological data to predict disease outbreaks. Satellite remote sensing data tracking regional climate patterns produce less precise, qualitative data that inform eco-climate trends with relevance to potential disease outbreaks. On the other hand, ground-based measurements for microlevel results of weather and habitation conditions are more precise and geographically localized.

Predictive surveillance can improve risk communication, providing geotargeted alerts that are tailored in terms of geographic scale (from local to regional), risk population, and condition or event.[105,106] Enhanced health communication and situation awareness increases community feedback, accessible through established surveillance channels (e.g., EBS), active vector surveillance, and social media sources.[106] Increased reliability and validity of the predictive model output can be achieved through adoption of shared standards across program components (environmental, vector, animal, and human).[105]

Outcomes of predictive surveillance are predicated on transdisciplinary, collaborative research.[106] Models in predictive surveillance are drawn from data melded from One Health disciplines. Predictive surveillance also incorporates climatological data to compute dynamic geotemporal estimates of disease transmission and epicenters of risk.[105,106,108] Prominent predictive surveillance initiatives include the United States Agency for International Development PREDICT project spearheaded by the University of California, Davis, School of Veterinary Medicine at their One Health Institute and the Armed Forces Health Surveillance Center's Global Emerging Infections Surveillance and Response System model for predictive surveillance.[105,107,109] Both organizations run partnerships that are multidisciplinary and integrate data, systems, and methods to produce outputs.[105] Additional information and examples of predictive surveillance systems are provided in Chapter 27.

Limitations of Predictive Surveillance

The biggest limitation of predictive surveillance is the lack of accurate data available to inform and refine models.[105,110] Strong relationships and collaborations are needed to establish data sharing networks between multidisciplinary partners.

Participatory Surveillance

Characteristics of Participatory Surveillance

Participatory surveillance uses direct engagement with community members at large to collect data and improve public health understanding of disease patterns and population health.[111] It is predicated on traditional concepts of epidemiology but recognizes the value of collective intelligence and awareness.[112] It uses community knowledge to develop epidemic intelligence in a participatory manner and complements these data with secondary information sources, observations, and laboratory diagnostics.[111]

Methods of participatory surveillance or participatory epidemiology include interviews, focus group discussions, subjective scoring of disease observations, and visualization tools (e.g., maps and calendars).[112] Participatory surveillance relies heavily on social networking to initiate a conversation between public health and consumer communities.[113] Through social networking sites, crowd-sourced information can inform public health programs that in turn can take action in the form of feedback or interventions.[113] This type of data not just benefits public health practice, but the immediate feedback to communities generates discussion and can influence behavior.[113]

"Lateral surveillance" uses surveillance tools to conduct peer-to-peer monitoring.[114] Using geospatial information gleaned from mobile devices, lateral surveillance websites can effectively harness users as informants for public health purposes.[115] Social networking tools can empower users to voluntarily assume an active role in PHS by providing them the platform and audience to initiate action, gather intelligence, and disseminate information.[115]

Applications that permit public input and feedback are useful to gather information that can characterize risk and be used for outreach, education, and intervention.[67] For example, mobile apps for health surveillance could be used to monitor attendees at mass gatherings; surveillance elements could be incorporated into the app, providing attendees services such as event maps (including clinics and first-aid locations) and itineraries in return for basic demographic information and simple health survey data (e.g., "are you or anyone in your party ill?"). This information could then be used as an early event detection indicator and the app could issue alerts in the event of a public health threat.

Researchers and public health professionals can use social networking data for PHS and research.[116] Web-based monitoring facilitates rapid event detection, characterizes global trends, and enriches predictive disease models and informs strategies for preparedness and response.[117] Implementation of participatory surveillance tools appear to require country-specific considerations.[117] Participatory approaches can be used for marginalized groups to improve the timeliness and sensitivity of event detection and therefore response.[118] Results of one study indicate that participatory members of an online community for diabetes (TuDiabetes.com) were significantly more forthcoming about reporting device-related adverse events on the website than to FDA.[67] Furthermore, all reports submitted through the online app contained complete outcome information, in stark contrast to the 22% completion rate for FDA reports.[67]

Influenza Surveillance

Participatory surveillance has the benefit of being able to access rich personal data beyond standard disease-specific and demographic variables, such as time-stamped records of activities, events, behaviors, and attitudes not available through more traditional surveillance systems. Analysis of these data can provide contextual cues to epidemiologic research, and informs disease forecasts.[117] Web-based participatory surveillance has been implemented in Europe to complement and overcome limitations in state-of-the-art influenza surveillance systems.[117] GrippeNet.fr is France's version of the European InfluenzaNet that uses a participatory approach for ILI surveillance.[116] The limitation to participatory surveillance is that participants self-select and are not representative of the general population. For instance, researchers found the GrippeNet.fr user group to be more educated, more frequently employed, and had higher rates of vaccination than the general population and was not representative in terms of age or sex.[116]

There is great potential in the stream of real-time event-based signals from online communities, mobile networks, and participatory surveillance systems.[119] Data visualization tools such as a digital public health dashboard offer a novel way to integrate traditional methods with emerging approaches to embrace new data streams.[119] Applications like FluNearYou solicit data from their subscribers in a short weekly survey about ILI symptoms. Users can see visualizations of influenza across the USA or Canada. Participants who participate receive more information about influenza activity in their communities as well as resources such as nearby vaccination locations.[120]

Limitations of Participatory Surveillance

There are several challenges associated with recruiting participants in this surveillance model. The initial challenge involves setting a strategy to attract the target, at-risk population and enticing them to join. Once there, users must be motivated to participate. Furthermore, a lack of participants and a self-selection bias can generate skewed results. There is also the potential for participants to intentionally corrupt data and influence other participants to do the same, invalidating the results.[121]

Selection of Surveillance Model

Figs. 3-1 to 3-4 depict the order of prominence of selected models of surveillance during various public health scenarios given the relative size of the bubble in a figure. In Fig. 3-1, IBS is most useful for routine surveillance. National surveillance of notifiable diseases are implemented and managed by Ministries of Health and ministries for animal (domestic and wildlife) health to continually monitor national health outcomes and risk factors public health events. Other surveillance models may play a minor role in conducting routine surveillance depending on the availability of resources and training.

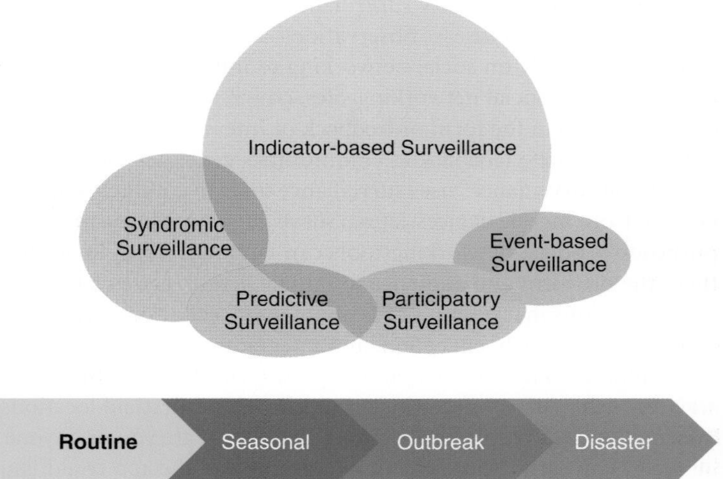

FIG. 3-1 Public health information useful to an epidemiologist during routine surveillance, by PHS model.

In Fig. 3-2, during optimal conditions for transmission of respiratory infections or other seasonal diseases, patients may inundate hospitals and clinics with symptoms such as cough, fever, and malaise. In this scenario, SS is very useful for early detection of potential seasonal disease outbreaks, which can prepare public health and clinical professionals alike for an endemic or pandemic outbreak of disease cluster. Predictive surveillance is also useful for identifying early warning signs for outbreaks, such as a surge in disease-related search terms on social media sites and search engines. At this point in time, the contribution of EBS and participatory surveillance models remains trivial, though as human behavioral integration with interactive media increases, we may see participatory surveillance as an increasing source of seasonal health data.

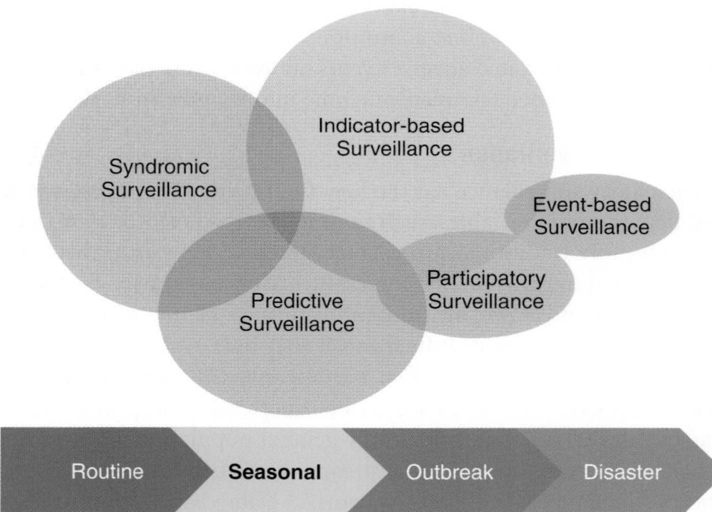

FIG. 3-2 Public health information useful to an epidemiologist during seasonal fluctuations of reportable diseases, by PHS model.

In Fig. 3-3, during active outbreaks, SS is important for timely situational awareness. Geocoding allows responders to locate and target disease hot spots first and dynamically adjust their approach according to real-time actionable information. Other models of surveillance are not as useful for facilitating effective response measures due to the lack of timely information among additional potential data quality issues.

Finally, in Fig. 3-4 we see that in disaster situations, EBS system for active assessment is extremely important, as is the increased volume of self-reports. IBS surveillance remains critical during disasters as there is increased risk of notifiable disease outbreaks due to the loss or reduction of sanitation, food and water levels, and health services. Such was the case following the 2010 earthquake in Haiti, when an outbreak of cholera ravaged the unfortunate populace.[122]

One Health Approach

One Health is a holistic approach to zoonotic disease surveillance. In the broadest sense, the **One Health approach** integrates the relationships among vectors, animals (domestic and wildlife), plants, and humans to develop surveillance systems that are attuned to real-world models of disease transmission. Data and research are blended from many disciplines, including environmental health, ecology, veterinary medicine, human medicine, public health, molecular biology, microbiology, and health economics. Collectively, these domains articulate the relationships among individual, population, and ecosystem health.[123] This approach recognizes the importance to plan and implement interventions that reduce disease transmissions by modulating nonhuman factors in our environment that lead to better health outcomes. Examples of interventions planned by the One Health Center organization include the following[124]:

- Improved water management in underserved regions to provide clean and ample water for better health outcomes
- Improved animal health to reduce risk of zoonotic disease transmission and enrich the quality of food
- Enhanced vector control
- Bioengineered food for better nutrition and food security

(See Chapter 14 for further discussion of One Health.)

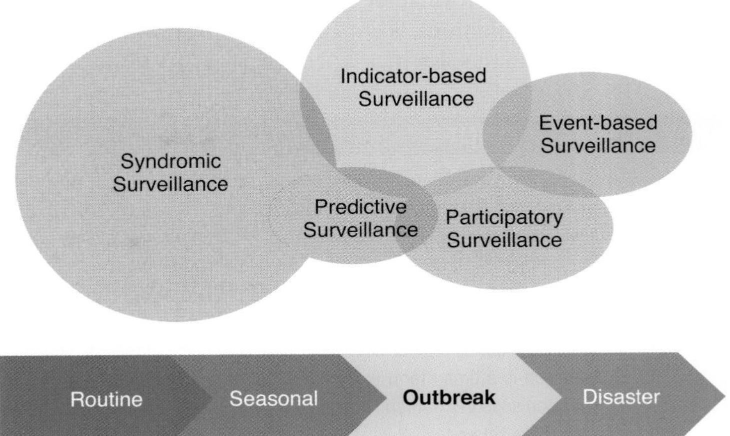

FIG. 3-3 Public health information useful to an epidemiologist during outbreaks, by PHS model.

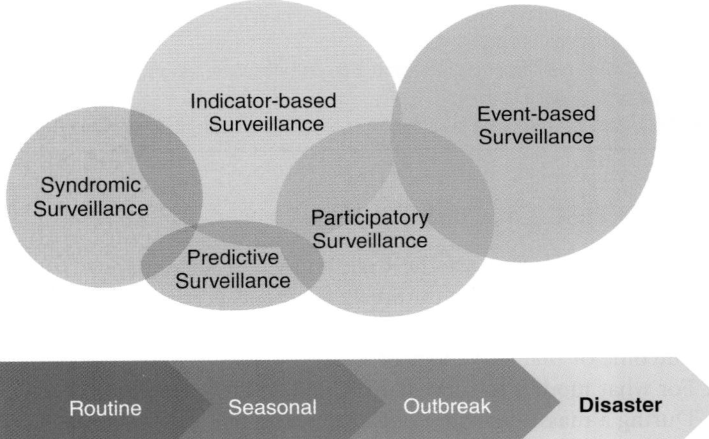

FIG. 3-4 Public health information useful to an epidemiologist during disasters, by PHS model.

CONCLUSIONS

Surveillance models, practices, methods, and technologies will continue to change over time as new diseases emerge and take priority for public health attention and response. Public health practitioners must constantly learn, evaluate, and test new surveillance methods to discover new ways to detect, report and respond to emerging health threats. These efforts are bolstered by the adaptation and widespread adoption of new technologies, methodologies, and policies that enable advances in new approaches such as One Health, integrated surveillance, and interoperable electronic tools.

Knowing the basics of the models of PHS will provide a foundation for learning about other PHS topics throughout this book, such as the reactive and proactive discussion in Chapter 5, the intersection of clinical medicine and public health discussed in Chapter 18, verification and validation issues discussed in Chapter 24, and new analytic approaches presented in Chapter 27. The awareness of different surveillance methods and approaches, as well as their benefits and limitations, is critical to deciding how to approach a public health problem or threat and gathering the appropriate data to solve it.

KEY SUMMARY POINTS

- Surveillance objectives, and therefore the modes of surveillance chosen, are defined by the information needs of surveillance, the stakeholders that are impacted, and the intended use of the data.
- Passive surveillance requires a predetermined list of conditions or events with defined case definitions and reporters (usually health care workers). This method of surveillance is the least burdensome but collects minimal information about a case.
- Sentinel surveillance is established by handpicking a group of voluntary health care facilities that report surveillance data regularly. Reporters in the network have a relatively large population served, well-trained staff, and a high-quality laboratory.
- Active surveillance requires regular field visits to review medical records and staff interviews to collect detailed data for research.
- Digital surveillance is a broad term to describe the surveillance activities that are conducted over electronic media, especially the internet. Digital surveillance supports traditional modes of surveillance, but has also enabled new modes of surveillance (e.g., predictive, participatory) and use of new data sets.
- Indicator-based surveillance is routine and structured.
- Event-based surveillance is sporadic and unstructured. It is complementary to IBS and is used for early detection of outbreaks.
- Community-based surveillance is the most effective type of surveillance to monitor diseases nearing eradication.
- Syndromic surveillance focuses on the early detection signals of conditions or events.
- Population-based surveillance is recommended by WHO to measure the efficacy of new vaccines, as it is very useful for determining a vaccine's overall effect on the population.
- Predictive surveillance uses integrated casual models of environmental, vector, animal, and human components to predict the locality and severity of disease or event.
- Participatory surveillance leverages peer networks and social media to monitor disease trends.

DISCUSSION QUESTIONS

1. Compare and contrast the basic modes of surveillance (passive, sentinel, and active). Which would be most appropriate for a polio outbreak; HIV; and pertussis?
2. In what situation would sentinel surveillance be preferable to passive surveillance and what would be the intended outcome of that surveillance?
3. For what models of surveillance (EBS, IBS, SS, etc.) would active surveillance be most useful and least useful?
4. During a massive cholera outbreak, what model(s) of surveillance would you use? Which data sources would be most useful? Which would be least useful? Why?
5. How can public health leverage participatory surveillance groups that are owned by patient groups? How can these communities be incentivized to contribute to public health initiatives?
6. In what ways can PHS be designed to account for a truly globalized population?
7. Discuss the pros and cons of different modes of surveillance in a health department with human and financial resource constraints. What criteria would you use to make decisions about what surveillance to conduct (or not to conduct)?

REFERENCES

1. Shangquan G. Economic globalization: trends, risks and risk prevention. United Nations, Department of Economics and Social Affairs, New York; 2000.
2. Frieden TR, Damon I, Bell BP, Kenyon T, Nichol S. Ebola 2014 — new challenges, new global response and responsibility. N Engl J Med 2014;371(13):1177–80.
3. Susser M, Susser E. Choosing a future for epidemiology: I. Eras and paradigms. Am J Public Health 1996;86(5):668–73.
4. Agyei-Mensah S, de-Graft Aikins A. Epidemiological transition and the double burden of disease in Accra, Ghana. J Urban Health 2010;87(5):879–97.
5. Thacker SB, Berkelman RL, Stroup DF. The science of public health surveillance. J Public Health Policy 1989;10(2):187–203.
6. Thacker SB, Stroup DF. Future directions for comprehensive public health surveillance and health information systems in the United States. Am J Epidemiol 1994;140(5):383–97.
7. Thacker SB, Qualters JR, Lee LM. Public health surveillance in the United States: evolution and challenges. MMWR Surveill Summ 2012;61(Suppl):3–9.

8. Berkelman RL, Stroup DF, Beuhler JW, Buehler JW. Public health surveillance. In: Detels R, McEwen J, Beaglehole R, Tanaka H, editors. 4th ed. Oxford, England: Oxford University Press; 2002. p. 759–78.
9. Amato-Gauci A, Ammon A. The surveillance of communicable diseases in the European Union—a long-term strategy (2008-2013). Euro Surveill 2008;13(26).
10. Thacker SB, Berkelman RL. Public health surveillance in the United States. Epidemiol Rev 1988;10:164–90.
11. Berkelman RL, Sullivan PS, Buehler JW, et al. Public health surveillance. In: Oxford Texbook of Public Health, 5th ed.; Oxford University Press, 2009. p. 699–715.
12. Shands KN, Schmid GP, Dan BB, Blum D, Guidotti RJ, Hargrett NT, et al. Toxic-shock syndrome in menstruating women: association with tampon use and Staphylococcus aureus and clinical features in 52 cases. N Engl J Med 1980;303(25):1436–42.
13. Jaffe HW, Choi K, Thomas PA, Haverkos HW, Auerbach DM, Guinan ME, et al. National case-control study of Kaposi's sarcoma and Pneumocystis carinii pneumonia in homosexual men: Part 1. Epidemiologic results. Ann Intern Med 1983;99(2):145–51.
14. Langmuir AD. The surveillance of communicable diseases of national importance. N Engl J Med 1963;268:182–92.
15. WHO. National Passive Surveillance. World Health Organization. <http://www.who.int/immunization/monitoring_surveillance/burden/vpd/surveillance_type/passive/en/>; October 2014.
16. WHO. WHO report on global surveillance of epidemic-prone infectious diseases. Geneva, Switzerland: WHO; 2000.
17. Hadorn DC, Haracic SS, Stärk KDC. Comparative assessment of passive surveillance in disease-free and endemic situation: example of Brucella melitensis surveillance in Switzerland and in Bosnia and Herzegovina. BMC veterinary research 2008;4(1):52.
18. Razuri H, Romero C, Tinoco Y, Guezala MC, Ortiz E, Silva M, et al. Population-based active surveillance cohort studies for influenza: lessons from Peru. Bull World Health Organ 2012;90(4):318–20.
19. Sandiford P, Annett H, Cibulskis R. What can information systems do for primary health care? An international perspective. Soc Sci Med 1992;34(10): 1077–87.
20. HHS. Vaccine adverse event reporting system. <https://vaers.hhs.gov/index>; October 2014.
21. Crosby C. Monitoring infections: active vs. passive surveillance. Infection Control Today. 2012.
22. WHO. Sentinel Surveillance. World Health Organization. <http://www.who.int/immunization/monitoring_surveillance/burden/vpd/surveillance_type/sentinel/en/>; October 2014.
23. Hampton LM, Zell ER, Schrag S, Cohen AL. Sentinel versus population-based surveillance of pneumococcal conjugate vaccine effectiveness. Bull World Health Organ 2012;90(8):568–77.
24. Laguna-Torres VA, Gómez J, Ocaña V, Aguilar P, Saldarriaga T, Chavez E, et al. Influenza-like illness sentinel surveillance in Peru. PloS one 2009;4(7):e6118.
25. Schrag SJ, Zell ER, Schuchat A, Whitney CG. Sentinel surveillance: a reliable way to track antibiotic resistance in communities? Emerg Infect Dis 2002;8(5):496–502.
26. Yukich JO, Butts J, Miles M, Berhane Y, Nahusenay H, Malone JL, et al. A description of malaria sentinel surveillance: a case study in Oromia Regional State, Ethiopia. Malar J 2014;13(1):88.
27. Thompson MG, Li DK, Shifflett P, Sokolow LZ, Ferber JR, Kurosky S, et al. Effectiveness of seasonal trivalent influenza vaccine for preventing influenza virus illness among pregnant women: a population-based case-control study during the 2010-2011 and 2011-2012 influenza seasons. Clin Infect Dis 2014;58(4):449–57.
28. Laupland KB, Lyytikainen O, Sogaard M, Kennedy KJ, Knudsen JD, Ostergaard C, et al. The changing epidemiology of Staphylococcus aureus bloodstream infection: a multinational population-based surveillance study. Clin Microbiol Infect 2013;19(5):465–71.
29. Clark SJ, Kahn K, Houle B, Arteche A, Collinson MA, Tollman SM, et al. Young children's probability of dying before and after their mother's death: a rural South African population-based surveillance study. PLoS Med 2013;10(3):e1001409.
30. Garcia-Abreu A, Halperin W, Danel I. Public health surveillance toolkit: a guide for busy task managers. Washington, DC: The World Bank; 2002.
31. WHO. Accelerated Disease Control. World Health Organization <http://www.who.int/immunization/monitoring_surveillance/burden/vpd/surveillance_type/active/en/>; October 2014.
32. Levitt A, Diop OM, Tangermann RH, Paladin F, Kamgang JB, Burns CC, et al. Surveillance systems to track progress toward global polio eradication - worldwide, 2012-2013. MMWR Morb Mortal Wkly Rep 2014;63(16):356–61.
33. Dunn J, Pryor J, Saketa S, Delai W, Buadromo E, Kishore K, et al. Laboratory-based Salmonella surveillance in Fiji, 2004-2005. Pac Health Dialog 2005;12(2):53–9.
34. WHO. Role of Laboratory in Disease Surveillance - Laboratory Training for Field Epidemiologists. Geneva, Switzerland; 2007.
35. WHO/Afro. Guide for establishing laboratory-based surveillance for antimicrobial resistance. Brazzaville: Republic of Congo; 2013.
36. CDC. National Notifiable Diseases Surveillance System (NNDSS) - carbon monoxide poisoning. Atlanta, GA: CDC; 2014.
37. Bauer N, Evans P, Leopold B, Levine J, White P. Current and future development and use of molecular subtyping by USDA-FSIS; 2014.
38. van de Ven JP, Smailhodzic D, Boon CJ, Fauser S, Groenewoud JM, Chong NV, et al. Association analysis of genetic and environmental risk factors in the cuticular drusen subtype of age-related macular degeneration. Mol Vis 2012;18:2271–8.
39. Haibe-Kains B, Desmedt C, Loi S, Culhane AC, Bontempi G, Quackenbush J, et al. A three-gene model to robustly identify breast cancer molecular subtypes. J Natl Cancer Inst 2012;104(4):311–25.
40. Buffler PA, Kwan ML, Reynolds P, Urayama KY. Environmental and genetic risk factors for childhood leukemia: appraising the evidence. Cancer Invest 2005;23(1):60–75.
41. Gerner-Smidt P, Kincaid J, Kubota K, Hise K, Hunter SB, Fair MA, et al. Molecular surveillance of shiga toxigenic Escherichia coli O157 by PulseNet USA. J Food Prot 2005;68(9):1926–31.
42. Swaminathan B, Barrett TJ, Hunter SB, Tauxe RV. PulseNet: the molecular subtyping network for foodborne bacterial disease surveillance, United States. Emerg Infect Dis 2001;7(3):382–89.
43. Unemo M, Fasth O, Fredlund H, Limnios A, Tapsall J. Phenotypic and genetic characterization of the 2008 WHO Neisseria gonorrhoeae reference strain panel intended for global quality assurance and quality control of gonococcal antimicrobial resistance surveillance for public health purposes. J Antimicrob Chemother 2009;63(6):1142–51.
44. Ammon A. Molecular typing for public health purposes. Euro Surveill 2008;13(19).
45. Niesters HG, Rossen JW, van der Avoort H, Baas D, Benschop K, Claas EC, et al. Laboratory-based surveillance in the molecular era: the TYPENED model, a joint data-sharing platform for clinical and public health laboratories. Euro Surveill 2013;18(4):20387.
46. Leekitcharoenphon P, Friis C, Zankari E, Svendsen CA, Price LB, Rahmani M, et al. Genomics of an emerging clone of Salmonella serovar Typhimurium ST313 from Nigeria and the Democratic Republic of Congo. J Infect Dev Ctries 2013;7(10):696–706.
47. Kuroda M, Ohta T, Uchiyama I, Baba T, Yuzawa H, Kobayashi I, et al. Whole genome sequencing of meticillin-resistant Staphylococcus aureus. Lancet 2001;357(9264):1225–40.
48. Ng PC, Kirkness EF. Whole genome sequencing. In: Barnes MR, Breen G, editors. Genetic variation. Humana Press, New York; 2010. p. 215–26.
49. WHO. Community-based surveillance and case containment activities. <http://www.who.int/dracunculiasis/eradication/strategy/en/>; October 2014.
50. Oum S, Chandramohan D, Cairncross S. Community-based surveillance: a pilot study from rural Cambodia. Trop Med Int Health 2005;10(7):689–97.
51. Kyei-Faried S, Appiah-Denkyira E, Brenya D, Akuamoa-Boateng A, Visser L. The role of community-based surveillance in health outcomes measurement. Ghana Med J 2006;40(1):26–30.

52. Definition provided by the chapter author.
53. CDC. NETSS. World Health Organization; 2013.
54. CDC. National electronic disease surveillance system. Atlanta, GA; 2007.
55. Klompas M, Haney G, Church D, Lazarus R, Hou X, Platt R. Automated identification of acute hepatitis B using electronic medical record data to facilitate public health surveillance. PloS one 2008;3(7):e2626.
56. Calderwood MS, Platt R, Hou X, Malenfant J, Haney G, Kruskal B, et al. Real-time surveillance for tuberculosis using electronic health record data from an ambulatory practice in eastern Massachusetts. Public Health Rep 2010;125(6):843–50.
57. Altamore R. Progress toward a reportable conditions knowledge management system (RCKMS). Meeting of the Council of State and Territorial Epidemiologists, Pasadena, CA, June 2013.
58. Denecke K, Krieck M, Otrusina L, Smrz P, Dolog P, Nejdl W, Velasco E, et al. How to exploit twitter for public health monitoring? Methods Inf Med 2013;52(4):326–39.
59. McNab C. What social media offers to health professionals and citizens. Bull World Health Organ 2009;87(8):566.
60. PatientsLikeMe. <https://www.patientslikeme.com/>; October 2014.
61. Rojahn SY. PatientsLikeMe gives Genentech full access. 2014.
62. Velasco E, Agheneza T, Denecke K, Kirchner G, Eckmanns T. Social media and internet-based data in global systems for public health surveillance: a systematic review. Milbank Q 2014;92(1):7–33.
63. Choudhury MD, Gamon M, Counts S, Horvitz E. Predicting depression via social media. In: Proceedings of the 7th International AAAI Conference on Weblogs and Social Media. Boston, MA; 2013.
64. Lamb A, Paul MJ, Dredze M. Separating fact from fear: tracking flu infections on Twitter. Proceedings of NAACL-HLT 2013, pg 789–795, Atlanta, GA, June 2013.
65. Neill DB. New directions in artificial intelligence for public health surveillance. IEEE Intelligent Systems 2012;27(1):56–59.
66. Dredze M. Social media and health research at Johns Hopkins University. 2013.
67. Mandl KD, McNabb M, Marks N, Weitzman ER, Kelemen S, Eggleston EM, et al. Participatory surveillance of diabetes device safety: a social media-based complement to traditional FDA reporting. J Am Med Inform Assoc 2013;21(4):687–91.
68. WHO/Wpro. A guide to establishing event-based surveillance. Geneva; 2008.
69. New Zealand Ministry of Health. Notifiable Disease Surveillance. <https://surv.esr.cri.nz/public_health_surveillance/notifiable_disease_surveillance.php>.
70. California Maternal Quality Care C. H1N1 and Pregnancy.
71. CDC. 2009 H1N1 Flu in the News. 2010.
72. Wane J, Nyatanyi T, Nkunda R, Rukelibuga J, Ahmed Z, Biedron C, et al. 2009 pandemic influenza A (H1N1) virus outbreak and response – Rwanda, October, 2009–May, 2010. PLoS One 2012;7(6):e31572.
73. Cox CM, Blanton L, Dhara R, Brammer L, Finelli L. 2009 Pandemic influenza A (H1N1) deaths among children—United States, 2009-2010. Clin Infect Dis 2011;52(Suppl. 1):S69–74.
74. Dalhatu IT, Medina-Marino A, Olsen SJ, Hwang I, Gubio AB, Ekanem EE, et al. Influenza viruses in Nigeria, 2009-2010: results from the first 17 months of a national influenza sentinel surveillance system. J Infect Dis 2012;206(Suppl. 1):S121–8.
75. WHO. International health regulations (2005). 2nd ed. Geneva: World Health Organization; 2008.
76. Thacker SB, Stroup DF. Public health surveillance. Oxford University Press, New York; 1998. p. 105–35.
77. NNDSS Home. <https://www.patientslikeme.com/>; October 2014.
78. WHO. WHO technical consultation on event-based surveillance — meeting report. Geneva, Switzerland; 2013.
79. M'Ikanatha NM , Lynfield R, Van Beneden CA, de Valk H. Infectious disease surveillance. Wiley, West Sussex, UK; 2013.
80. Severi E, Kitching A, Crook P. Evaluation of the health protection event-based surveillance for the London 2012 Olympic and Paralympic Games. Euro Surveill 2014;19(24).
81. Clingingsmith D, Khwaja AI, Kremer M. Estimating the Impact of the Hajj: Religion and Tolerance in Islam's Global Gathering. Harvard Kennedy School Faculty Research Working Paper Series 2008; RWP08–022.
82. Li W. Implementation of a mobile-based surveillance system in Saudi Arabia for the 2009 Hajj. Online J Public Health Inform 2013;5(1):e137.
83. Al-Tawfiq JA, Memish ZA. Mass gathering medicine: 2014 Hajj and Umra preparation as a leading example. Int J Infect Dis 2014;27:26–31.
84. FBI. Amerithrax or Anthrax Investigation. 2011.
85. Bush L, Malecki J, Wiersma S, Cahill K, Fried R, Grossman M, Borkowsky W. Update: Investigation of anthrax associated with intentional exposure and interim public health guidelines, October 2001. MMWR Morb Mortal Wkly Rep 2001;50(41):889–93.
86. Henning KJ. What is syndromic surveillance? MMWR Morb Mortal Wkly Rep 2004;53(Suppl):5–11.
87. Kleinman K, Lazarus R, Platt R. A generalized linear mixed models approach for detecting incident clusters of disease in small areas, with an application to biological terrorism. Am J Epidemiol 2004;159(3):217–24.
88. Buehler JW, Sonricker A, Paladini M, Soper P, Mostashari F. Syndromic surveillance practice in the United States: findings from a survey of state, territorial, and selected local health departments. Int Soc Dis Surveill 2008;6(3):1–20.
89. Henning KJ. Overview of syndromic surveillance what is syndromic surveillance. MMWR Morb Mortal Wkly Rep 2004;53:5–11.
90. HHS. Syndromic Surveillance Data Submission. 2012.
91. CMS. Eligible professional meaningful use menu set measures measure 10 of 10. 2013.
92. Pavlin JA. Implementing syndromic surveillance systems in the climate of bioterrorism. In: M'Ikanatha N, Lynfield R, Van Beneden CA, de Valk H, editors. Blackwell Publishing Ltd, Oxford, UK; 2007. p. 351–60.
93. Yih WK, Caldwell B, Harmon R, Kleinman K, Lazarus R, Nelson A, et al. National Bioterrorism Syndromic Surveillance Demonstration Program. MMWR Morb Mortal Wkly Rep 2004;53(Suppl):43–9.
94. NCI. SaTScan. 2014.
95. Dorea FC, Lindberg A, McEwen BJ, Revie CW, Sanchez J. Syndromic surveillance using laboratory test requests: a practical guide informed by experience with two systems. Prev Vet Med 2014;116(3):313–24.
96. Dorea FC, Sanchez J, Revie CW. Veterinary syndromic surveillance: current initiatives and potential for development. Prev Vet Med 2011;101(1–2):1–17.
97. Dórea FC, Lindberg A, McEwen BJ, Revie CW, Sanchez J. Syndromic surveillance in veterinary medicine using laboratory submission data - lessons learned from two systems. Society for Veterinary Epidemiology and Preventive Medicine. Madrid, Spain; 2013.
98. Dupuy C, Bronner A, Watson E, Wuyckhuise-Sjouke L, Reist M, Fouillet A, et al. Inventory of veterinary syndromic surveillance initiatives in Europe (Triple-S project): current situation and perspectives. Prev Vet Med 2013;111(3–4):220–9.
99. Behavioral Risk Factor Surveillance System. BRFSS frequently asked questions (FAQs), <http://www.cdc.gov/brfss/about/brfss_faq.htm-1/>; 2015.
100. WARFS - World Alliance for Risk Factor Surveillance. Welcome, <http://www.warfs.info/>; 2015.
101. Baldissera S, Campostrini S, Binkin N, Minardi V, Minelli G, Ferrante G, et al. Features and initial assessment of the Italian Behavioral Risk Factor Surveillance System (PASSI), 2007-2008. Prev Chronic Dis 2011;8(1):A24.
102. Powell-Griner E. Uses and limitations of the behavioral risk factor surveillance system data. Section on Survey Research Methods, American Statistical Association. American Statistical Association, Alexandria, VA; 1998 (219–23). <http://www.amstat.org/>.
103. Luckerson V. Landline phones are getting closer to extinction. Time Magazine, July 8, 2014. <http://time.com/2966515/landline-phones-cell-phones/>; October 2014.

104. Meldrum A. Mobile phones the talk of Africa as landlines lose out. The Guardian, May 5, 2004. <http://www.theguardian.com/media/2004/may/05/citynews.newmedia>; October 2004.
105. Witt CJ, Richards AL, Masuoka PM, Foley DH, Buczak AL, Musila LA, et al. The AFHSC-Division of GEIS operations predictive surveillance program: a multidisciplinary approach for the early detection and response to disease outbreaks. BMC public health 2011;11(Suppl. 2):S10.
106. Lwin MO, Vijaykumar S, Fernando ONN, Cheong SA, Rathnayake VS, Lim G, et al. A 21st century approach to tackling dengue: crowdsourced surveillance, predictive mapping and tailored communication. Acta Tropica 2013;130C:100–7.
107. Krist AH, Woolf SH, Johnson RE, Rothemich SF, Cunningham TD, Jones RM, et al. Patient costs as a barrier to intensive health behavior counseling. Am J Prev Med 2010;38:344–8.
108. Atkinson J-AM, Gray DJ, Clements AC, Barnes TS, McManus DP, Yang YR. Environmental changes impacting Echinococcus transmission: research to support predictive surveillance and control. Glob Chang Biol 2013;19: 677–88.
109. Sanchez JL, Johns MC, Burke RL, Vest KG, Fukuda MM, Yoon IK, et al. Capacity-building efforts by the AFHSC-GEIS program. BMC Public Health 2011;11(Suppl. 2):S4.
110. Moloney JM, Skelly C, Weinstein P, Maguire M, Ritchie S. Domestic Aedes aegypti breeding site surveillance: limitations of remote sensing as a predictive surveillance tool. Am J Trop Med Hyg 1998;59:261–4.
111. Ameri AA, Henderick S, Jones B, Mariner J. Introduction to participatory epidemiology and its application to highly pathogenic avian influenza participatory disease surveillance a manual for participatory disease contributors. 2009.
112. Jost CC, Mariner JC, Roeder PL, Sawitri E, Macgregor-Skinner GJ. Participatory epidemiology in disease surveillance and research. Rev Sci Tech 2007;26(3):537–49.
113. Ulrich T. Participatory surveillance in public health: sharing is caring; 2013.
114. Andrejevic M. The work of watching one another: lateral surveillance, risk, and governance. Surveill Soc 2005;2(4):479–97.
115. Albrechtslund A. Online social networking as participatory surveillance. First Monday, [S.l.], Mar. 2008. ISSN 13960466. <http://firstmonday.org/ojs/index.php/fm/article/view/2142/1949>; October 2014.
116. Debin M, Turbelin C, Blanchon T, Bonmarin I, Falchi A, Hanslik T, et al. Evaluating the feasibility and participants' representativeness of an online nationwide surveillance system for influenza in France. PloS one 2013;8(9):e73675.
117. Paolotti D, Carnahan A, Colizza V, et al. Web-based participatory surveillance of infectious diseases: the Influenzanet participatory surveillance experience. Clin Microbiol Infect 2014;20(1):17–21.
118. Mariner JC, Hendrickx S, Pfeiffer DU, Costard S, Knopf L, Okuthe S, et al. Integration of participatory approaches into surveillance systems. Rev Sci Tech 2011;30(3):653–9.
119. Kostkova P. A roadmap to integrated digital public health surveillance: the vision and the challenges. London: Proceedings of the 22nd International Conference on World Wide Web; 2013. p. 687–94.
120. Healthmap, Boston Children's H, American Public Health A, Skoll Global Threats F. About - flu near you, <https://flunearyou.org/>; 2013.
121. Nsoesie E. Digital disease detection: a look at participatory surveillance of dengue, <http://www.healthmap.org/site/diseasedaily/article/digital-disease-detection-look-participatory-surveillance-dengue-51314/>; 2014.
122. Walton DA, Ivers LC. Responding to cholera in post-earthquake Haiti. N Engl J Med 2011;364(1):3–5.
123. One Health I. About the One Health initiative. <http://www.onehealthinitiative.com/about.php>; October 2014.
124. Global Health I. One Health: water, animals, food and society. <http://www.ucghi.universityofcalifornia.edu/coes/one-health/index.aspx>; October 2014.

CHAPTER

4

Integrated versus Vertical Public Health Surveillance Systems

Vivek Singh, Rajeev Gera, Paige Ryland

Shared problems present you with better shared solutions and they present a better chance for revival to survive future problems.

Frank Matobo

KEY WORDS

Integrated surveillance
Vertical surveillance
Integrated disease surveillance and response (IDSR)

INTRODUCTION

The debate about the benefits of integrated versus vertical public health surveillance has been raised time and again by public health professionals, governmental agencies, and private health organizations. Available resources, surveillance goals, and organizational structures all determine which type of public health surveillance will be implemented—integrated or vertical.

Vertical surveillance is a type of surveillance that focuses on a single disease or injury. Information is collected and fed back into the specific disease control program.[1] The surveillance of acute flaccid paralysis (AFP), for example, guides the Global Polio Eradication Initiative (GPEI) in different countries and, similarly, certain tuberculosis and HIV-prevention programs have dedicated surveillance components that guide their programming.

Integrated surveillance is a type of surveillance that uses a common approach to provide a universal surveillance service using similar structures and techniques.[1] Integrated public health surveillance thus provides universal surveillance services for multiple diseases, health-related events, or risk factors. The East Africa Integrated Disease Surveillance Network, for example, includes priority disease surveillance for multiple diseases including cholera, polio, malaria, and typhoid.[2]

This chapter discusses the factors that drive the decision to use integrated or vertical surveillance, examples of both, and the outcomes each type of design has on health systems. We will show that as public health surveillance continues to transform, integrated surveillance systems will be essential for creating the interoperable infrastructure needed to strengthen the field.

VERTICAL SURVEILLANCE

By focusing only on a single disease or injury, vertical surveillance is very resource intensive, and is also very effective in guiding a disease control program. Vertical systems are more common when a high profile disease is identified for control, elimination, or eradication. This tends to occur when the number of cases is very high and a concentrated effort is needed. This chapter points out that the transformation of public health surveillance should not lead us away from vertical surveillance entirely. The following sections offer examples of times when vertical surveillance may be most useful.

Vertical Surveillance Programs Set Up for Accelerated Response to Diseases Marked for Elimination or Eradication

When 166 WHO member states resolved to eradicate paralytic poliomyelitis by 2000 at the 41st World Health Assembly (WHA) in 1988, polio was endemic in 125 countries on five continents with an estimated 350,000 annual cases. By 2002, the number of endemic countries dropped to seven and the number of cases decreased by more than 99%. This extraordinary progress was possible because of actions based on the vertical program for AFP surveillance. Timely detection and investigation of all cases of AFP and the examination of stool samples collected from the AFP cases and from environmental sites in an accredited WHO Global Network laboratory guided the response.[3,4] When the poliovirus resurged globally, spreading from endemic countries like Nigeria and India, it was the AFP surveillance system that could track the global movement of the virus by using advancements in laboratory surveillance that relied on molecular genetic techniques.[5-7] Genetic mapping of the poliovirus showed that the Hajj pilgrimage to Saudi Arabia was a major route of the global spread of the disease. Accordingly, in 2005, Saudi Arabia made it mandatory for people under the age of 15 traveling from polio-affected countries to be immunized against the disease before traveling for Hajj, which led to a subsequent major decline in the global spread of polio.[8] As we approach the end game for polio eradication, the role of AFP surveillance will become even more important for understanding the patterns of movement, pathogenesis, and virology of the infection for the remaining viruses.[9,10]

The AFP surveillance system, one of the fundamental pillars of the GPEI and a vertical surveillance system, has set high standards in disease surveillance, especially in countries where disease surveillance is still nascent. Guidelines; standard operating procedures; monitoring of data timeliness, completeness, and accuracy; and support from the laboratory network have all contributed in making the AFP surveillance system a benchmark in disease surveillance in countries like India. There have been substantial gains in the last decade in the GPEI when India, one of the major polio endemic countries, was declared polio free in March 2014 after 3 consecutive years without detection of wild poliovirus and maintaining WHO-prescribed AFP surveillance standards.

The lessons of the AFP surveillance system from India are being transferred to other polio endemic countries like Nigeria, Afghanistan, and Pakistan. WHO surveillance officers from India are being deployed to the remaining endemic countries to share their lessons and provide technical support to the program. Countries can transfer the health systems level lessons from the gains made with AFP surveillance for polio eradication to strengthen IDSR and vertical surveillance for other priority disease like measles.[11] The gains made from the GPEI in the strengthening of health systems should also be utilized systematically to strengthen the overall vaccine-preventable diseases programs and service delivery through the primary health care system.[12,13]

Guinea worm is another disease marked for eradication. As for polio eradication, vertical surveillance for Guinea worm eradication has proven necessary and effective. The approach for Guinea worm employs a community-based eradication strategy that relies on village volunteers. This means asking a single volunteer in each community to routinely look for symptomatic persons in his or her community for very little in return in terms of incentive. It can be a very expensive and very fragile system. When cases become rare, volunteers must remain focused on just Guinea worm instead of diverting attention to other diseases. It can be very difficult to keep village volunteers actively engaged in the search for symptomatic persons when they may have not found a case in months. Adding additional tasks to these volunteers would only distract them from the goal at hand: eradication of Guinea worm. The program has been largely successful but not without critics.

These types of disease environment typically draws the attention of funding organizations, which perpetuate the use of vertical surveillance systems by funneling money into surveillance activities for a single disease such as polio or HIV/AIDS.

Vertical Surveillance Programs Set Up after Disasters or Mass Gathering Events

Natural and man-made disasters disrupt routine surveillance systems and pose a challenge for disease control in the early recovery phase. Countries rich and poor are struck by the challenge of postdisaster surveillance, and need-based, context-specific, postdisaster surveillance system plans are needed during the interdisaster phase.[14,15]

On May 12, 2008, an earthquake with a magnitude of 8.0 struck the northwestern area of China's Sichuan Province. Over 80,000 people were killed and 5 million more left homeless. The earthquake disrupted the Chinese information system for disease control and prevention through which routine disease surveillance information was being collected. To track the epidemic-prone diseases and respond to potential outbreaks postdisaster, the Chinese Center for Disease Control and Prevention (China CDC) developed an emergency reporting system using mobile phones.[16] The mobile-based surveillance system not was only effective in postdisaster disease surveillance and response but also led to wider adoption of mobile technology for routine surveillance.

The 2012 London Olympic and Paralympic Games were one of the largest mass gathering events in British history. The United Kingdom's Health Protection Agency set up multisource surveillance systems for monitoring disease and health-related events during the games. These systems included not only enhancements of the existing systems but also systems created especially for the games.[17,18] These enhanced and newly established surveillance systems are ready for future reactivation should the need arise.

IMPEDIMENTS AND LIMITATIONS TO GOALS OF VERTICAL SURVEILLANCE

Vertical surveillance, used in programs like the AFP surveillance for polio eradication, is capable of strengthening additional public health surveillance systems if it provides the framework for strengthening surveillance for other diseases and health-related events.[19,20] These positive impacts of the polio eradication campaign are dependent on the initiative of policy makers. Polio surveillance activities—and other vertical surveillance—can provide support for surveillance of other diseases, especially those that are vaccine preventable, but many opportunities to do so remain missed. Identification and documentation of best practices and political commitment for scaling up could lead to significant positive impacts.[21]

GOALS FOR VERTICAL SURVEILLANCE

Short-term goals:

- Use the guiding principles and practices of the surveillance network used for successful disease control programs, like polio and tuberculosis, to guide programs for other diseases in the low- and middle-income countries (LMICs).

Medium-term goals:

- Develop strategies for convergence of surveillance resources of tuberculosis, HIV, and malaria disease control programs for integrating disease surveillance—a core component of the health systems in LMICs.
- Develop interoperability standards for different information sources and systems to integrate public health surveillance systems.

Long-term goals:

- Build health system capacity to initiate a public health surveillance system in any public health emergency situation—man-made or environmental.

INTEGRATED SURVEILLANCE

Integrated surveillance relies on existing resources and capacity, promoting the most effective use of health resources.[1] An integrated system, therefore, requires a high level of coordination but is more cost-effective and efficient than a vertical system. It is more common to find integrated surveillance systems at the local level where the number of cases is likely small for most diseases.[1] The following sections offer examples of times when integrated surveillance may be most useful.

Integrated Disease Surveillance and Response Programs in Different Regions of the World

Integrated disease surveillance takes different shapes and forms in different places depending on resources and program objectives. Examples found on two different continents highlighting the different outcomes integrated systems experience from place to place are shown below.

Integrated disease surveillance and response (IDSR) evolved as a strategy for integrated disease surveillance in African countries in the 1990s in response to the emergence of severe outbreaks of largely preventable diseases. IDSR is a comprehensive regional framework for strengthening national public health surveillance and response systems in Africa. In 2006, WHO/AFRO member states recommended to implement International Health Regulations (IHR 2005) using the IDSR framework, especially to strengthen core capacities for surveillance and response. The IDSR framework illustrates the functions, activities, and skills required to implement an integrated, coordinated, comprehensive surveillance, and response system.[22]

IDSR was adopted by African member states as a comprehensive regional framework for strengthening national public health surveillance and response systems in Africa. An evaluation of the strategy in four countries in the WHO African region for the period 1998–2005 showed that in spite of major challenges in strengthening laboratory networks and extending the strategy to subnational levels, the integration of the surveillance function of most of the categorical disease control programs led to improved outbreak response.[23] Evaluation of IDSR in Uganda showed that in a 5-year period, from 2001 to 2007, the strategy led to a decrease in the case fatality rate for two target priority diseases, cholera from 7% to 2% and meningococcal meningitis from 16% to 4%, most likely due to improved outbreak response.[24]

The WHO South East Asia Region adopted a strategic plan for integrated disease surveillance in 2002.[25] In line with the WHO strategic plan in the region and in an effort to improve the surveillance and response infrastructure in the country, India launched the Integrated Disease Surveillance Project (IDSP) in 2004 and scaled up across the entire country in a phased manner by 2007.[26] Recent assessment of the functions of IDSP in India showed major gaps in the structural integration of surveillance systems and, contrary to its original purpose, it is functioning as an isolated program.[27] Another assessment of core and supplementary surveillance system attributes and functions affecting the outcome of the IDSP in one state in India found weak laboratory and outbreak detection capacity of the system.[28] These findings from the assessment of IDSP in India are quite contrary to the findings from Africa and highlight the challenges of effective implementation of IDSR.

An Opportunity for Integrated Surveillance

In many LMICs there is a significant burden of both noncommunicable disease (NCD) and communicable disease (CD), which can stretch the already overburdened and strained health systems. Fundamental data on NCD and CD comorbidity in vulnerable populations are needed, yet surveillance systems rarely address these conditions simultaneously. Integrated surveillance of NCD and CD comorbidity (e.g., diabetes and tuberculosis) would generate the empirical data needed to better understand the dual disease burden. Convergence of NCD and CD surveillance, especially in LMICs, calls for realignment of efforts to combine NCD and CD screening. This effort is especially needed for vulnerable populations such as rural to urban migrants who experience high disease burden from both NCD and CD.[29] Also, as the migrant population changes its lifestyle (from rural to urban) and diet, a range of cardiovascular risk factors are affected, adding to other NCD risk factors like tobacco use, which is known to be elevated in this group. Again, the working and living conditions of these migrants put them at higher risk for CD like tuberculosis infection. Although certain risk factors for NCD (e.g., obesity) are commonly associated with increased affluence, a study in India has shown that risk factors for NCDs are also present among those of lower socioeconomic status.[30] Based on a resolution in the 64th WHA, the WHO Secretariat developed a draft "Global action plan for the prevention and control of NCDs for the period 2013–2020,"[31] building on what has already been achieved through the implementation of the 2008–2013 action plan. The provisions of this global action plan provide an opportunity to utilize the current focus of the world health community to mainstream NCD surveillance into an integrated disease surveillance strategy to generate vital information for better control and response to NCD.

IMPEDIMENTS AND LIMITATIONS TO GOALS OF INTEGRATED SURVEILLANCE

Several impediments and limitations exist in creating efficient and effective surveillance programs. First, donor-driven strategies undermine the collaboration that is key to establishing a well-functioning integrated surveillance system. Donor agencies focusing on a single disease are more interested in strengthening a vertical system at the expense of an integrated system by funneling all resources into activities related to a particular disease. To ensure sustainability and a strong health system, stakeholders need to agree to a common set of priorities and goals.

Second, surveillance systems often suffer from a lack of proper coordination. For successful collaboration to occur, both inter- and cross-sectoral communications are necessary, as many sectors are involved in the collection and communication of data in an integrated system.

Another limitation faced by integrated surveillance systems is the lack of adequate resources. An effective surveillance system that has the capacity to generate real-time, high-quality information for guiding appropriate action requires substantial resources. Government agencies, especially in LMICs that have high disease burden, often do not have enough resources to invest in building and maintaining an IDSR system even though doing so will conserve more resources than vertical surveillance when seen over time.

Finally, surveillance is not always seen as a priority. Due to limited resources and competing priorities, surveillance often does not get the attention and resources it requires. The usefulness of a robust surveillance system is often not appreciated by decision-makers. It is not perceived as a vital component of disease prevention and control programs. When it is recognized as an important step in disease control and prevention, limited resources may still restrict priorities. For example, if a country has limited resources, it may only be able to devote resources to a small number of diseases, which would not require an integrated surveillance system.

GOALS FOR INTEGRATED SURVEILLANCE

Short-term goals:

- Use an IDSR framework to establish guidelines that will meet the surveillance, response, and laboratory core capacity requirements of the IHR (2005).
- Use the PHEIC reporting requirements under the IHR (2005) to strengthen early warning signals through IDSR.
- Create reports for donors and governments highlighting the importance of strong integrated surveillance to motivate their commitment to support such programs.

Medium-term goals:

- Develop strategies to integrate NCD risk factor surveillance into integrated disease surveillance systems.
- Develop interoperability standards for different information sources and systems for integrated public health surveillance systems.

Long-term goals:

- Use readily available, informal data sources to complement integrated systems.

- Reevaluate and redesign lists of diseases under surveillance on an annual or as needed basis.
- Improve the efficiency of surveillance systems as more efficient technology becomes available.
- Continue to use public health surveillance data to improve public health programs.
- Promote workforce growth to meet the needs of integrated surveillance across the globe.

ESTABLISHING INTEGRATED SURVEILLANCE SYSTEMS

Establishing an integrated surveillance system begins as with any other program: with an analysis of current capabilities, weaknesses, and gaps. Based on the results of that analysis, a plan of action is developed for implementation. IDSR programming in the African region is completing these plans for 43 countries in an effort to help countries meet the IHR (2005) requirements.[26]

IDSR was implemented because vertical systems, occurring in tandem for various diseases, were putting stress on health systems by spreading resources thin, resulting in poor health outcomes.[25,32]

WHO surveillance guidelines exist for vertical programs but are harder to find for developing an integrated system to meet IHR (2005) requirements.[11] In addition to planning for the core functions of surveillance—detection, registration, reporting, confirmation, analyses, and feedback[33]—an integrated system necessitates a high-level process for coordinating these activities across all levels (local, regional, national). This coordination includes ensuring that staff members have the proper training for the role(s) they perform, needed resources are available, systems are interoperable, and there is a plan for monitoring and evaluation.

WHEN TO USE INTEGRATED OR VERTICAL SURVEILLANCE

There are arguments for and against both types of surveillance systems. Not surprisingly, public health professionals working with integrated surveillance systems tend to be the most critical of vertical systems. They argue that a vertical system, focusing too much on a single disease, weakens overall surveillance efforts by depleting the available financial, logistical, and human resources. On the other hand, advocates of vertical systems argue that the goal of any accelerated disease control, elimination, or eradication program cannot be achieved without establishing a dedicated, focused surveillance system that can stand up to the requirements of such a control program. What both arguments fail to explain, however, is that health agencies deciding which type of surveillance system to implement will need to consider their resources and surveillance goals. The goals of surveillance may be varied, but if the health system resources needed to perform the surveillance are absent, both vertical and integrated systems will fail to meet their objectives.

Vertical and integrated surveillance systems serve different and distinct functions in PHS. The same health-related event or disease can be a part of integrated disease surveillance or the focus of a vertical surveillance system. For example, AFP is a reportable condition as part of an integrated surveillance strategy in many countries without polio, whereas in polio endemic countries—and in India, which was recently declared polio free in March 2014—AFP surveillance is a vertical strategy that guides the polio eradication efforts.[34,35] However, the very elements of vertical programs that ensure success can be tailored to improve integrated systems.

It is important for health managers to make the right choice for their health surveillance objectives. Deciding which option is best should include considering the point of view of public health systems strengthening. This means considering how the type of surveillance chosen will help or hurt the overall public health system. In a well-functioning health system, an integrated surveillance system is expected to detect all cases and outbreaks of notifiable diseases, analyze the information, and respond in an appropriate amount of time. When a disease is marked for eradication or elimination and every case must be found and investigated, the same integrated system should be able to respond to the needs of the program with a high level of sensitivity by including additional data elements and collection methods.

It is important to note that there is a degree of verticality within integrated systems. Because each individual notifiable disease or health condition within an integrated system has specific requirements from identification to response that require special focus within the integrated system, one can imagine an integrated surveillance system as made up of several coordinated vertical systems.

PUBLIC HEALTH SURVEILLANCE SYSTEMS AND HEALTH SYSTEM STRENGTHENING

Perhaps the most important aspect of any surveillance system is the human dimension required for success. In countries with systems of surveillance supported by a strong workforce, a weak health system may be buoyed by their capacities. This is echoed by WHO's building blocks for health strengthening, which include the importance of a health care workforce for strengthening health systems.[36] Importantly, they note that a "well-performing" health workforce is one with available, competent, responsive, and productive workers. Surveillance demands a lot from its workforce. Amos et al.[37] write that appropriate assessment, diagnosis, investigation, specimen handling, laboratory processing, and data handling are all required for good surveillance and must be operational 24 h a day wherever a patient is located. One way to develop the capacity needed for surveillance and, following, health system strengthening is the use of the field epidemiology training program (FETP) and the field epidemiology and laboratory training program (FELTP).[38] The benefit of competent surveillance staff to a health system may come from both vertical and integrated systems. Additionally, other windfalls from surveillance programs, such as the development of new technology or an improved utilization of resources, are likely to trickle back to the overall strengthening of the health system. (For more information about workforce needs in public health surveillance, see Chapter 9.)

All WHO member states revised the WHO IHR at the 2005 WHA. These became a binding instrument of international law and entered into force on June 15, 2007. The stated purpose and scope of the IHR are "to prevent, protect against, control, and provide a public health response to the international spread of disease in ways that are commensurate with and restricted to public health risks, and which avoid unnecessary interference with international traffic and trade."[39] Of particular interest are the PHEICs defined in the Chapter 3. The IHR (2005) require member states to strengthen the core surveillance and response capacities of their health systems at all levels of health care service delivery. Their adoption highlights the need for the IDSR strategy, which can aid countries in meeting the surveillance and response core capacity requirements.[40] By meeting these core capacities, it is hoped that a strong global surveillance network will be able to prevent the spread of PHEICs.

The continuing evolution of, and advancements in, the information, communication, and technology fields, especially the increasing reach of mobile technology, provides an opportunity to more easily coordinate an integrated public health information and surveillance system. With an integrated system, a wide range of diverse individual information systems will continue to exist but these systems must be interconnected, comparable, and easy to use. For this to happen, users and providers must agree on standards and guidelines, which will ease the coordination of systems. Advancements in health informatics approaches can be used to integrate health information sources and surveillance systems.

KEY SUMMARY POINTS

- Integrated and vertical surveillance systems should be judged based on their usefulness for the context in which they are to be applied.
- Advocates for integrated surveillance reason that resources, human resources, and logistical support are best utilized to strengthen the overarching integrated surveillance system rather than individual vertical health surveillance initiatives.
- Vertical surveillance systems may be necessary for diseases or health-related events that are marked for elimination or eradication or for those that show up as an emergency for a short duration.
- The signing of IHR (2005) demonstrates member states' understanding in the importance of strengthening overarching surveillance, laboratory, and response core capacities.
- Designing and conducting both vertical and integrated surveillance systems should use a health systems strengthening perspective.
- One of the largest challenges in integrated surveillance is that donors undermine the investment in the collaboration that is necessary for an integrated surveillance system to function, but investors are readily available to fund vertical disease specific initiatives.
- IDSR systems require both systematic situation analysis and stakeholder participation to be successful.

DISCUSSION QUESTIONS

1. List some of the regional and global integrated surveillance systems. Also, list some of the regional and global vertical surveillance systems?
2. What are the differences between a vertical and an integrated disease surveillance system in terms of system planning, design, and operation?
3. What are the commonalities between a vertical and an integrated disease surveillance system in terms of system planning, design, and operation?
4. What are the factors that determine whether a vertical or an integrated surveillance system is used to collect information on a disease or health-related event?
5. What are the effects of a vertical disease surveillance system on the overall health system?
6. What are the effects of an integrated disease surveillance system on the overall health system?
7. What advances in information and communication technology can be utilized for the integration of public health surveillance systems?
8. What opportunities do the IHR (2005) provide for strengthening countries' integrated disease surveillance systems?
9. What kind of a surveillance system design is needed to tackle the growing burden of NCD in many countries?

REFERENCES

1. Garcia-Abreu A, Halperin W, Danel I. Public health surveillance toolkit: a guide for busy task managers. Washington, DC: The World Bank; 2002.
2. Ope M, Sonoiya S, Kariuki J, Mboera LE, Gandham RN, Schneidman M, et al. Regional initiatives in support of surveillance in East Africa: the East Africa Integrated Disease Surveillance Network (EAIDSNet) experience. Emerg Health Threats 2013;6:3–4.
3. De Gourville E, Dowdle WR. The role of surveillance in polio eradication and identification of emerging viral encephalitis. Arch Virol Suppl 2004;(18):13–20.
4. Hovi T, Shulman LM, van der Avoort H, Deshpande J, Roivainen M, EM DEG. Role of environmental poliovirus surveillance in global polio eradication and beyond. Epidemiol Infect 2012;140(1):1–13.
5. Zarocostas J. Polio-endemic countries pledge to boost eradication efforts in 2004. Lancet 2004;363(9404):215.
6. Raufu A. Nigeria apologises to neighbours for spread of polio. BMJ 2004;329(7462):365.
7. de Gourville E, Duintjer Tebbens RJ, Sangrujee N, Pallansch MA, Thompson KM. Global surveillance and the value of information: the case of the global polio laboratory network. Risk Anal 2006;26(6):1557–69.
8. Saudi Arabia requires people aged under 15 years travelling from polio-affected countries to be immunized against the disease. Wkly Epidemiol Rec 2005;80(33):288.
9. Abraham T. Polio eradication: a complex end game. BMJ 2012;344: e2398.
10. Minor PD. The polio-eradication programme and issues of the end game. J Gen Virol 2012;93(Pt 3):457–74.
11. Perry HN, McDonnell SM, Alemu W, Nsubuga P, Chungong S, Otten Jr MW, et al. Planning an integrated disease surveillance and response system: a matrix of skills and activities. BMC Med 2007;5:24.
12. Closser S, Rosenthal A, Parris T, Maes K, Justice J, Cox K, et al. Methods for evaluating the impact of vertical programs on health systems: protocol for a study on the impact of the global polio eradication initiative on strengthening routine immunization and primary health care. BMC Public Health 2012;12:728.
13. Loevinsohn B, Aylward B, Steinglass R, Ogden E, Goodman T, Melgaard B. Impact of targeted programs on health systems: a case study of the polio eradication initiative. Am J Public Health 2002;92(1):19–23.
14. Arima Y, Matsui T, Partridge J, Kasai T. The great East Japan earthquake: a need to plan for post-disaster surveillance in developed countries. Western Pac Surveill Response J 2011;2(4):3–6.
15. Mohamad N, Abu Bakar NH, Mohamed NA, Baharudin KA, Noh AY, Ahmad R, et al. Post-impact disaster surveillance - a medical reconnaissance team at tsunami-struck Sri Lanka. Malays J Med Sci 2007;14(1):79–83.
16. Yang C, Yang J, Luo X, Gong P. Use of mobile phones in an emergency reporting system for infectious disease surveillance after the Sichuan earthquake in China. Bull World Health Organ 2009;87(8):619–23.
17. Harcourt SE, Fletcher J, Loveridge P, Bains A, Morbey R, Yeates A, et al. Developing a new syndromic surveillance system for the London 2012 Olympic and Paralympic Games. Epidemiol Infect 2012;140(12):2152–56.
18. Elliot AJ, Morbey RA, Hughes HE, Harcourt SE, Smith S, Loveridge P, et al. Syndromic surveillance - a public health legacy of the London 2012 Olympic and Paralympic Games. Public Health 2013;127(8):777–81.
19. Centers for Disease Control and Prevention. Expanding poliomyelitis and measles surveillance networks to establish surveillance for acute meningitis and encephalitis syndromes—Bangladesh, China, and India, 2006-2008. MMWR Morb Mortal Wkly Rep 2012;61(49):1008–11.
20. Centers for Disease Control and Prevention. Acute flaccid paralysis surveillance systems for expansion to other diseases, 2003-2004. MMWR Morb Mortal Wkly Rep 2004;53(47):1113–6.
21. Closser S, Cox K, Parris TM, Landis RM, Justice J, Gopinath R, et al. The impact of polio eradication on routine immunization and primary health care: a mixed-methods study. J Infect Dis 2014;210(Suppl. 1):S504–13.
22. Global Health Protection & Security. What Is integrated disease surveillance and response (IDSR)? <http://www.cdc.gov/globalhealth/healthprotection/ghsb/idsr/what/default.html/>; 2015.
23. Nsubuga P, Brown WG, Groseclose SL, Ahadzie L, Talisuna AO, Mmbuji P, et al. Implementing integrated disease surveillance and response: four African countries' experience, 1998-2005. Global Public Health 2010;5(4):364–80.
24. Lukwago L, Nanyunja M, Ndayimirije N, Wamala J, Malimbo M, Mbabazi W, et al. The implementation of integrated disease surveillance and response in Uganda: a review of progress and challenges between 2001 and 2007. Health Policy Plan 2013;28(1):30–40.
25. World Health Organization. Asia WHOROfS-E. Regional strategy for integrated disease surveillance. New Delhi; 2003.
26. Suresh K. Integrated Diseases Surveillance Project (IDSP) through a consultant's lens. Indian J Public Health 2008;52(3):136–43.

27. Phalkey RK, Shukla S, Shardul S, Ashtekar N, Valsa S, Awate P, et al. Assessment of the core and support functions of the Integrated Disease Surveillance system in Maharashtra, India. BMC Public Health 2013;13:575.
28. Singh V, Mohan J, Rao UP, Heymann D, Dandona L. An evaluation of the key indicator based surveillance system for international health regulations (IHR) -2005 core capacity requirements in India. Online J Public Health Inform 2014;6(1):e121.
29. Remais JV, Zeng G, Li G, Tian L, Engelgau MM. Convergence of non-communicable and infectious diseases in low- and middle-income countries. Int J Epidemiol 2013;42(1):221–7.
30. Vellakkal S, Subramanian SV, Millett C, Basu S, Stuckler D, Ebrahim S. Socioeconomic inequalities in non-communicable diseases prevalence in India: disparities between self-reported diagnoses and standardized measures. PLoS One 2013;8(7):e68219.
31. World Health Organization. Global action plan for the prevention and control of NCDs 2013-2020. World Health Organization. 2013. p. 55.
32. Nsubuga P, White ME, Thacker SB, Anderson MA, Blount SB, Broome CV, et al. Public health surveillance: a tool for targeting and monitoring interventions. In: Jamison DT, Breman JG, Measham AR, Alleyne G, Claeson M, Evans DB, et al., editors. Disease control priorities in developing countries. 2nd ed. Washington, DC: World Bank; 2006.
33. McNabb SJ, Chungong S, Ryan M, Wuhib T, Nsubuga P, Alemu W, et al. Conceptual framework of public health surveillance and action and its application in health sector reform. BMC Public Health 2002;2:2.
34. World Health Organization. Technical guidelines for integrated disease surveillance and response in the African region. Brazzaville: Republic of Congo and Atlanta, USA; 2010. p. 1–398.
35. Banerjee K, Hlady WG, Andrus JK, Sarkar S, Fitzsimmons J, Abeykoon P. Poliomyelitis surveillance: the model used in India for polio eradication. Bull World Health Organ 2000;78(3):321–9.
36. World Health Organization. Everybody's business: strengthening health systems to improve health outcomes, WHO's framework for action. Geneva; 2007.
37. Amos B, Kisakye A, Makewa D, Mudhune S, Mwamtemi H, Nansera D, et al. Behind the data: establishing the network for surveillance for pneumococcal diseases in the East African region, netSPEAR. Clin Infect Dis 2009;48(Suppl. 2):S162–71.
38. Nsubuga P, Nwanyanwu O, Nkengasong JN, Mukanga D, Trostle M. Strengthening public health surveillance and response using the health systems strengthening agenda in developing countries. BMC Public Health 2010;10(Suppl. 1):S5.
39. World Health Organization. International health regulations (2005). Geneva; 2008.
40. Kasolo F, Yoti Z, Bakyaita N, Gaturuku P, Katz R, Fischer JE, et al. IDSR as a platform for implementing IHR in African countries. Biosecur Bioterror 2013;11(3):163–9.

CHAPTER

5

Reactive versus Proactive Public Health Surveillance

Richard V Birtwhistle, Kieran Moore

The result of the inquiry, then, is, that there has been no particular outbreak or prevalence of cholera in this part of London except among the persons who were in the habit of drinking the water of the above-mentioned pump-well. I had an interview with the Board of Guardians of St James's parish, on the evening of the 7th inst. [7 September], and represented the above circumstances to them. In consequence of what I said, the handle of the pump was removed on the following day.

John Snow (1854, letter to the editor of the Medical Times and Gazette)

KEY WORDS

Active surveillance
Canadian Primary Care Sentinel Surveillance Network
Google Flu Trends
Passive surveillance
Pharmacosurveillance
Predictive modeling
Proactive surveillance
Reactive surveillance

INTRODUCTION

Given current public health threats, including emerging infectious diseases (e.g., H7N9, MERS-CoV, H5N1, and Ebola virus), extreme weather events, and an ever-increasing burden of chronic disease, it is essential that public health practitioners have valid, reliable, and accessible surveillance information at their fingertips to increase their awareness and understanding of these problems and respond in a timely and effective way. Surveillance systems need to be integrated and fuse data from multiple sources with an emphasis on real-time information, especially to detect emergent public health threats and enable evidence-informed public health action.

Traditionally, public health surveillance has been considered either passive or active.[1] National notifiable disease surveillance systems rely on data submitted by providers to track these diseases.

Access to electronic, real-time information about the health of the population provides the opportunity for an active surveillance system that can automatically alert public health practitioners of a potential threat or use predictive modeling to enable health system preparedness and response.

In this chapter, we will update the definition of active surveillance to include both reactive and proactive approaches and provide examples of how both of these methods are being used in public health (Fig. 5-1).

PASSIVE SURVEILLANCE

Presently, most surveillance is passive and relies on receiving paper or faxed reports from hospitals, clinics, laboratories, public health units, or other sources. Passive surveillance is described in more detail in Chapter 3.

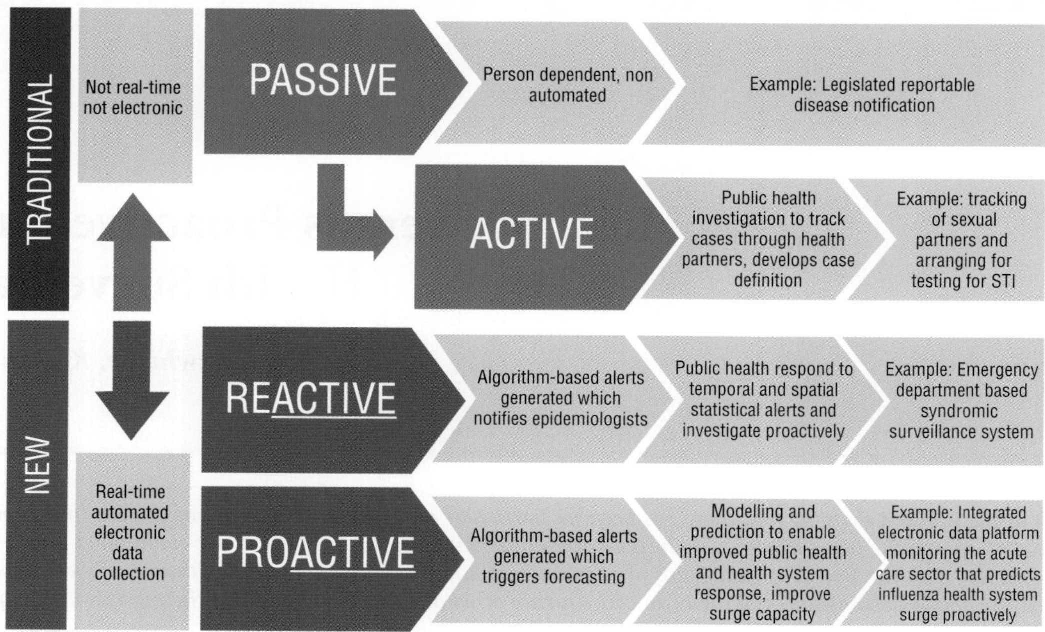

FIG. 5-1 Descriptions of passive, reactive, and proactive surveillance systems.

An example of this method is a national influenza surveillance system such as Canada's Respiratory Virus Detection Surveillance System, which relies on the collection and aggregation of results from laboratories across the country and provides weekly summaries of the number of tests performed and samples tested positive for various influenza strains and other respiratory viruses.[2] At a national level, this typically can take weeks for data to be received, analyzed, and communicated to stakeholders. While laboratory-based passive surveillance is simple, acceptable, and flexible, it tends to lack sensitivity and is often not timely or representative (as it is dependent upon persons getting tested).[1]

A noninfectious disease example of passive surveillance is a cancer registry, such as the Provincial Ontario Cancer Registry in Canada that collects data from cancer-related hospital discharge and day surgery records, pathology reports received (largely electronically) from hospitals and other laboratories, consultation and treatment records from cancer treatment centers, and death certificates.[3]

ACTIVE SURVEILLANCE

As outlined in Chapter 3, active surveillance is a type of surveillance that is dynamically seeking data from participants in the surveillance system on a regular basis. It is the ongoing, systematic collection of information so that a disease or infection can be tracked over time, or a new public health threat can be detected at the earliest possible time. This should allow for rapid effective interventions. Active surveillance systems have the benefit of being acceptable and sensitive, may be more representative and they help ensure that data will be reported in a timely manner.[1] These systems have typically been used during mass gatherings, high-risk event outbreaks, or epidemics for case finding.

Traditional active surveillance systems are typically initiated on alerts from passive systems and are labor intensive. Public health offices may be required to contact and work with health partners to follow up the event in question and then analyze the data using standard outbreak response protocols. However, there are now new electronic data sources that have not been available to public health in the past that will create more dynamic approaches to active surveillance. We are entering a new era that provides opportunities for both ongoing reactive and proactive surveillance.

Reactive Surveillance

Definition of Reactive Surveillance

Reactive surveillance is a type of active surveillance in which health system electronic data or other complementary data are systematically collected in as close to real time as possible and regularly monitored automatically resulting in spatial and/or temporal anomaly detection.

This occurs through computer-based algorithms that identify abnormal changes in time or per geographic location compared to what is expected. These automated, statistically generated alerts allow epidemiologists or public health clinicians to review the alert and decide whether further investigation is necessary. Often these systems need additional contextual data or intelligence to strengthen the investigation and potential response. This contextual data may include confirmed diagnoses, laboratory testing, or prescribed medications.

Advantages and Disadvantages of Reactive Surveillance

The clear advantage of reactive surveillance is the real-time nature of the data collection and analysis. Timely data that flow automatically from a variety of sources can be linked for a more complete picture of the disease and need for further investigation and response. There are few disadvantages to this approach, however; it requires resources to build the system, ensure data quality, and develop the surveillance algorithms. It also requires a clear process for public health personnel to interpret and act on the signals without creating too many false-positive or false-negative events. It may require specific nontraditional public health skill sets and be difficult to sustain.

Examples of Reactive Surveillance. Examples of reactive surveillance are influenza surveillance monitoring of emergency department visits[4,5] for influenza-like illness (ILI) and Google Flu Trends.[6]

In chronic disease, reactive surveillance can occur through the ongoing collection of primary care electronic medical record health data on individual patients, which can be extracted and analyzed to look for trends in incidence and prevalence of chronic diseases such as diabetes, risk factors such as tobacco use, and demographic changes or changes in the management of chronic diseases. The use of this data source is early in its development but holds potential for both further expansion in reactive surveillance and implementation in proactive surveillance.[7]

Proactive Surveillance

Definition of Proactive Surveillance

Proactive surveillance is a type of active surveillance using routinely collected real-time data as a predictive tool to model potential health system outcomes and enhance system preparedness and response.

Advantages and Disadvantages of Proactive Surveillance

Like reactive surveillance, the main advantage of proactive surveillance is the real-time nature of the data collection and analysis. Once the data are collected and linked, big data analytics can be applied and models developed, which provide an early warning for future events or uncover novel risk factors for disease prevention. The disadvantages are similar to reactive surveillance methods. Developing these models and data analytics requires skill and the ability to distinguish a signal from noise.

Examples of Proactive Surveillance. An example of proactive surveillance is in predicting the occurrence of influenza in a community or health region and its impact on the health care system. This proactive modeling may allow for timely preparation, prevention, and response strategies. An example of this is the ILI mapper (http://www.kflaphi.ca/ILI-Mapper/) produced by Kingston, Frontenac and Lennox & Addington (KFL&A) Public Health Informatics. This local public health agency in Ontario, Canada, projects weekly influenza activity by health region into four categories and provides level-specific prevention and response activity.[8] This modeling activity can result in timely interventions to minimize the impact of a surge, such as implementation of public education utilizing computer-based self-treatment guidelines or nurse helplines to advice on appropriate health-seeking behavior and appropriate use of health care services. From a health systems perspective, proactive surveillance may predict the optimum time to open alternative influenza assessment centers to provide early care to vulnerable populations in a less costly setting, thereby decreasing the impact of the high surge of patients on the acute care sector during severe influenza seasons or a pandemic. This proactive modeling was integrated into the response in Ontario, Canada, during the 2009 H1N1 pandemic.[9,10] The system enabled KFL&A to be the first in Ontario to establish flu assessment centers in the community to minimize the impact of the surge in health-seeking behavior on the acute care sector. The timing of the opening and closing of the clinics was based on local surveillance data to maximize effectiveness and efficiency. Proactive surveillance can also help focus immunization and communication strategies as well as prepare laboratory systems for surges in sample submission through testing prioritization to improve turnaround times. The system is now in place on a provincial basis for all participating hospitals and regions. The color-coded predictive tool has associated recommendation for action by the health system at each level of influenza-like activity.

FUTURE VISION

Future areas of work and research on reactive and proactive surveillance include sophisticated predictive modeling using "big data" for outbreaks[11]; chronic disease development and burden of illness; health system utilization and detection of high cost and high frequency users; pharmacosurveillance[12]; and health impacts of environmental air pollution particulates.[13] Additionally, work should utilize a vulnerability lens in surveillance systems through the real-time application of deprivation indices (e.g., the social and material deprivation index created by Pampalon et al.[14] in Canada).

Furthermore, given increasing utilization of the internet and social media, these data sources should be reviewed for surveillance opportunities. Most sites have analytic engines that can be used to monitor traffic and measure effectiveness of population health communication strategies. Content can also be monitored by using keyword searches that can be a proxy for infectious or chronic disease by grouping the key words into syndromes, natural language processing, and infectious or chronic disease syndromes. There are several advantages of using internet and social media sources: the data have a wide population reach, can provide national or international coverage, can be collected and analyzed in real time, and can be analyzed with a level of spatial identification. These systems would also be inexpensive to maintain.[15,16] Additionally, these data sources may be a good surveillance tool for monitoring knowledge, attitudes, and behaviors for chronic disease risk factors, e.g., immunization, smoking, eating habits, and drug use.

Increasingly, linked electronic health data are used in health systems settings and surveillance of chronic disease management. These linkages can be used, for example, to identify people at high risk of hospitalization.[17] Primary care electronic health record (EHR) data linked with emergency room and hospitalization data can be used for this purpose. Once health care providers identify these individuals, using EHR data, more intensive treatment or additional community services can be provided to prevent or delay hospitalization.

Each available electronic data set may identify various components of an individual's health record such as diagnosis, laboratory tests, or prescribed medications and, if unique identifiers exist, can provide linked data that provide a much richer picture of the individual's health. For example, a nurse may use helpline "reasons for call" data in conjunction with primary care, emergency department management systems, and pharmacy and hospital surveillance data, complemented by Google Flu and laboratory data for a clearer infectious disease surveillance picture. Creating a real-time dashboard fusing these data sources can provide a more complete picture of the individual's health status and help monitor the overall health system. This will also provide public health decision-makers with an overall view of health system activity and synergistic data elements for disease detection. Each data element complements the next and predicts overall health system activity.

A real-life example of using EHR data to improve individual health is that of a parent who calls a nurse helpline. The parent calls the helpline for a child's respiratory infection and is referred to a primary care provider. The child is seen and considered to be ill, and the provider refers the child to a local emergency department, where a viral respiratory swab is taken. The laboratory result is positive for influenza A. All of these data elements may be used in a proactive or reactive surveillance system.

These integrated models help to detect outbreaks of respiratory infection in the community, which is important from a public health perspective, but these data also can provide health system management. This approach can improve the surveillance system's sustainability, as it also is important for system management. Additionally, it is more cost-effective and efficient to integrate these functions. Legislation is needed to address data elements and privacy concerns for data access and monitoring.

Once the right comprehensive data sets are available in real time, more sophisticated predictive modeling can be incorporated. **Predictive modeling** is a name given to a collection of mathematical techniques having in common the goal of finding a mathematical relationship between a target, response, or "dependent" variable and various predictor or "independent" variables with the goal in mind of measuring future values of those predictors and inserting them into the mathematical relationship to predict future values of the target variable.[18] Retrospective validation with historical data can be performed to look at the correlation of various data sets and their predictive capacity. Their reliability can then be prospectively validated and improved. Due to the annual epidemic of influenza and its year-to-year variability, this is the best infectious disease for testing system outbreak detection and predictive capacity.

GOALS TO ACHIEVE

- Short-term:
  - Increase effective use of EHRs in practice with data quality and discipline among users. Health care professionals should use the EHR in the same consistent manner so that essential data elements are properly coded. Many EHR systems have back-end coding systems that are very primitive, and physicians are not interested in coding. Therefore, EHR vendors will have to improve disease-coding algorithms using coding systems such as SNOMED CT or ICD-10-CM.
  - Ensure consistency and standardization of case and syndromic definitions for public health purposes. Notably, develop standardized syndromes for infectious and chronic diseases for acute care surveillance.
  - Develop tools, metrics and outcomes that provide practitioners with information about their care of individual patients and practice population to enhance practice and that enable the continuous quality improvement of initiatives.
  - Develop methods for routine data linkage that comply with privacy legislation and provide timely information for public health surveillance.
  - Develop appropriate and tailored spatial and temporal detection tools.
- Mid-term:
  - Review pertinent privacy laws to ensure ongoing sustained data access and the ability to link data longitudinally.
  - Build partnerships for data sharing and a secure, dependable means for ongoing data transmission.
  - Develop an ongoing, reliable, and validated review process for syndrome and diagnostic coding methodologies and data classification methods.
  - Customize spatial and temporal anomaly detection methods for each data stream.
- Long-term:
  - Validate reliable real-time electronic data sources that enable analysis and prospective modeling. Integrate these data into a meaningful, comprehensive, functional, and easily understood dashboard for decision-makers.
  - Foster legislation and privacy protection to allow data sharing among health system partners to better protect the public's health and manage the health system.

- Develop analytic predictive tools for areas such as health system utilization beyond outbreak detection methods, pharmacosurveillance, and assessment of risk factors in chronic disease development.
- Expand the system to include monitoring of the health of the population during extreme weather events, detection and monitoring of terrorist events, and overall emergency preparedness.

These goals are ambitious and they require commitment and investment in software development and infrastructure from both the public and private sectors in order to be accomplished. An early need will be to incorporate an evaluation framework for active surveillance systems to be able to show improved population health outcomes and economic value. These approaches may also result in sharing data across jurisdictions and organizations, which is privacy sensitive, and for both the public and privacy commissioners, appropriate safeguards must be in place that will insure minimal risk of a privacy breach.

CURRENT BEST PRACTICES

Surveillance Using EHR Data

The promise of using EHR data for Meaningful Use (MU) and public health purposes is emerging slowly as EHR use by physicians expands in clinical care.[19] MU programs exist in some jurisdictions to incentivize the use of the EHRs to achieve core patient based objectives. The use of EHR data for acute infectious and chronic disease surveillance is described below.

The **Canadian Primary Care Sentinel Surveillance Network** (CPCSSN), established in 2008 with funding from the Public Health Agency of Canada, is a primary care research initiative, which is the first pan-Canadian multi-disease electronic medical record surveillance system.[20] They collect health information from electronic medical records in the offices of participating primary care providers.[7] CPCSSN merges data from primary care practices in 10 practice-based research networks across Canada. Currently about 650 primary care practitioners contribute de-identified patient health data on 850,000 patients. These data are extracted quarterly from the electronic medical records of participating primary care practices; cleaned, coded, and stored in a secure data repository. The eight chronic diseases that are monitored currently by CPCSSN are diabetes, hypertension, epilepsy, dementia, depression, chronic obstructive pulmonary disease (COPD), osteoarthritis, and Parkinsonism. Case definitions have been validated for all of these conditions.[21,22] CPCSSN collects information related to each patient's encounter with the practice, health conditions, risk factors, referrals, laboratory investigations, procedures, medications, and physiological data such as height and weight. The regular extraction of these data allows for timely reporting on trends in individual and population risk factors, the development of chronic diseases, and changes in chronic disease management.

Others have also developed innovative ways of using EHRs for public health surveillance. Klompas and colleagues[23] have developed an Electronic Medical Record Support for Public Health Surveillance (ESP) that uses electronic patient data from large multispecialty practices in several states in the USA to provide surveillance information on infectious diseases and diabetes. The ESP system has been used to identify and electronically report patients with notifiable diseases such as Lyme, active versus latent tuberculosis, and hepatitis. The system has been expanded to include methods to monitor diabetes incidence, prevalence, and complications in a specific patient population. The system potentially identifies health disparities and opportunities for intervention.

EHR data can also be used for pharmacosurveillance. **Pharmacosurveillance** is a term to refer to the monitoring of drug safety, for example, by means of spontaneous adverse-effect reporting systems, case–control, and cohort studies.[24] The Mini-Sentinel system in the USA, as described by Behrman and her colleagues,[25] is a system that provides tools for individual health plans to analyze patient data related to the safety of approved medical products. This system allows each health plan organization to remain in control of their patient data and transmit only aggregate data to the Federal Drug Agency to answer specific questions about a particular set of medical products. Data from millions of patients, not previously available, are analyzed to look for potential adverse effects of medical products.

Syndromic Surveillance

Syndromic surveillance has been previously discussed in Chapter 3. It is an important component of reactive and proactive surveillance. The following is an example of this approach.

Example of Syndromic Surveillance

Since 2005, KFL&A Public Health, located in Kingston, Ontario, Canada, has operated an acute care enhanced surveillance system (ACES) on behalf of the province of Ontario.[26] ACES uses real-time or near real-time emergency department and hospital admission data to detect potential threats to public health and health system utilization patterns. Advanced natural language processing algorithms are used to reduce free-text chief complaints, entered by emergency department triage nurses, into a series of discrete syndromes. The admission diagnosis is used to monitor inpatient patterns by syndrome relevant to inpatient utilization. Admission diagnoses are also grouped into syndromes of interest from a public health perspective, such as pneumonia, meningitis and encephalitis, trauma, and sepsis. Time–space series aberration detection methods are continuously run to test for current emergency room visit volumes that are statistically in excess of an expected number of visits, given each hospital's historical emergency department visit and admission patterns. When an excess volume of visits is detected overall or for a particular syndrome, alerts are automatically generated, notifying local epidemiologists in the associated health unit for further investigation. Data integrated into this system include absenteeism from large health system employers, mortality data from municipal registries, and local viral and bacterial laboratory data.

Another example of a syndromic surveillance system is the Electronic Surveillance System for the Early Notification of Community-based Epidemics (ESSENCE), which was originally developed for the US military and then adapted to provide early warning of abnormal health conditions in the National Capital Area of the USA.[27,28] It is now used by numerous state public health agencies. The system combines clinical data (e.g., emergency room syndromes, private practice billing codes grouped into syndromes, and veterinary syndromes) and nonclinical data (e.g., absenteeism, nurse hotline calls, prescription medications, and over-the-counter medications). Both temporal and spatial-temporal algorithms are used by the system, including autoregressive modeling looking for differences between expected and predicted counts, exponentially weighted moving average, and a variant of the scan statistic that includes multiple data sources.

Google Flu Trends is a web service operated by Google that provides near real-time estimates of flu activity for a number of countries and regions around the world, based on aggregated search queries.[29] Some of these estimates have been validated through comparison with official historic influenza data from the relevant country or region.[29] This analysis is available for over 25 countries.[30] The analysis is timely and has been shown to predict regional outbreaks 10 days before they are reported by the US Centers for Disease Control and Prevention using passive data system and analysis.[6] The data and analysis are updated daily, whereas most health agencies update their analyses weekly, based on week-old data. This system can be characterized as a reactive surveillance system; however, in the future, modeling and prediction could be also incorporated to serve as a proactive surveillance system. However, it is necessary to continuously modify, customize, and validate the algorithms used by this system. As Cook and her colleagues[31] have demonstrated, internet search behavior changed during the H1N1 pandemic, limiting the effectiveness of Google Flu Trends; Olson and colleagues[32] also have noted that flaws within the models have misrepresented historical influenza seasons.

Methods in Air Quality Health Monitoring

A current example of proactive surveillance is monitoring particulate matter of 2.5 micrometers size (PM 2.5) released from burning fossil fuels from transportation, industry, electricity generation, or forest fires.[33] There is a direct, linear, and causal relationship between this exposure, exacerbations of asthma and COPD, and an increased risk of cardiovascular illness.[34] The PM 2.5 level can be monitored via a distributed sensor system or through satellite imaging using a measurement called aerosol optical depth, which relates to the amount of aerosol particles in the air between the ground and the satellite. These systems can also predict the movement of the particulate matter in the atmosphere given current wind and weather patterns.

Modeling air movement allows officials to issue potential warnings for vulnerable populations under this airshed distribution and to implement interventions to minimize exposure. For example, in the event of a forest fire, public health officials may monitor particulate matter and air movement and enact interventions if a certain threshold is reached. Interventions may include evacuating vulnerable populations, maximizing medication to stabilize preexisting medical conditions before exposure occurs, or providing high-efficiency particulate air filters to at-risk homes.

Affected populations can be monitored on an ongoing basis through real-time acute care sector surveillance for diseases related to the respiratory track or cardiovascular disease. This monitoring can also be used on a population level to monitor the effectiveness of implemented interventions and for spatial correlation analysis.

Air quality health index (AQHI) systems are another proactive surveillance method used in population health to predict health impacts of increasing pollutants in the air. This system monitors data more locally from the ground level.[13] The AQHI is calculated on the basis of the relative risks of a combination of common air pollutants known to harm human health detected at a local level, mainly urban settings in Canada. These data are provided to the public through a web portal and through community partners, much like the weather is reported, and use a numbered scale from 1 to 10.

The AQHI is designed to provide an air quality rating, a category to describe the level of health risk associated with the index, and health messages for the general and at-risk populations, such as suggestions on how individuals can adjust activity levels depending on their health risk from air pollution. The system is mainly targeted at minimizing the acute impacts of specific air pollutants in at-risk populations. It was created on the basis of retrospective statistical relationships between air pollution and mortality. The system is a significant improvement over air quality monitoring, as it correlates with health events. The AQHI has the necessary infrastructure to proactively inform populations at risk.[13,34]

METHODS ANOMALY DETECTION TOOLS

Once electronic data sets are reliable, available in real time, and validated, then appropriately tailored anomaly detection tools can be created. These need to be customized for each data set and updated regularly.[32] Any modification of the data stream or addition of hospitals data sets needs revalidation and an assessment of representativeness. Hospitals in different jurisdictions, whether rural or urban, have different health system utilization patterns that need to be taken into consideration during anomaly detection and when setting baseline alerts. These quality assurance processes need to be incorporated into these systems in an ongoing systematic basis. This will allow for the potential transition from passive to active surveillance systems with proactive-predictive capacity. Analytical toolkits used in many real-time surveillance systems currently include standard techniques such as cumulative sum methods, moving window approaches (e.g., exponentially weighted moving averages) and spatial scan statistics (e.g., SatScan, www.satscan.org), Poisson regression modeling, and other basic anomaly detection methods. Multiple methods are often used within one system to detect slow- versus fast-moving health events. Recent and more advanced methods include multiresolution spatial cluster detection, arbitrarily shaped spatial clusters, tests for space–time clustering, and more recent techniques in time series wavelets.

In public health surveillance, often spatial clustering of anomalous events and time series aberration techniques fail to detect interesting and potentially informative anomalies. For example, time series aberration techniques may mask truly anomalous events if the geographic scale is too large, resulting in missing a localized event. Conversely, purely spatial techniques over too long or too short a time window can mask potentially important time series anomalies. An accepted approach to public health surveillance anomaly detection is predicated on a rigorous examination of three approaches: (1) those that are purely temporal; (2) those that are purely spatial; and (3) those that detect spatiotemporal anomalies. Each anomaly detection method must be tailored for each data set, to ensure appropriate detection of signal from noise, and then investigated and verified by a person familiar with the data and their limitations and strengths. Thus, a system requires a team-based approach where epidemiologists and public health responders work directly with the spatial and temporal anomaly detection experts to ensure that there is a common understanding of the strengths, weaknesses, and limitation of the automated system. All data elements should be easily visualized through epidemic curves or maps to enable human decision-making and to allow for the visualization of multiple complementary data sets to improve situational awareness and cross validation.

Evaluation of all methods on known historical data is helpful, but using recent outbreaks with gold standard level data is essential. Gold standard data examples may include confirmed laboratory testing, diagnostic imaging, or physician diagnosis. The work by Olson and colleagues[32] on evaluating Google Flu Trends emphasizes that all anomaly detection methods require continued model fitting and ongoing evaluation, refinement, and improvement.

Active surveillance systems require customized temporal and spatial detections methods for each syndrome irrespective of whether they are infectious or noninfectious. An understanding of the epidemiology of the disease process will inform this work. Hence, the need for a team-based approach with input from medical, epidemiological, statistical, and spatial experts to ensure that the system detects aberrations appropriately. All systems will require ongoing monitoring of the data by experts familiar with the systems and data sources independent of the alerts as a safety measure.

KEY SUMMARY POINTS

- Electronic health records have created the possibility for improved public health surveillance to become an active process with both reactive and proactive approaches. Public health does not need to depend on passive surveillance systems through traditional reportable disease data sources.
- Automated alerts are the key feature of both reactive and proactive surveillance systems. Alerts initiate event investigation by public health practitioners in reactive systems, while the alerts trigger and refine forecasting in proactive systems.
- Improving reactive and proactive surveillance systems in innovative ways, such as pharmacosurveillance, should be a priority for the public and private sectors.
- Predictive modeling helps with health system planning and encourages health promotion and prevention strategies.
- Appropriate legislative and privacy frameworks need to be in place when using EHRs.
- Efforts to continue EHR adoption across the health system is vital and should concentrate on ensuring high-quality data through the use of international standards and data consistency among users.
- Internet and social media data are potential sources of surveillance data to provide a comprehensive image of the population's health and health system utilization.
- Developing a dashboard for decision-makers to merge analysis and modeling can manage complex and varying multisourced data streams long term.
- For anomaly detection, there is a need to contextualize each data source for spatial and temporal detection of anomalies. There needs to be a process for interpretation and verification of the syndrome alerts.

DISCUSSION QUESTIONS

1. What are potential advantages and disadvantages for clinical practices to provide real-time clinical data for public health surveillance? How can public health, governmental, and societal support be developed for these systems?
2. Given the global transmission of diseases, how can these less traditional types of surveillance affect international disease patterns?
3. What public health infrastructure is necessary to respond to events identified by the types of surveillance systems described in this chapter?
4. What are some innovative uses of electronic health records?
5. In systems that automatically detect potential public health events and threats, to what extent should thresholds be set to increase sensitivity at the risk of missing events?
6. How do we properly use internet and social media data, given changing utilization, query patterns, and possible influence by media, marketing, and entrepreneurial forces?
7. Provide examples of appropriate circumstances for both passive and active surveillance.

REFERENCES

1. Rosenau MJ, Maxcy KF, Last JM. Public health and preventive medicine. 12th ed. Norwalk, Conn: Appleton-Century-Crofts; 1986.
2. Squires S, Winchester B, Zabchuk P, Li Y, Vanderkloot M, Tam T, et al. Respiratory virus surveillance FluWatch Project. Can Commun Dis Rep 2000;26(6):45–7.
3. Ontario CC. Ontario Cancer Registry, 2012, <https://http://www.cancercare.on.ca/ocs/csurv/stats/ocr/>; 2013.
4. van Dijk A, Aramini J, Edge G, Moore K. Real-time surveillance for respiratory disease outbreaks, Ontario, Canada. Emerg Infect Dis 2009;15(5):799–801.
5. Heffernan R, Mostashari F, Das D, Kulldorff M, Weiss D. Syndromic surveillance in public health practice, New York City. Emerg Infect Dis 2004;10(5):858–64.
6. Carneiro HA, Mylonakis E. Google trends: a web-based tool for real-time surveillance of disease outbreaks. Clin Infect Dis 2009;49(10):1557–64.
7. Birtwhistle R, Keshavjee K, Lambert-Lanning A, Godwin M, Greiver M, Manca D, et al. Building a pan-Canadian primary care sentinel surveillance network: initial development and moving forward. J Am Board Fam Med 2009;22(4):412–22.
8. KFLA. ILI Mapper, <http://www.kflaphi.ca/ILI-Mapper/>; 2014.
9. Masotti P, Green ME, Birtwhistle R, Gemmill I, Moore K, O'Connor K, et al. pH1N1 - a comparative analysis of public health responses in Ontario to the influenza outbreak, public health and primary care: lessons learned and policy suggestions. BMC Public Health 2013;13(1):687.
10. Hall GG, Perry AG, VanDijk A, Moore KM. Influenza assessment centres: a case study of pandemic preparedness to alleviate excess emergency department volume. CJEM 2013;15(4):198–205.
11. Hay SI, George DB, Moyes CL, Brownstein JS. Big data opportunities for global infectious disease surveillance. PLoS Med 2013;10(4):e1001413.
12. Harpaz R, DuMouchel W, LePendu P, Bauer-Mehren A, Ryan P, Shah NH. Performance of pharmacovigilance signal-detection algorithms for the FDA adverse event reporting system. Clin Pharmacol Ther 2013;93(6):539–546.
13. Stieb DM, Burnett RT, Smith-Doiron M, Brion O, Shin HH, Economou V. A new multipollutant, no-threshold air quality health index based on short-term associations observed in daily time-series analyses. J Air Waste Manag Assoc 2008;58(3):435–50.
14. Pampalon R, Hamel D, Gamache P, Philibert MD, Raymond G, Simpson A. An area-based material and social deprivation index for public health in Québec and Canada. Can J Public Health 2012;103(8 Suppl. 2):S17–22.
15. Brownstein JS, Freifeld CC, Madoff LC. Digital disease detection—harnessing the Web for public health surveillance. N Engl J Med 2009;360(21):2153–5, 2157.
16. Eysenbach G. Infodemiology and infoveillance: framework for an emerging set of public health informatics methods to analyze search, communication and publication behavior on the Internet. J Med Internet Res 2009;11(1):e11.
17. Pacala JT, Boult C, Boult L. Predictive validity of a questionnaire that identifies older persons at risk for hospital admission. J Am Geriatr Soc 1995;43(4):374–77.
18. Dickey DA. Introduction to Predictive Modeling with Examples. Proceedings of 2012 SAS Global Forum, paper 337.
19. Blumenthal D, Tavenner M. The "meaningful use" regulation for electronic health records. N Engl J Med 2010;363(6):501–4.
20. Canadian Primary Care Sentinel Surveillance Network About CPCSSN, <http://cpcssn.ca/about-cpcssn/>; 2015.
21. Kadhim-Saleh A, Green M, Williamson T, Hunter D, Birtwhistle R. Validation of the diagnostic algorithms for 5 chronic conditions in the Canadian Primary Care Sentinel Surveillance Network (CPCSSN): a Kingston Practice-based Research Network (PBRN) report. J Am Board Fam Med 2013;26(2):159–67.
22. Williamson T, Green ME, Birtwhistle R, Khan S, Garies S, Wong ST, et al. Validating the 8 CPCSSN case definitions for chronic disease surveillance in a primary care database of electronic health records. Ann Fam Med 2014;12(4):367–72.
23. Klompas M, Murphy M, Lankiewicz J, McVetta J, Lazarus R, Eggleston E, et al. Harnessing electronic health records for public health surveillance. Online J Public Health Inform 2011;3(3).
24. World Health Organization. Introduction to Drug Utilization Research. Geneva;2003. p. 48.
25. Behrman RE, Benner JS, Brown JS, McClellan M, Woodcock J, Platt R. Developing the Sentinel System—a national resource for evidence development. N Engl J Med 2011;364(6):498–9.
26. Moore KM, Edgar BL, McGuinness D. Implementation of an automated, real-time public health surveillance system linking emergency departments and health units: rationale and methodology. CJEM 2008;10(2):114–9.
27. Lombardo J, Burkom H, Elbert E, Magruder S, Lewis SH, Loschen W, http://www.ncbi.nlm.nih.gov/pubmed/?term=Sari J%5BAuthor%5D&cauthor=true&cauthor_uid=12791777 et al. A systems overview of the Electronic Surveillance System for the Early Notification of Community-Based Epidemics (ESSENCE II). J Urban Health 2003;80(2 Suppl. 1):i32–42.
28. Lombardo JS, Burkom H, Pavlin J. ESSENCE II and the framework for evaluating syndromic surveillance systems. MMWR Morb Mortal Wkly Rep 2004;53(Suppl):159–65.
29. Google Flu Trends FAQ, <http://www.google.org/flutrends/about/faq.html/>; 2015.
30. Google Flu Trends, <http://www.google.org/flutrends/about/faq.html/>; 2011, [2013].
31. Cook S, Conrad C, Fowlkes AL, Mohebbi MH. Assessing Google flu trends performance in the United States during the 2009 influenza virus A (H1N1) pandemic. PLoS One 2011;6(8):e23610.
32. Olson DR, Konty KJ, Paladini M, Viboud C, Simonsen L. Reassessing Google Flu Trends data for detection of seasonal and pandemic influenza: a comparative epidemiological study at three geographic scales. PLoS Comput Biol 2013;9(10):e1003256.
33. Rappold AG, Stone SL, Cascio WE, Neas LM, Kilaru VJ, Carraway MS, http://www.ncbi.nlm.nih.gov/pubmed/?term=Szykman JJ%5BAuthor%5D&cauthor=true&cauthor_uid=21705297 et al. Peat bog wildfire smoke exposure in rural North Carolina is associated with cardiopulmonary emergency department visits assessed through syndromic surveillance. Environ Health Perspect 2011;119(10):1415–20.
34. To T, Shen S, Atenafu EG, Guan J, McLimont S, Stocks B, et al. The air quality health index and asthma morbidity: a population-based study. Environ Health Perspect 2013;121(1):46–52.

CHAPTER

6

New Public Health Surveillance Evaluation Model

Ngozi Erondu

As the importance of health in the global agenda grows, so does the responsibility to measure accurately its complex dimensions and to assess the effects of increasing investments on population health. The present burst of political and financial will to improve global health has to be matched by an adequate response from the community of experts in constructing a firm foundation of metrics and evaluation.

Dr Christopher JL Murray

KEY WORDS

Surveillance system evaluation
Triggers
Data quality monitoring
ECDC
The European Surveillance System (TESSy)

WHY WE NEED TO EXAMINE THE PROCESSES OF PUBLIC HEALTH SURVEILLANCE

Public health surveillance is a multitiered system that relies on a network of health system players to fulfill core surveillance functions (detect, confirm, notify, respond[1]) in order to produce useful data to guide decision-making in nearly every disease program. This system is inherently fragile; if any one step is not accomplished, or if the entire process is not properly resourced and maintained, the surveillance system will diminish.[2] Globally, communicable disease detection is conducted at the local or peripheral level, which is the patient's first point of contact with the public health system. To successfully monitor priority diseases, each person who exhibits clinical symptoms meeting the case definition for a priority or reportable disease must first be diagnosed by a clinician and then reported to the appropriate public health authority. Furthermore, at this first point of contact, the provider must adequately collect and send the necessary specimens (e.g., blood samples for suspected measles or stool samples for suspected poliomyelitis) to the laboratory for analysis and confirmation of the disease agent (e.g., bacteria strain or virus type). Several presuppositions underlie this process:

(1) There are policies in place that establish national priority and reportable diseases.
(2) There are enough health workers at the local health facilities to adequately serve the population.
(3) These health workers are aware of national reportable and priority diseases and are able to identify each disease based on standard case definitions.
(4) There are appropriate tools and mechanisms to register and report suspected cases of notifiable diseases.
(5) Health workers have been trained to collect appropriate specimens for laboratory analysis.
(6) There are materials and mechanisms in place to store and send the specimens to a diagnostic laboratory.

(7) There is an accessible diagnostic laboratory equipped to analyze the specimens and confirm the presence of disease.

The tasks in this list formulate various public health surveillance work processes needed to operate a disease surveillance system. Additionally, there are several inputs that must be identified in order for these tasks to occur, including human and financial resources. These inputs will change depending on work tasks and must be thoughtfully identified and considered to ensure that the system is able to meet the needs of the population. This process–task–input relationship is the substructure of all health systems and should be analyzed at all administrative and jurisdictional levels.

This chapter examines how communicable disease surveillance systems (CDSS) are currently evaluated through two angles: first, by presenting traditional evaluation methods to understand what one should look for when planning to evaluate a surveillance system, and second, by proposing a new process-focused surveillance evaluation framework for improving public health practice performance. A practical application of this framework is presented at the end of the chapter through a case study of developing an evaluation plan for a meningitis disease surveillance system in Chad. Further steps on how to conduct an evaluation of a surveillance system are detailed in Chapter 7.

THE PROCESS–TASK–INPUT RELATIONSHIP

All levels of the health system, from high-level policy to the health practitioner, contribute toward successfully implementing the surveillance system. Therefore, it is vital to understand the different players and their roles. The astute practitioner is key for timely detection of reportable diseases. Laboratory confirmation is also necessary to identify pathogens, develop vaccines, and rapidly respond to an outbreak and prevent further transmission.

Fig. 6-1 illustrates the process–task–input relationship by examining the process "complete high school." In this example, this is just one process of many needed to qualify for a specific occupation. A process, which in this example is "*complete high school*," is a high-level activity that must be achieved. It is then disaggregated into discrete work tasks. Tasks are chronological steps needed to fulfill the attribute listed. This example demonstrates a set of activities, 2a and 2b, which are separate tasks but can be performed concurrently. Finally, the inputs needed to complete each task are identified. Inputs are composed of associated costs for human labor, materials, and other items needed to fulfill a task.

The interdependent work processes of surveillance can be achieved through adequate financial resources and a skilled workforce. Such a system is vulnerable because the entire process could be obstructed by a "weak link" or an

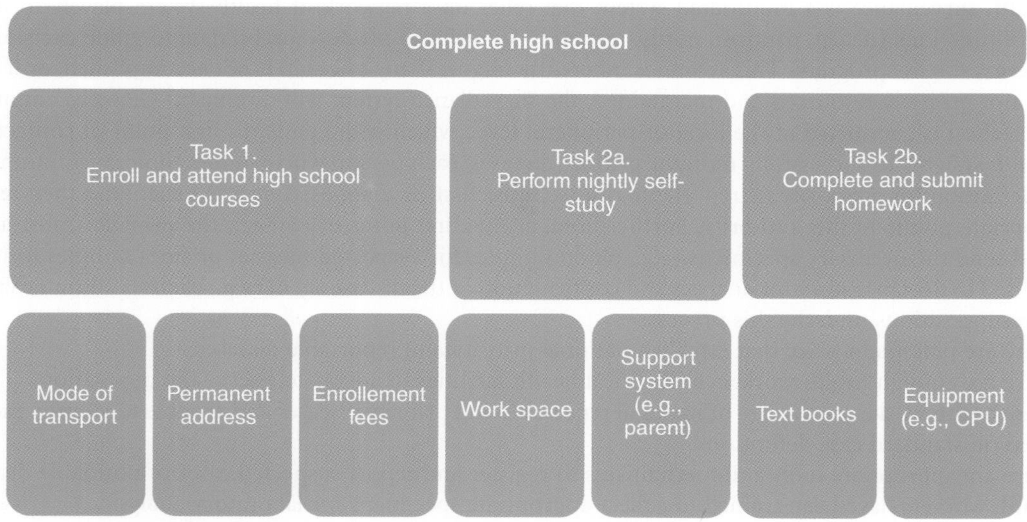

FIG. 6-1 Process–task–input relationship for completing high school.

outright gap. Comprehensive budget development and program planning for surveillance can decrease the probability of failure in any of these processes by supporting and increasing opportunities to prevent or respond quickly to public health threats. A strong public health surveillance system (PHSS) serves as an early warning and alert system to detect disease outbreaks and inform appropriate response measures[3]; conversely, a weak system can obstruct this process and negatively impact a population with a high disease burden, long-term sequelae, or even preventable deaths. Surveillance systems can be strengthened by program planning that understands the work processes needed to run the system and that provides adequate resources to fill system gaps and support surveillance practitioners. Program evaluation is a method to identify and assess system gaps. Several evaluations have been conducted on PHSS and their findings provide some insight on how to assess work processes for improved system performance.

REVIEW OF COMMUNICABLE DISEASE SURVEILLANCE SYSTEM EVALUATIONS

Looking for gaps in a surveillance system goes beyond comparing a standard set of surveillance processes to the specific system being examined. A structured and purposeful evaluation study can be used to understand the input constitution of unique systems (as described in Chapter 7).

Surveillance system evaluations are essential to developing program budgets and identifying the processes that must be supported for effective surveillance. Certain work processes are repeated for every disease program, and surveillance systems can benefit greatly from consolidating repeated tasks into discrete program components that are easier to manage. For example, in a country where priority diseases include bacterial meningitis, acute flaccid paralysis, yellow fever, and measles, surveillance staff can be taught to collect routine data for all four diseases using one data collection form instead of four separate forms. This creates efficiencies in reporting data. In this example, efficiency can be defined by the quantity of inputs needed to perform the work process of disease reporting.

Combining the work tasks of several diseases also results in conducting one training for priority disease detection and reporting versus several disease-specific trainings. Moreover, one data manager can be hired to analyze reportable diseases from one form as opposed to several data managers for each disease program. This type of task sharing and application of establishing surveillance cross-cutting services is known as *integrated surveillance* and contrasts the more widely used vertical disease surveillance (see Chapter 4 for a detailed discussion on vertical and integrated surveillance systems). Evaluating a surveillance system by examining work processes and potential overlaps can highlight areas of sensible input investment for each task. In order to understand the work processes, this chapter now turns to understanding how evaluations identify and describe gaps in the surveillance system.

Since 1988, the year US Centers for Disease Control and Prevention (CDC) first published *Guidelines for Evaluating Surveillance Systems,*[4] there have been several evaluations specifically examining CDSS. Twenty-one evaluations have been identified in the published and available literature that provide information about CDSS work processes and gaps.

Most of these evaluation studies organized evaluation questions and indicators around specific system attributes or by categorized activities. Depending on the disease, governmental structure, or even political system, certain system evaluation methods are more applicable than others in a specific country. For example, half of the developing economy country studies evaluated their systems through the organization of core activities and support functions, while none of the high-income counties assessed their systems this way. Understanding the circumstances of a country is the first step in ascertaining the system processes.

While no surveillance system can operate without financial input, most studies do not assess resource allocation or any cost component. However, related surveillance costs are mentioned in two studies. Wuhib et al.[5] did not collect data on any surveillance-associated costs but described observed factors that influenced costs, such as paper-driven reporting, lack of allocated funding, and use of human resources for outbreak investigations. Carrieri et al.[6] included a brief summary about ad hoc resources acquired to support a newly implemented computerized surveillance network for communicable diseases in Italy. Neither of these studies obtained actual costs or made any evidence-based conclusions as to the systems' cost-effectiveness. Fig. 6-2 illustrates the number of studies that used each methodology.

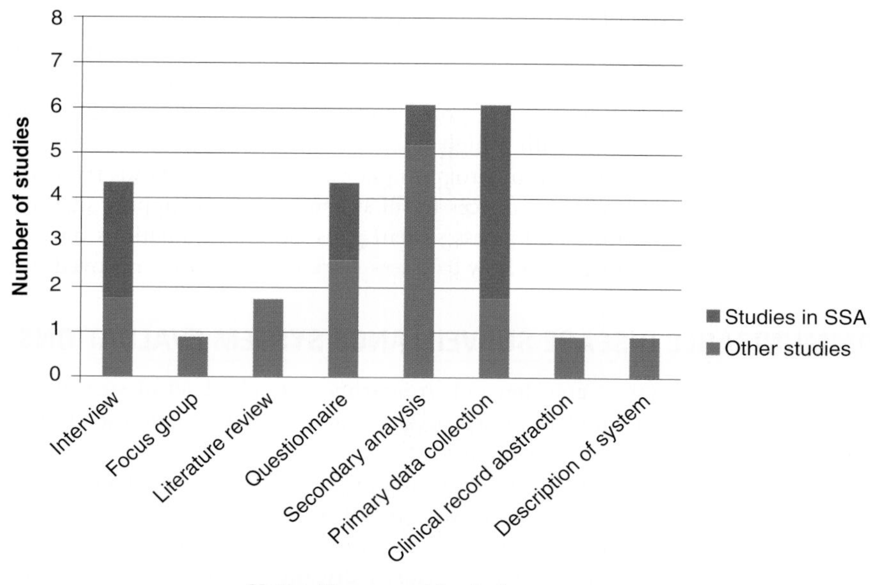

FIG. 6-2 Type and frequency of methods used for the CDSS evaluation literature review.

Several factors are identified as having a direct or indirect impact on CDSS performance. Many studies cite lack of standardized procedures or case definitions as a limiting factor for accurate case detection. Several studies list lack of clinician reporting as a major factor affecting CDSS performance, though the reason for this differed across studies. Lack of regular supervisor feedback was frequently mentioned as a cause of low motivation among health staff to fully participate in surveillance activities. This factor was often stated as essential, with one study concluding that feedback is one of the most important tools to develop health workers' skills and improve performance.[7] In studies conducted in sub-Saharan Africa, the factors affecting case detection included level of community involvement, training of subnational health levels on integrated disease surveillance and response (IDSR), strength of clinical and laboratory network, and need for clear disease system objectives.[7-11]

Limitations of Current Communicable Disease Surveillance System Evaluations

Reviewing these studies illuminates CDSS evaluation methods and factors affecting surveillance performance. The way these methods are incorporated into evaluation plans is highly dependent on understanding how the PHSS operates in a specific country. These studies highlighted the major factors in surveillance performance, including timely feedback, regular supervision, perceived complexity of case definition, and attitudes about reporting. These factors are directly linked to program planning and a high-level commitment to the surveillance system effectiveness. It is important to point out that none of the studies cite operational or environmental factors (e.g., "condition of roads" or "data transmission method") as direct or indirect factors affecting CDSS performance. Finally, while many of the studies mention the need for support or reinforcement of skills, capabilities, or human resources, none undertakes a detailed assessment or review of CDSS costs. These omissions are important to underscore as they influence public health budget development and program planning. Understanding the direct and indirect factors impacting surveillance systems is integral to process mapping. When funding is allocated for disease-specific surveillance, gaps between these vertical systems impede overall performance.

These studies benefit from existing frameworks that provide general descriptions, definitions, and other important guidance about what functioning CDSS should achieve.[3, 12, 13] While overall system performance is important, other information, such as program integration and collaboration, program planning priorities, costs, and specific training needs, are difficult to ascertain with this traditional evaluation perspective.

INTRODUCING THE WORK PROCESS ANALYSIS FRAMEWORK TO EVALUATE SURVEILLANCE SYSTEMS

The work process analysis (WPA) framework for public health performance builds on the structural parameters provided by past CDSS evaluations and existing frameworks by examining public health practice processes and causal effects. The **WPA framework** is a methodological framework for evaluating and improving public health practice performance by identifying existing and missing processes and determining causal effects.[14]

In contrast to the information provided by the traditional evaluation methods reviewed above, the WPA aims to collect and assess additional information that directly impacts the surveillance practitioner and consequently affects surveillance performance.

The WPA framework's objective is to define and assess discrete public health processes by linking work tasks to program indicators and outcomes. Assessing discrete tasks allows for a more granular understanding of work processes throughout the administrative levels of the public health system. This novel framework provides results that better inform public health program management and generate cost estimates to inform prioritization of surveillance activities.

The WPA consists of the following tools:

- Logic model: A **logic model** frame is used to separate surveillance components into individual program and evaluation elements, including inputs, outputs, intermediate outcomes, and long-term outcomes. The logic model is also a yardstick for ideal implementation of the surveillance system and depicts the standard system components identified by authoritative sources (e.g., World Health Organization, CDC).[14]
- Comprehensive performance indicators: **Performance indicators** are items of information collected at regular intervals to track the performance of a system.[15] Indicators that assess surveillance performance should include international, national, and disease-specific measures. The indicators can be used to develop complementary evaluation tools, such as interview questions and study questionnaires, data abstraction forms, and checklists.
- Work process tree: A **work process tree** is a diagram that incorporates work processes identified through the established guidance and evaluation data collected from system stakeholders. Work process trees are composed of sequential tasks needed to complete a given surveillance activity and inform graphical representations that illustrate gaps in the surveillance system. This tool also provides the basis for inputs that can be used for an ingredient-style costing approach.[14]

Beyond understanding surveillance systems' performance, this approach to evaluating PHSS can provide decision-makers and program implementers with a complete strategic framework that identifies gaps in the system, estimates costs to calculate return on investment of proposed interventions (see Chapter 8), and lays out how to fill those gaps. Many countries can use the results of this evaluation to solicit donor funding to continue strengthening surveillance activities.

The following example illustrates the use of the WPA framework to develop an evaluation plan for a disease surveillance system (Fig. 6-3).

A Case Study to Demonstrate the Steps for Developing an Evaluation Plan for Meningitis Surveillance in Chad Using Work Process Analysis

Step 1. Describe Evaluation Purpose and Identify Stakeholders

Chad is a landlocked country in central Africa with an estimated population of 12.6 million.[16] According to the *Human Development Index*, Chad is currently listed as the fourth least developed country in the world.[17] For the last 25 years, meningitis outbreaks in Chad and other countries in the sub-Saharan Africa "meningitis belt" have been managed by using a polysaccharide vaccine that offered limited protection. A new meningococcal A conjugate vaccine, MenAfriVac (Serum Institute, India), was introduced in Chad in late 2011, and immunization campaigns were implemented for those aged 1–29 years.[18]

The introduction of MenAfriVac provides an opportunity to evaluate and strengthen meningitis surveillance in this region. MenAfriVac has been shown to reduce the rate of NmA meningococcal infection and induce herd immunity.[19] A more accurate and efficient surveillance system is needed to monitor possible epidemiologic shifts and measure the impact of the new vaccine.

Example of how to apply WPA Framework:

The WPA framework does not replace existing evaluation methods but supplements the traditional approach with tools that produce task-specific information. For example, rather than stopping at the evaluation finding: *clinician reporting is an obstacle to the surveillance system,* the WPA framework goes several steps further than traditional evaluations to understand the 'why' behind the finding.

Using a logic model, 'physician reporting' is divided into separate processes. Next, indicators are translated to work tasks and included in an evaluation questionnaire. A work process tree is used to assign inputs to each work task. One such task is *'physician sends weekly surveillance data to district level'*; an input needed for this task is *'internet access'*.

When the evaluation is conducted, physicians are then asked if they have access to the Internet. If the majority of the responses reveal Internet access is low or non-existent, public health program managers can develop a plan to fill this gap. The plan may be to advocate for funding to equip clinics with Internet or it may propose a different method to send weekly reports.

FIG. 6-3 Example of how to apply WPA framework.

Following a surveillance scale up in several districts to assess the effectiveness of the new vaccine,[19] the Chadian government, along with other countries in the meningitis belt, is considering how to implement a more sensitive meningitis surveillance system.[20] An evaluation study was authorized to help the primary stakeholders, the Chadian government and international funding partners, understand the current performance and cost of their meningitis surveillance system as well as the incremental costs needed to shift to a stronger system. The expected study results will equip policy makers and external stakeholders with information to determine the most feasible and effective meningitis surveillance strategy for Chad.

Step 2. Create an Evaluation Blueprint with a Logic Model and Indicators

Understanding the current meningitis surveillance guidance and how it is implemented in Chad was the starting point to create the evaluation plan. Conducting a literature review, like the one presented earlier in the chapter is highly valuable when beginning to construct an evaluation plan. To serve the Chadian context, existing national guidelines, policies, and regional guidance were included in the review. Additionally, local surveillance experts were consulted to detail the flow of epidemiologic and laboratory surveillance data, which is captured in Fig. 6-4. All of the information was then imported into a logic model framework, which aligns corresponding meningitis surveillance activities to outputs and outcomes. Indicators are concurrently identified through the literature and policy reviews. These indicators are mapped to the logic model and the evaluation blueprint is established. This logic model portrays the activities of the "ideal meningitis system for Chad," which follows established standards and policies for meningitis surveillance; it is used to reveal gaps in current system components (Fig. 6-5).

Step 3: Design Evaluation Study Using a Work Process Tree

The evaluation's primary focus is on surveillance activities at the subnational (i.e., health facility and district) level. This evaluation uses a descriptive, cross-sectional, and retrospective study design. The three objectives for this evaluation are (1) conduct a systematic evaluation and costing of the meningitis surveillance system; (2) apply the WPA framework to assess operational and financial gaps in the meningitis surveillance system; and (3) examine factors that influence surveillance performance. Table 6-1 lists the objectives and the evaluation questions developed to meet these objectives.

In order to fulfill the second objective, both existing meningitis surveillance strategies in Chad are included: enhanced surveillance, the baseline strategy that assesses population-based data from weekly aggregate reporting, and case based surveillance, which collects data on each suspected case at the individual level and links them to epidemiological and microbiological case data.

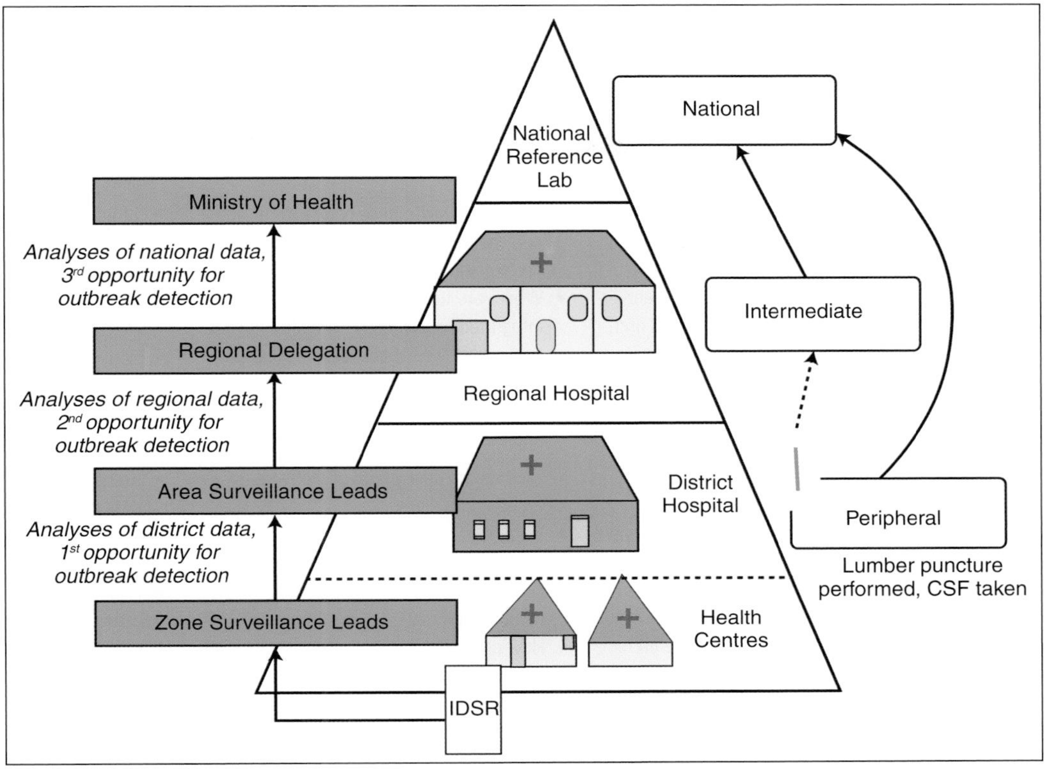

FIG. 6-4 Chadian meningitis surveillance system activities.

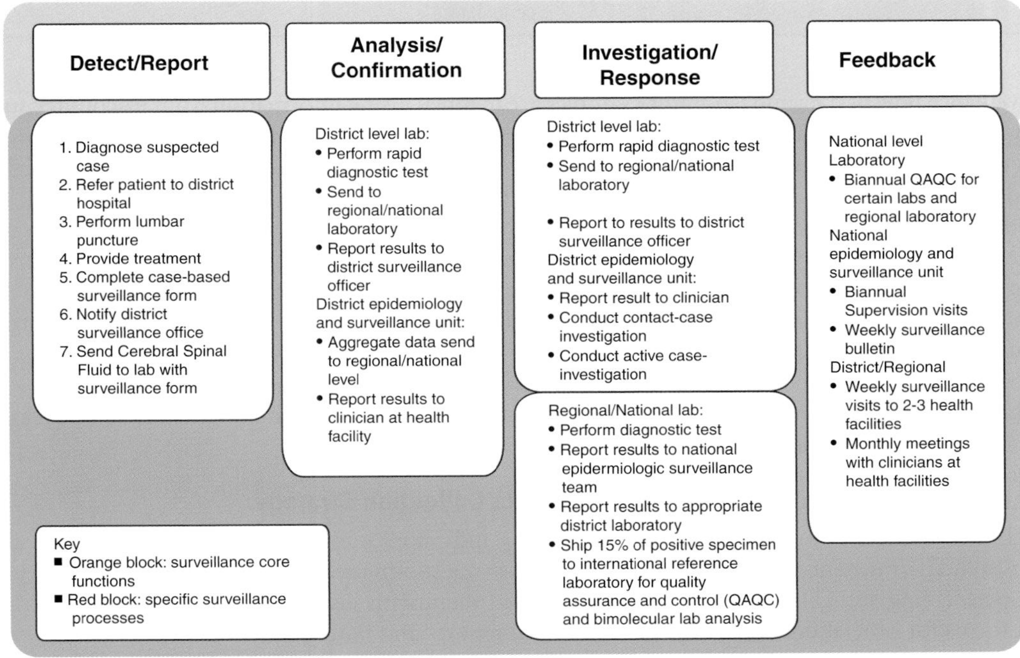

FIG. 6-5 Logic model of functional activities of meningitis surveillance in Chad.

TABLE 6-1 **Evaluation Objectives and Study Questions**

OBJECTIVE	SPECIFIC OBJECTIVE	EVALUATION QUESTION(S)	DATA COLLECTION METHOD(S)
1. **Apply WPA framework to assess operational and financial gaps in the meningitis surveillance system (MSS)**	a. Map meningitis surveillance components into logic model and work process tree framework b. Collect information about what is needed to achieve an optimal and feasible MSS in Chad c. Measure gap between current system and desired optimal and feasible MSS d. Assess areas for program integration opportunities	• What are the activities and costs to achieve an optimal and feasible MSS in Chad? • What is the difference between current and desired MSS in Chad, by cost and performance? • Where are the opportunities to strengthen integrated work processes with other vaccine preventable diseases surveillance? • What are the incremental costs of improving the current system to a desired optimal and feasible MSS?	• Literature review • Key informant interviews • Structured interviews
2. **Conduct a systematic evaluation and costing of the meningitis surveillance system**	a. Assess identified surveillance system attributes b. Assess core activities and support functions c. Measure performance of current system using identified indicators d. Explore relationships between performance and cost	• What is the description of the MSS in Chad? • What is the MSS performance of selected health facilities in Chad? • How much does surveillance costs by health facility? • How does cost impact performance?	• Review of surveillance data sources, reports, budgets, and related documents • Active case search • Structured interviews • Inventory of materials and supplies
3. **Examine the factors that influence surveillance performance**	a. Document factors observed at health facilities and attained through health staff interviews b. Compare funding factors across health facility	• What are the factors associated with low-, medium-, and high surveillance performance? • What factors impact surveillance and how? • How does funding affect surveillance performance?	• Observations • Key informant interviews

The surveillance flow of data and laboratory samples are mapped, using information from in-country surveillance players (Fig. 6-6). In-country surveillance experts provide the system flow that illustrates which work processes are assigned to each level of the public health system. Using a work process tree, necessary human and financial resources are mapped to each work task in the surveillance system. Once parallel players and tasks are identified, study participant and site selection criteria are defined. The study sites were selected through a consultation with in-country surveillance experts. For this evaluation, relevant study participants in each district include a district laboratory manager, at least one district surveillance officer, and one lead health personnel at each health facility. Additional identified actors germane to this evaluation include other government and nongovernmental players who participate in meningitis surveillance in Chad. Three criteria were defined for health facility selection:

(1) The health facility must be accessible to the evaluation team during the rainy season.
(2) The health facility must have had at least one suspected case of bacterial meningitis in the last year.
(3) Both rural and urban health facilities must be included.

Step 4: Develop Data Collection Instruments and Data Collection Strategy

Data collection instruments were developed by converting indicators into interview questions about surveillance program costs and performance (Figs. 6-6 and 6-7). Interview questionnaires also include data on resource quantities needed for performing surveillance functions per suspected meningitis case. Other cost data are included in data abstraction forms for official documents, such as financial reports and budgets.

Most of the quality indicators are based on the diagnostic outcome for a suspected case of meningitis. This process starts when a lumbar puncture (i.e., a spinal tap) is performed to retrieve cerebral spinal fluid (CSF), the biological specimen from which meningitis bacteria can be easily identified in laboratory diagnostic tests. Since meningitis surveillance relies heavily on the laboratory to correctly identify strain and serotype, laboratory materials, equipment, and corresponding human resources were considered in the evaluation plan. Data tools were developed to conduct inventories and capture costs associated with analysis of CSF for meningitis surveillance.

Resource provisions
- Human
- Consumables
- Capital
- Funds

Core surveillance functions
- Detection
- Report
- Analysis
- Feedback
- Investigation
- Response

Resource provisions
- Training
- Supervision
- Communication
- Co-ordination

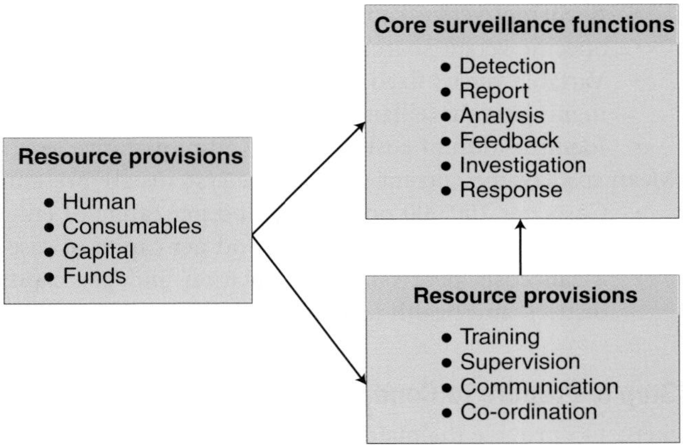

FIG. 6-6 Cost included in data collection tools. Source: Zana C Somda, Meltzer MI, Perry HN. *SurvCost* 1.0: a manual to assist country and district public health officials in estimating the cost of the implementation of Integrated Disease Surveillance and Response systems (Beta test version). Centers for Disease Control and Prevention, National Center for Prevention, Detection and Control of Infectious Diseases, Division of Emerging Infections and Surveillance Services, U.S. Department of Health and Human Services; 2007.

Step 5: Create a Preliminary Data Analysis Plan

Analysis of the evaluation findings will provide comparisons of surveillance costs and performance across regional, district, and health facility study units. Presentation tables using IDSR categorizations of surveillance functions and activities are useful to illustrate results (Fig. 6-6).

Quality indicators collected at all health levels will be used to compare performance and understand the costs of upgrading systems to optimum operational standards. Following are the main indicators in assessing system quality for this evaluation:

1. Percentage of meningitis cases with a positive CSF test for any bacterium: combines the percentage of the population served by health facilities included in surveillance, the percentage of patients with a lumbar puncture, the percentage of CSFs transported to the lab, and the percentage with a positive laboratory test (at a local or reference laboratory).
2. Percentage of outbreaks reported to the national level within 2 days of surpassing the alert threshold and percentage of epidemics identified at national level but missed at district level: average of the two percentages.
3. Percentage of surveillance reports sent from health facilities to the district and the percentage of reports then sent to the national level in a timely manner: average of the two percentages.

The expected cost estimation summaries are defined in the preliminary data analysis plan. The total cost estimates at each administrative level are converted to costs per 100,000 population and costs per capita. Total costs are analyzed according to the following:

- Administrative levels
- Activities (both core activities and support functions, as defined in Fig. 6-6)

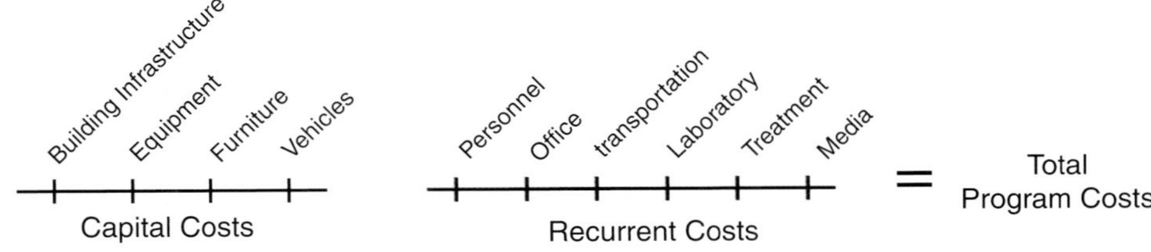

FIG. 6-7 Structure used to present surveillance activity performance and costs.

- Recurrent versus capital costs
- Specific versus shared costs—to inform the level of funding that is not supported by other programs
- Variable versus fixed costs—to identify cost categories, which are likely to rise proportionally to variation in meningitis surveillance activities
- Identification of cost drivers by administrative level and by activities

Mean costs of the current surveillance systems are presented as follows:

- Costs per 100,000 population and per capita of enhanced meningitis surveillance
- Costs per 100,000 population and per capita of case-based surveillance
- Mean costs per 100,000 population and per capita according to administrative level—national, regional, district, and health facility

Step 6: Prepare to Conduct the Evaluation

Steps 1–5 provide the major segments of the evaluation plan, which can also be used as the protocol for the evaluation study. At this point, the following components of the evaluation have been put in place:

1. The objective and aims of the evaluation are clear and defined
2. A meningitis surveillance system logic model is developed and will be revisited to illustrate gaps in current surveillance system once the evaluation is completed
3. The evaluation is accepted and approved by in-country stakeholders
4. The evaluation plan includes appropriate participants and sites to provide feedback on surveillance system performance
5. Data collection instruments are designed to reflect indicators and provide relevant information identified in preliminary data analysis plan

The next step, in this case study, was to develop a timeline to conduct the evaluation and confirm this with stakeholders. Chad, like most countries, required authorization from an institutional review board or ethics committee before any type of research involving human subjects can be conducted. Time for submitting the protocol for institutional review board review should always be considered when developing the evaluation timeline.

Finally, before performing the actual evaluation, all evaluation instruments were field tested to ensure that the questions were valid, reliable, and appropriate for the population. Field tests should be conducted in a population that closely resembles the study population, such as an adjacent district, which was the case in this study.

Designing this evaluation using the aforementioned steps created a clear platform for analyzing and interpreting results to directly answer evaluation questions. From this study, the researchers were able to provide the Chadian government and other stakeholders with evaluation results that

1. Identify the gaps in surveillance functions in each district by comparing current surveillance activities against the evaluation logic model as a consensus standard;
2. Present district surveillance performance according to costs that highlights specific areas of investment need for overall system improvement; and
3. Provide cost estimates per surveillance function and support activity that can be used in all meningitis belt countries to estimate cost per 100,000 population of upgrading their system.

These types of results cannot be obtained using traditional evaluation frameworks for PHSS. The data collected elucidates the specific needs of the Chadian meningitis and PHSS, and also provides generalizable data that are useful to the region and similar environments. The unique benefit of the WPA evaluation design is affirmed by the quality of pertinent information that is produced for improving program management and functionality of the PHSS.

CONCLUSION

Day-to-day surveillance is an amalgam of well-defined work processes, which occur primarily at the subnational health levels. The literature review presented at the beginning of this chapter reveals the need for these levels to be well supported and strengthened. In order to accomplish this, gaps in the system must be identified first and contextual factors that impact surveillance performance must be understood. Then, participants in the surveillance process must be equipped with information that they can use to drive program changes.

The case study presented walks through the practical steps of creating an evaluation plan to assess performance and costs of a CDSS. The WPA framework can be used to assess any program or process within the PHSS because it is a work-process-centered approach. The information generated from this framework can be used to request resources to improve specific parts of the system. Including surveillance players at all levels helps evaluations capture how various factors affect their work and sheds light on how to better streamline work activities. Readers should note that these steps underscore the importance of truly understanding a system before evaluating it. While regional strategies are used in most instances to guide surveillance functions, country health structures and surveillance nuances must be studied to accurately guide surveillance system program planning. Furthermore, national surveillance officials and experts should be consulted during the early stages of an evaluation plan's development, specifically to validate the WPA tools (logic model, indicators, and work process tree).

Finally, while this case study looked at meningitis surveillance specifically due to the introduction of a new meningitis vaccine, it is important to approach surveillance, especially in resource-limited countries, using the more efficient and resource-sharing strategy of integrated surveillance (see Chapter 4).

KEY SUMMARY POINTS

- Disease surveillance includes an interdependent network of surveillance players, work processes, and public health competencies.
- Gaps in surveillance work processes can diminish the quality and utility of surveillance data.
- Contextual factors, costs, and areas of program integration are usually not captured in traditional surveillance system evaluations.
- The WPA evaluation framework guides program improvement by focusing on understanding a system's work processes.
- Logic models, indicator databases, and work process trees are complementary tools to describe a surveillance system's architecture and provide the blueprint for an evaluation plan.
- Evaluation plans should include guidance and participation of a country's surveillance players.
- A clear understanding and mapping of a country's surveillance system should be completed before an evaluation is conducted.
- Evaluation plans should include the costs and performance data that will be collected from which areas of the health system.
- Surveillance activities should be conducted in an integrated way across disease programs as to prevent unnecessary overburdening of human and financial resources.

DISCUSSION QUESTIONS

1. Which types of methods can be used to assess surveillance program attributes for surveillance system performance?
2. Which types of information must be gathered in order to understand how a surveillance system works in one country? Where would you go to get this information?
3. List some advantages and disadvantages of the work process analysis evaluation approach presented in this chapter.
4. Review the logic model presented in Fig. 6-7. What ways can you use this to assist stakeholders in understanding and supporting the evaluation study?
5. Once the evaluation is completed, what are the next steps to improve the surveillance system?
6. Review Fig. 6-6 and give a scenario illustrating how the listed surveillance functions can be used to collect data across disease programs in a way that saves the surveillance program time and money.

REFERENCES

1. World Health Organization, Prevention USCfDCa. Technical guidelines for integrated disease surveillance and response in the African region. 2nd ed. Brazzaville: Republic of Congo and Atlanta, Georgia, USA; 2010.
2. Berkelman RL, Bryan RT, Osterholm MT, LeDuc JW, Hughes JM. Infectious disease surveillance: a crumbling foundation. Science 1994;264(5157):368–70.
3. WHO. Communicable disease surveillance and response systems: guide to monitoring and evaluating. Geneva; 2006.
4. Klaucke DN, Buehler JW, Thacker SB, Parrish RG, Trowbridge FL, Berkelman RL. The Surveillance Coordination Group. Guidelines for evaluating surveillance systems. MMWR 1988;37(Suppl. 5):1–18.
5. Wuhib T, Chorba TL, Davidiants V, Kenzie WRM, McNabb SJN. Assessment of the infectious diseases surveillance system of the Republic of Armenia: an example of surveillance in the Republics of the former Soviet Union. BMC Public Health 2002;2:3.
6. Carrieri MP, Salmaso S, Bella A, D'Ancona F, Demicheli V, Marongiu C, et al. Evaluation of the SIMI system, an experimental computerised network for the surveillance of communicable diseases in Italy. Eur J Epidemiol 2000;16(10):941–7.
7. Rumisha SF, Mboera LE, Senkoro KP, Gueye D, Mmbuji PK. Monitoring and evaluation of integrated disease surveillance and response in selected districts in Tanzania. Tanzan Health Res Bull 2007;9(1):1–11.
8. CDC. Assessment of infectious disease surveillance—Uganda, 2000. MMWR Morb Mortal Wkly Rep 2000;49(30):687–91.
9. CDC. Evaluation of meningitis surveillance before introduction of serogroup a meningococcal conjugate vaccine - Burkina Faso and Mali. MMWR Morb Mortal Wkly Rep 2012;61(50):1025–8.
10. Sahal N, Reintjes R, Eltayeb EM, Aro AR. Assessment of core activities and supportive functions for the communicable diseases surveillance system in Khartoum state, Sudan, 2005-2007. East Mediterr Health J 2010;16(12):1204–10.
11. Nsubuga P, Brown WG, Groseclose SL, Ahadzie L, Talisuna AO, Mmbuji P, et al. Implementing integrated disease surveillance and response: four African countries' experience, 1998-2005. Glob Public Health 2010;5(4):364–80.
12. German RR, Lee LM, Horan JM, Milstein RL, Pertowski CA, Waller MN, et al. Updated guidelines for evaluating public health surveillance systems: recommendations from the Guidelines Working Group. MMWR Recomm Rep 2001;50(RR-13):1–35 quiz CE1–7.
13. McNabb SJ, Chungong S, Ryan M, Wuhib T, Nsubuga P, Alemu W, et al. Conceptual framework of public health surveillance and action and its application in health sector reform. BMC Public Health 2002;2:2.
14. Definition provided by the chapter author.
15. Performance indicators. England: Routledge; 1990.
16. Central Intelligence Agency. The world factbook, <http://www.cia.gov/library/publications/the-world-factbook/geos/cd.html/>; 2013. [updated May 15, 2013; cited July 7, 2012].
17. Malik K. Human development report 2013: the rise of the South. New York: United Nations Development Programme (UNDP); 2013.
18. African Meningococcal Carriage Consortium. Chad, <http://www.menafricar.org/countries/chad/>. [updated June 6, 2013; cited April 29, 2013].
19. Daugla DM, Gami JP, Gamougam K, Naibei N, Mbainadji L, Narbe M, et al. Effect of a serogroup A meningococcal conjugate vaccine (PsA-TT) on serogroup A meningococcal meningitis and carriage in Chad: a community study [corrected]. Lancet 2014;383(9911):40–7.
20. Djingarey MH, Barry R, Bonkoungou M, Tiendrebeogo S, Sebgo R, Kandolo D, et al. Effectively introducing a new meningococcal A conjugate vaccine in Africa: the Burkina Faso experience. Vaccine 2012;30(Suppl. 2):B40–5.

CHAPTER

7

New Matrix for Evaluation of Public Health Surveillance Systems

Isabelle Devaux, on behalf of the working group surveillance system quality and ECDC experts

It all depends on how we look at things and not how they are in themselves...

Carl Jung

KEY WORDS

Work Process Analysis Framework
Work process tree
Logic model
Performance indicators

INTRODUCTION

Public health surveillance data are used for multiple purposes and actions, including response to public health events,[1] program planning and evaluation, and formulating research hypotheses.[1] A public health surveillance system (or health information system) is usually created and operated within a legislative framework that can apply at different levels (locally, nationally, or internationally) to serve the health system of a community.

This framework usually starts with objectives, defines a list of diseases or health-related events[1] under surveillance according to agreed upon case definitions and specifies the stakeholders and community related to the surveillance process. Public health surveillance systems are characterized by specific attributes (e.g., sensitivity) and components (e.g., population and geographic areas that they cover, type of surveillance) that have to be considered to assess their performances and to specifically evaluate if the system can address its objectives and/or if it is "fit for purpose."

This chapter aims to review the current international guidelines used for evaluation of public health surveillance systems and to introduce a novel approach to evaluation developed by a group of surveillance experts from 16 European Union countries. Such an approach is supported by examples of evaluation of data quality using European data sets for tuberculosis and hepatitis B and is further described in the European Centre for Disease Prevention and Control (ECDC) handbook "Data quality monitoring and surveillance system evaluation."[2]

The main goal of communicating this evaluation approach is to provide practical material for public health students and professionals who have to perform evaluations of surveillance systems.

CURRENT INTERNATIONAL GUIDELINES FOR EVALUATION OF PUBLIC HEALTH SURVEILLANCE

The purpose of evaluating public health surveillance systems is to ensure that human and financial resources are used efficiently to perform tasks that can address the objectives of surveillance for the disease(s), population, and geographic area covered by the system. Several dimensions of a public health surveillance system can be evaluated:

- The legislative framework defining public health functions (mandatory notification, response to public health emergencies, etc.);
- The performance of case/event reporting processes within the organization of public health services, using surveillance attributes;
- The capacity to detect event(s)/case(s) and address the appropriate response;
- The contribution and added value of public health surveillance to the stakeholders participating in the processes; and
- The general public health importance and benefit of surveillance activities (role of surveillance for disease prevention, monitoring impact of public health events).

Surveillance system evaluations perform comprehensive measurements of relevant attributes (over time or in a single effort) in order to verify whether the system is still "fit for purpose" and recommend improvements.[2]

The guidelines for evaluating public health surveillance systems from the Centers for Disease Control and Prevention (CDC), first published in 1988[1] and updated in 2001,[3] have been used internationally as one of the main references to perform these types of evaluations by a generation of public health professionals. They specify surveillance attributes and practical approaches to the evaluation of surveillance system performance. The guidelines from the World Health Organization (WHO), published in 2006,[4] specify the processes of monitoring the quality of surveillance information by using indicators and evaluation processes. Finally, guidelines were developed by the European Commission in the early 2000s to prepare for the evaluation of European disease-specific networks for their integration into the surveillance system of the ECDC.[5] **The European Centre of Disease Prevention and Control** (ECDC) is a European Union agency, founded in 2005, which aims to strengthen Europe's defenses against infectious diseases.[6]

The existing guidelines of CDC, WHO, and the European Commission are generic; they do not suggest targeted evaluation questions and associated objectives and they should be completed using protocols that specify objectives and evaluation approach(es) to be performed.

The CDC guidelines set up concepts for the definitions of surveillance attributes and evaluation of performances of surveillance systems, but their application is context specific. There is a need to provide more detailed specification and examples of application of these concepts.

Existing evaluation guidelines mainly apply to disease-specific evaluations, whereas surveillance systems often address several diseases/conditions that require evaluation. The guidelines do not necessarily take into account an integrated approach to surveillance including the multiple dimensions (stated above) of a public health surveillance system that need to be considered before starting an evaluation process.

Furthermore, public health informatics concepts and practices have changed since the development of the original evaluation guidelines, and existing guidelines do not account for new technologies and standards requirements (e.g., HL7). These new environments need to be taken into account for evaluation of public health surveillance systems (see Chapter 22 on surveillance informatics).

NEW METHODOLOGICAL APPROACH FOR EVALUATIONS OF SURVEILLANCE SYSTEMS

To address some of the limitations of the current international surveillance evaluation guidelines, there was a need to further define concepts, describe methodologies, and provide practical examples for how to monitor data quality and conduct evaluations of public health surveillance systems. A working group of experts from 16 European countries developed a framework (or matrix) to create strategies for the evaluation of surveillance systems. This framework is described in the ECDC handbook, "Data Quality Monitoring and Surveillance Systems Evaluation. A Handbook of Methods and Applications."[2,7,8] This section of the ECDC handbook specifies the definitions of surveillance system attributes and describes a methodological approach for the evaluation of surveillance systems.

Definitions of Surveillance Attributes for Evaluation

Specific definitions of surveillance system attributes used in this evaluation framework are available in the ECDC handbook.

These definitions are based on the concepts used in previous guidelines except for data quality, for which we define an external and internal dimension of completeness and validity (Table 7-1). Internal completeness or validity is calculated within a data set whereas external completeness or validity implies the comparison of the surveillance data set to a reference source. External completeness is equivalent to sensitivity of case reporting.

Definitions of sensitivity, specificity, and predictive value (positive and negative) are further specified in Table 7-2.

Several factors may affect sensitivity of surveillance along the case ascertainment and reporting processes. Cases may not be reported to the surveillance system for different reasons: asymptomatic cases, cases not seeking medical attention, undiagnosed cases, too specific case definition, when a test is not available at certain points of the health care system, or if a case is not classified (case definition not applied). The sensitivity of a case-based reporting system depends on the sensitivity of the case definition, which should be constructed to address agreed surveillance objectives. For event-based surveillance, sensitivity represents the proportion of outbreaks occurring in a community that are picked up by the surveillance system.

The positive predictive value (PPV) (proportion of real cases reported through the surveillance system ("true positives") (a) divided by the total number of cases reported to the surveillance system ($a + b$)) is directly linked to the laboratory diagnosis of a case and reflects the probability that a case reported in the surveillance system is

TABLE 7-1 Internal and External Dimensions of Completeness and Validity

	COMPLETENESS	VALIDITY
Internal	Proportion of missing (unknown or blank) records or values within a data set.	Extent of errors within the system.
External	Relates to whether the data available to the surveillance system reflects the true number of cases diagnosed with notifiable conditions. External completeness is equivalent of sensitivity of case reporting.	Verify if the information collected represents the "true" incidence, whether there is no bias in the data collected. Require comparison to a gold standard.

TABLE 7-2 Sensitivity, Specificity, PPV Positive, and Negative Predictive Value of a Case Reporting System

	CASES (CONDITION PRESENT)/OUTBREAK	NONCASE (CONDITION NOT PRESENT)/NO OUTBREAK	
Reported	a True case True outbreak	b False case False outbreak	$a + b$
Not reported	c False noncase False "no outbreak"	d True noncase True "no outbreak"	$c + d$
	$a + c$ Total cases Total outbreaks	$b + d$ Total noncases Total "no outbreak"	$N = a + b + c + d$

Notes: Sensitivity = $[a / (a + c)] \times 100$; PPV = $[a / (a + b)] \times 100$; Specificity = $[d / (b + d)] \times 100$; Negative predictive value = $[d / (c + d)] \times 100$; N: population under surveillance.

indeed a real case. For event-based surveillance, PPV reflects the probability that a detected outbreak is really an outbreak.

Proposed Steps for the Evaluation of Public Health Surveillance Systems

The steps for evaluating public health surveillance systems included in this new framework are as follows:

Step 1: Describe the system
Step 2: Plan the evaluation
Step 3: Run the evaluation
Step 4: Identify gaps
Step 5: Create an action plan and follow-up

For step 1, elements of surveillance systems were reviewed and documented as part of one chapter of the manual for surveillance system quality.[7,8] As described in a simplified flowchart from the CDC guidelines,[1] the main elements of a surveillance system are as follows:

- capacity to define and confirm a case or health-related event,
- description of the reporting process by the data providers,
- data management and analysis steps operated by public health authorities, and
- feedback information for data providers and the concerned population.

To augment the CDC guidelines, ECDC included further elements to be considered for the description of a surveillance system[7,8] that can be identified using a checklist (Table 7-3). This checklist allows a surveillance officer to get a quick overview of the surveillance system and related processes to be evaluated.

TABLE 7-3 Checklist to be used for the Description of a Surveillance System

ELEMENT OF THE SURVEILLANCE SYSTEM	CHECKS	COMMENT
Surveillance objectives defined	Yes ☐ No ☐	
List of disease under surveillance	Defined by regulatory process ☐ Defined by public health authorities ☐ Not defined ☐	
Case definitions for surveillance	Defined by regulatory process ☐ Defined by public health authorities ☐ Not defined ☐	
Population under surveillance	Defined by size ☐ Defined by risk group ☐	
Geographic coverage defined	Yes ☐ No ☐	
Type of surveillance defined	Passive ☐ active ☐ Compulsory ☐ voluntary ☐	
Specification of the information/data to be reported	Case-based aggregated ☐ Variable specification ☐ Frequency of data collection ☐ Frequency of data analysis and reporting ☐	
IT components	Paper-based vs. electronic ☐ Data entry using Excel/Access ☐ Data entry is web-based ☐ Architecture of the database described ☐	

A Trigger-Oriented Approach to Select Appropriate Evaluation Protocols

A novel concept of identifying triggers of evaluation to select the appropriate evaluation protocol is a breakthrough new element in this evaluation framework. A **trigger** is a term for an event that is the cause of a particular action, process, or situation—in the use for this chapter; a trigger prompts a surveillance system evaluation.[9]

In step 2, the planning phase, objectives of surveillance system evaluation are triggered by events or specific issues/questions to be addressed within the scope of the surveillance processes. An evaluation of a surveillance system usually does not occur by chance, but it is planned to address specific issues or triggers. Based on experts' discussions and a literature review, ECDC identified categories of triggers that can be used to initiate an evaluation of a surveillance system (Fig. 7-1). The ability to identify what is triggering an evaluation is important because the evaluation objectives and methods should be tailored according to the triggers identified.

The following triggers can be cited as examples:

1. Conducting an evaluation of the surveillance system as part of an agreed routine process.
2. Measuring the impact related to a change in policy. For example, a policy change can be the introduction of a new vaccination schedule/new vaccine, a change in hospital control practices to reduce health-care-associated infections, introduction of a target for disease elimination, or introduction of a target for reducing the burden of disease in a certain group (e.g., in children). Also, a change in case definition can have an impact on case classification and calculation of incidence.
3. Surveillance systems may have to be adapted to respond to an outbreak situation. For example, during the VTEC outbreak in Germany, the timeliness of the surveillance system was increased as well as addition of syndromic surveillance.
4. If a special event is planned like a mass gathering, some components of the surveillance system should be enhanced and evaluated *a priori*.

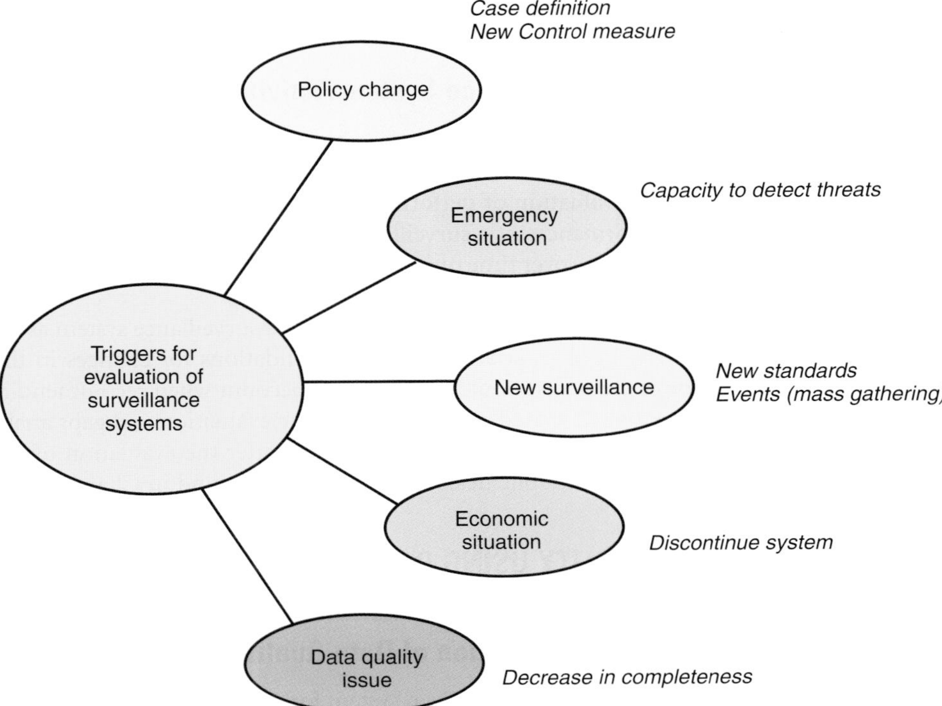

FIG. 7-1 Planning a trigger-oriented approach to the evaluation of surveillance systems.

5. Due to economic constraints, the evaluation of the cost of surveillance is an important element to consider.
6. Through data quality monitoring, it is possible to identify issues concerning the performances of the surveillance system. Subsequent evaluation can be performed. **Data quality monitoring** is the monitoring of the "quality" of data collected, which includes accuracy and validity, reliability, confidentiality and security, legibility, currency and timeliness, accessibility, meaning or usefulness, and completeness.[10]
7. Impact of technological innovation needs to be evaluated.
8. Change in the size of population under surveillance will have an impact on disease incidence.

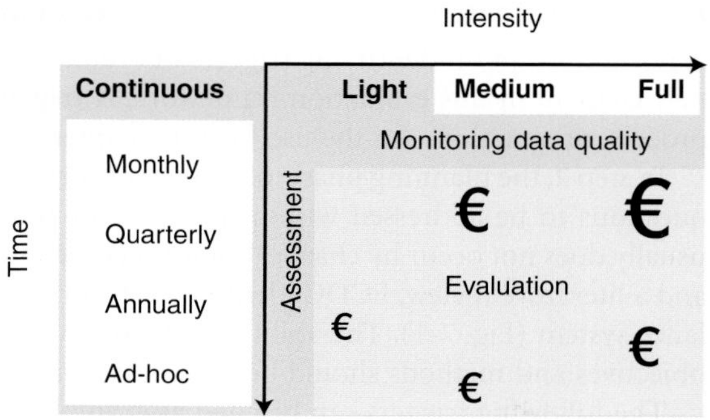

After having identified the possible reason(s) that can trigger a surveillance evaluation, it is important to define the evaluation model (or type of evaluation) that is required to address the specific questions triggering the evaluation. In Fig. 7-2, the evaluation model includes two dimensions: the frequency of the evaluation (*y*-axis) and the level of the protocol to be developed (*x*-axis). The choice of evaluation protocol depends not only on the triggers but also on its cost.

Intensity

Continuous	Light	Medium	Full
	Monitoring data quality		
Monthly		€	€
Quarterly			
Annually	€	Evaluation	€
Ad-hoc		€	

Time; Assessment

FIG. 7-2. Cost of surveillance system evaluation by time and intensity to aid in the *Selection of appropriate evaluation model.* Source: Surveillance system quality manual.

ECDC defines three levels of protocols—light, medium, and full—which correspond to the increasing number and/or level of complexity of the surveillance attributes, resources, stakeholders, and time necessary to perform the evaluation. The focus of the evaluation depends on the triggers and will be characterized by a specific type of protocol, including selected attributes for the performances of the system to be evaluated. A decision tree can be developed, starting from the triggers, taking into account the parameters defining the type of protocol to guide decisions for the evaluation, as part of a planning phase. An added value of the trigger-oriented approach is that it allows for optimization of resources, better definition of evaluation methods and therefore more efficiency and effectiveness.

Evaluating Performance and Cost of Surveillance System Activities

After identifying the type of evaluation to be performed, it is necessary to engage a team and stakeholders to be consulted during the evaluation process.

Step 3 includes two main components: evaluation of performances and evaluation of cost of the activities of a surveillance system. The evaluation of performances of a surveillance system involves performing a comprehensive measurement of relevant surveillance attributes (over time or in a single effort) in order to verify whether the system is still "fit for purpose" and to give recommendations for guiding improvements.

Step 4 identifies gaps by interpreting performance using the attributes of a surveillance system as well as the cost. Approaches for a gap analysis can be developed in addition to recommendations for changes in the surveillance system to address its objectives. Economic elements should be taken into account when recommending continuity/discontinuity of systems and/or system activities. Based on the results of the evaluation and gaps analysis, an action plan (step 5) should be suggested to assess the impact of changes initiated after the evaluation of the surveillance system. (Further discussion of the economics of public health activities can be found in Chapter 8.)

EXAMPLE OF EVALUATING DATA QUALITY USING DATA FROM THE EUROPEAN SURVEILLANCE SYSTEM (TESSy)

Description of TESSy and Rationale for Evaluation of Data Quality

The European Surveillance System is a flexible metadata-driven system for collection, validation, cleaning, analysis, and dissemination of data. Its key aims are data analysis and production of outputs for public health action. All

European Union Member States (28) and EEA countries (3) report their available data on communicable diseases (52) to the system.[11]

The reporting of these 52 diseases and conditions to the ECDC has been agreed upon by a commission decision[12] and complies with European case definitions updated in 2012.[13] For each disease/condition, standards for surveillance have been defined, including surveillance objectives and a metadataset with detailed specification of variable definitions and coding systems. One of the main objectives with the launch of TESSy in 2008 was the standardization and harmonization of surveillance processes across diseases and European countries[14]; however, issues with data quality and comparability still remain.

A data collection schedule has been established on an annual basis for diseases/conditions to be reported to TESSy. Data collected in TESSy are validated and analyzed for the production of disease-specific surveillance reports as well as the ECDC annual epidemiological report.[15] Data validation processes were developed with setting up of automated validation rules as part of the data upload to TESSy, but this does not replace systematic feedback and exchange of information on data quality with the data providers. As part of the surveillance report production process, the validation can last up to 6 weeks after finishing data collection. During this period, the epidemiologist and data manager verify completeness and validity of the data and go back to the data providers to correct information if needed.

As specified in the current ECDC long-term surveillance strategy, 2014–2020,[16] data quality monitoring processes need to be further improved through the management of European data. This requires the development of data quality standards for European Union surveillance to further address surveillance objectives. The evaluation of data quality in TESSy is a collective approach, which aims at enhancing understanding to correct data-related specific issues across the reporting process.

Planning the Evaluation of TESSy Data for Selected Diseases

One of the main triggers to evaluate data quality in TESSy was the need to set up a data quality monitoring system to identify and characterize specific data quality issues and possibly address them on a continuous basis. We evaluated the internal completeness and validity of TESSy data for selected diseases (see examples below). We set up disease-specific evaluation teams, drafted protocols, and planned the evaluation according to the following steps:

- Identify types of analyses and variables used for these analyses in surveillance reports.
- Define data quality indicators (completeness, validity) by surveillance objectives and types of analyses.
- Specify the calculation of completeness and validity by variables or groups of variables, using data quality indicators.
- Measure and interpret results.

We used TESSy data sets from 2007 to 2012 for tuberculosis (TB) and hepatitis B. Data quality indicators were linked to surveillance objectives, program monitoring targets, and key surveillance outputs.

Example of Evaluation of Tuberculosis Data Quality

ECDC reviewed the tables of the latest tuberculosis surveillance report[17] and identified the types of analyses used across the report or surveillance indicators (below), whereas the main objective of analysis of surveillance data is to produce surveillance indicators within a specific timeframe; a completeness analysis will provide a background of the data available to produce the surveillance report.

- History of TB: History can be defined by previous treatment or previous diagnosis of TB, which allows stratified analysis of patients with previous TB, as opposed to newly treated patients. It also discriminates previous treatment history by previous treatment completion (relapses from previous failures and defaulters).
- Origin of TB cases: Origin can be defined either by country of birth or citizenship, whether the patient was born in or is a citizen of the reporting country. The origin of the patient is necessary to perform analysis among migrants.
- Multidrug-resistant (MDR) tuberculosis: MDR TB is defined as resistance to isoniazid and rifampicin while extensively drug-resistant (XDR) tuberculosis is defined as MDR plus resistance to a fluoroquinolone and one or more of the following injectable drugs: amikacin, capreomycin, and kanamycin.

- Site of disease: Site is defined by major site and minor site (it is possible to consider more than one localization).
- Treatment outcome monitoring: Outcome of treatment is measured in periods of after 12 months, after 24 months for MDR-TB cases, and after 36 months for XDR-TB cases.
- Patients with HIV and TB coinfections.

Data quality indicators comply with program indicators and targets defined in the framework action plan to fight tuberculosis in the European Union.[18] Completeness indicators were defined as the number of data fields with a value other than "UNK" (unknown) and missing (numerator) divided by the total number of data fields for all cases or a subgroup of cases (denominator).

Results of the analyses for key indicators are displayed in Table 7-4 and include proposed associated actions. The completeness of previous TB data was high across all countries. The completeness of culture results was calculated for new pulmonary cases only and was above 80% in almost all countries.

One of the possible follow-up actions to improve completeness of culture results could be to improve the linkage between notification and laboratory data. All countries using case-based data do not report the completeness of laboratory-confirmed cases with drug sensitivity testing results. Countries should be encouraged to report case-based data to ECDC for the monitoring of drug sensitivity. Although the completeness of treatment outcome monitoring is high, it is important to ensure continuity of cohort monitoring across reporting years.

Examples of the Evaluation of Hepatitis B Data Quality

An algorithm was developed for the reporting of cases of hepatitis B to implement the new European Union hepatitis B case definition,[12] and classify cases as acute or chronic. As further described in the ECDC hepatitis B and C surveillance report,[19] this information is collected in TESSy with a completeness of 90% in 2012. Missing or unknown information may be explained by the complexity of serological markers in differentiating between acute and chronic infections, the limitations of testing capacities in some countries, and differences in surveillance policies.[20] The completeness of the vaccination status is 23% overall. Country of birth or country of nationality could potentially be some information of interest for interpretation of the epidemiology, as the incidence of hepatitis B infection is expected to be higher in patients originating from high endemicity countries. However, the completeness of such information is low at only 21% complete for country of birth and 7% complete for country of nationality in 2011. The completeness of the transmission mode is only 9%.[17] These preliminary results on the evaluation of hepatitis B surveillance data quality confirm that improved understanding of testing and surveillance policies will aid the interpretation of surveillance data to provide better information for planning services. Also, consideration should be given to alternative epidemiologic methods such as prevalence surveys and sentinel surveillance.[21]

TABLE 7-4 **Completeness Analysis for Key TB Indicators**

QUALITY INDICATOR	RESULTS	SUGGESTED INTERVENTIONS
Completeness of previous TB history	Previous treatment or diagnosis: 91%	Optimal
Completeness of culture result reported (new pulmonary cases)	87% in all European Union countries	Improve linkage notification and laboratory data
Completeness of laboratory-confirmed cases with DST results	Two countries not reporting, 80% for all other countries	Support countries to report DST on case-based data
Completeness of TOM among TB cases reported in previous year	94% (excluding 3 countries not reporting)	Improve cohort monitoring

Notes: DST, drug sensitivity test; TOM treatment outcome monitoring.

CONCLUSIONS AND RECOMMENDATIONS

This chapter summarizes an approach for the evaluation of public health surveillance systems developed by an international working group from 16 European countries. More information is available in the ECDC handbook.[2] The method described in this chapter does not replace already existing international guidelines published by the WHO or the CDC. Rather, it is complementary to supporting practical issues identified when planning and conducting evaluations of public health surveillance systems. It can be qualified as a novel approach to surveillance system evaluation, as it focuses on triggers to evaluation and also includes new attributes for evaluation of surveillance systems such as its cost. The surveillance officer and the team in charge of conducting and evaluation can focus on the development of an appropriate protocol and planning to address the issues that have triggered the evaluation.

This chapter focuses on completeness and validity as attributes for data quality; however, timeliness is also important. As discussed in Chapter 24, "a surveillance system that puts a premium on timeliness will always tend to present analysts with data whose quality is uncertain."

Evaluation of external completeness and sensitivity of surveillance data refer to the capacity of a reporting system to detect cases of notifiable diseases. Underreporting occurs when patients affected by the notifiable condition visit physicians or health care facilities but, once diagnosed, are not properly reported by the health care provider to the local public health unit. The evaluation of the "real" burden of disease requires specific studies to estimate under-ascertainment of cases of infectious diseases or the number of infected individuals who are not diagnosed and hence, not identified by the health care systems.[21] Sensitivity and PPV are reversely linked, and both are associated to timeliness (see Chapter 24 for more detail).

It is important to plan and perform the evaluation of a surveillance system according to a stepwise process. The preparation step and, in particular, formulation of triggers are necessary for conducting an evaluation of a surveillance system. Further examples of triggers are provided in Chapter 24. The type of protocol to be developed for an evaluation (light, medium, or full) could be further specified by the development of templates associated with the case studies.

The method proposed in this chapter for evaluation of surveillance systems has been applied to European data sets of selected infectious diseases (TB and hepatitis are provided as examples). The types of indicators that are defined at a European level would be different than the ones to be defined at a national or subnational level due to the nature of the data set (comparability issues when pulling data produced by different surveillance systems) and the analysis to be performed (defined by different objectives at international, national, and local levels).

The evaluation of TESSy data quality is in line with the ECDC's long-term surveillance strategy. It was triggered by the need to set up a data quality monitoring system, and was developed according to a stepwise approach. From the examples provided in this chapter, it is clear that the results of the evaluation of TB completeness indicators comply with international targets and the evaluation of hepatitis B surveillance reveals difficulties related to the implementation of case definitions.

KEY SUMMARY POINTS

- The CDC guidelines for evaluation of public health surveillance systems have been used internationally for decades. A working group of experts from 16 European countries developed a manual to further guide public health professionals to set up data quality monitoring systems and conduct evaluations of public health surveillance systems.
- Data quality is defined mainly by completeness and validity, and is related to other surveillance systems' attributes including timeliness, sensitivity, specificity, and positive predictive value.
- Five steps are proposed for evaluation of a public health surveillance system: (1) describing the surveillance system, (2) planning the evaluation, (3) implementing the evaluation, (4) identifying gaps, and (5) proposing an action plan.
- Most recently, the evaluation of TESSy was triggered due to the need to set up a data quality monitoring system to provide regular feedback to the ECDC networks participating in the surveillance processes of communicable diseases in Europe.

DISCUSSION QUESTIONS

1. When performing an evaluation of a surveillance system or component of surveillance, what is most important to characterize?
2. What types of evaluations or evaluations of what surveillance system characteristics would provide informed decisions for policy makers about a surveillance system?
3. What is the main goal of evaluating any surveillance system?
4. When evaluating a surveillance system, what types of stakeholders should be provided with feedback?
5. What surveillance attribute is considered essential to be evaluated to verify that the system is "fit for purpose" and possibly address fundamental public health functions for society?
6. Describe a trigger for evaluation and design the appropriate methods to perform the surveillance system's evaluation.

REFERENCES

1. Klaucke DN, Buehler JW, Thacker SB, Parrish RG, Trowbridge FL, Berkelman RL, The Surveillance Coordination Group. Guidelines for evaluating surveillance systems. MMWR 1988;37(Suppl. 5):1–18.
2. European Centre for Disease Prevention and Control. Data quality monitoring and surveillance system evaluation - A handbook of methods and applications. Stockholm: ECDC; 2014.
3. German RR, Armstrong G, Birkhead GS, Horan JM, Herrera G. Updated guidelines for evaluating public health surveillance systems. MMWR 2001;50:1–35.
4. World Health Organization. Communicable disease surveillance and response systems: Guide to monitoring and evaluating. World Health Organization epidemic and pandemic alert and response; 2006.
5. Ruutu P, Breuer T, Desenclos J-C, et al. A framework and recommendations for evaluating surveillance systems within the community network for communicable diseases, Basic Network for Surveillance of infectious diseases in European Union. European commission: Directorate General Health & Consumer protection; 2001.
6. Official Journal of the European Union. Regulation (EC) No 851/2004 of the European Parliament and of the Council of 21 April 2004, establishing a European centre for disease prevention and control. <http://ecdc.europa.eu/en/aboutus/Key%20Documents/0404_KD_Regulation_establishing_ECDC.pdf>.
7. Devaux I. Data quality monitoring and evaluation of public health surveillance in European Countries. International society for disease surveillance webinar; 2012.
8. Devaux I. An electronic manual and resource e-library to monitor and evaluate surveillance systems' quality. ESCAIDE; 2012.
9. Trigger. Oxford Dictionaries.
10. World Health Organization. Improving Data Quality: A Guide for Developing Countries. Philippines: 2003. <http://www.wpro.who.int/publications/pub_9290610506/en/>.
11. The European Surveillance System (TESSy), <http://ecdc.europa.eu/en/activities/surveillance/Pages/index.aspx>; 2015.
12. Commission decision of 22 December 1999 on the communicable diseases to be progressively covered by the community network under Decision No 2119/98/EC of the European Parliament and of the Council. Official Journal of the European Union 1999.
13. Commission implementing decision of 8 August 2012 amending decision 2002/253/EC laying down case definitions for reporting communicable diseases to the community network under decision No 2119/98/EC of the European parliament and of the council. Official Journal of the European Union 2012.
14. Amato-Gauci A, Ammon A. The surveillance of communicable diseases in the European Union—a long-term strategy (2008-2013). Euro Surveill 2008;13(26).
15. European Centre for Disease Prevention and Control. Annual Epidemiological Report 2013. Reporting on 2011 surveillance data and 2012 epidemic intelligence data.Stockholm: ECDC; 2013. <http://ecdc.europa.eu/en/publications/Publications/annual-epidemiological-report-2013.pdf>.
16. European Centre for Disease Prevention and Control. Long-term surveillance strategy 2014-2020. Stockholm: ECDC; 2013.
17. European Centre for Disease Prevention and Control/WHO Regional Office for Europe. Tuberculosis surveillance and monitoring in Europe 2014. Stockholm: European Centre for Disease Prevention and Control, 2014.
18. European Centre for Disease Prevention and Control. A framework action plan to fight tuberculosis in the European Union. Stockholm; 2008.
19. European Centre for Disease Prevention and Control. Hepatitis B and C surveillance in Europe. 2012. Stockholm: ECDC; 2014.
20. Duffell E, van de Laar M. Under ascertainment of Hepatitis B and C in Europe. 2013.
21. European Centre for Disease Prevention and Control. Methodology protocol for estimating burden of communicable diseases. Stockholm: ECDC; 2010.

CHAPTER

8

Economics of Public Health Surveillance

Rebecca Katz, Julie E Fischer

The first wealth is health.

Ralph Waldo Emerson

KEY WORDS

Socioeconomic determinants of health
Return on investment
Cost analyses
Global public good
Results-based financing (RBF)
Cost–benefit analysis
Cost-effectiveness

BACKGROUND AND CURRENT ENVIRONMENT

A body of evidence built over decades clearly links health and wealth. Studies spanning all regions of the world have demonstrated that low national income levels generally correlate with indicators of poor population health, such as high infant mortality rates and shorter life expectancies. Conversely, child survival rates can be predicted to rise with increasing per capita national income levels before reaching a plateau at higher income levels.[1]

In the mid-twentieth century, concepts based on demographic transition theory characterized the connection between economic growth and improved health status as a straightforward, almost inevitable progression. Influential work published in the 1970s extrapolated from historical data to propose that the improved standards of living afforded by wealth, particularly nutrition, played a far more significant role in reducing premature mortality than medical or public health interventions.[2] Other key research postulated that economic transition organically precipitates epidemiologic transition, with declining mortality from "pestilence and famine" leading to longer life expectancies and a gradual stabilization of fertility rates, followed by a gradual shift in disease burden as chronic "man-made" diseases replace infectious diseases as the major risks for disability and death.[3]

This focus on the socioeconomic determinants of health helped bolster arguments for free-market reforms as the paramount instrument of development assistance by the 1990s.[4] Some contemporary researchers suggested that this approach might underrate the importance of investments in basic public services and health technologies.[5] Even as international development institutions required recipient governments to reduce public spending as a condition of aid, some advocates and researchers argued that these policies would undermine essential public health services that prevent disease and disability and help offset the hazards of urbanization and industrialization.[6]

Researchers began to scrutinize more nuanced relationships between specific socioeconomic determinants and health outcomes and to invert the core question about the health–wealth link: if increased wealth improves population health, can interventions that improve population health status conversely accelerate socioeconomic development? **Socioeconomic determinants of health** are the complex, integrated, and overlapping social structures and economic systems that are responsible for most health inequities. These social structures and economic systems include the social environment, physical environment, health services, and structural and societal factors.

Social determinants of health are shaped by the distribution of money, power, and resources throughout local communities, nations, and the world.[7]

In 2002, a panel commissioned by the Director General of the World Health Organization (WHO) reported that very modest per capita investments in essential health services and effective interventions for priority diseases and conditions (e.g., HIV/AIDS, malaria, tuberculosis, vaccine-preventable diseases, and tobacco-related conditions) might not only save millions of lives but also could free billions of dollars in capital to accelerate economic growth in low- and middle-income regions.[8] Studies cited the benefits of improved population health on worker productivity and capacities for educational attainment, with implications for increased savings, attractiveness for foreign investment, and access to global markets.[9]

At the same time, high-profile outbreaks of emerging infectious diseases, such as severe acute respiratory syndrome (SARS) and highly pathogenic H5N1 avian influenza, coupled with evidence that developing regions face a "dual disease burden" of communicable and noncommunicable conditions, underscored the seriousness of transboundary health risks in an era of interdependent economies and rapid international trade and travel. Researchers and practitioners increasingly adopted a multidisciplinary approach to global health, rather than technical public health interventions focused on specific populations or areas.[10] Their work collectively underpins current concepts of the health–wealth relationship as mutually reinforcing.

Improved health status leads to increased economic potential and thus to expanded health and educational opportunities—a virtuous cycle concept that might apply to poorer areas within wealthy countries as well as to low- and middle-income nations.[11] Conversely, poor health status erodes earning potential at the individual and household levels and economic development at the national level. This perpetuates a vicious cycle in which the lack of resources to secure safe water, adequate nutrition, and essential health services leaves populations even more vulnerable to the spread of infectious diseases. Recent research suggests that national socioeconomic indicators might even be used to forecast the likelihood of infectious disease outbreaks.[12]

Informed decision-making to reinforce the virtuous health–wealth cycle relies on the ability to detect threats to population health and identify effective interventions. Public health surveillance supplies this information. For chronic communicable and noncommunicable diseases, periodic reporting on disease distribution and risk factors can help decision-makers target prevention and control resources efficiently. Rapid detection, verification, and early warning of emerging and epidemic-prone infectious diseases can allow timely responses that prevent further spread of disease.

The use of public health surveillance data for effective decision-making can avert disease, disability, and deaths. In turn, this can save direct costs to health systems, indirect costs to potentially affected individuals and households (such as lost wages), and, ultimately, the costs of societal and market disruptions. At the same time, perceptions that a reported health event poses an unmanageable risk to public safety may damage national economic interests by disrupting trade, travel, and public trust.[13]

FUTURE DIRECTIONS IN THE ECONOMICS OF SURVEILLANCE

In the last 2 decades, dramatic increases in global health assistance and a new emphasis on collective investments in global health security, as demonstrated by the adoption of the revised International Health Regulations in 2005, have raised the stakes for demonstrating the value of strengthening health systems.[14] Development assistance for health rose from approximately US$5.59 billion worldwide in 1990 to approximately US$26.87 billion in 2010, with philanthropic foundations and public–private partnerships contributing a growing share of funding.[15]

The engagement of new payers/donors in global health—including nongovernmental organizations, public–private partnerships, and "super-empowered" philanthrocapitalists—has translated to changing expectations for measurements of impact and effectiveness, often on the part of actors looking to apply models or experiences from the business paradigm to public health actions. This includes a new emphasis on measuring results rather than tracking process indicators, as illustrated by proposals that external partners "pay for performance" in development assistance, linking financing to the achievement of predetermined outcomes such as a reduction in disease burden.[16] For example, the innovative aid mechanism called results-based financing (RBF) has been tested extensively in maternal–child health programs, offering households or health care providers incentives to increase the utilization of essential health services such as antenatal care. **Results-based financing** is any program that rewards the delivery of one or more outputs or outcomes by one or more incentives, financial or otherwise.[17] The full monetary or nonmonetary transfer is made only after the recipient achieves a predetermined goal, from increased service coverage to a measureable reduction in targeted conditions (e.g., neonatal deaths within the catchment area).[18]

Governments have also imposed new demands for demonstrations of efficiency or effectiveness of publicly funded programs. As in most countries, domestic public health surveillance in the USA primarily relies on public funding, which generally takes the form of federal block grants administered by state and local agencies. During periods of constrained economic growth (particularly in the early 1990s and starting again in 2009), the US government implemented new policies that require agencies and organizations to calculate the costs and values of federally funded programs using a range of new methodologies. This puts pressure on state-level health departments to apply costing calculations to health surveillance activities. In turn, states apply many of the same requirements to local health actors.[19]

Short-Term Goals in Economics and Surveillance

In the short term, stakeholders ranging from WHO to local health agencies require new tools to calculate the costs and benefits of public health surveillance programs, particularly of integrated surveillance systems that cut across jurisdictional levels and disease-specific programs (Box 8-1). **Cost–Benefit analysis** is the comparison of costs and achieved benefits, where both costs and benefits are expressed in monetary terms. The usual rule in cost–benefit analysis is for the benefit to cost ratio (B/C) to exceed unit or for $(B - C) > 0$.[20]

For researchers, this means creating a conceptual framework for assigning cost values to cases and deaths averted for multiple endemic, epidemic-prone, and emerging diseases within a population, as well as to broader economic and societal benefits. Models are needed to understand the economic impact of early detection and warning of animal and human health events, including positive effects (e.g., preventing market disruptions or erosion of social institutions) and potential negative effects (e.g., behavioral changes that undermine trade and travel).

This need places new demands on health economists and on the public health community to identify use cases: what are the right scenarios to use in estimating whole-of-society costs and benefits of detecting disease events promptly? What inputs, outputs, and outcomes can be used to predict the costs of surveillance successes and failures, with and without factoring in response capabilities?

Long-Term Goals in Economics and Surveillance

The influx of global health stakeholders from the private sector has encouraged an approach to health evaluation that borrows from the business world—the concept of return on investment (ROI). **Return on investment** is a financial ratio that measures the benefit or gain generated relative to the amount of money invested.[21]

BOX 8-1 US Guidance for Cost–Benefit Analysis of Regulations

For the past 40 years, the US government has required that Federal agencies apply a variety of analytical methods to evaluate the economic impact of new, proposed, and existing regulations. These requirements often take the form of executive orders (EO), instructions issued by the president to Federal agencies that can have the force of law under authorities granted by the Constitution or delegated by legislation. The examples below illustrate how EO and similar guidance that apply to federally funded programs can pertain to health actions, including disease surveillance activities.

1993 Executive Order 12866. Directed Federal agencies to estimate and report the expected benefits of proposed major regulations in conjunction with their estimated costs.

2003 Office of Management and Budget (OMB) Guidance. Required Federal agencies to supplement cost–benefit analyses with cost-effectiveness analyses for economically significant health and safety regulations.

2011 Executive Order 13563. Reiterated EO 12866 and the need to select regulatory approaches to maximize net benefits, as determined through cost–benefit analyses. Also, directed agencies to use the best available techniques to quantify both current and future benefits, and to review previous regulations.

2011 Executive Order 13579. Encouraged, but did not require, independent regulatory agencies to apply the principles in EO 13563.

This approach encompasses traditional cost–benefit analyses. The ROI considers the costs averted by program implementation as well as the program costs:

ROI = (Costs averted by program – Program costs)/Program costs

In this approach, any result greater than zero reflects a net savings or gain. As models are developed to predict the costs and benefits of building national surveillance capabilities across programmatic siloes more reliably, researchers will be able to calculate with increasing confidence the ROI offered by the use of surveillance data, as well as the opportunity costs of action—and of inaction.

Impediments and Limitations

The economic benefits of using public health surveillance data to prevent new cases and to make the best use of finite resources can be extrapolated for specific conditions or diseases where the baseline incidence can be reliably predicted. However, persistent gaps in baseline data and limitations in standard methodologies have hampered systematic analysis of the value of national public health surveillance systems. To calculate benefits in terms of the number of cases and deaths averted, researchers must often rely on modeling or expert opinions derived from limited data.

The conceptual foundations to help researchers determine how best to identify, evaluate, and measure the benefits of avoiding outbreaks, including the potential disruption of trade and services and less tangible outcomes such as lost public trust, remain uneven. An even more fundamental challenge lies in the linkage between surveillance and response, and the near impossibility of considering either in isolation.[22]

Measuring the outputs and outcomes of disease- or condition-specific programs is far more straightforward than measuring the impact of integrated surveillance systems that collect information on multiple diseases or conditions simultaneously. Early evidence points to the cost-effectiveness of such integrated surveillance programs,[23] but analysis that would allow measurement of performance across programmatic siloes, across institutions, and at the population level is still evolving.

CALCULATING THE COSTS OF SURVEILLANCE

Public health surveillance systems serve as tools to detect priority diseases or events within a relevant time frame for effective public health actions. Surveillance systems incorporate several general elements: standardized guidance to allow prompt case detection; systematic recording and confirmation of cases by trained personnel; mechanisms for reporting data; data analysis and sharing of results; and processes to assure the timeliness and reliability of reporting. The direct costs of conducting public health surveillance encompass the fixed and recurrent costs required to carry out these steps, which include the following:

- Human resources, or the number and type of personnel and the percentage of their working hours dedicated to surveillance activities;
- Materials and equipment, such as computer hardware and software, phones, or printed materials such as casebooks and reporting forms;
- Infrastructure, including the use of buildings or office space where needed; and
- Tools and services, including planning, training, oversight, travel, transport, and access to utilities and communications services.[24]

The full costs of implementing a public health surveillance system depend on preexisting infrastructure, workforce, tools, and the scope of the surveillance efforts. The costs of building and sustaining surveillance systems obviously tend to be higher where the planners must create systems for managing flows of information and materials, rather than incurring the marginal costs of building on existing capacities. The direct costs of integrated disease surveillance carried out at local, intermediate, and national levels may be incurred across thousands of sites in the context of other ongoing surveillance and health service activities.[25]

The process of costing surveillance activities involves the logical, if not simple, listing or mapping of the surveillance system's objectives to identify the inputs needed to carry out each step. The sources of information used to calculate costs can affect total cost estimates. For example, when considering surveillance activities supported through external assistance, international partners may place a different value on goods, services, or human resources than the local market rates.[22]

Options for Analyzing the Benefits of Surveillance

Researchers often employ one of three basic analytical methods to evaluate the benefits of public health interventions: cost–benefit (or benefit–cost), cost–utility, and cost-effectiveness. A **cost analysis** is the act of breaking down a cost summary into its constituents and studying and reporting on each factor.[26] All three methods seek to identify the most efficient means of achieving desired objectives, or stated more specifically, of minimizing resource consumption while maximizing the desired outcomes given a fixed expenditure of resources. These methods can be applied retrospectively, to evaluate programs or policies, or prospectively, to assist in planning and decision-making.

- Cost–benefit analysis: These methods assign a monetary value to health improvements to allow comparison of costs and benefits of policy interventions expressed in units of money/currency. The money scale allows an evaluation of the desirability of various options (with the caveat that not all stakeholders agree on the ethical foundations for valuation of life).
- Cost–utility analysis: These methods yield a ratio of monetary units per unit of *utility*. Utility is generally measured on a scale ranging from no utility to complete utility. (For health status, the extremes are commonly death and perfect health.)
- Cost-effectiveness analysis: **Cost-effectiveness analysis** is a form of economic evaluation where costs are expressed in money terms but consequences are expressed in physical units.[20] It is used to compare different ways of achieving the same objective. Costs in this method are measured in monetary units and compared to nonmonetary effectiveness measures such as final health outcomes (e.g., years of life saved) or intermediate outcomes (e.g., behavioral change expected) to produce improved health (e.g., reduced smoking or increased exercise). Because results of cost-effectiveness analysis are expressed as a ratio, costs and benefits must be defined consistently. In analyzing health interventions, costs may include direct health care costs (e.g., services, drugs, and facility costs), direct non-health-care costs (e.g., transportation, child care, and home modifications), the informal caregiver time, and patient time.

When considering the economics of public health surveillance, it is important to remember that there is no absolute threshold for determining when an action is cost-effective or worth the investment. Commonly, public health interventions are defined as cost-effective in the range of US$50,000–100,000 per life year saved, with a typical value of US$60,000–80,000. For surveillance efforts, especially those that span more than one disease or condition, the challenge is identifying the denominator: the number of years of life that have been saved by detecting a public health threat.

The Cost of Surveillance Failures

For all of these methods, the major challenge in evaluating the impact of public health surveillance is determining what outcomes to measure (Box 8-2). When evaluating the benefits of surveillance for a specific disease or condition, researchers can use historical data to model or predict the number of cases that might have occurred without any interventions and to estimate the number of cases or deaths averted as a result of surveillance activities. Such calculations inevitably rely on some degree of conjecture but can then be applied, with various methods for estimating the costs of illness and deaths, to develop a defensible and understandable estimate. For example, during an outbreak of food-borne illnesses, historical data on outbreaks and the characteristics of pathogens and information on food distribution can be used to estimate the number of cases averted through

BOX 8-2 Basic Concepts and Methods in Cost Analyses

The goal of this family of analyses is to determine the best approaches to minimize resource consumption in achieving the objective or maximize the amount of objective achieved.

Life cycle costs model—Estimates costs of achieving and sustaining a capability (including use, maintenance, and rehabilitation or replacement).

Cost–benefit analysis—Costs and benefits are measured in monetary units.

Cost-effectiveness analysis—Costs are measured in monetary units, while effectiveness is measured in either final or intermediate health outcomes.

$$\frac{\text{Cost(New)} - \text{Cost(Old)}}{\text{Effect(New)} - \text{Effect(Old)}}$$

Cost–utility analysis—To determine which of the alternative interventions, designed to achieve the same or different objectives, produces the most utility for a given level of expenditure, or costs the least to achieve a given level of utility.

Sensitivity analysis—A test of whether uncertainty about the value of a variable (or variables) significantly influences the conclusion of an analysis.

Return on investment—The efficiency of an investment or efficiency of a number of different investments. To calculate ROI, the benefit of an investment is divided by the cost of the investment

$$\text{ROI} = \frac{(\text{Gain from investment} - \text{Cost of investment})}{\text{Cost of investment}}$$

Opportunity cost—The cost of a missed opportunity; the cost associated with forgoing one option to pursue another.

rapid detection and reporting that trigger quick actions, such as risk communications, recalls, or other measures to prevent further exposures.

When applied to national surveillance systems, particularly those that integrate routine indicator-based surveillance for numerous priority diseases and conditions and include an early warning function for epidemic-prone diseases, the question of what outcomes to measure becomes significantly more complex. Models need to predict the cases and deaths averted for multiple diseases in multiple areas across a period of time, and calculations should consider not only the costs of illness and health services but also the costs averted by avoiding disruptions to trade, travel, and essential services.[21] Taken together, these require a significant amount of modeling and extrapolation, and the data needed to determine the baselines and outcomes are often fragmented, at best.

One strategy used to calculate the value of public health surveillance for emerging and epidemic-prone infectious diseases is to use information from past public health crises as a benchmark. For example, the SARS coronavirus most likely emerged in November 2002, causing an outbreak of atypical pneumonia in China's Guangdong Province before transmission in a business hotel in Hong Kong and through air travel that helped spread the disease among international travelers.[27] The SARS outbreak ultimately spread to more than two dozen countries, causing an estimated 8096 cases and 774 deaths by mid-2003.[28] The Asia Development Bank determined that the SARS outbreak weakened gross domestic product (GDP) for 2003 transiently but dramatically in East and Southeast Asia, resulting in losses of about US$18 billion in nominal GDP terms—or about US$2 million for each known case in the region—by comparing pre- and post-SARS economic forecasts. When considering the overall costs of government expenditures and revenue losses incurred by businesses, the tourism industry, and other service sectors, the Bank estimated overall costs to the region of about US$60 billion.[29] The economic impact of the SARS outbreak helped catalyze adoption of the revised International Health Regulations, illustrating how information on the financial impact of a public health event—regardless of the uncertainty in economic or costing models—can help mobilize resources for strengthening and maintaining capacities for public health surveillance.[30]

The Value of Surveillance as a Global Public Good

Another mechanism for determining the value of public health surveillance is to consider surveillance as a global public good. A public good is a product or service that is nonexcludable and nonrival in consumption: no individual can be restricted from using the good, and consumption or access by one individual or group does not reduce consumption or access by another. In other words, no one can be excluded from their benefits and their consumption by one person does not diminish consumption by another.[31] Public goods become global (sometimes called international public goods) in nature when the benefits flow to more than one country and no country can effectively be denied access to those benefits. Classic examples such as lighthouses, clean air, and water represent services whose benefits span borders and cannot be denied to or "used up" by a specific person or group.[32]

As tangible items, such as clean air, and intangible services, such as financial stability, represent global public goods, their opposites, such as transnational pollution and financial crises, have been termed "global public bads." These "bads" include infectious diseases that have the potential to spread to vulnerable populations across borders.[32] Thus, control of communicable diseases—and by extension, public health surveillance actions to help detect disease risks and spread—has been recognized generally as a global public good that merits collective action by government and nongovernmental actors.[33] These collective actions cannot depend on typical market forces; by nature, they require cooperation and information sharing across borders, which may in some cases directly undermine the interests of reporting governments while benefiting populations that have not invested directly in the disease surveillance infrastructure.[34]

This underscores, rather than eliminates, the need for economic tools and analysis to help determine the real costs of investing in public health surveillance systems and the potential benefits of detecting and responding to infectious diseases effectively. One of the greatest challenges in establishing the value of public health surveillance is that, as systems become more effective at detecting cases and collecting information that can be used for action, the number of cases of epidemic-prone diseases should naturally decrease, and support for surveillance programs can wane in parallel. As governments and major funders and implementers of global health initiatives face competing priorities in public health, evidence is needed to encourage decision-makers to maintain momentum for integrated, global surveillance of emerging health threats. This requires a clear understanding of the opportunity costs of disease surveillance failures and the full benefits of successes—and new cooperation across public health disciplines to translate the economics of public health surveillance into effective policies.

KEY SUMMARY POINTS

- The relationship between health and wealth is mutually reinforcing. Informed decision-making to reinforce this health–wealth cycle relies on nations' abilities to detect health threats through public health surveillance and identify interventions to mitigate their consequences.
- Public health surveillance data are used to support appropriate actions to avert and mitigate disease, disability, and deaths, reducing direct and indirect costs to health systems.
- New donors and actors in global health has changed expectations for measurements of impact and effectiveness, including an emphasis on measuring results, rather than process indicators, and looking at programs using the concept of ROI.
- Program funders increasingly require cost–benefit analyses, which require creating conceptual frameworks for assigning cost values to cases and deaths averted for diseases as well as broader economic and societal benefits.
- There is no standard methodology for analyzing the value of national public health surveillance systems.
- Researchers have attempted to calculate benefits associated with numbers of cases and deaths averted by creating models that often rely on limited data.
- Cost–utility and cost-effectiveness analyses may be applied more easily than cost–benefit analysis to evaluate programs or policies related to disease surveillance, although the major challenge for all methods is determining what outcomes to measure.
- One strategy used to calculate the value of public health surveillance is to use information from past public health events as benchmarks for impact.
- Public health surveillance can be categorized as a global public good, with benefits that extend across countries, populations, and possibly even generations.

DISCUSSION QUESTIONS

1. From an economics perspective, why is effective disease surveillance important?
2. How have expectations changed for assessing public health programs?
3. What is return on investment and how does it apply to disease surveillance?
4. How are costs associated with public health surveillance calculated? What types of costs need to be considered?
5. What are the benefits associated with public health surveillance, and how would you assign costs to them?
6. What are cost-effectiveness and cost–utility analyses, and how might you measure effectiveness and utility associated with disease surveillance?
7. How can historical data be used to calculate the value of public health surveillance?
8. Can you think of any other challenges associated with assessing the economic benefit of surveillance?
9. What do you believe should be the top research priorities for economic analysis of public health surveillance in the future?

REFERENCES

1. O'Hare B, Makuta I, Chiwaula L, Bar-zeev N. Income and child mortality in developing countries: a systematic review and meta-analysis. J R Soc Med 2013;106(10):408–14.
2. McKeown T. The Modern Rise of Population. Academic Press, New York, NY; 1976.
3. Omran AR. The epidemiological transition: a theory of the epidemiology of population change. Milbank Mem Fund Q 1971;49:509–38.
4. Paloni A, Zanardi M. The IMF, World Bank and policy reform. vol. 48. London and New York: Routledge Studies in Development Economics; 2006.
5. Preston SH. The changing relation between mortality and level of economic development. Int J Epidemiol 2007;36:484–90.
6. Szreter S. The population health approach in historical perspective. Am J Public Health 2003;93(3):421–31.
7. WHO. Closing the gap in a generation: health equity through action on the social determinants of health. Final Report of the Commission on Social Determinants of Health. Geneva: World Health Organization; 2008.
8. Health CoMa. Macroeconomics and health: investing in health for economic development. Geneva: World Health Organization; 2001.
9. Bloom DE, Canning D. Population health and economic growth (Commission on Growth and Development Working Paper No. 24). Washington, DC: World Bank; 2008.
10. Koplan JP, Bond TC, Merson MH, Reddy KS, Rodriguez MH, Sewankambo NK, et al. Towards a common definition of global health. Lancet 2009;373:1993–5.
11. Mirvis DM, Bloom DE. Population health and economic development in the United States. JAMA 2008;300(1):93–5.
12. Chan EH, Scales DA, Brewer TF, Madoff LC, Pollack MP, Hoen AG, et al. Forecasting high-priority infectious disease surveillance regions: a socioeconomic model. Clin Infect Dis 2013;56(4):517–24.
13. Cash RA, Narasimhan V. Impediments to global surveillance of infectious diseases: consequences of open reporting in a global economy. Bull World Health Organ 2000;78:1358–67.
14. Katz R, Haté V, Kornblet S, Fischer JE. Costing framework for International Health Regulations (2005). Emerg Infect Dis 2012;18:1121–7.
15. Schmidt M. Return on Investment (ROI) Explained: Definition, Meaning, and Example Calculations. Encyclopedia of Business Terms and Methods. Solution Matrix Ltd, Boston, MA; 2015. <https://www.business-case-analysis.com/return-on-investment.html>; 23 September 2015.
16. Birdsall N, Savedoff WD. Cash on delivery: a new approach to foreign aid. Washington DC: Center for Global Development; 2010.
17. Fritsche GB, Soeters R, Meessen B. Performance-Based Financing Toolkit. World Bank, Washington, DC; 2014. p. 6-12. <https://openknowledge.worldbank.org>; 23 September 2015.
18. Bank W. Using results-based financing to achieve maternal & child health: progress report. Washington DC: World Bank; 2013.
19. Copeland CW. Cost-benefit and other analysis requirement in the rulemaking process. Washington DC: Congressional Research Service; 2011.
20. World Health Organization. Health systems strengthening glossary, <http://www.who.int/healthsystems/hss_glossary/en/index2.html/>; 2011. [accessed 2015].
21. Schmidt M. Return on Investment (ROI) Explained: Definition, Meaning, and Example Calculations. Encyclopedia of Business Terms and Methods. Solution Matrix Ltd, Boston, MA; 2015. <https://www.business-case-analysis.com/return-on-investment.html>; 23 September 2015.
22. Anker M. Evaluating the costs and benefits of national surveillance and response systems. Geneva: World Health Organization; 2005.
23. Somda ZC, Perry HN, Messonier NH, Djingarey MH, Ki SO, Meltzer MI. Modeling the cost-effectiveness of the integrated disease surveillance and response (IDSR) system: meningitis in Burkina Faso. PLoS One 2010; 5(9):e13044.
24. German RRC. Recommendations from the guidelines working group. MMWR 2001;50(RR13):1–35.
25. Somda ZC, Meltzer MI, Perry HN. SurvCost 1.0: A manual to assist country and district public health officials in estimating the cost of the implementation of integrated disease surveillance and response systems (Beta test version). Atlanta, Georgia: Centers for Disease Control and prevention, National Center for Prevention, Detection and Control of Infectious Diseases (NCPDCID), Division of Emerging Infections and Surveillance Services (DEISS), U.S. Department of Health and Human Services; 2007.
26. Baltussen R, Adam T, Tan-Torres Edejer T, Hutubessy R, Acharya A, Evans DB, Murray CJL. Part One: Methods for generalized cost-effectiveness analysis. In: Adam T, Baltussen R, Tan-Torres Edejer T, Evans DB, Hutubessy R, Acharya A, Murray CJL, editors. Making Choices in Health: WHO Guide to Cost Effectiveness Analysis. World Health Organization, Geneva; 2003. p3–15.
27. Group SARSSE. Consensus document on the epidemiology of severe acute respiratory syndrome (SARS). Geneva: Department of Communicable Disease Surveillance and Response; 2003.
28. World Health Organization. Summary of probable SARS cases with onset of illness from 1 November 2002 to 31 July 2003, <http://www.who.int/csr/sars/country/table2004_04_21/en/>; 2004. [Accessed 01.03.2014].
29. Asian Development Bank. Asian Development Outlook 2003. Manila. 2003. 75–92.
30. Katz R, Fischer J. The revised international health regulations: a framework for global pandemic response. Global Health Governance 2010;3.
31. World Health Organization. Global public goods, <http://www.who.int/trade/glossary/story041/en/>;2010, [accessed 2015].
32. Kaul I, Grunberg I, Stern MA. Global public goods: international cooperation in the 21st century. New York: United Nations Development Programme; 1999. p. 2–16. [Chapter 1: Defining global public health goods].
33. Smith RD. Global public goods and health. Bull World Health Organ 2003;81(7):475.
34. Zacher M. Global epidemiological surveillance: international cooperation to monitor infectious diseases. In: Kaul I, Grunberg I, Stern MA, editors. Global public goods: international cooperation in the 21st century. New York: Oxford University Press; 1999. p. 266–84.

CHAPTER

9

Supply and Demand of the Public Health Workforce

Peter Nsubuga, Jeffrey Engel

The issue of workforce training and competency is central to the success of any public health system. Governmental public health agencies have a responsibility to identify the public health workforce needs within their jurisdictions and to implement policies and programs to fill those needs.

IOM Report of 2003, "Who Will Keep the Public Healthy? Educating Public Health Professionals in the 21st Century"

KEY WORDS

Workforce
Field epidemiologists
Competency
Workforce capacity
Field Epidemiology and Laboratory Training Program
EIS
Epidemiologist
CSTE

INTRODUCTION

This chapter will discuss how a well-functioning workforce can be used to operate a robust public health surveillance and response system. A public health surveillance and response system is a type of health information system with the addition of service through response; it is assumed that this system will be well led, well financed, and equitable. **Public health** is an organized effort by society, primarily through its public institutions to improve, promote, protect, and restore the health of the population through collective action.[1] It includes services such as health situation analysis, health surveillance, health promotion, prevention, infectious disease control, environmental protection, and sanitation, disaster and health emergency preparedness and response, and occupational health, among others.[2]

There is a growing gap between the supply of health care professionals and the demand for their services, and it is recognized as a key issue for health and development worldwide. As a result of this shortage, many health programs have consistently experienced shortages of suitable health personnel, especially in developing countries, which have the highest disease burden and where the 2015 Millennium Development Goals (MDGs) are not being achieved (see Chapter 29).

According to the World Health Organization (WHO), there is an estimated global shortage of 4.3 million health workers, including 2.4 million physicians, nurses, and midwives.[3] This deficiency translates to over 1 billion people without access to health care. Although many countries are affected by this shortage, 57 countries have been identified as "in crisis." Of these, 36 are in sub-Saharan Africa. In a number of countries, there are underemployed and unemployed health professionals in addition to the shortages of available personnel, further contributing to the labor shortage. This is the context in which public health surveillance and response systems operate in the developing world.

In the developed world, using the USA as an example, the public health enterprise is distributed among federal, state, territorial, local, and tribal agencies. Compared to sub-Saharan Africa, public health epidemiologists, who are central to the public health surveillance workforce, number an order of greater magnitude, hence are counted per 100,000 people versus 1,000,000 people. The vast clinical enterprise in the USA, predominately in the private sector, will not be discussed in this chapter except in the context of data sharing.

This chapter will look at the current status of the global public health workforce and an in-depth look at the most recent US public health workforce capacity national assessment.

THE GLOBAL PUBLIC HEALTH WORKFORCE

Workforce is a term for all the people working or available to work in a country, industry, or on a project.[4] The professions that contribute to the public health workforce are varied and include nurses, physicians, laboratory scientists, environmental scientists, epidemiologists, managers, social workers, and others. Because of these underlying differences in skill sets, the training required to perform public health functions, including public health surveillance, is often learned on the job or through specific competency-based training programs. **Competency** is a term for the measurable or observable knowledge, skills, abilities, and behaviors critical to successful job performance.[5] Workforce competencies are the particular skills and abilities necessary to succeed in that sector of the workforce. They must be defined for each job description according to tiers, or levels, of the job function in hierarchical order.

One example in a developing context is the operation of public health surveillance and response systems in Africa, which are inherently a function of the government, conducted primarily through ministries of health and local government staff or equivalent ministries.[6] In countries where One Health (see Chapter 14) is practiced, the ministries in charge of veterinary services, usually the ministries of agriculture and wildlife, play an additional role.[7] In some countries there is some participation in the public health surveillance system (and response, to a lesser degree) from the nongovernmental sector, particularly nonprofit organizations (often religion or mission affiliated-health facilities). However, there is usually very limited participation by private for-profit health units in public health surveillance and response. The staff who participate in public health surveillance and response have varying levels of prior training before they start working in governmental health facilities—ranging from basic at the peripheral levels to advanced training at the higher administrative levels (e.g., district, province or state, and national agencies). Some countries have community health workers (sometimes referred to as village health workers or extension workers), who may be paid or unpaid volunteers, who also conduct public health surveillance for priority health conditions as part of their duties.[7]

The paucity of health care staff in developing countries is well known. Public health duties are performed in addition to the clinical duties that these few staff must perform, and some of the clinical duties (e.g., delivering babies) are urgent. Moreover, in the past, each disease control program designed and implemented its own public health surveillance system using the same few staff at the frontline, thereby contributing to their workload, which led to poor outcomes, for the clinical and public health systems. In recognition of this issue, WHO's Africa Regional Office (WHO-AFRO) developed and implemented the Integrated Disease Surveillance and Response (IDSR) strategy in 1998 with the support of several partners.[8-11]

Africa has very few professionals trained in epidemiology, particularly in field epidemiology, which emphasizes public health surveillance and response. **Epidemiologists** are public health professionals who investigate patterns and causes of disease and injury in humans. They seek to reduce the risk and occurrence of negative health outcomes through research, community education, and health policy.[12] The proposed target for the ideal number of trained field epidemiologists for a country is 3–5 trained field epidemiologists per million residents, preferably working in suitable designated public health units, with background training as physicians or nurses, laboratory scientists, or veterinarians.[13]

TRAINING THE GLOBAL PUBLIC HEALTH WORKFORCE

Competency-based field epidemiology training programs provide an opportunity to learn public health surveillance and response through workplace-based education. These programs involve applied (i.e., field-based) projects after short classroom or didactic courses.[14] They typically offer training through service provision, which provides an immediate public health purpose to the trainees. Training is also combined with mentoring and supervision, providing trainees with immediate reinforcement of the concepts. Experienced field supervisors, through regular feedback, follow-up, and recommendations, mentor the trainees while they are working in field. **Field epidemiologists** are public health epidemiologists who, when a problem is unexpected, must travel to and work in the field to solve the problem, and the extent of the investigation is likely to be limited because of the imperative for timely intervention.[15] This aspect of the training is critical, for it ensures high-quality training and builds stronger relationships between mentors and trainees as they progress. These components distinguish this form of training from more traditional university-only or classroom-only settings. Competency-based training requires more resources than purely classroom-based work, but the investment produces a cadre of graduates who have unique experiences and skills critical for performing essential public health functions, including public health surveillance.[16]

Field Epidemiology and Laboratory Training Program

The US Centers for Disease Control and Prevention (CDC)'s Epidemic Intelligence Service (EIS) program is one strategy used to strengthen US public health surveillance and response over the more than 60 years of EIS's existence. **Epidemic Intelligence Service** is a US 2-year postgraduate training program of service and on-the-job learning for health professionals interested in the practice of applied epidemiology.[17] EIS officers are on the public health frontlines, conducting epidemiologic investigations, research, and public health surveillance both nationally and internationally. Several countries have taken the EIS model and adapted it to fit their contexts. **Field Epidemiology and Laboratory Training Program (FELTP)** is a program that focuses on assisting countries to build sustainable capacity for detecting and responding to health threats and to develop expertise so disease outbreaks can be detected locally and prevented from spreading.[18] In Africa, the EIS model led to the FELTPs, which train program participants in applied epidemiology while developing a workforce that can operate public health- and laboratory-based surveillance systems. The CDC works with regional partners and ministries of health to develop such programs, which are modeled after the CDC's EIS.

Some countries have included veterinarians as a specific track in their FELTPs to address animal–human issues. Some countries have developed strategic plans to use FELTPs as the anchor for developing a holistic national and subnational public health surveillance and response workforce that includes epidemiologists and public health laboratory scientists trained in a combination of degree and non-degree granting courses.[16, 19, 20]

For example, Nigeria has developed a workforce development plan with the 2-year FELTP at the apex.[21] The FELTP is a partnership between the Federal Ministry of Health, the Federal Ministry of Agriculture, and universities, which grant Masters of Public Health (Field Epidemiology or Laboratory Management and Epidemiology) degrees. The plan is a four-tier pyramid plan, which, in addition to the FELTP at the top, also includes 3-month mid-level courses in the middle, a 1-week fundamental short course at the base, and an additional base of online certificate courses. FELTP trainees are exceptionally suited to support public health emergency response activities initiated at the Federal Ministry of Health and the state levels as part of their training. Trainees are located at the federal level, which allows the 2-year residents to support the national Emergency Operations Center and obtain hands-on training in coordinating emergency response activities. The trainees are trained in public health evaluation and can provide a needed service through postemergency response evaluations to improve the public health surveillance and response system.

THE VISION FOR A GLOBAL PUBLIC HEALTH WORKFORCE

Public health surveillance and response in the developed and developing world should aim for a state where forecasting and predicting potential threats is the norm rather than the exception. In order for this vision to be achieved there should be an increased focus on training and retaining public health professionals who will sustain the public health system. Training should be implemented through competency-based approaches that work for the diverse

Level	Structure	Staffing	Number	Duties
National N= 1	Multi-disease Surveillance, Response, and Public Health Laboratory Group	Field Epidemiologists (FELTP graduates), includes veterinarians	At least 10 Total = 10	Multi-disease surveillance and response for IDSR, IHR, NCDs, key programs
		Public Health Laboratory Scientists (FELTP graduates)	At least 5 Total = 5	Public health laboratory network for IDSR, IHR, NCDs
Regional N= 10	Regional Multi-disease Surveillance, Response, and Public Health Laboratory Unit	Field Epidemiologists (FELTP graduates), includes veterinarians	At least 2 per region Total = 20	Regional multi-disease surveillance and response
		Public Health Laboratory Scientists (FELTP graduates)	At least 1 per region Total = 10	Regional public health laboratory network development
District N =100	Complimentary structures	FELTP short course graduates	At least 2-3 per district Total = 200-300	IDSR development at district level; Public health response
Total FELTP 2-year graduates = at least 45, total short course graduates at least 200				

FIG. 9-1 Public health staffing for a country with 100 districts.

nature of the public health workforce.[22] Beyond training, there is the often poorly understood need to develop a public health system in which trained public health professionals can be hired to implement public health surveillance and response tasks in a sustainable manner. To do this effectively, countries need to develop positions, at all levels of the administrative or health system, for suitably trained public health workers. An illustrative example of a public health structure that can be achieved through competency-based training for a country with 100 districts, 10 regions, and one national level is shown in Fig. 9-1. An FELTP should be operating for approximately five years in order to achieve this critical mass.

PUBLIC HEALTH WORKFORCE CAPACITY IN THE USA

For the developed world, as in the USA, teams of epidemiologists, laboratorians, and their support staff perform the work of public health surveillance. In 1994, the US Public Health Functions Steering Committee identified the core functions of a public health system: (a) prevent epidemics and the spread of disease; (b) protect against environmental hazards; (c) prevent injuries; (d) promote and encourage healthy behaviors; (e) respond to disasters and assist communities in recovery; and (f) assure the quality and accessibility of health services.[23] These core functions would be carried out through the ten Essential Public Health Services for a healthy population, which are as follows:

1. *"monitoring health status to identify community health problems;*
2. *diagnosing and investigating health problems and health hazards in the community;*
3. *informing, educating, and empowering people about health issues;*
4. *mobilizing community partnerships to identify and solve health problems;*
5. *developing plans and policies that support individual and community health efforts;*
6. *enforcing laws and regulations that protect health and ensure safety;*
7. *linking people to personal health services and assuring provision of healthcare when otherwise unavailable;*

8. *assuring a competent public health workforce;*
9. *evaluating effectiveness, accessibility, and quality of personal- and population-based health services; and*
10. *promoting research which provides insights and innovative solutions to health problems.*"[23]

This section will focus on the US epidemiologist workforce distribution, capacity and competency assessments, and the alignment with the Essential Public Health Services. The US Department of Labor, Bureau of Labor Statistics' Standard Occupational Classification system defines an epidemiologist as a medical scientist who investigates and describes the determinants and distribution of disease, disability, or health outcomes; and may develop the means for prevention and control.[24] Epidemiologists exist across the public health enterprise of the federal, state, territorial, and local (including cities, counties, and tribes) public health government agencies. This governmental workforce, informally known as applied public health epidemiologists, is differentiated from academic and private sector epidemiologists who conduct research, teach, or carry out surveillance and analytics for specific populations, such as for health insurance companies or health care providers.

US Federal Workforce Capacity Efforts

Workforce capacity is a term for a country or organization's ability to ensure sufficient staffing levels to accomplish its work processes and successfully deliver its products or services to the targeted group or population.[25] At the federal level, the majority of applied public health epidemiologists are uniformed officers of the US Public Health Service Commissioned Corps, or civilian employees, in the US Department of Health and Human Services, the Department of Agriculture, and the Environmental Protection Agency; many fewer are employed in other departments of the executive branch of the federal government. The CDC serves as the lead agency for public health surveillance within the Department of Health and Human Services; however, federal epidemiologists perform important surveillance activities in other health agencies, including the Food and Drug Administration, Health Resources and Services Administration, and Centers for Medicare and Medicaid Services, among others. The CDC epidemiology workforce is composed of highly educated and trained professionals with a minimum of a graduate school degree (MPH, MSPH, PhD, or DrPH) and/or a clinical professional degree (MD, DO, DVM, DDS, RN, or PharmD). Furthermore, these epidemiologists may have completed CDC's prestigious 2-year EIS program.[26] The CDC, within its centers, institutes, and offices, and its skilled workforce, guides national public health surveillance programs and aggregates and analyzes state jurisdictional reports to monitor the nation's health.

The US Public Health Workforce in a Federated Model

Despite this leadership role, the CDC, as part of the federal government, has constitutional limitations on public health surveillance activities. Only the states have authority to collect identifiable data from individuals suspected or identified as having reportable diseases or conditions, and states voluntarily notify the CDC, hence the origin of the National Notifiable Disease Surveillance System.[27] In the hierarchy of the public health enterprise, local jurisdictions, even large cities, investigate and report cases to their state, a work flow that further emphasizes the central role of the state health department and its workforce in national surveillance.

The applied epidemiology workforce in government public health agencies in the USA is classified by experience, professional degree, and capacity to perform specific job duties (i.e., competencies). The classification levels have been identified as tiers: Tier 1, entry-level or basic; Tier 2, mid-level; Tier 3a, supervisor or program manager; and Tier 3b, senior scientist or subject matter expert, with competencies at each tier.[28] The competencies for training programs or fellowships for applied epidemiologists are listed in Box 9-1, summarized from various sources.[28, 29]

ASSESSING US NATIONAL PUBLIC HEALTH WORKFORCE CAPACITY AND COMPETENCY

Beginning in 2001, assessments of state-level epidemiology workforce capacity within the USA have been performed periodically by the **Council of State and Territorial Epidemiologists** (CSTE). CSTE is an organization of member

BOX 9-1 Core Competencies for Training of Applied Epidemiologists in Government Public Health Agencies

Epidemiologic methods

Design a surveillance system for a public health issue and identify surveillance data needs
Evaluate an existing surveillance system and identify key surveillance findings
Design data collection tools to address a health problem
Collect health data and create and manage a database
Analyze and characterize epidemiologic data with statistical software
Apply epidemiologic principles to make recommendations on data validity
Interpret data and findings and recommend control measures, prevention programs, or other public health interventions
Apply understanding of causes of disease in practicing epidemiology
Apply knowledge of laboratory resources to support epidemiologic practice
Understand types of study design and design an epidemiologic study

Communication

Write surveillance and field investigation reports
Present epidemiologic data using graphic software
Demonstrate the skills and principles of risk communication and be able to communicate epidemiology findings orally and in writing to nonprofessional audiences
Present research results in a scientific poster, report or manuscript
Present data orally using appropriate media

Public health practice, policy, and legal issues

Have an understanding of public health law
Apply privacy laws to protect confidentiality including the Health Insurance Portability and Accountability Act of 1996 (HIPAA)
Distinguish between public health practice and research
Understand policies designed for the protection of human subjects and the role for an institutional review board (IRB) process
Know the essential public health functions
Practice culturally appropriate epidemiologic activities and effectively negotiate culturally sensitive issues
Understand the roles of local, state, and federal public health agencies
Understand the diversity of epidemiology and how it is used in different program areas
Understand role in bioterrorism and emergency preparedness and response

states and territories representing public health epidemiologists. CSTE works to establish more effective relationships among state and other health agencies.[30] It also provides technical advice and assistance to partner organizations and to federal public health agencies such as the CDC.

Detailed questionnaires sent to state epidemiologists' offices inquire about the number, category, funding sources, and other descriptive factors of the epidemiology workforce in state health departments. Structured around the 10 essential public health services and estimates of capacity in eight program areas (bioterrorism and emergency response; chronic diseases; environmental health; infectious diseases; injury; maternal and child health; occupational health; and oral health), enumerations, trends, and workforce gaps in epidemiology and surveillance have been determined.[31]

Results from the Council of State and Territorial Epidemiology Capacity Assessment (2009–2013)

Recent assessments of the 50 states and the District of Columbia performed in 2009[31] and 2013[32] were analyzed in three groupings by small (<2.65 million people), medium (2.65–6 million), and large (>6 million) populations. In the 4-year interval between 2009 and 2013, the median number of epidemiologists rose in small jurisdictions (from

1.41 to 2.57 epidemiologists per 100,000 people) and in large jurisdictions (from 0.54 to 0.59); in medium jurisdictions, the median fell from 1.1 to 1.04 epidemiologists per 100,000 people. The overall US estimate rose from 0.77 to 1.04 epidemiologists per 100,000. Assessments on capacity in different program areas from 2004 to 2013 are shown in Fig. 9-2.[32] The state health department epidemiologist workforce representation by highest obtained degree was compared from 2009 to 2013 with results presented in Fig. 9-3.[32]

Local US Public Health Workforce Capacity

The local epidemiology workforce was assessed in a 2010 CSTE enumeration analysis, along with the 50 states and the District of Columbia.[33] The 3754 applied epidemiologists identified throughout the USA resulted in an overall rate of 1.22 epidemiologists per 100,000 people. In a two-grouping analysis by population, these epidemiologists were not distributed equally; smaller (<5 million people) states reported more epidemiologists per 100,000 people than the larger (>5 million) states (1.48 vs. 1.14). However, the five largest cities had more epidemiologists than either state grouping (2.10 per 100,000).

US Workforce Capacity and Competency

The results of these assessments were used to examine alignment and gaps with the aforementioned Essential Public Health Services,[24] in particular essential services 1, 2, 9, and 10, which rely heavily on epidemiologic and surveillance functions. The majority of the 50 states and the District of Columbia responded that they had at least substantial capacity to perform services 1 and 2 (health monitoring and diagnosis and investigation), but less than substantial capacity to perform services 9 and 10 (assess personal and population-based health services and research for new solutions to health problems).[32]

By program area, more than half of the respondents had substantial to full capacity in infectious disease, bioterrorism and emergency response, maternal and child health, and chronic disease. In contrast, more than half reported

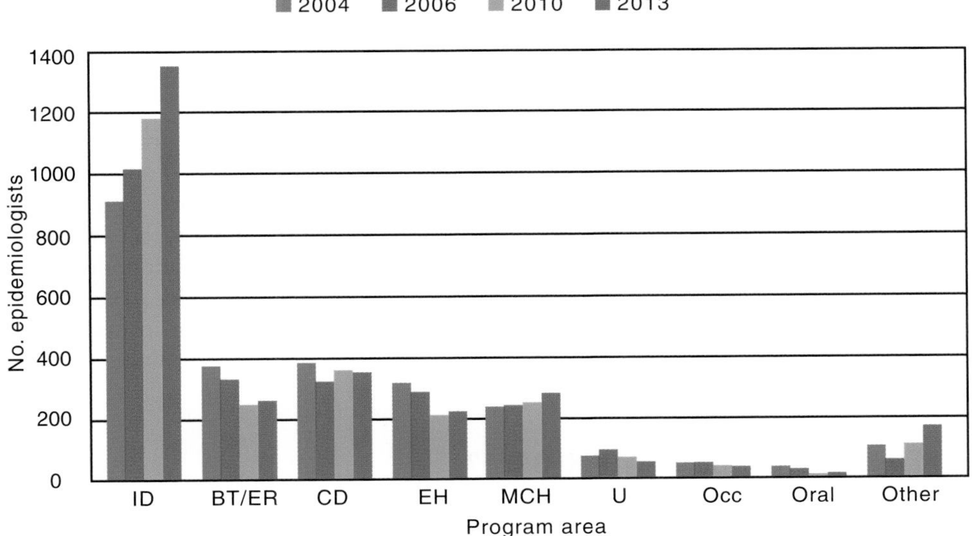

ID=infectious diseases; BT/ER=bioterrorism and emergency response; CD=chronic disease; EH=environmental health; MCH=maternal and child health; IJ=injury and violence prevention; Occ=occupational health; Oral=oral and dental health; Other includes mental health, substance abuse, and other non-categorized

FIG. 9-2 Trends in epidemiology capacity by program area in the USA, 2004–2013.

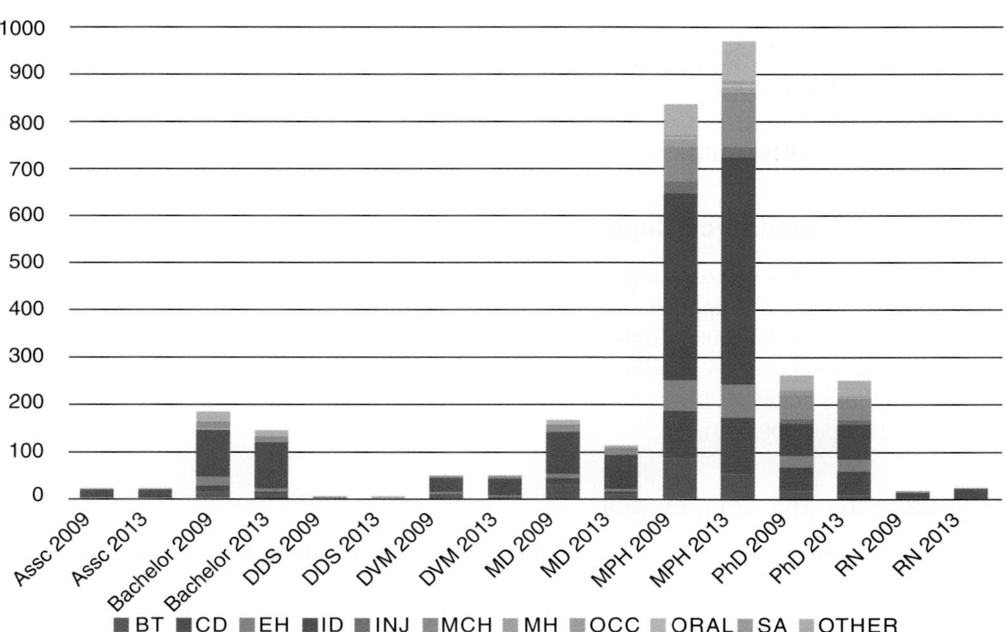

ID=infectious diseases; BT/ER=bioterrorism and emergency response; CD=chronic disease; EH=environ mental health; MCH=maternal and child health; IJ=injury and violence prevention; Occ=occupational health; Oral=oral and dental health; Other includes mental health, substance abuse, and other non-categorized

FIG. 9-3 Highest degree obtained by epidemiologists in various programs in state health departments: 2009 to 2013 comparison.

minimal to no capacity in environmental health, injury, occupational health, substance abuse, and oral health.[32] The 36 states (representing 68% of the US population) that responded in 2008 as needing additional epidemiologists to fully carry out the four essential services stated that an additional 1490 epidemiologists were needed, more than double the 1470 enumerated in the same 36 states.[32]

In addition to these measured capacity needs, there is an emerging competency gap growing in workforce development of applied epidemiologists, notably in the field of public health informatics. Public health informatics is broadly defined as the systematic application of knowledge about systems that capture, manage, analyze, and use information to improve population health.[34] Practically, this translates into the application of information technology (IT) into public health practice and is especially relevant to surveillance. The rapid adoption of electronic health records (EHRs) in clinical care, exponential IT improvements (speed, storage, messaging, security, standardization, and interoperability), and advances in health policy have led to a virtual revolution in health data acquisition, exchange, analysis, and reporting. These developments promise to vastly improve sensitivity, specificity, completeness, and timeliness of public health surveillance systems.

HOW PREPARED IS THE CURRENT WORKFORCE?

Government public health epidemiologists and informaticians are transforming surveillance systems by establishing ongoing, bidirectional, and timely electronic data flow with point-of-care and clinical data sources, involving leveraging EHRs from clinical encounters to automatically report legally mandated reportable events to public health. Syndromic surveillance involves collecting real-time encounters with emergency medical services by utilizing natural language algorithms that define syndromes rather than definitive diagnoses. These informatics capabilities stem from public health's use of EHRs, as determined by US Centers for Medicare and Medicaid Services.[35] Global health security is increasingly becoming important, as the world realizes that it is interconnected; a disease occurring in one country is often only an airplane ride away from another.[22] Also, as the climate changes and the population expands, diseases and their associated vectors are moving from endemic regions to other new regions.

In light of these issues, a public health surveillance and response workforce that is trained to detect, respond, and predict the occurrence of priority diseases is more important than ever. Efforts are being made to prepare the current and future public health workforce to adopt and utilize modern information system tools and public health informatics competencies are being defined.[36] There is no official classification of the informatician in the 2010 US Department of Labor Standard Occupational Classification.

One of the most widely implemented newer functionalities utilized by epidemiologists is automated electronic laboratory reporting of reportable conditions to public health electronic disease surveillance systems. In a 2010 assessment, 22 (45%) states in the USA reported receiving between 50% and 99% of positive reportable infectious disease laboratory results electronically.[37] Here, the epidemiologist, working as an informatician and/or with ICT specialists, develops, implements, and maintains messaging from public and private sector (mainly hospital) laboratory information systems. When fully operational, public health receives notification in real-time of an abnormal laboratory report of a disease or condition that is reportable in that jurisdiction, and thus an epidemiologist can initiate an investigation or associate the report to an existing case. New skill sets for epidemiologists include an understanding, including in-depth programming skills, of machine language translation and messaging into standard surveillance forms that reside on public health agency internet-based platforms. These skill sets are being offered by more schools of public health, fellowships, and on-the-job training experiences.[38]

The Emerging Field of Public Health Informatics

The US public health informatics field was greatly accelerated in 2009 by the passage of the Health Information Technology for Economic and Clinical Health Act (HITECH).[39] Under the HITECH Act, nearly US$26 billion was allocated to the federal Department of Health and Human Services to promote and expand the adoption of health information technology. The Office of the National Coordinator (ONC) for HIT was created in 2004 and its activities were accelerated by the HITECH mandate. Most HITECH resources were used to incentivize the clinical care sector by supporting training on and implementation of EHRs to eligible providers, mainly physicians and hospitals. Importantly, however, led by ONC, significant policy was directed to population health and public health practice by the meaningful use rules that predicate incentive payment to providers for adoption of the EHR.[40]

Beginning in 2013, the EHR meaningful use requirements in the public health surveillance domain were incorporated into the certification and attestation process of EHR implementation and have heralded a new era of information sharing and integration between the clinical and public health sectors. These requirements include a technical interoperable platform between the provider and the public health agency that allow electronic reporting of immunizations to state immunization registries, cancer diagnoses to state cancer registries, select clinical data elements (e.g., age, gender, address, chief complaint, and vital signs) to syndromic surveillance systems, and electronic laboratory reporting of positive results of nationally notifiable conditions. A meaningful use requirement of automated case reporting that would interface with the EHR clinical decision support functionality to prompt the provider to transmit to public health an entire medical record visit of a patient presenting with a reportable disease is in development.

These meaningful use requirements have provided new opportunities to public health epidemiologists for more sensitive, specific, complete, and timely surveillance of reportable conditions, immunization rates, preparedness and response, and outbreak detection and management. These requirements have also revealed a widening gap in public health work force capacity and competency in the emerging field of public health informatics. In fact, a decade before the HITECH Act, the CDC and its partners had started system upgrades to the National Notifiable Disease Surveillance System, began electronic laboratory reporting, initiated syndromic surveillance (also known as BioSense) and developed workforce competency recommendations.[37] Simultaneously, states were upgrading information systems including immunization and cancer registries and electronic disease surveillance systems. However, the HITECH Act was a one-sided stimulus package to the clinical sector; hence, in the years following its implementation, public health agencies have fallen further behind. In the 2013 CSTE Epidemiology Capacity assessment, one third of states had no functional electronic laboratory reporting, considered a core function of modern public health informatics and surveillance.

Academic centers have begun to address the public health informatics workforce gap. However, a search of the Association of Schools and Programs in Public Health database showed only four schools or programs offering an accredited public health informatics certificate.[41] Furthermore, there has been no formal evaluation of these certificates answering questions like how well prepared graduates are for the workplace or assessing alignment of curriculum with the needs of employers, especially government public health agencies. The CDC has led the nation in providing or funding postgraduate fellowships and on-the-job training opportunities in public health informatics, but similar to academic programs, these efforts are too recent to have undergone evaluation.

In 2013, the African One Health e-Surveillance Initiative, led by the African Field Epidemiology Network, developed a pilot project to help African countries develop strategic plans for sustainable electronic surveillance within the IDSR framework. This pilot project was designed to provide countries with a tailored roadmap to develop and enhance public health infrastructure and workforce through the integration of electronic tools. The objective of the pilot project was to develop and recommend country-specific strategic plans for implementing One Health e-Surveillance that abides by IDSR and International Health Regulations (IHR) (2005) strategies and guidelines by using regional and national country-level workgroups. Future efforts that engage at the local level in developing nations will be critical for the success of addressing the remaining gaps and obstacles faced by many countries when it comes to implementing e-Surveillance. Centers for training the workforce need to be established at the local and regional levels to have an immediate and long-lasting effect. Any surveillance system, but especially electronic surveillance systems, cannot function properly without a robust and competent workforce at the helm.

REMAINING WORKFORCE CHALLENGES AND RECOMMENDATIONS

There are many challenges in implementing health ICT into the public health surveillance workflow; these can be categorized into three areas: governance, funding, and workforce.[36] Governance refers to the authority and accountability structure that oversees the electronic transmission of identifiable patient information between the public and private sectors and the appropriate and legal use of this information (see Chapter 13).[42]

The funding of the necessary infrastructure, platforms, and software needed within governmental public health agencies is formidable. Related to needing adequate infrastructure, platforms, and software, the new workforce must include information technologists, epidemiologists with new competencies, and public health informaticians (a hybrid of the first two); this staffing structure may be a significant barrier for many jurisdictions.

To address these gaps within the USA, the following actions are recommended:

1. Epidemiology training at all levels should incorporate the information sciences and systems skills necessary to connect with clinical information systems.
2. Public health surveillance workflows should integrate with local, regional, and state clinical provider networks by adopting and implementing interoperable platforms and instituting public–private governance structures over health data, including confidentiality and security safeguards.
3. Fiscal policies should budget sustainable support of public health informatics within government public health agencies with public funds.
4. All sectors should share accountability for the new information-sharing infrastructure, ultimately by demonstrating improvement in population health and overall cost savings to society.
5. The workforce training pipeline, particularly in schools and programs of public health, should align epidemiology curriculum, informatics certification and accreditation standards with the needs of government public health employers, notably training epidemiologists to understand, utilize and collect public health meaningful use business and technology requirements.

6. As the HITECH Act provided jumpstart funding for EHR implementation to the clinical sector, similar public funding is needed to upgrade the public health sector, both for technology infrastructure and workforce development.

To address gaps in workforce, developing nations should address the following recommendations:

1. Consider implementing a four-tier pyramidal workforce development program for their public health surveillance and response staff. The four-tiers comprise a 2-year FELTP at the apex and shorter competency-based field epidemiology training programs below (e.g., 1-year diploma, 3-month certificate), with a base of 2-week certificate level applied epidemiology training programs for the frontline workers.
2. Trained workforce should be deployed and supported through multidisease surveillance and response units at all levels of the health system. These units should have a One Health approach to public health surveillance and response to address the increasing incidence of zoonotic diseases as well as the unaddressed problem of noncommunicable diseases and other public health problems.
3. Public health staff in developing nations should be obtained from personnel with differing but complementary background training (e.g., physicians, nurses, clinical officers, veterinarians, laboratory scientists, social workers) to address the multifaceted nature of the public health problems that are faced by developing nations.

Developing nations should also incorporate public health and use FELTPs or equivalent applied epidemiology and public health laboratory leadership training programs to develop multidisease surveillance and response capabilities.

KEY SUMMARY POINTS

- Public health professionals, especially in international settings, are stretched thin and often do not have the skills or time to adequately address public health, epidemiology, and surveillance needs.
- Competency-based field epidemiology training programs provide an opportunity for public health surveillance and response education by providing workplace-based learning through applied (i.e., field-based) projects after short classroom or didactic courses.
- The proposed target for the ideal number of trained field epidemiologists for a country is 3–5 trained field epidemiologists per million people, preferably working in suitable designated public health units, with background training as physicians or nurses, laboratory scientists, or veterinarians.
- In 2013, the overall US estimate of epidemiologists in state health departments rose to 1.04 per 100,000 people.
- There is an emerging competency and capacity gap in the field of public health informatics. There should be an increased focus on training and retaining public health professionals who will sustain the public health system through increased surveillance and informatics-related competencies.
- Funding the necessary infrastructure, platforms, and software for modern public health practice, and training the public health workforce to use such infrastructure, platforms, and software, is essential for improving public health.
- At the international level, governance deals with the regulation of political exchanges between countries, which leads governments to form connected sets of both formal and informal rules that direct behavioral roles, restrain activity, and shape expectations of sovereign states.
- The World Health Assembly (WHA) constituted of WHO member states (currently 196), has the authority to adopt regulations and resolutions, which are then implemented by countries with the support of the WHO secretariat. For over 40 years, the WHO's IHR have been the primary legally binding global agreement addressing the risks of the international spread of infectious disease. Under the IHR (2005), countries must report "an extraordinary event" which is determined, as provided in the Regulations, and refers to a "public health emergency of international concern (PHEIC)."
- Experience has shown that a weakness in one country's capacities to detect and respond to emerging events is a threat to all others. International organizations share a responsibility in supporting member states in the strengthening of capabilities for early warning and rapid response, by acting both at local and global levels.
- The provision of appropriate tools and rapid access to subject matter experts and networks for event-based surveillance and laboratories, continues to be crucial for providing a coordinated analysis and response (i.e., GOARN, EDPLN).
- Under the IHR (2005), states have made great strides in capacity building. Maintaining high quality and adequate capacities over time is a priority.

DISCUSSION QUESTIONS

1. Compare and contrast the public health surveillance workforce in the developing world and in the developed world. What are the similarities and differences in training, competency, and capacity?
2. Using examples such as Middle East Respiratory Syndrome coronavirus or a cardiovascular disease, estimate the public health workforce and associated competencies needed to implement a new surveillance system for an emerging public health threat in a defined population. What kinds of skills, roles, and public health professionals would be needed?
3. What issues go into developing a public health surveillance and response workforce for a country?
4. How can existing public health practitioners be trained for the new competencies needed for modern informatics and surveillance responsibilities in a public health agency?
5. What specific challenges can you identify in funding the necessary infrastructure, platforms, and software in public health agencies?

REFERENCES

1. La salud pública en las Americas: nuevos conceptos, análisis del desempeño y bases para la acción. Revista do Instituto de Medicina Tropical de São Paulo 2003;45:102.
2. World Health Organization. WHO | Health systems strengthening glossary, <http://www.who.int/healthsystems/hss_glossary/en/index2.html/>; 2011 [2015].
3. WHO. The World Health Report 2006 - working together for health. World Health Organization; 2006.
4. Workforce. American heritage dictionary of the English language. 5th ed. Houghton Mifflin Harcourt; 2011.
5. Resources WSH. Competencies, <http://www.hr.wa.gov/WorkforceDataAndPlanning/WorkforcePlanning/Competencies/Pages/default.aspx/>; 2015.
6. Nsubuga P, Eseko N, Tadesse W, Ndayimirije N, Stella C, McNabb S. Structure and performance of infectious disease surveillance and response, United Republic of Tanzania, 1998. Bull World Health Organ 2002;80(3):196–203.
7. Becker KM, Ohuabunwo C, Ndjakani Y, Nguku P, Nsubuga P, Mukanga D, et al. Field epidemiology and laboratory training programs in West Africa as a model for sustainable partnerships in animal and human health. J Am Vet Med Assoc 2012;241(5):572–9.
8. Perry HN, McDonnell SM, Alemu W, Nsubuga P, Chungong S, Otten Jr MW, et al. Planning an integrated disease surveillance and response system: a matrix of skills and activities. BMC Med 2007;5:24.
9. McNabb SJ, Chungong S, Ryan M, Wuhib T, Nsubuga P, Alemu W, et al. Conceptual framework of public health surveillance and action and its application in health sector reform. BMC Public Health 2002;2:2.
10. Lukwago L, Nanyunja M, Ndayimirije N, Wamala J, Malimbo M, Mbabazi W, et al. The implementation of integrated disease surveillance and response in Uganda: a review of progress and challenges between 2001 and 2007. Health Policy Plan 2013;28:30–40.
11. Nsubuga P, Brown WG, Groseclose SL, Ahadzie L, Talisuna AO, Mmbuji P, et al. Implementing integrated disease surveillance and response: four African countries' experience, 1998-2005. Global Public Health 2010;5(4):364–80.
12. Statistics USBoL. Epidemiologists, <http://www.bls.gov/ooh/life-physical-and-social-science/epidemiologists.htm/>; 2015.
13. Nsubuga P, Nwanyanwu O, Nkengasong JN, Mukanga D, Trostle M. Strengthening public health surveillance and response using the health systems strengthening agenda in developing countries. BMC Public Health 2010; 10(Suppl. 1):S5.
14. Nsubuga P, White M, Fontaine R, Simone P. Training programmes for field epidemiology. Lancet 2008;371(9613):630–1.
15. Field epidemiology. 2nd ed. New York, NY: Oxford University Press; 2002.
16. Nsubuga P, Johnson K, Tetteh C, Oundo J, Weathers A, Vaughan J, et al. Field epidemiology and laboratory training programs in sub-Saharan Africa from 2004 to 2010: need, the process, and prospects. Pan Afr Med J 2011;10:24.
17. Prevention CfDCa. Epidemic intelligence service, <http://www.cdc.gov/eis/index.html/>; 2015.
18. Prevention CfDCa. Global Health | Field epidemiology training program, <http://www.cdc.gov/globalhealth/fetp/>; 2015.
19. Kariuki Njenga M, Traicoff D, Tetteh C, Likimani S, Oundo J, Breiman R, et al. Laboratory epidemiologist: skilled partner in field epidemiology and disease surveillance in Kenya. J Public Health Policy 2008;29(2):149–64.
20. Gitta SN, Mukanga D, Babirye R, Dahlke M, Tshimanga M, Nsubuga P. The African field epidemiology network—networking for effective field epidemiology capacity building and service delivery. Pan Afr Med J 2011;10(Suppl. 1):3.
21. Nigeria FELTP. About Us, <http://www.nigeria-feltp.net/about.php/>.
22. Nsubuga P. Gaps and priorities in US contribution to global disease challenges.
23. Committee PHFS. Public health in America: the essential public health services. In: US Public Health Services PHFSC, editor. Washington, D.C: US Public Health Services, Public Health Functions Steering Committee; 1995.
24. United States Depart of Labor BoLS. Standard Occupational Classification. 2010.
25. Workforce Capacity, <http://www.baldrige21.com/BALDRIGE_GLOSSARY/BN/Workforce_Capacity.html/>; July 2015.
26. Thacker SB, Dannenberg AL, Hamilton DH. Epidemic intelligence service of the Centers for Disease Control and Prevention: 50 years of training and service in applied epidemiology. Am J Epidemiol 2001;154(11):985–92.
27. Centers for Disease Control and Prevention. National Notifiable Disease Surveillance System (NNDSS), <http://wwwn.cdc.gov/nndss/>; April 2014.
28. Lichtveld M, Boulton M, Lemmings J, Gale J. From competencies to capacity: assessing the national epidemiology workforce. Public Health Rep 2008; 123(Suppl. 1):128–35.
29. Epidemiologists CoSaT. Applied epidemiology core competencies. <http://www.cste.org/default.asp?page=CoreCompetencies>.
30. Epidemiologists CoSaT. About CSTE, <http://www.cste.org/?page=About_CSTE/>; April 2014.
31. Epidemiologists CoSaT. National assessment of epidemiology capacity. 2009.
32. Epidemiologists CoSaT. National assessment of epidemiology capacity. Atlanta, GA USA: Council of State and Territorial Epidemiologists; 2013.
33. Epidemiologists CoSaT. Epidemiology enumeration assessment. 2010.
34. Prevention CfDCa, Savel TG, Foldy S. The role of public health informatics in enhancing public health surveillance. MMWR Surveill Summ 2012; 61(Suppl.):20–4.
35. Centers for Medicare and Medicaid Services. Regulations and guidance. <http://www.cms.gov/Regulations-and-Guidance/Legislation/EHRIncentivePrograms/Meaningful_Use.html>; April 21, 2014.

36. Smith PF, Hadler JL, Stanbury M, Rolfs RT, Hopkins RS. "Blueprint Version 2.0": updating public health surveillance for the 21st Century. J Public Health Management Practice 2013;19(3):231–9.
37. Epidemiologists CoSaT. National electronic disease surveillance system assessment. 2010.
38. The Association of Schools and Programs of Public Health academic program finder. <http://www.aspph.org/program-finder>; September 19, 2014.
39. Congress U. American Recovery and Reinvestment Act, Health information technology for economic and clinical health act or the "HITECH Act", <http://www.healthit.gov/sites/default/files/hitech_act_excerpt_from_arra_with_index.pdf/>; May 2014.
40. Services CfMaM. Public health registry tip sheet, <http://www.cms.gov/Regulations-and-Guidance/Legislation/EHRIncentivePrograms/Downloads/PublicHealthRegistry_Tipsheet-.pdf/>; 2004 [Accessed September 18, 2014].
41. Prevention CfDCa. Competencies for public health informaticians 2009. 2009.
42. The Office of the National Coordinator for Health Information Technology. Governance Framework for Trusted Electronic Health Information Exchange. <http://www.healthit.gov/sites/default/files/GovernanceFrameworkTrustedEHIE_Final.pdf>; May 2, 2014.

2

SECTION

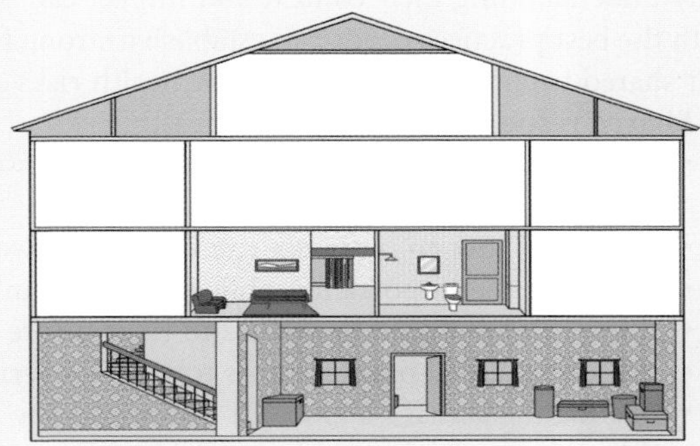

Governance Unlocks Transformation

Affan T Shaikh

Section Outline

Relating to the vision of making a PHS house for the twenty-first century, governance represents an integral part of that structure—the framework and roof. As shown here, threats posed by new, emerging, or re-emerging infectious diseases transcend economic, geological, sociological, and political boundaries. They present a serious threat and require an efficient, effective, and equitable global response. To support varied functions of PHS across multiple actors and sectors, governance acts as a framework ensuring lessons learned over the years from global public health crises such as the SARS pandemic, H1N5 influenza, and threats of deliberate epidemics are leveraged to support future holistic, flexible capacity to detect and respond to PH crises. Building on this framework will take initiative and cooperation from the international community. The creation and adoption of a global governance model for PHS will need to steer communities, countries, or groups of countries in the management of PHS, yet still balance the rights of sovereign nations and the global community with shared responsibilities to safeguard populations. The roof of the house represents the international regulations and treaties needed to facilitate and protect the functions of PHS. Without these protections, the structure would be exposed to the elements, preventing effective, efficient, and equitable PHS. The need to create this vision of governance is as pressing as ever. But we first need to understand the context and development of existing international governance documents that guide PHS in light of global health security concerns, as well as the ethical and moral considerations. Only when fully understanding their context and impact can we move forward to create governance models for PHS equipped with the best practices needed to establish a strong framework and roof for our PHS house; only then can we weather our shared twenty-first century public health risks and threats.

Shared responsibility to public health risks:

- Describe recent outbreaks and the weaknesses they have demonstrated in national and international public health surveillance systems.
- Describe how an outbreak can impact the world economy.
- Describe the importance, obligation, and authority mandated by domestic and global PHS governance.
- Identify global alert systems and their future to protect global health security.
- Describe global best practices for PHS governance.
- Define the statist vs. globalist points of view for global health surveillance.
- Identify appropriate ethical considerations on both the individual and population levels.
- Identify why countries may be hesitant to share data and samples and how these barriers should be removed.
- Identify gaps and impediments in the governance for domestic and global PHS and propose interventions.

CHAPTER

10

Policies, Standards, and Best Practices for Public Health Surveillance

Stella Chungong, Rajesh Sreedharan, Jun Xing, Stephane de la Rocque

Alone we can do so little; together we can do so much.

Helen Keller

KEY WORDS

Standards
Governance
Public health emergency of international concern
World Health Assembly (WHA)
OIE
FAO
IHR focal points
Asia Pacific Strategy for Emerging Diseases (APSED)
GOARN
INFOSAN
GLEWS
Terrestrial Animal Health Code
International Health Regulations (2005)

INTRODUCTION

Global standards for public health surveillance governance have been defined and influenced by many factors over time. The issue of surveillance is not new; it dates back to the mid-fourteenth century in the Republic of Venice where three keepers were designated to detect and keep away ships with passengers infected with Black Death (pneumonic plague), perhaps the first official public health measure in the prevention of disease spread. Varying surveillance measures were put in place in subsequent centuries in Europe and the USA. These measures or **standards** are the established, accepted, and evidence-based technical specifications for responding to public health issues.[1]

William Farr, who worked at the General Register Office in the UK and became the first Compiler of Scientific Abstracts in 1866, is recognized as the founder of the modern concept of surveillance for his routine of recording causes of death in England and Wales.[2, 3] The twentieth century witnessed the further expansion and refinement of disease surveillance. Data collection, analysis, and information dissemination methods and other methodological elements are greatly diversified to respond to different needs. Although public health surveillance has greatly improved with the use of modern technology—the most notable advances being, mobile communication, computerized data management, modeling—the last decades have witnessed new challenges resulting from the rapid expansion of global travel and trade as well as emerging and re-emerging infectious diseases. This, along with challenges in early/timely detection and reporting of public health events, has led to major disease outbreaks, which may have been controlled through early detection and rapid response. In some member states (MS), the main difficulties are due to a lack of timeliness in detection, investigation, flow of information, response, civil unrest, and limited human and logistical capacities.[4] As demonstrated in recent history, the delay in timeliness in detecting a Marburg virus outbreak that occurred in Angola in 2005 resulted in 124 cases of which 117 were fatal.[5] In 2003, an *Escherichia coli* outbreak could not be timely investigated in Democratic Republic of Congo (DRC) due to insecurity.[6]

Insecurity also delayed a Rift Valley fever outbreak investigation in Afmadow, Somalia, in 2006.[7] Delay in data analysis and reporting led to late detection and, therefore, delayed response to a measles outbreak in Kinshasa (DRC) in 2002 and Chad in 2005.[8, 9]

Fragmented approaches to public health surveillance, varying reporting and notification standards, differing risk assessment, and the need to establish common references for the surveillance of diseases have fostered the move toward global standards. While routine surveillance including specific disease surveillance and indicator- and event-based surveillance have been put in place in many countries, globally applicable standards are required.

The first human outbreak of avian influenza A (H5N1) resulted in six deaths in 1997 in the Special Administrative Region of Hong Kong. This outbreak prompted an acute awareness of the reality that a virus previously confined to wild and domestic avian species can begin to infect humans with devastating consequences; it raised the need for intensive public health surveillance, enhanced preparedness, and response capacities.[10] The experience with H5N1, and the emergence of severe acute respiratory syndrome (SARS) in Hong Kong years later in 2003, was a clarion call that the threat of a major, novel pandemic was real and that a global approach to pandemic preparedness and response were imperative. Both the scientific and political communities were in agreement that the challenges of ascertaining information about an emerging disease event and the coordination of a global response to contain and mitigate against a pandemic required a new instrument.

INTERNATIONAL STANDARDS FOR DISEASE SURVEILLANCE

The World Health Organization (WHO) constitution not only states that governments have a responsibility for the health of their peoples that can be fulfilled only by the provision of adequate health and social measures but also recognizes that unequal development in different countries in the promotion of health and control of disease, especially communicable disease, is a common danger. The constitution mandates WHO to, among other tasks, establish and revise international nomenclatures of diseases, of causes of death, and of public health practices as necessary and to propose conventions, agreements and regulations, and make recommendations with respect to international health matters.

The **World Health Assembly (WHA)**, constituted of WHO Member States (currently 194), has the authority to adopt regulations and resolutions, which are then implemented by countries with the support of the WHO Secretariat.[11] A number of resolutions have been adopted over the years with regard to global surveillance. One of the most significant instruments adopted by the WHA is the **International Health Regulations (IHR)**.[12] The IHR evolved from efforts to address the threat posed by the international spread of epidemics. The more recent international sanitary agreements grew out of international conventions dating to the last half of the nineteenth century and the public health institutions founded in the first half of the twentieth century.[13] In 1951, the 4th WHA adopted the International Sanitary Regulations (ISR), the first of these WHO global agreements. In 1969, the ISR were replaced by the IHR, which, until 2007, focused mainly on obligations of WHO MS to report human cases and related information to WHO for "quarantinable" diseases. MS were also responsible for implementing public health response measures primarily relating to a few "quarantinable" diseases; by 1981 these were cholera, plague, and yellow fever. Following a 10-year negotiation process, the IHR (2005) were adopted in May 2005 and came into force in June 2007. The revised IHR (2005) present a fulfillment of the WHO constitution mandate as a binding international legal instrument to 196 MS party to this framework for global surveillance and response aiming to prevent and respond to acute public health risks that have the potential to cross borders and threaten and pose a public health threat to people worldwide. The revised version of the IHR (2005) differs from its 1969 predecessor in several important ways.

Under the IHR (2005), one of the new key definitions is an "extraordinary event", which is determined, as provided in the IHR (2005), and refers to a "**public health emergency of international concern**" (PHEIC).[12] Declaration of a PHEIC would imply a situation that is

- serious, sudden, unusual, or unexpected;
- carries implications for public health beyond the affected State's national border; and
- may require immediate international public health action.

Since the IHR (2005) entered into force on June 15, 2007, the WHO Director General has thrice declared a PHEIC: the first for the 2009 influenza pandemic, the second for polio on May 5, 2014, and the third for the 2014 Ebola outbreak. These declarations are examples of when WHO, through the director general, is advised by a committee of experts to take appropriate public health actions including issuing temporary recommendations that should be taken by countries on areas of travel, surveillance, clinical management, and infection control. The IHR Emergency Committee concerning Middle East respiratory syndrome coronavirus (MERS-CoV), technical consultation on global standards and tools for influenza surveillance, and the consultation on event-based surveillance are other examples of committees and task forces that provide evidence-based guidance on surveillance. The IHR Emergency Committees called for under the IHR play an important role in the provision of advice to the Director General on public health measures, including for surveillance.

Other major changes regarding surveillance within the IHR (2005) include the requirement for the development of national capacities for surveillance and response, including at Points of Entry, obligations to report or notify through a designated **IHR national focal point**,[12] and expansion of the scope of surveillance beyond infectious disease. Events for notification under the IHR (2005) could be infectious with epidemic and pandemic potential but may include emergencies due to contamination with toxins, chemicals, or radioactive material, or to industrial leaks or intentional release. Annex 2 of the IHR (2005) comprises a decision-making algorithm for the identification of events requiring notification (Fig. 10-1).

CURRENT ADOPTION OF THE IHR (2005)

The IHR (2005) aim to provide a global alert and response system built on partnership, quality, and transparency, which is based on:

- Strong national public health systems able to maintain active surveillance of diseases and public health events, rapidly investigate reports, assess public health risk, share information, and implement public health control measures.
- An effective international system that supports disease control programs to contain specific public health threats, continuously assesses the global picture of public health risks (e.g., global risk assessment), and rapidly responds to events with unexpected, international spread.

This is achieved through a number of national and international efforts, processes, and networks. Technical consultation groups on global standards and tools for surveillance bring together experts and networks globally and are usually convened by WHO for the development of guidance material. The consultations on tools for influenza surveillance and on event-based surveillance are examples of committees and task forces that provide evidence-based guidance on surveillance.[14-16]

Regional Successes

At the regional level, the WHO regional offices work collaboratively with MS and institutions, using relevant instruments, initiatives, and strategies to guide public health surveillance. In the Western Pacific Regional Office (WPRO) and the South East Asia Region (SEARO), WHO works through the **Asia Pacific Strategy for Emerging Diseases (APSED)**, a common strategic framework to strengthen regional capacity to manage and respond to emerging disease threats.[17] In the WHO African Region (AFRO), the integrated disease surveillance and response (IDSR) framework is implemented by 43 of the 46 countries. This particular framework is noteworthy for containing guidance to improve the capacity to "detect, confirm, and respond to high-priority communicable and noncommunicable diseases."[18] The WHO Regional Office for Europe (WHO/Europe) has worked with MS and with the European Centre for Disease Prevention and Control (ECDC) on several initiatives on cross-border and international threats to health. The WHO regional offices for the Americas (PAHO) and the Eastern Mediterranean region (EMRO) continue to implement emerging infectious disease strategies in support of surveillance and response.

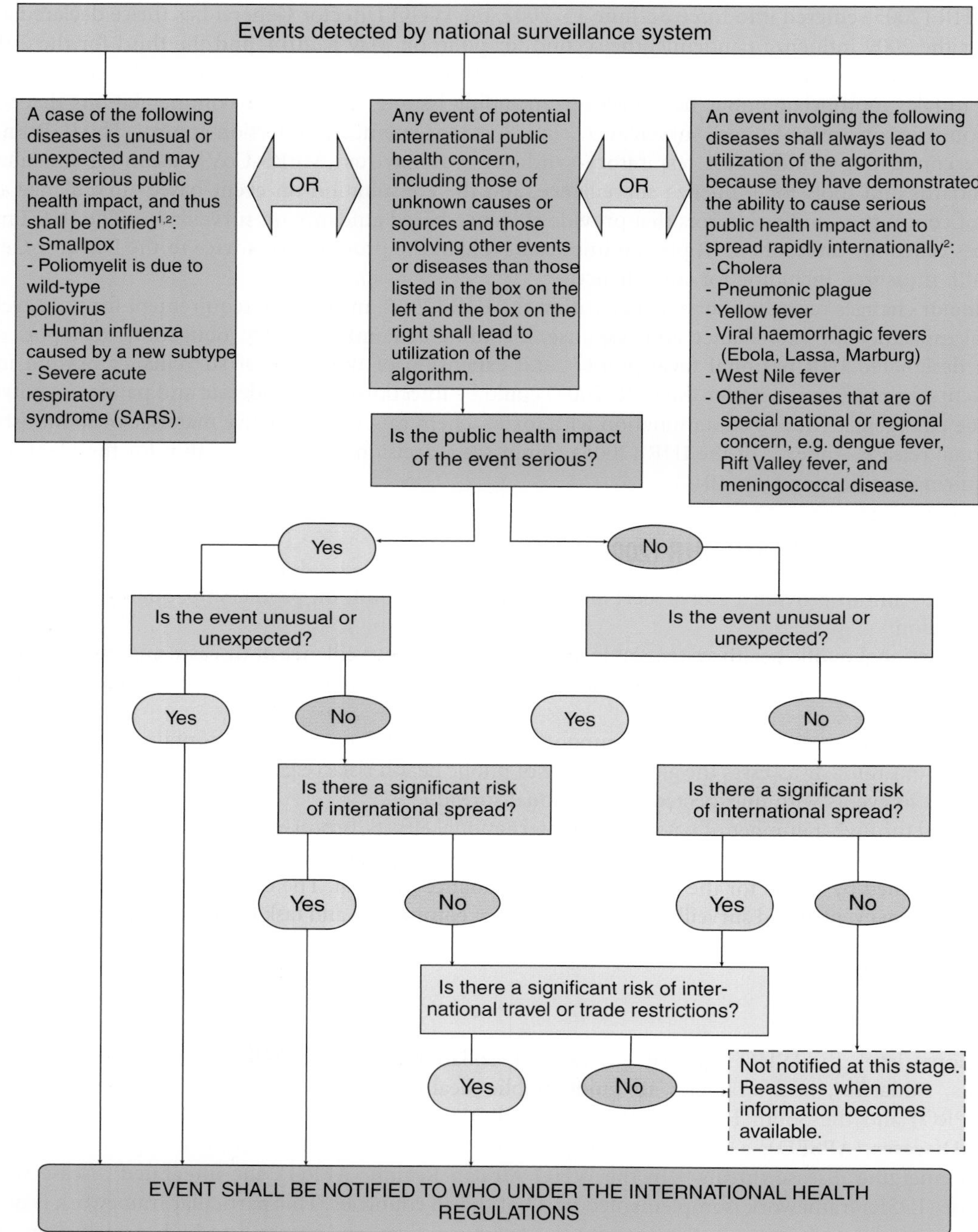

FIG. 10-1 Decision instrument for the assessment and notification of events that may constitute a public health emergency of international concern. http://www.who.int/ihr/revised_annex2_guidance.pdf?ua=1

Global real-time risk assessment, verification, and information sharing that guide response are key in public health surveillance. The provision of appropriate tools and rapid access to subject matter experts and networks for event-based surveillance, a flexible operational platform for coordination of response, and rapid information sharing has also been crucial. The WHO Event Management System (EMS) and Event Information Site (EIS) for IHR national focal points are tools that facilitate public health surveillance risk assessment, timely communications, and information sharing on events. The Global Outbreak Alert and Response Network (**GOARN**), the secretariat of which is hosted in WHO, is a collaboration of existing institutions and networks that pools human and technical resources for the rapid identification, confirmation, and response to outbreaks of international importance. The network contributes to global health security through the prompt identification, confirmation and response to international outbreaks combating the spread of outbreaks, providing technical assistance, and capacity building.[19]

Formal and informal networks also support public health surveillance. The IHR (2005) take into account the mandate for WHO to use information about health events coming from sources other than official government notifications, a departure from the limited liberties allowed in 1969. Fig. 10-2 shows some of these networks.

Laboratory Support

The role of the laboratory in surveillance cannot be overemphasized. The support in diagnosis and sharing of information about disease pathogens is important for the confirmation and control of outbreaks. It is critical in novel outbreaks where knowledge needs to be quickly gathered and analyzed for understanding an unfolding event. For example, the support to the Malaysian government in 1999 was the key when 257 cases of febrile encephalitis were detected in Kampung Sungai Nipah, Malaysia. The Australian Animal Health Laboratory and the US Centers for Disease Control and Prevention (CDC) teamed up to identify the Nipah Virus (NiV) as the cause of the outbreak.[20] In another example, in 2003, Singapore health authorities requested the support of WPRO and the CDC to investigate what eventually became known as SARS. An important laboratory network used in the

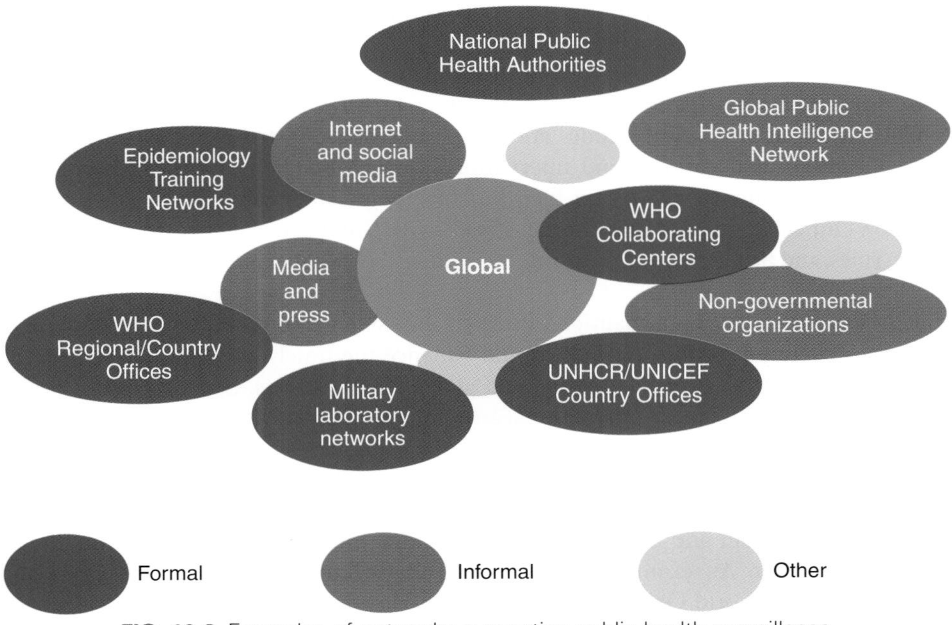

FIG. 10-2 Examples of networks supporting public health surveillance.

identification of unknown diseases is the Emerging and Dangerous Pathogens Laboratory Network (EDPLN).[21] The network comprises high-security Biosafety level (BSL)-3 and BSL-4 human and veterinary diagnostic laboratories that share knowledge, materials, and experimental results in real time to support international diagnostic responses. The network also supports transfer of technologies, practices, and trainings to regional networks and national laboratories.[22]

The pandemic influenza preparedness (PIP) framework for the sharing of influenza viruses, and access to vaccines and other benefits is another important framework adopted by the 64th WHA.[23] The framework's aim is to allow for the global sharing of influenza viruses with human pandemic potential, access to vaccines, and sharing of other benefits in a fair, transparent, equitable, and efficient approach within an effective system.[18]

GOVERNANCE IN PUBLIC HEALTH SURVEILLANCE

The global nature of threats to human health from diseases that respect no boundaries requires an effective and integrated public health surveillance and response system if the goals of timely detection and effective and appropriate response are to be achieved. At its core, **governance** constitutes the structures, rules, and processes used by society to shape and apply power to identify and achieve objectives.[24]

In the globalized context, governance includes, but is not equivalent to government. The literature identifies three broad spheres of governance: national, international, and global.[25] National governance, which is normally hierarchical, refers to how a country organizes power within its jurisdiction from the lowest administrative structure, up to the central government. The rules of operation at the national level are based on the constitution, legislation, and administrative regulations. Public health surveillance responsibility is usually at the subnational level (state or province) with government, health partners (including private practitioners), and civil society as stakeholders.

At the international level, governance deals with the regulation of political exchanges between countries, which leads governments to form connected sets of both formal or informal rules that direct behavioral roles, restrain activity, and shape expectations of sovereign states.[26] Governments govern their relations through jointly developed instruments and institutions such as international laws and international governmental organizations that allow the identification of common interests, negotiations, and cooperation between various stakeholder states and international organizations.

In global governance, states and nonstate actors interact to influence the exercise of political power within and between countries. The participation of nonstate actors highlights that sovereign states are not the only actors in governance. International laws or codes are global governance instruments used by nonstate actors that can reach beyond the traditional national and international governance boundaries.[27] Governance at each level identifies the goals (what), defines the reason for their pursuits (why), and lays out strategies and mechanisms, and builds capacities (how) for achieving and maintaining stated goals. Governance is affected through binding laws and nonbinding norms, rules, and principles that moderate individuals, corporates, and states' behaviors to meet common goals.

Current public health surveillance is a coalition of surveillance systems of states, organizations, and regional and subregional networks structured to fill specific gaps and enhance the timely and effective sharing of information and collaboration in response to national, regional, and global health threats. Effective public health surveillance and response requires states to implement international and global governance approaches within their jurisdictions, from the local to the central levels, through formal legal rules and informal means of partnership. How states adapt and apply the hard and soft governance laws for high-priority global threats to health is complex.

The current trends and drivers of emerging and re-emerging human and zoonotic diseases, including food-related health threats, have driven human and animal health state actors, international governmental organizations, and nonstate actors closer together. An example of this is, WHO working closely with the Food and Agriculture Organization (**FAO**)[28] and the World Organisation for Animal Health (**OIE**)[29] collaboration network (OFFLU) in coordinating efforts to timely detect and track important animal influenza viruses.[30]

FUTURE INVESTMENTS

Experience has shown that a weakness in one country's capacities to detect and respond to emerging events is a threat to all others. International organizations share a responsibility in supporting MS in the strengthening of capabilities for early warning and rapid response, by acting both at local and global levels. The ability to minimize the harmful impact of emerging diseases relies on the capacity to rapidly detect unusual events and implement containment and control measures as early as possible.

Investing in Building Countries' Capacity for Surveillance and Response

WHO convened five meetings of stakeholders in 2012 to discuss mapping of unmet needs to accelerate IHR implementation in several regions. This forum allowed countries to define needs and map resources needed to meet the IHR requirements and provide the opportunity for all stakeholders to propose recommendations and solutions to address the challenges and bridge the gaps identified. This helped in setting the stage for further discussions on future strategies for collaboration, partnership, and the mobilization of technical and financial resources required to meet core capacities.

The lack of sufficient human and financial resources remained major obstacles to building and maintaining the necessary capacities for effective surveillance, early detection, and rapid response. Various technical capacities were identified as priorities. Among other needs, countries requested building and strengthening subregional, regional, and global capacity for surveillance and response.

Strengthening Public Health Surveillance

Strengthening public health surveillance, global risk assessment, and reporting and verification is critical for prompt global response. As required by the IHR (2005) and delineated in Annex 1 of the IHR (2005), State Parties should utilize existing national structures and resources to meet their core competencies with regard to surveillance, reporting, notification, verification, response and collaboration activities as well as activities concerning designated airports, ports, and ground crossings. At the local community level and/or primary public health response level, the capacities include to detect events involving disease or death above expected levels and to report all available essential information immediately to the appropriate health care response, and finally to implement preliminary control measures. Capacities needed at the intermediate public health response level include to confirm the status of reported events and support additional control measures, to assess reported events immediately and if urgent enough report to the national level. Finally, the capacities needed at the national level fall under: (1) assessment and notification and (2) public health response. The national assessment and notification capacities include:

- to assess all reports of urgent events within 48 h; and
- to notify WHO immediately through the national IHR focal point when required IHR (2005) reporting criteria.

The national public health response capacities include

- to determine rapidly the control measures to prevent spread;
- to provide support through specialized staff, laboratory analysis, and logical assistance;
- to provide on-site assistance as required to supplement local investigations;
- to provide a direct operational link with senior health and other officials;
- to provide direct liaison with other relevant government agencies;
- to provide means of communication links to key affected areas; and
- to establish, operate, and maintain a national public health emergency response plan.

Workshops held in Washington DC and Geneva in June and August of 2010, respectively, focused on capacity building and implementation of the IHR (2005). As Katz et al. report, workshop participants identified a number of challenges to IHR (2005) implementation including gaps in resources, particularly human resources, meeting obligations at Points of Entry, safe and effective transportation of specimens and samples, need for better laboratory infrastructure, developing local-level capacity, and a need to focus on developing basic public health infrastructure before focusing specifically on IHR (2005) compliance.[31]

Strengthening Global and Regional Networks

The IHR have encouraged countries to develop and strengthen capacities to detect and respond to all public health threats. Though many reporting networks exist and are obliged to report under regional or subregional agreements for particular diseases or agents, additional instruments may need to be put in place to encourage international notification and reporting of potential PHEICs.

Formal and informal networks play an important role for early detection of potential public health threats[1] and for countries with limited resources, bilateral agreements for resource sharing and support during an event can provide cost-effective solutions to strengthening national surveillance systems.

Intersectoral Coordination and Collaboration

Recognizing that about 60% of human pathogens and the large majority of emerging diseases in humans are of animal origin, with most of them originating in wildlife and many amplifying in livestock,[32] outbreaks of zoonoses are good examples where the intersectoral collaboration in the IHR framework can be explored. The IHR (2005) are not restricted to the public health sector and encourage a coordinated and integrated response to risks—they constitute a privileged platform for the implementation of cross-sectoral approaches.

Zoonotic diseases have increased in human and animal public health importance over the last two decades[33] and both the animal and human health authorities have a stake in, and responsibility for, their control. Practically, the ability to stop the spread of pathogens relies on the capacity to detect unusual events early and rapidly implement control measures. This necessitates the coordinated involvement of multiple actors standing in a variety of sectors and at different levels of implementation. Although substantial improvements in coordination have been made, many countries still need large, long-term investments in the development of infrastructure, human resource, and legislation to meet the challenges posed by emerging diseases.

Both WHO and OIE work closely with national authorities under legally binding frameworks, the IHR and the Terrestrial and Aquatic Animal Health Codes, respectively. For OIE, the obligations to disclose all relevant information about animal diseases are set out in the OIE Organic Statutes. Each MS must report the occurrence of animal diseases, the emergence of new diseases, and significant epidemiologic events within 24 h of the event.[34] This also includes diseases transmissible to humans and intentional introduction of pathogens. The World Animal Health Information System (WAHIS) allows immediate notification and dissemination of near real-time warnings on exceptional events of domestic and wild animal disease. The official notification of events to OIE facilitates the activation of the OIE-FAO Crisis Management Center—Animal Health (CMC-AH). When appropriate, the CMC-AH offers a mechanism for the provision of rapid technical advice and support to countries requesting assistance. The CMC-AH links with other mechanisms developed jointly by WHO, OIE, and/or FAO, including the Global Early Warning System (GLEWS) and the International Food Safety Authorities Network (INFOSAN).

GLEWS is a joint system that builds on the added value of combining and coordinating the alert and disease intelligence mechanisms of OIE, FAO, and WHO, enhancing the early warning capacity for the benefit of the international community. Through GLEWS, the verification process of the three organizations is combined and coordinated, and sharing assessments for an on-going outbreak enables a joint and comprehensive analysis of the event and its possible consequences. Disease intelligence generated by GLEWS directly feeds into and informs the respective response mechanisms of the three organizations.[35]

INFOSAN is an initiative that promotes, through designated contact points, the rapid exchange of information during food-safety-related events; the sharing of information about important food-safety-related issues of global interest; the enhancement of partnerships and collaboration between countries; and the strengthening of each country's capacity to manage food safety risks.[36] As such, INFOSAN complements and supports the IHR.

Alignment of Standards between Sectors

The best systems are only as strong as their weakest components and the timely notification of a disease is dependent on the ability of countries to detect diseases at an early stage. (OIE: Notification of animal and human diseases—Global legal basis)

Given that the notification systems of both WHO and OIE have the necessary instruments and legally binding obligations for a fast and efficient distribution of information globally on human and animal diseases, the priority is to focus efforts on the strengthening of governmental public health and veterinary services.[34]

Common references, standards, and global mechanisms are needed to ensure that all countries have minimum requirements that, when met, protect all countries from public health disasters. These references and standards have been democratically adopted by State Parties of WHO through the IHR (2005) and by OIE MS through the **Terrestrial Animal Health Code**.[37] Using these standards, international organizations have developed guidance materials and appropriate tools to assist countries in the strengthening of their operational capacities for the detection of and response to emergencies.

To be effective against emerging zoonotic diseases, institutions need to not only be efficient in their operations but also seek strong synergies with other services. This translates into concrete action to improve governance mechanisms, develop and promote policies, design and implement systems and processes, strengthen surveillance and response capacities, and target investments at the national, regional, or international level.[38]

Promoting Good Governance among Health Systems at the Interface Between Human and Animal Health

A joint tripartite concept note described areas of common interest when "address[ing] health risks at the animal–human–ecosystems interfaces."[39] Although numerous coordination mechanisms had already been developed at the technical level, the tripartite note still recognized "*a need to strengthen animal and human health institutions*," and suggested that "*protocols and standards … should be jointly developed*" to achieve coherence of any related global standard-setting activities and to address gaps in the capacities of countries. The three organizations agreed to search for alignment and coherence of related global standard setting activities, in the respect of existing structures and mechanisms.

An overarching concept is that preventing and controlling emerging infectious diseases at both animal and human levels is an international public good, which requires strong political and financial commitment at the national, regional, and international levels. Furthermore, a long-term vision is needed to build sound and sustainable infrastructures and those actions should build on existing approaches and mandates of international institutions and other partners. Changes are best based on strong, functional systems for human and animal endemic disease; they do not necessarily demand integration or fusion among various specialized stakeholders or agencies at the national level, but rather improved communication, coordination, and collaboration.

CONCLUSION

The IHR (2005) are one of the most successful and comprehensive internationally binding instruments to require signatory MS to improve disease surveillance and response capacities. While there have been successes in global disease surveillance as demonstrated, some challenges remain. Transparency and trust are key elements of success. Under the IHR (2005), MS have made great strides in capacity building. Maintaining high quality and adequate capacities over time is a priority.

The use of global information technology and improvement of interoperability between systems could improve disease surveillance.

The role of nonstate actors will continue to be important as they increase in number and reach. Although setting policies, developing standards, and exercising governance can be challenging, these are crucial in achieving integrated global disease surveillance.

KEY SUMMARY POINTS

- At the international level, governance deals with the regulation of political exchanges between countries, which leads governments to form connected sets of both formal and informal rules that direct behavioral roles, restrain activity, and shape expectations of sovereign states.
- The WHA, constituted of WHO member states (currently 196), has the authority to adopt regulations and resolutions, which are then implemented by countries with the support of the WHO secretariat. For over 40 years, the WHO's IHR have been the primary legally binding global agreement addressing the risks of the international spread of infectious disease. Under the IHR (2005), countries must report "an extraordinary event", which is determined, as provided in the regulations, and refers to a "public health emergency of international concern (PHEIC)".
- Experience has shown that a weakness in one country's capacities to detect and respond to emerging events is a threat to all others. International organizations share a responsibility in supporting member states in the strengthening of capabilities for early warning and rapid response, by acting both at local and global levels.
- The provision of appropriate tools and rapid access to subject matter experts and networks for event-based surveillance and laboratories, continues to be crucial for providing a coordinated analysis and response (i.e., GOARN, EDPLN).
- Under the IHR (2005), states have made great strides in capacity building. Maintaining high quality and adequate capacities over time is a priority.

DISCUSSION QUESTIONS

1. How can sociocultural behaviors and practices be integrated into governance and disease surveillance specifically, to enhance prediction, timely detection, and effective response to public health threats?
2. What are the effective mechanisms to ensure the functional maintenance of national capacities as required under the IHR (2005)?
3. Is public health governance a recognized entity by State Parties or is it assumed?
4. How can State Parties build good public health governance capacity?
5. What would it take to build a dedicated (even a regional) Public Health Leadership Institute in less-resourced settings?
6. How can the perception of public health surveillance as a "medical/treatment" issue be change to "preventive health" issue involving the multiple sectors, beyond the health sector?
7. What is the best way to optimize the use of real-time health threats surveillance data as a governance tool?
8. Is the language used by public health surveillance experts friendly to the general public or does it impede implementation and effectiveness of approaches, and their timely detection and effective response?
9. Does political leadership appreciate public health surveillance as an ingredient of economic development?
10. Are the current myriad of surveillance and response systems too fragmented and cocooned as organizational entities with separate and hierarchical structures and mandates to meet the needs of the twenty-first century?
11. How well are the regulations, tools, and protocols internationally developed for public health surveillance known at the subdistrict levels of State Parties? How well are they adapted for local use and action?

REFERENCES

1. Last JM. A dictionary of public health. Oxford University Press; Oxford, UK, 2007.
2. Galbraith N. Communicable disease surveillance No. 2. In: Recent advances in community medicine. London: Churchill Livingstone; 1982. p. 127–42.
3. Langmuir AD. William Farr: founder of modern concepts of surveillance. Int J Epidemiol 1976;5(1):13–8.
4. Bruckner C, Checchi F. Detection of infectious disease outbreaks in twenty-two fragile states, 2000-2010: a systematic review. Confl Health 2011;5:13.
5. CDC. Outbreak of Marburg virus hemorrhagic fever—Angola, October 1, 2004-March 29, 2005. MMWR Morb Weekly Rep 2005;54(12):308–9.

6. Koyange L, Ollivier G, Muyembe JJ, Kebela B, Gouali M, Germani Y. Enterohemorrhagic Escherichia coli O157, Kinshasa. Emerg Infect Dis 2004; 10(5):968–9.
7. WHO. Outbreaks of Rift Valley fever, in Kenya, Somalia and United Republic of Tanzania, December 2006-April 2007. Wkly Epidemiol Rec 2007;82(20): 169–78.
8. WHO. Epidemics of meningococcal disease. Wkly Epidemiol Rec 2001; 76(37):282–8.
9. Grais RF, Dubray C, Gerstl S, Guthmann J.P, Djibo A, Nargaye KD, et al. Unacceptably high mortality related to measles epidemics in Niger, Nigeria, and Chad. PLoS Med 2007;4(1):e16.
10. Claas EC, Osterhaus AD, van Beek R, De Jong JC, Rimmelzwaan GF, Senne DA, et al. Human influenza A H5N1 virus related to a highly pathogenic avian influenza virus. Lancet 1998;351(9101):472–7.
11. WHO. World Health Assembly, <http://www.who.int/mediacentre/events/governance/wha/en/>; [updated April 23, 2015; cited 2015].
12. WHO. International health regulations (2005). 2nd ed. Geneva: World Health Organization; 2008.
13. Eylenbosch WJ, Noah ND, editors. Historical aspects. In: Surveillance in health and disease. Oxford, UK: Oxford University Press; 1988. p. 3–8.
14. WHO. WHO technical consultation on event-based surveillance, <http://www.episouthnetworkorg/sites/default/files/meeting_report_ebs_march_2013_final.pdf/>; 2008.
15. WHO. WHO global technical consultation: global standards and tools for influenza surveillance, <http://www.who.int/influenza/resources/documents/technical_consultation/en/>; 2011a. [Geneva, Switzerland, 8-10 March 2011 Report No: WHO/HSE/GIP/20111.].
16. WHO. IHR Emergency Committee concerning Middle East respiratory syndrome coronavirus (MERS-CoV), <http://www.whoint/ihr/ihr_ec_2013/en/>; 2014.
17. Emerging Disease Surveillance and Response. Asia pacific strategy for emerging diseases (APSED, 2010), <http://www.wpro.who.int/emerging_diseases/APSED2010/en/>. [updated May 16, 2013; cited 2015].
18. WHO. Pandemic influenza preparedness framework for the sharing of influenza viruses and access to vaccines and other benefits, <http://www.whoint/influenza/resources/pip_framework/en/>; 2011b.
19. WHO. Global Outbreak Alert and Response Network (GOARN), <http://www.who.int/ihr/alert_and_response/outbreak-network/en/>. [updated June 08, 2015; cited 2015].
20. WHO. Labs form a new front against deadly pathogens. Bull World Health Organ 2009;87(4):248–9.
21. Hottes AK, Rusek B, Sharples F, Committee on Anticipating Biosecurity Challenges of the Global Expansion of High-Containment Biological Laboratories, National Academy of Sciences, National Research Council. Biosecurity challenges of the global expansion of high-containment biological laboratories. Washington, DC: National Academies Press; 2013. p. 216.
22. WHO. WHO emerging and dangerous pathogens laboratory network (EDPLN), <http://www.whoint/csr/bioriskreduction/laboratorynetwork/en/>; 2014.
23. WHO. World Health Assembly. Pandemic influenza preparedness: sharing of influenza viruses and access to vaccines and other benefits. 2011c.
24. Bevir M. Governance. Encyclopedia of governance [Internet]. Sage Publications; Thousand Oaks, California, 2007. p. 365–82.
25. Fidler D. Architecture amidst anarchy: global health's quest for governance. Glob Health Governance 2007;1(1):1–17.
26. Keohane R. After hegemony: cooperation and discord in the world political economy. Princeton University Press; Princeton, New Jersey, 1984. p. 320.
27. IOM (Institute of Medicine) NNRC. Sustaining global surveillance and response to emerging zoonotic diseases. National Academies Press; Washington DC, 2009. p. 340.
28. Food and Agriculture Organization of the United Nations. About FAO, <http://www.fao.org/about/what-we-do/en/>. [cited 2015].
29. The World Organisation for Animal Health. The World Organisation for Animal Health (OIE), <http://www.oie.int/about-us/>. [cited 2015].
30. OFFLU. OFFLU OIE/FAO Network of expertise on animal influenza: mission and objectives; 2014.
31. Katz RL, Fernandez JA, McNabb SJ. Disease Surveillance, capacity building and implementation of the International Health Regulations (IHR[2005]). BMC Public Health 2010;10(Suppl1):S1. doi:10.1186/1471-2458-10-S1-S1.
32. Jones KE, Patel NG, Levy MA, Storeygard A, Balk D, Gittleman JL, et al. Global trends in emerging infectious diseases. Nature 2008;451:990–4.
33. FAO. World livestock 2013 - changing disease landscape. Rome: Food and Alimentation Organisation of the United Nations; 2013.
34. OFFLU. Notification of animal and human diseases global legal basis. Paris, France: World Organisation for Animal Health; 2012.
35. About GLEWS: The Joint FAO-OIE-WHO global early warning system for health threats and emerging risks at the human-animal-ecosystems interface, <http://www.glews.net/about-glews/>. [cited 2015].
36. World Health Organization. International food safety authorities network (INFOSAN). World Health Organization; Geneva, Switzerland, 2007.
37. Terrestrial Animal Health Code: The World Organisation for Animal Health (OIE), <http://www.oie.int/international-standard-setting/terrestrial-code/>. [cited 2015].
38. World Health Organization. WHO-OIE operational framework for good governance at the human-animal interface: bridging WHO and OIE tools for the assessment of national capacities. 2014.
39. FAO, WHO. Sharing responsibilities and coordinating global activities to address health risks at the animal-human-ecosystems interfaces. A Tripartite Concept Note. 2010.

CHAPTER

11

Keeping Our World Safe by Integrating Public Health Surveillance and Health Security

David L Heymann, Edmund Howard

Unprecedented technological capabilities combined with unlimited human creativity have given us tremendous power to take on intractable problems like poverty, unemployment, disease, and environmental degradation. Our challenge is to translate this extraordinary potential into meaningful change.

Muhammad Yunus

KEY WORDS

Global public health security
Emerging infectious diseases
Response
Biological weapons
ProMED-mail
Participatory surveillance
HealthMap
GPHIN
Digital search surveillance

INTRODUCTION

This chapter traces the evolution of global health security from its origins, rooted in attempts to stop the international spread of infectious disease outbreaks at international borders, to the current understanding that the best means of prevention is rapid detection and response where outbreaks originate. The chapter shows how emphasizing **global public health security**—characterized as the need to reduce the vulnerability of people around the world to emerging and remerging risks to health[1]—has shifted from attempts to prevent international spread through measures at international borders to strong national disease alert and response capacities. It traces the evolution of global public health surveillance from passive country reporting to active surveillance that feeds genetic and other surveillance information into global databases, internet-based searching for infectious disease events, and attempts to develop disease alert systems based on individual self-reporting of predefined syndromes of infections that could signal infectious disease outbreaks.

STRENGTHENING PUBLIC HEALTH SECURITY WITH ACTION AT BORDERS

As cross-border trade, pilgrimage, and war occurred and intensified throughout the history, so did the international spread of infectious diseases. By the fourteenth century it was understood that the waves of epidemic disease, such as plague, were seeded by international travel, and prevention against importation of disease soon became an important part of national security efforts (Fig. 11-1). Defense mechanisms against the international spread of disease were first developed by individual countries, and then by groups of countries, as they attempted to prevent cross-border disease importation.[2]

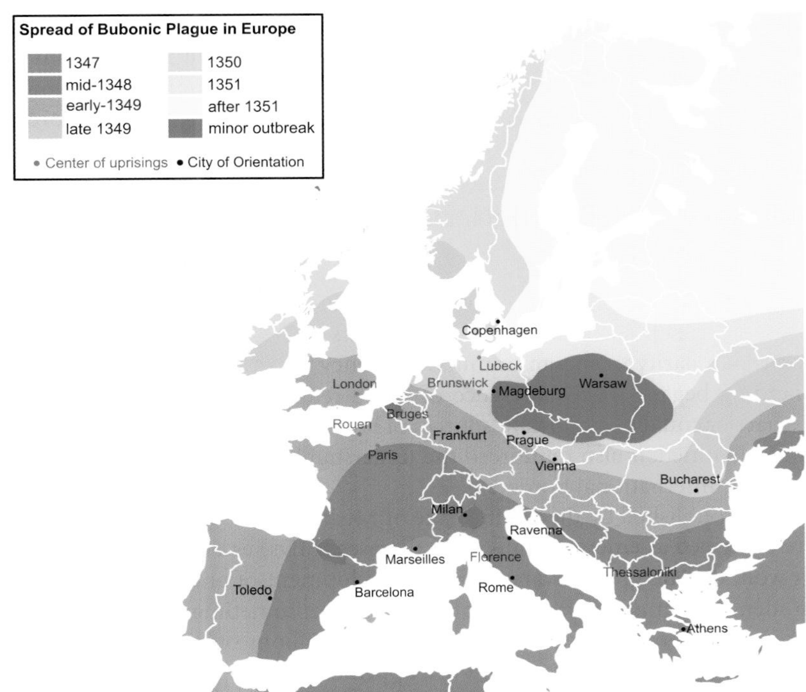

FIG. 11-1 Plague in the middle ages. *Source:* https://en.wikipedia.org/wiki/Black_Death_migration.

An early national attempt is recorded in the archives of the city-state of Venice in the fourteenth century, where quarantine measures were imposed in an attempt to stop the spread of bubonic plague.[3] Pandemic waves of plague continued during the following centuries, and then in the early nineteenth-century cholera pandemics, originating in southeast Asia, were added to the list of global concerns and quarantine measures adopted as the main strategy for attempting to stop their spread across international borders.[4] As new technologies were developed, policies such as the obligatory telegraphic notification of first cases of cholera and plague were adopted; and as understanding of the etiology of infectious diseases evolved, the length of quarantine was varied depending on the presumed cause of an epidemic and its incubation period.

As travel between Europe and North America intensified in the nineteenth and early twentieth centuries, it was understood that smallpox and yellow fever, in addition to cholera and plague, were often carried by international travelers.[5] The Pan American Sanitary Bureau (now called the Pan American Health Organization) and its European counterpart, the Office International d'Hygiène Publique, were created in the early twentieth century. These organizations served to coordinate reporting and international border actions aimed at vector control in an effort to better prevent the international spread of four infectious diseases—cholera, plague, smallpox, and yellow fever.

By 1951, 3 years after its founding, the World Health Organization (WHO) agreed on the necessity of continued international collaboration to ensure a "maximum of protection against the transmission of pestilential diseases with a minimum of interference of travel and trade" and adopted the international sanitary regulations.[6] These regulations continued to focus on the reporting of cholera, plague, smallpox, and yellow fever and also epidemic typhus and relapsing fever. Rooted firmly in preceding international agreements, they required reporting by all WHO member states when and where these diseases were occurring and the implementation of applying measures to prevent the spread of disease by vectors on public conveyances and at international border posts. They also clearly outlined the maximum set of measures that could be undertaken at international borders to prevent importation of disease from areas with reported cases.

In 1969, WHO member states agreed to a revised set of international sanitary regulations—the International Health Regulations (IHR)—aimed at better ensuring public health security with minimal interruption in travel and trade.[7] In addition to requiring reporting of four infectious diseases (cholera, plague, yellow fever, and smallpox), the IHR also aimed at implementing measures on public conveyances and at international borders that would prevent the proliferation and spread of the infection.

STOPPING THE SPREAD OF EMERGING INFECTIOUS DISEASES REQUIRES MORE THAN ACTION AT BORDERS

The discovery of acquired immunodeficiency syndrome (AIDS), first identified in 1981, caught the world unprepared for new infectious diseases. Once the social and economic impacts of AIDS were fully understood, its wide geographic spread recognized, and its similarity to simian immunodeficiency viruses clearly demonstrated, a new era in infectious disease understanding began.[8] The occurrence of AIDS reinforced the understanding that breaches in the animal/human species barrier could be important sources of human infection. Because it had silently spread to many continents before it was identified, it also reinforced the understanding that the spread of infectious diseases could not effectively be stopped at international borders.

Soon afterward, a report published by the US Institute of Medicine in 1992, citing the emergence of AIDS, called attention to what were described as emerging infectious diseases (EIDs) as evidence that the fight against infectious diseases was far from won, despite great advances in the development of anti-infective drugs and vaccines.[9] Since then, EIDs have been identified at an average rate of one per year, sometimes becoming pandemic and spreading throughout the world in a matter of weeks or months, placing millions of persons, or entire populations, at risk. **EIDs** are broadly defined as infections that have newly appeared in a population or have existed but are rapidly increasing in incidence or geographic range.[10] EIDs can encompass:

- a recognized infection spreading to new areas or populations;
- the discovery that a known disease is caused by infection;
- a previously unrecognized infection appearing in areas where the habitat is changing (e.g., deforestation);
- a new infection resulting from change(s) in existing microorganisms (e.g., mutation); and
- a recognized infection, re-emerging in a form resistant to treatment, or as a result of a breakdown in public health prevention measures.

EIDs can be caused by bacteria, viruses, parasites, and fungi. They have risen significantly over time and are dominated by zoonoses (60.3%); the majority of these (71.8%) originate in wildlife.[11]

In many instances, identification of an EID occurs many years after a breach in the species barrier, such was the case for AIDS; it was thought to have breached the species barrier toward the end of the nineteenth or beginning of the twentieth century.[12] During the past 40 years, EIDs that have been identified and linked to an animal source range from Ebola and Marburg hemorrhagic fevers to AIDS, severe acute respiratory syndrome (SARS), influenza A (H5N1), paramyxovirus infections (Hendra and Nipah viruses), variant Creutzfeldt–Jakob disease/bovine spongiform encephalopathy (vCJD/BSE), and foodborne infections caused by verocytotoxin-producing *Escherichia coli* O157.[13,14] Recently the emergence of Middle East respiratory syndrome corona virus (MERS-CoV) has also been linked to a possible animal source—dromedary camels—as has the emergence of influenza A (H7N9)—linked to chickens as the probable source.[15,16]

Humans are often the sentinel population in which a newly emerged animal infection is first recognized, and there are generally three pathways that a newly emerged infection can take in human populations: no further transmission (e.g., rabies and leptospirosis), limited human-to-human transmission (e.g. influenza A [H5N1 and H7N9], Ebola and MERS-CoV), or sustained human-to-human transmission, leading to endemicity (e.g., HIV). Other infections have emerged in recent decades in new forms with the evolution of multidrug-resistant staphylococcal species and multidrug-resistant and extensively drug-resistant (MDR and XDR) tuberculosis (TB), while others, such as cholera, West Nile, dengue, and chikungunya, have emerged in geographic areas where they had not previously been recorded.[17]

HUMAN AND ECONOMIC COSTS OF EIDS

Emerging infections are threats to public health security. They cause human suffering, illness, and death, and they require medical care, which is sometimes costly because of the requirement for special procedures and protracted hospitalization. Their control may require the culling of animals being raised commercially for food or other animal products, with loss of profit. And finally, emerging infections sometimes cause economic loss because of barriers to trade and travel when there is a perceived, often misguided, fear of their international spread through travel, tourism and/or trade. In economic terms, EIDs are estimated to have caused damage worth hundreds of billions of dollars in the last 20 years through both direct impact on health systems and indirect impact from decreased travel and trade, the latter often unwarranted (Fig. 11-2).[18,19]

Influenza A (H1N1)

During 2009, a total of 70,715 Mexicans, of whom 1316 died, were reported with confirmed influenza A (H1N1) infection in the initial outbreak after the emergence of the virus from swine.[20] By the end of 2009, more than 208 countries and territories had reported laboratory-confirmed cases of pandemic influenza A (H1N1) to WHO, and there had been at least 12,799 deaths worldwide.[22] When Mexico first reported human infections with the H1N1 influenza virus, it was hypothesized, from genetic sequence information that had been accumulated by the US Centers for Disease Control and Prevention (CDC) and other institutions, that the virus had undergone several different mutations in pigs before finally mutating in such a manner that it could successfully breach the species barrier between pigs and humans.[23] Because it spread easily from human to human, it caused a major influenza outbreak in Mexico that spread globally within weeks, causing a pandemic (Fig. 11-3).

Many countries activated their influenza pandemic plans after WHO declared in April 2009 that influenza A (H1N1) was a public health emergency of international concern (PHEIC) and later that year declared it a pandemic. Though at no time did WHO recommend any decrease in pork trade or travel, there were still major economic losses

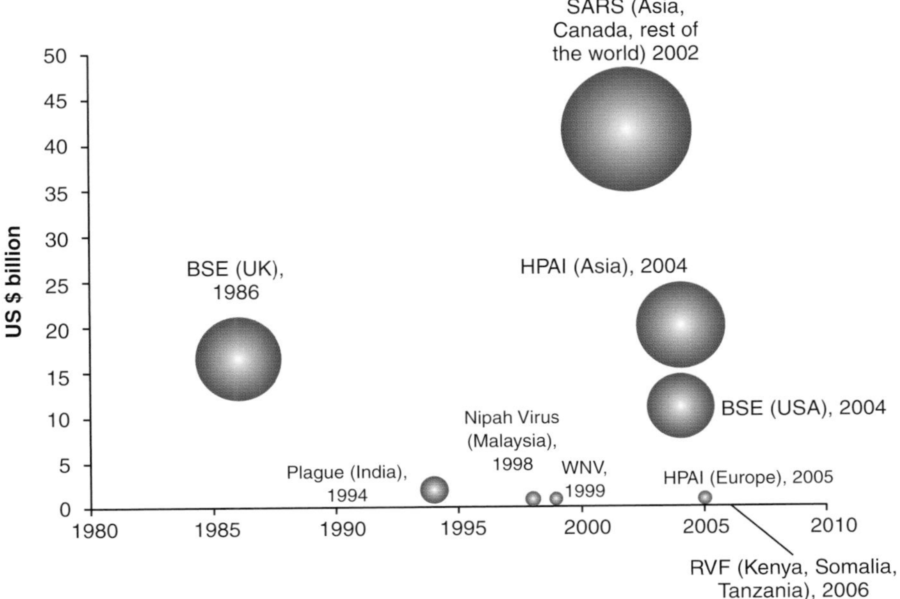

FIG. 11-2 Estimated cost of selected emerging zoonotic diseases (1986–2006).

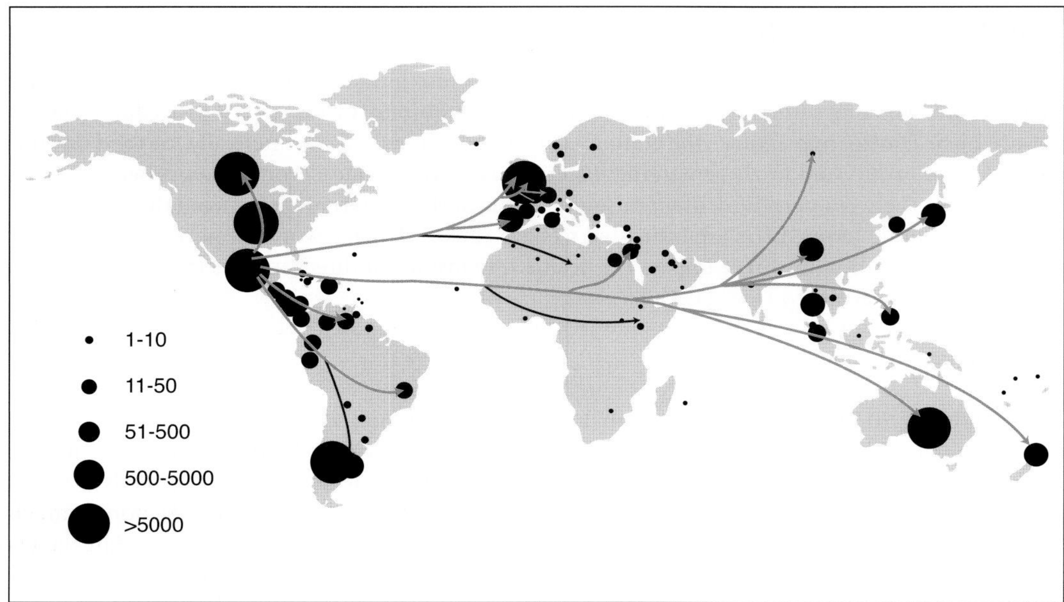

FIG. 11-3 Spread of influenza A (H1N1), April–July 2009.

related to influenza A (H1N1) in Mexico in both these sectors.[24] These losses occurred because of an unwarranted perception among tourists and travel agencies that the risk of becoming infected with the virus was somehow greater in Mexico than elsewhere, even though the virus had spread throughout the world, and by a misunderstanding among pork markets that pandemic transmission was being amplified by infected pigs, despite the fact that it was being caused by human-to-human transmission, in which pigs no longer played a role.[25]

Because of the resulting decrease in overseas visitors to Mexico, thought to be approximately 1 million, there was an estimated economic loss of approximately US$2.8 billion.[24] Because of unnecessary trade bans on Mexican pork products, there was a major decrease in demand from the pork industry that contributed to a pork trade deficit of an estimated US$27 million.[24] In countries other than Mexico there were official recommendations, apparently based on this same misunderstanding that likewise caused negative economic impact. In Egypt, for example, slaughter of pigs was ordered by the Egyptian Government early in the pandemic, even though the H1N1 virus had already been demonstrated to be highly transmissible from human to human, and despite the recommendation of the World Organization for Animal Health (OIE) that the culling of pigs was not scientifically justifiable.[25]

Countries around the world were affected as the influenza A (H1N1) pandemic spread, and most economies suffered. In Spain, for example, the direct economic impact of illness from influenza A (H1N1) on health services utilization, and indirect costs from work absenteeism, has been estimated at €6236 per hospitalized patient.[26] In Canada, it is estimated that the cost of the increased patient load to hospitals caused by influenza A (H1N1) between April and December 2009 was Canadian $200 million.[27]

Variant Creutzfeldt–Jakob disease

Another example of the human and economic costs of EIDs is vCJD, a human infection that emerged in the UK in the mid-1990s. vCJD required the culling of infected animals that can be a continued source of human infection. The infection known as vCJD in humans is caused by the same infectious agent that causes BSE, also known as "mad cow disease" in cattle. From cattle, it can spread to humans through meat and other cattle products that were infected with the causative agent of BSE.[28] vCJD does not spread from one human to another, and each human infection is thought to occur independently, either from infected cattle or products made from them. There is a potential for iatrogenic human-to-human transmission in blood transfusion, surgical and other skin-penetrating equipment, and organ transplants. Since first being identified, 225 human cases of vCJD have been reported from 12 countries, and each case has been fatal within a short period from onset.[29]

BSE was first identified in cattle that developed severe neurological symptoms in the UK during the 1980s.[30] In order to rid cattle of infection, culling of herds with infected cattle was required. When it was understood that humans could be infected with BSE from cattle and cattle products in 1996, culling activity increased, and the economic loss in the UK during the following year was estimated to be US$1.5 billion.[31] Trade of British beef and other cattle products was banned in many countries, markedly decreasing British exports and adding greatly to the costs already associated with culling. In the 12 countries where BSE and vCJD had spread from the UK through cattle or bovine products, herds of cattle infected with BSE were culled at a considerable economic loss to each of these countries as well.[29]

PUBLIC HEALTH SURVEILLANCE

The 2009 pandemic of influenza A (H1N1) was first identified through the Global Influenza Surveillance and Response System (GISRS), a laboratory-based surveillance network that aims to better understand influenza epidemiology, provide information necessary to prepare seasonal influenza vaccines, and detect novel influenza virus strains that could have pandemic potential.[32] GISRS is thus a guarantor of global public health security, and the guiding principle of that network—collection of data for action—was developed during the early twentieth century in the yellow fever laboratory surveillance network, established in Africa and South America in 1928 by the Rockefeller Foundation.

The yellow fever laboratory network's objective was to examine cross-immunity to various strains of the yellow fever virus found in monkeys and thus to better understand the potential usefulness of a yellow fever vaccine that was under early development. Blood specimens were collected from monkeys in sub-Saharan Africa and Brazil, and a central coordinating laboratory demonstrated that the African and Brazilian strains were closely related. With this evidence, vaccine development was justified, and an eventual attenuated yellow fever virus vaccine was developed. The yellow fever laboratories remain today as the WHO Collaborating Centre network on Yellow Fever ensuring a continual collection of data for action.

Global Influenza Surveillance in Humans

GISRS, which identified the influenza A (H1N1) pandemic, was established in 1952 by WHO, based on the yellow fever laboratory network model, in order to provide the information required for timely recommendations for the most effective seasonal influenza control measures. GISRS consists of health facilities where health workers collect nasal swab specimens from patients with influenza-like illness (ILI), and three different types of quality-assured national laboratories where nasal swab specimens are analyzed (Fig. 11-4). National laboratories around the world receive nasal specimens collected from patients with ILI. The specimens are tested for influenza virus, and a representative sample of influenza virus isolates is sent to a WHO Collaborating Centre for Reference and Research on Influenza for genetic sequencing.

The six WHO Collaborating Centres for Reference and Research on Influenza also identify suitable viruses for vaccine use, report on antiviral susceptibility, and provide training and quality assessment to national laboratories. GISRS also consists of four essential regulatory laboratories with a critical role in developing, regulating, and standardizing influenza vaccines and ensuring the development of seasonal and pandemic influenza vaccines by processing influenza viruses to further select, develop, and distribute seed influenza viruses.

The WHO Collaborating Centres analyze approximately 200,000–250,000 seasonal influenza specimens each year, the results of which are reviewed twice a year to determine which circulating seasonal influenza strains are

The WHO Global Influenza Surveillance Network (GISN), July 2008

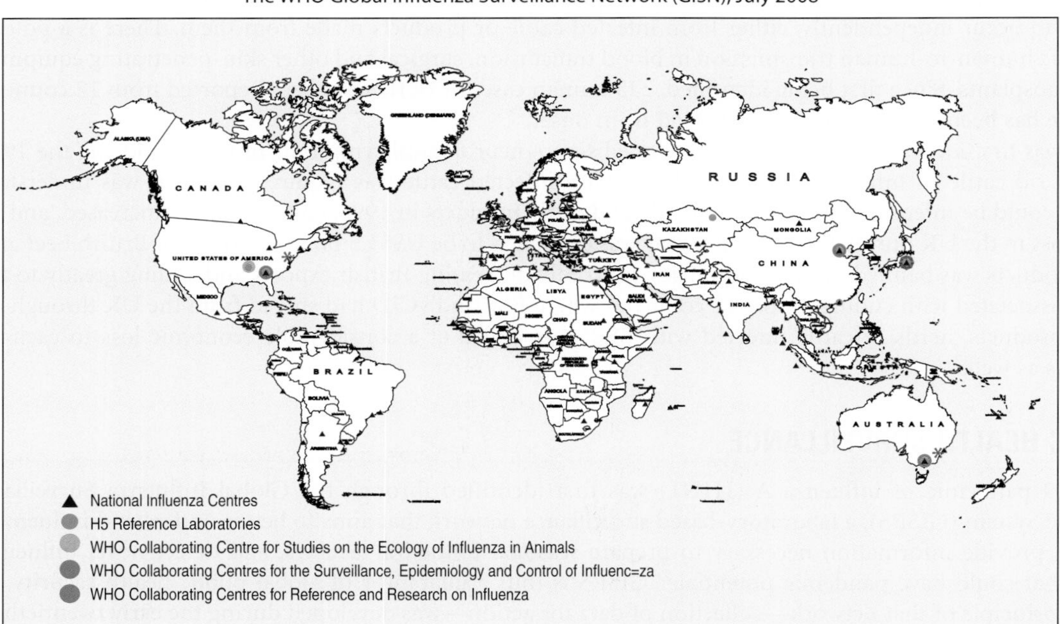

FIG. 11-4 Global influenza surveillance and response system.

predominant and therefore appropriate components of seasonal vaccines. WHO then makes a recommendation, based on these data, on the influenza strains to be included in the vaccine for the coming influenza season in the northern and southern hemispheres. These recommendations are made 6 months in advance of expected seasonal outbreaks; however, the final decision on the composition of vaccines in each country is the responsibility of relevant national authorities.

GISRS is also called into action to support the surveillance of novel influenza viruses that emerge in human populations. There is generally at least one novel influenza virus identified by GISRS in human populations each year, and though all influenza viruses are thought to have pandemic potential, a novel influenza virus only occasionally causes a pandemic.

FluNet is a web-based data collection and reporting tool—a global interactive database—for influenza virological data associated with GISRS.[33] It is used to track the movement of influenza viruses globally and to interpret epidemiologic data collected about influenza outbreaks. FluNet uses data from the GISRS laboratories and other national influenza reference laboratories, and the data are publicly available in real time. Results are presented in various formats including tables, maps, and graphs, depending on the data query. FluNet includes a data query function that permits browsing, viewing, querying, and searching the FluNet database. Data query outputs are presented as reports, charts, or maps or downloaded as spread sheets. FluNet also features interactive mapping showing FluNet data for selected geographic areas, a map library to view and download ready-made FluNet maps, and remote data entry for participating laboratories (Fig. 11-5).

Global Influenza Surveillance in Animals

Animal influenza is a threat to humans when it emerges at the animal/human interface and when it threatens animal health and welfare and food production. The OIE and the Food and Agriculture Organization of the United Nations

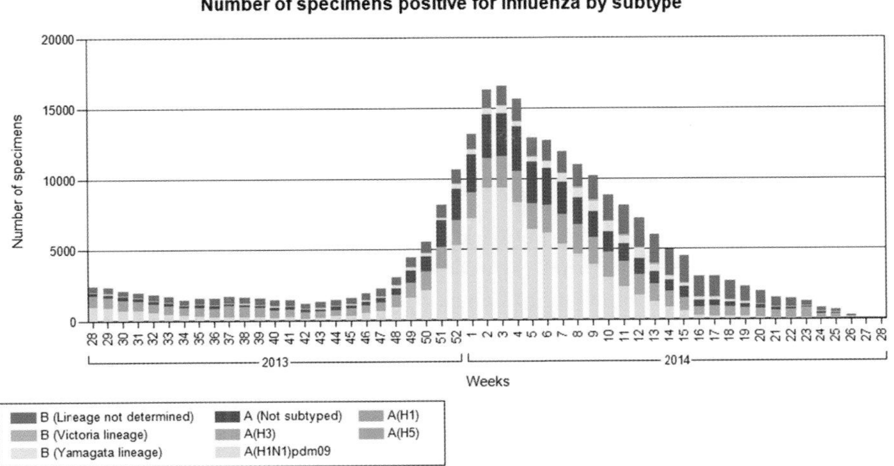

FIG. 11-5 FluNet: influenza laboratory surveillance information, GISRS.

(FAO) have established a global surveillance and expertise network for animal influenza, OFFLU, in order to better understand animal influenza viruses and their risks to both animals and humans.[34] OFFLU seeks to generate and gather information to prepare animal vaccines to prevent swine, avian, and other animal influenza; to detect antigenic drift (simple mutation) or shift (reassortment or recombination) of influenza viruses in animals that require rapid containment and/or control; to contribute genetic information and virus strains for the preparation of human influenza vaccines against potential emerging human pandemic viruses; and to inform and support rapid response for containment of influenza outbreaks in animals including development of diagnostic tests and guidelines to ensure that existing diagnostic reagents are sensitive to circulating field viruses. OFFLU has two major surveillance networks, swine and poultry (see Fig. 11-6).

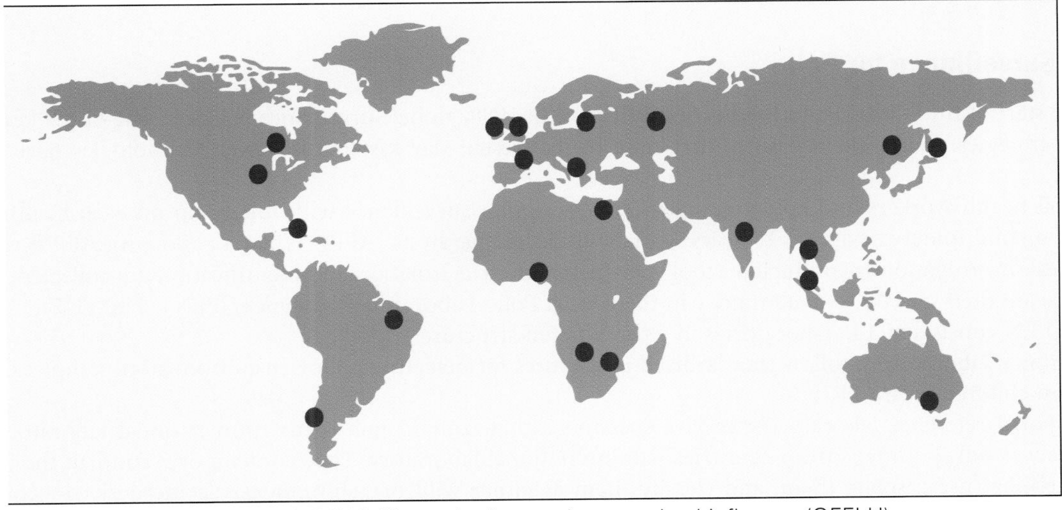

FIG. 11-6 OIE/FAO Network of expertise on animal influenza (OFFLU).

Laboratories in OFFLU's swine influenza network screen nasal specimens from swine to provide information about the origins, evolution, and spread of influenza viruses in swine. Genomic information is used to provide information about reassortment and recombination, antiviral resistance, and virulence; it is used to prepare specific nucleic acid-based diagnostic tests for surveillance that are then made widely available to veterinary laboratories. The laboratories receive specimens from targeted animals, such as those that fit the case definition for ILI or those with epidemiologic links to other animals that fit the case ILI definition.

Poultry Influenza Surveillance

Laboratories of the OFFLU's poultry influenza network screen specimens collected from living poultry and tissue specimens collected postmortem. As with swine, farmed poultry with severe respiratory symptoms or from flocks with clinical signs or suggestive lesions of avian influenza, and any poultry in markets or at slaughter with signs of disease consistent with avian influenza upon antemortem examination, are tested for disease. In some instances, statistically representative risk-based serological surveys are conducted to complement surveillance, as are outbreak investigations when necessary.

Animal–Human Surveillance

OFFLU and other animal surveillance systems provide data in freely accessible digital databases. Countries use this information in various ways as they link animal and human surveillance and risk assessment in national One Health activities (see Chapter 14). The UK Human Animal Infections and Risk Surveillance (HAIRS) Group, founded in 2004, includes three components: human surveillance (Public Health England), veterinary surveillance (Animal Health Veterinary Laboratories Agency), and food/environment surveillance (Department for the Environment, Food and Rural Affairs).[35] Each month the three agencies in England—with representation from Scotland, Wales, and Northern Ireland—review known animal infectious disease surveillance results from OFFLU and other animal surveillance systems, including those of the European Commission, and assess their risk to humans.

If more information is required for risk assessment by the HAIRS collaborative group, the collection of this information is assigned to one of the agencies in the group and then reviewed virtually as soon as it becomes available. If risk assessment suggests that an animal infection is of potential significance, it is included in the group's monthly summary of notable events/incidents of public health significance and is regularly followed until preventive action is required or it is no longer considered a risk. An annual HAIRS Group report is prepared each year summarizing the group's work.

Global Surveillance for Polio

From the start of the Global Polio Eradication Initiative in 1988, global surveillance has been one of the key underpinning strategies. It has evolved since that time to its present day system, as newer technologies have become available.

Clinical health workers and epidemiologists conduct polio surveillance with follow-up on each health facility report of a child under the age of 15 years with acute flaccid paralysis (AFP). When a child with AFP is reported, an outbreak investigation is conducted, stool specimens for virus isolation and identification are collected, and the specimens are then sent on to a laboratory in the Global Polio Laboratory Network (GPLN) (Fig. 11-7).

The GPLN consists of 145 laboratories in a three-tiered structure:

- National laboratories: follow standardized procedures for detecting polioviruses from stool samples collected from children with AFP.
- Regional reference laboratories: receive specimens that contain poliovirus from national laboratories, and receive stool specimens from countries with no national laboratory. They confirm or reconfirm the presence of polioviruses, isolate them, and classify them as either wild or Sabin, or as vaccine-derived—circulating polioviruses that could have originated from vaccine.

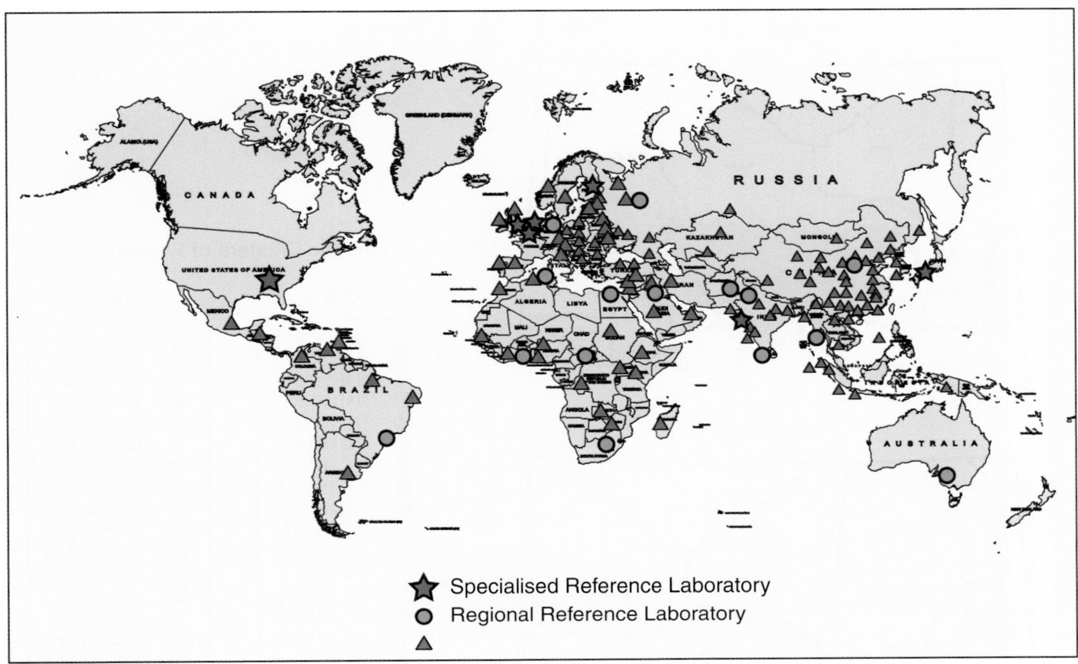

FIG. 11-7 Global polio laboratory network.

- Global specialized laboratories: genetically sequence each wild and vaccine-derived poliovirus sent from regional reference laboratories. Genetic sequence information from these laboratories is used to better understand the epidemiology of each poliovirus by comparative analysis with a global database that organizes genetic data by country or region of origin. From this comparison, it is understood where the genetic ancestors of the virus have most recently been circulating, thus giving an indication of the source of the current case or outbreak (Fig. 11-8).

All GPLN laboratories are continually monitored for adherence to quality indicators and have annual accreditation assessments. Each year, the GPLN tested over 150,000 stool samples from nearly 90,000 cases of AFP and other sources. The GPLN also carries out a research agenda aimed at improving laboratory diagnostics for polio.

The global surveillance system for polio is unique in that it is itself quality controlled, using minimum levels of acceptability that have been developed for monitoring the effectiveness of polio surveillance operations, two of which are listed below:

- At least one case of AFP detected per 100,000 children under 15 years of age in polio-free regions, and two per 100,000 in endemic regions (Fig. 11-9)
- At least 80% of children with AFP have two stool specimens collected at least 24 h apart and within 14 days after the onset of paralysis (Fig. 11-10)

Environmental Surveillance for Polio

Environmental surveillance for polio is the systematic testing of sewage or other environmental samples for the presence of poliovirus. It has varying sensitivity and provides information about both wild and Sabin polioviruses in human fecal material. At times it confirms wild poliovirus infections when AFP has not been reported. Genetic sequencing of the poliovirus demonstrates its geographic origin when compared to national and global databases of poliovirus sequence information.

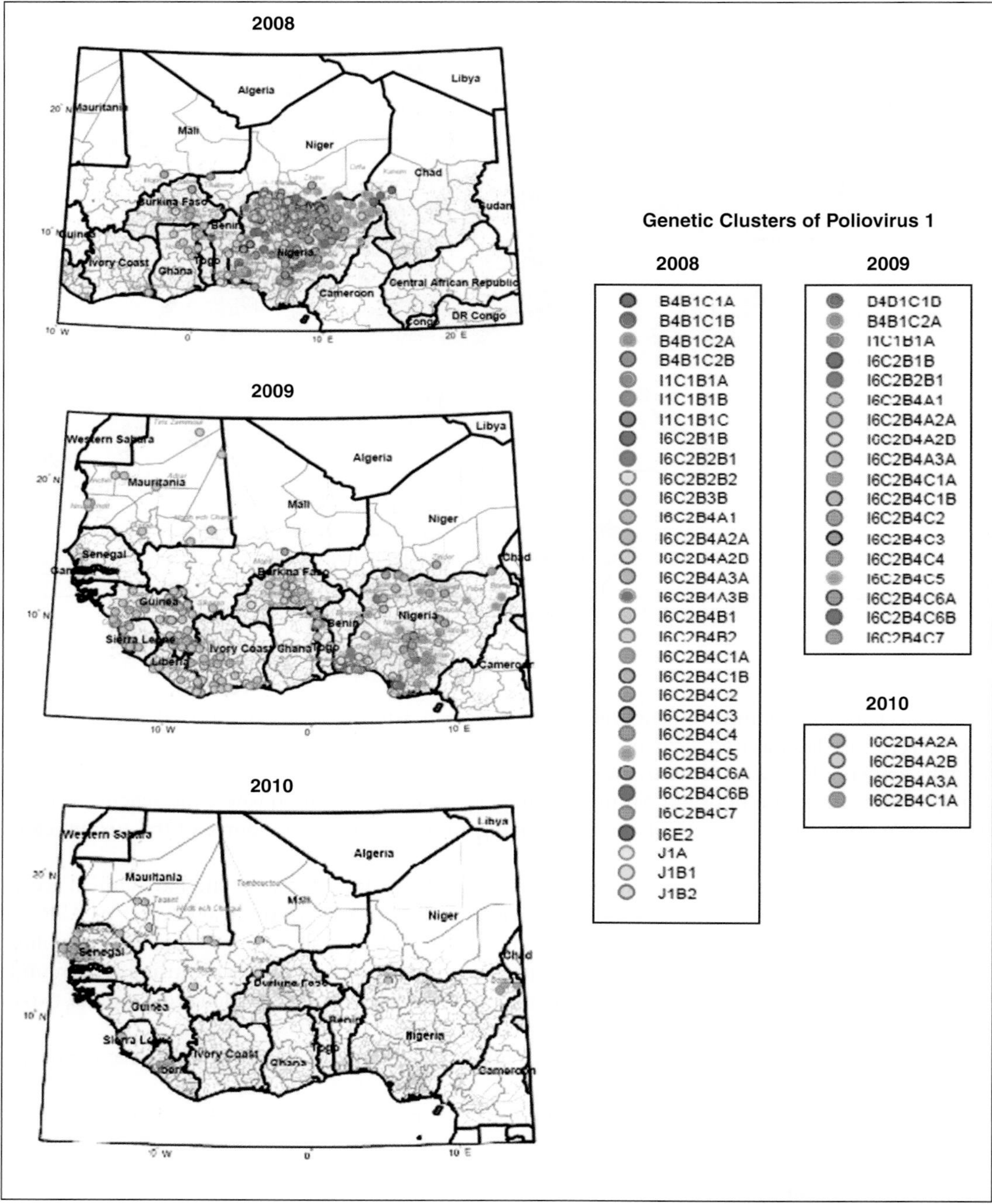

FIG. 11-8 Changing genetic diversity, wild poliovirus type 1, West Africa 2008–2010.

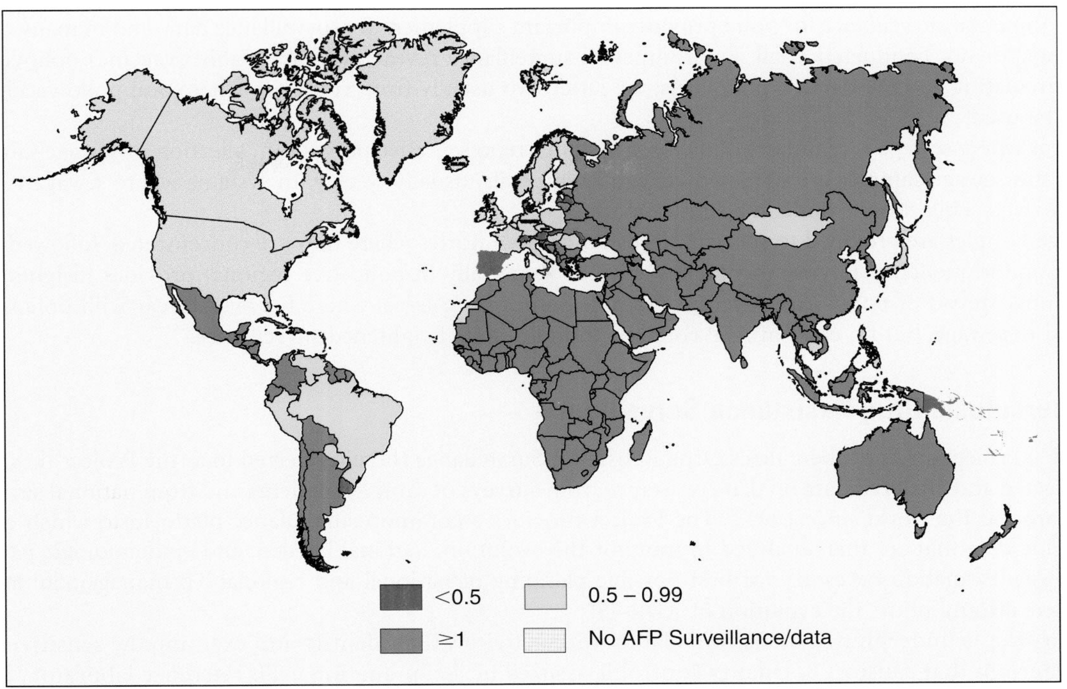

FIG. 11-9 Non-polio acute flaccid paralysis rate, May 2013–April 2014.

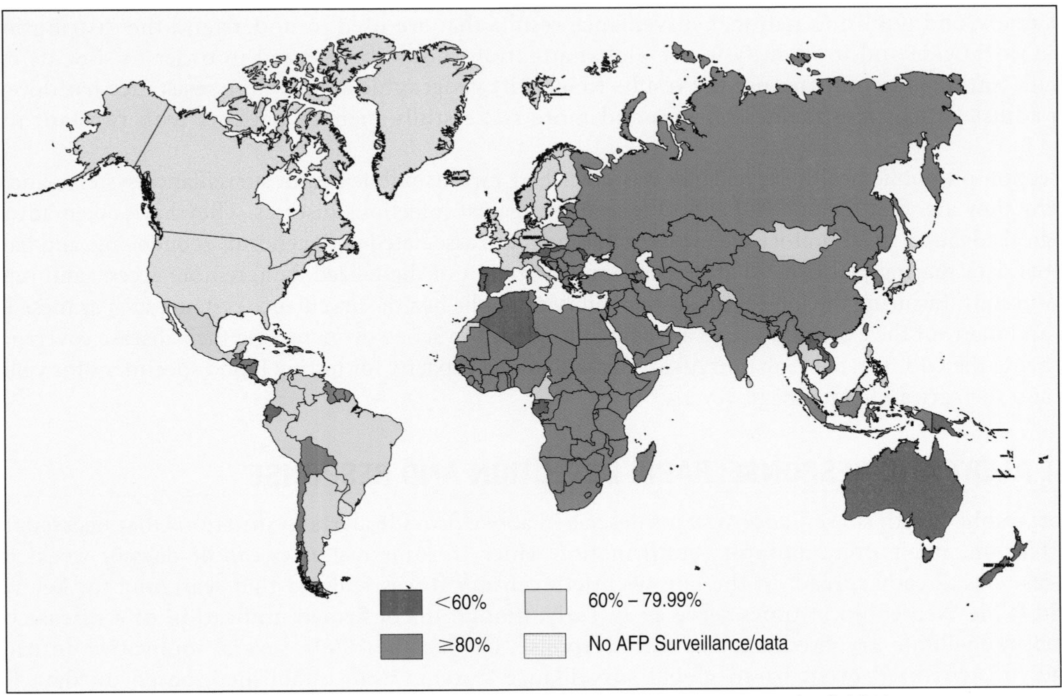

FIG. 11-10 Adequate stool collection percentage, May 2013–April 2014.

Environmental surveillance for polio provides important supplementary surveillance data, and in many countries it is ad hoc, or not conducted at all. Environmental surveillance reveals wild and Sabin (vaccine) polioviruses, as well as circulating vaccine-derived poliovirus, the latter two usually from countries where oral polio vaccines continue to be used.

In areas where sewage is maintained in closed systems, representative points for collection of sewage samples are selected and sewage samples are obtained at regular intervals, usually weekly. In systems where sewage is in open canals or rivers, collection is done in a similar manner.

Sewage samples are provided to specialized reference laboratories where they are concentrated, followed by virus isolation and sequencing. Environmental surveillance (especially in polio-free regions) provides insights into the international spread of poliovirus. A recent example comes from Israel where for over 1 year wild poliovirus was identified in sewage, but no cases of AFP could be found despite heightened surveillance.[36]

Antituberculosis Drug Resistance Surveillance

The Global Project on Antituberculosis Drug Resistance Surveillance (herein referred to as the Project) has periodically collected and analyzed data on drug resistance from surveys of sampled patients and from national surveillance systems around the world since 1994.[37] The Project provides a common surveillance platform to which countries can provide data that are then analyzed to monitor the evolution, national burden, and epidemiologic patterns of MDR-TB—information necessary for best possible planning of national and regional TB management strategies. The Project also monitors the evolution of XDR-TB.

The Project is underpinned by national laboratory activities that identify and examine the sensitivity of the mycobacterium that causes TB. Quality control is assured by a supranational TB reference laboratory network that continuously assesses the drug-susceptibility testing and other laboratory processes. The Project also supports countries by providing technical assistance in design and implementation of antituberculosis drug resistance surveys that supplement information obtained from existing surveillance systems. Globally, the Project analyzes, maps, and publishes national surveillance results that are used to understand the distribution of TB resistance worldwide and to identify where global attention should be focused in order to slow its evolution and spread. Nationally, countries use the results to identify geographic areas where resistance has developed in order to adjust patient treatment strategies and more successfully manage patients with resistant infections (Fig. 11-11).

This section on public health surveillance has described various public health surveillance systems and demonstrated why they are vital for our global health security against infectious diseases. They have taken advantage of technological advances in laboratory diagnosis including those associated with genomic sequencing, and have developed global data sharing platforms that permit standardization of digitalized data, remote access, and rapid comparison of results. Ensuring the long-term sustainability of public health surveillance systems such as these is of high priority; and many of the existing systems are being broadened in scope by increasing their disease coverage; a good example being the GPLN in sub-Saharan Africa that has added capacity for testing blood specimens for yellow fever, measles, and the African hemorrhagic fevers.[38]

GLOBAL ALERT AND RESPONSE: RAPID DETECTION AND RESPONSE

The global public health surveillance systems described above provide alerts to situations that necessitate public health attention, albeit after laboratory confirmation which in some instances can be days or weeks later and after disease has already spread. In the late twentieth century it was realized that searching for key words on the World Wide Web could at times serve as an early, though unconfirmed, indication of a disease outbreak and therefore facilitate preparedness and early response. During the 1990s, several innovative, informal, and sometimes unstructured event-based global surveillance systems were established, based on data from the internet and the World Wide Web.

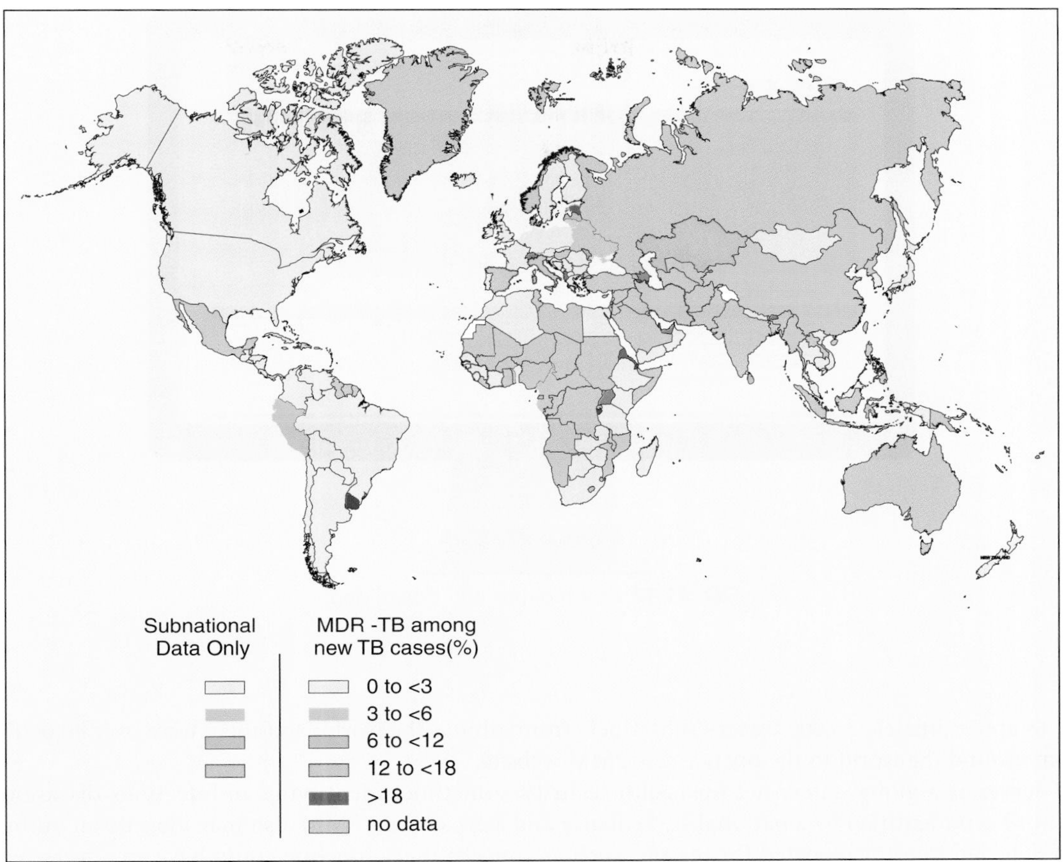

FIG. 11-11 Percentage of new TB cases with MDR-TB, 1994–2010.

PARTICIPATORY SURVEILLANCE

ProMED-mail

One early event-based system was **ProMED-mail (PMM)**, a listserv established in 1994 as a mechanism to identify emerging disease outbreaks.[39] PMM receives reports of public health events in humans, animals, and plants from its subscribers who report information from many different sources including personal observation, written or electronic reports, the news media, and various open websites.[40] PMM is moderated by a group of medical epidemiologists, and many of them are clinicians, epidemiologists, microbiologists, virologists, and government civil servants, although the PMM listserv also includes members of the general population and international organizations. PMM also receives input from a specially selected group of voluntary reporters who actively search for and report public health events in real time.

Each report from a listserv subscriber, or elsewhere, is reviewed by one of the PMM moderators, who makes an initial assessment. Relevant subject matter experts then further examine reports considered potentially valid. Moderators often attempt to validate the report with additional questions to the reporter or to others who may have information. The reports that are accepted after this vetting process are placed in a standard format with references from the medical literature that provide information about the suspected etiology. They are then provided to the listserv, where discussion among listserv subscribers often ensues and where the events are archived for future public searching (Fig. 11-12). At the end of the first 10 years of PMM, an average of seven reports were being provided

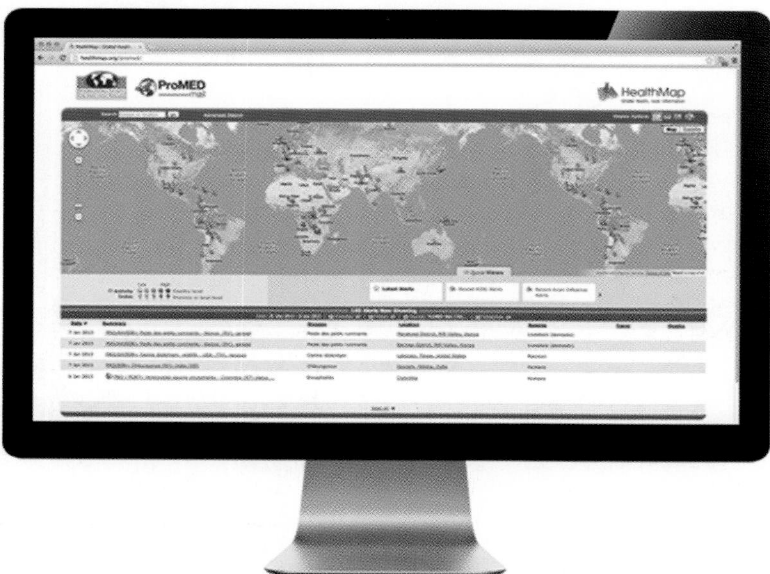

FIG. 11-12 ProMed-mail and HealthMap.

each day to approximately 35,000 listserv subscribers from around the world; and there were over 40,000 monthly visits from around the world to the open access PMM website.

PMM serves as a global safety net for health security, sometimes identifying an infectious disease outbreak that has not been identified by a national surveillance and alert system. PMM also may identify an outbreak that has been detected but not reported for reasons such as concern that reporting could have an adverse economic impact.

Flu Near You

Flu Near You is a free, participatory surveillance system open to anyone over 12 years of age living in the USA or Canada.[41] To register, a potential participant provides basic data, including age, sex, and email address. Once registered, participants are asked to complete a brief survey via email every week that seeks information about 10 symptoms linked to influenza, and other information such as whether the registered participant has had an influenza vaccination. Once weekly data have been submitted by a participant, a map appears that shows how many people have influenza symptoms in the immediate geographic area and nationally and permits comparison of the agglomerated self-reported data against two other influenza databases, Google Flu Trends and CDC. Flu Near You also provides links to information such as where a participant can obtain an influenza vaccination. Other countries, including the UK, have adopted similar participatory influenza surveillance systems, adding greater understanding to the epidemiology of influenza around the world (Fig. 11-13).

Flu Near You and other participatory surveillance systems are still in an early stage of development and evaluation, but they hold the potential to provide more timely and sensitive information for national and global alert. Because they provide feedback directly to participants, they may be able to strengthen prevention by also providing information such as why vaccination is important, and where it can be obtained. They also have the potential to guide participants who seek medical advice to health facilities where clinical assessment and management are available.

DIGITAL SEARCH SURVEILLANCE

HealthMap

HealthMap is an electronic computer-based mechanism that collects online information about outbreaks from real-time surveillance reports of PMM, and from many other open electronic sources as well.[42] Other sources of information that HealthMap uses include GeoSentinel, a clinician-based sentinel surveillance system of international travelers; *EuroSurveillance*, a peer-reviewed European information publication on communicable disease surveillance and control; commercial news aggregation services such as Google News, Moreover, Baidu News, and SOSO Info; and several international organizations and academic institutions. HealthMap was founded in 2006 and is maintained by epidemiologists and software developers.

The information acquired and processed by HealthMap is displayed using open source software tools from Google. The software tools permit HealthMap to organize and display public health events by time, geographic location, and etiology. The open access website and other digital display mechanisms of HealthMap provide real-time displays of information that map current infectious disease outbreaks in humans and animals. The system is fully automated and runs 24 h a day, monitoring, organizing, integrating, filtering, and visualizing online information in nine different languages. Fig. 11-12 shows how HealthMap reports are integrated with PMM, but they can also be accessed independently. HealthMap also uses innovative information such as that from Flu Heat You.

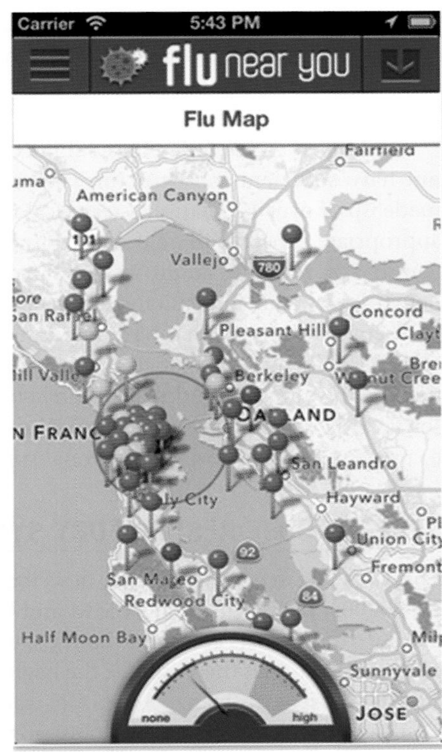

FIG. 11-13 Flu Near You and HealthMap.

Syndromic Surveillance

Syndromic surveillance (SS) is the collection, analysis and interpretation of signs and symptoms (syndromes) that could indicate an infectious disease, and provide early indication of an outbreak. In some countries, signs and symptoms are reported through routine or sentinel disease reporting sites, while in others they are proactively collected by periodically and remotely scanning digital records, permitting real-time syndromic surveillance. Digital records that are used include databases at sites such as emergency departments or outpatient clinics, and some systems are fully automated.

Prior to establishing syndromic surveillance, baselines of syndromes included in the system must be established using historical data, and once established, they serve as a threshold. When a particular syndrome passes this threshold, a standard investigation protocol is usually implemented to determine what type of response is required.

The Global Public Health Intelligence Network

The **Global Public Heath Intelligence Network (GPHIN)**, developed in 1999, is a secure, nonpublic web application that collects information about public health events of potential international significance.[43] Unlike PMM, GPHIN has restricted access limited to organizations with an established public health mandate. GPHIN provides information only to its subscribers. Email alerts are sent automatically to subscribers at the time of new postings.

GPHIN scans the internet to gather information from multiple news aggregators in real time, 24 h a day. It searches using key words that could indicate outbreaks caused by infectious diseases and environmental, radioactive, and natural disasters in six major languages.

Based on a memorandum of understanding between WHO and GPHIN, information is reported to WHO every 24 h for validation through the WHO network of regional and country offices. Any public health events that are validated are discussed in confidence with the countries involved, and WHO support is provided through the Global Outbreak Alert and Response Network (GOARN), if requested.[44]

GOARN was developed as a support mechanism to countries that have confirmed public health events but do not have sufficient infrastructure and/or capacity to respond without external support. The GOARN network is made up of over 120 national technical institutions that support WHO in responding to outbreaks by ensuring that appropriate experts can be provided to countries if requested. Once a request for support has been received from a country or multiple countries, WHO provides terms of reference for experts required to all institutions in the network by email, and suitable experts who are proposed by the network's institutions are then recruited by WHO and sent to countries that have requested support.

GOARN enhances global health security by providing technical experts and other support to strengthen the national response to outbreaks of infectious diseases in countries that have insufficient national capacity. By doing so GOARN helps ensure effective outbreak investigation and the implementation of containment measures necessary to prevent national and international spread.

SEVERE ACUTE RESPIRATORY SYNDROME AND GLOBAL ALERT AND RESPONSE

The alert and response systems described above played important roles in the identification and response to the 2002–2003 SARS outbreak.[45] PMM and GPHIN first identified and reported an outbreak of highly fatal respiratory disease from reports coming from the Guangdong Province of China as early as late 2002. GISRS was alerted because of the concern that this could be the beginning of an influenza pandemic caused by a mutation event of the influenza A (H5N1) virus. Influenza A (H5N1) was first identified in humans by the GISRS when it emerged in 1997 in Hong Kong as a small and highly fatal cluster of respiratory infections, carried to Hong Kong by infected poultry from the Guangdong Province in China.

Outbreak Detection

Occasional reports of high mortality respiratory illness in the Guangdong Province continued to be detected by PMM and GPHIN, and in February 2003, GSIRS identified influenza A (H5N1) in a father and his child who had recently returned from China with influenza symptoms, adding to the concern that an influenza pandemic was possibly beginning. Shortly afterward, a medical doctor who had been treating patients with highly lethal respiratory illness in the Guangdong Province entered Hong Kong, while ill, to attend a wedding. Upon arrival in Hong Kong he spent the night in a hotel, and is thought to have infected other hotel guests staying overnight on the same floor, who unknowingly spread the infection as they returned to their home countries while still in the incubation period of disease (Fig. 11-14).

A businessman, who had stayed on the same hotel floor as the medical doctor, traveled from Hong Kong to Vietnam, where he subsequently became seriously ill with respiratory symptoms requiring ventilator support (Fig. 11-15). GISRS was unable to identify an influenza virus in specimens taken from this patient, and he became the first reported human outside of China with an infection that we now know was caused by the SARS coronavirus. Other hotel guests traveled by air to other Asian countries, North America, and Europe, where they, like the businessman in Vietnam, became sick. They in turn spread infection to hospital workers and other close contacts, beginning local outbreaks. The index case of this international cluster of cases, the medical doctor from Guangdong, also spread infection to health workers in the Hong Kong Hospital where he had been admitted, setting up a major focus of transmission in Hong Kong.

Once the extent of international spread was understood, technical experts from GOARN-associated partners were solicited. Public health institutions and NGOs from multiple countries responded to the GOARN request to provide technical support at WHO headquarters, and in the countries where outbreaks were occurring.

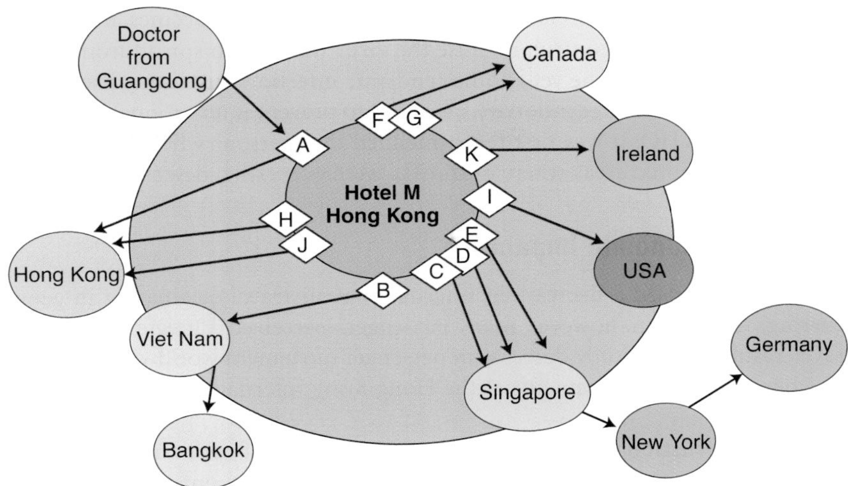

FIG. 11-14 International spread of SARS coronavirus, 2003.

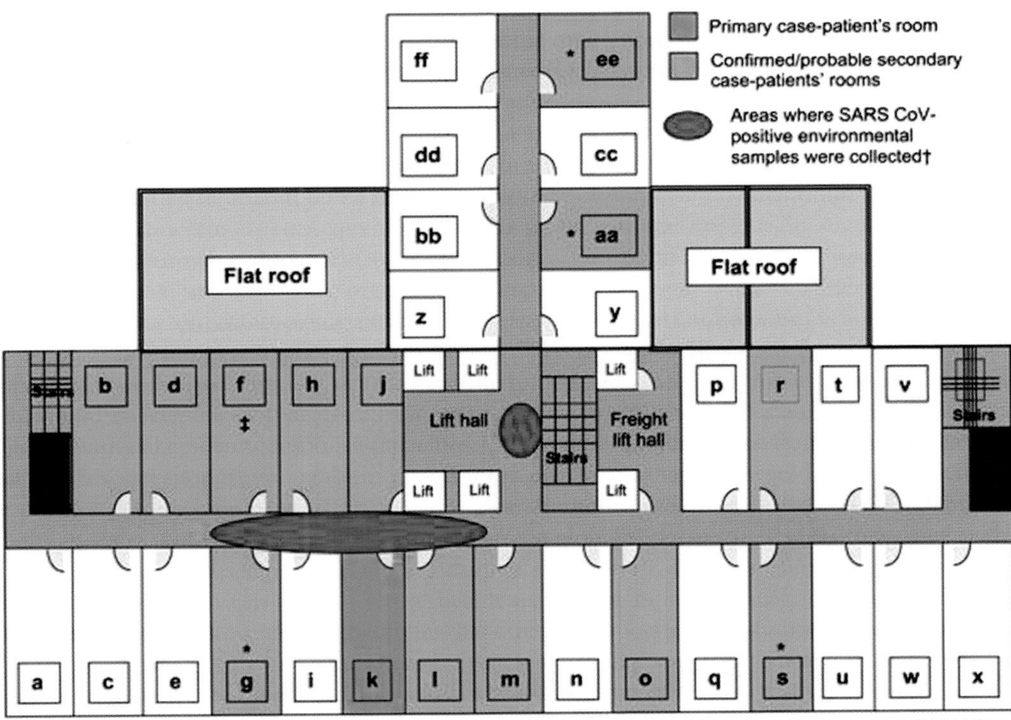

FIG. 11-15 Layout of ninth floor of Hotel Metropole, where superspreading event of SARS occurred, Hong Kong, 2003. Braden CR, Dowell SF, Jernigan DB, Hughes JM. Emerg Infect Dis 2013;19:864–9. <http://wwwnc.cdc.gov/eid/article/19/6/13-0192-f1.htm>.

SARS had never before been identified in humans, and thus there were no vaccines, medicines, or predetermined measures that could be used for disease control. Because the virus was able to spread from human to human, there was concern that, like HIV, it would become yet another endemic infection, sustaining itself indefinitely in humans, or in an animal infected from humans. Precautionary measures to prevent international spread of the infection were immediately recommended by WHO. It was first recommended that persons who were ill with similar symptoms, and who had contact with geographic areas where outbreaks were occurring, defer travel until they were well.

Outbreak Mitigation and Economic Impact

These precautionary measures caused a decrease in international air travel originating in geographic areas where outbreaks were occurring. In addition, however, many passengers perceived a greater risk of travel and postponed or cancelled their travel, resulting in a steady decrease in passenger movement worldwide. This decline is most clearly shown in Fig. 11-16, where passenger movements at the Hong Kong International Airport decreased soon after the outbreak was announced.

Overall, the Hong Kong International Airport experienced a decrease of approximately 70% in passenger movements in April 2003 compared with the previous year, and aircraft movements decreased by an estimated 30%. During this same period, restaurants, hotels, and retail sales decreased, often due to panic and misperception of the risk of transmission, which resulted in people avoiding populous gatherings and decreasing consumer activities (Fig. 11-17).

When SARS spread throughout a major housing complex in Hong Kong among persons who had not been in direct face-to-face contact with each other, it was hypothesized that SARS might also be spreading through a secondary factor, such as an insect or water. This hypothesis led to stronger precautionary recommendations, including postponement or cancellation of travel to areas where outbreaks of SARS were occurring and a human contact could not be identified as a source of infection for each person in the outbreak.

The Aftermath of SARS

The SARS outbreak ended in July 2003, with 8096 cases reported from 29 countries, of which 774 (9.6%) were fatal (Fig. 11-18).

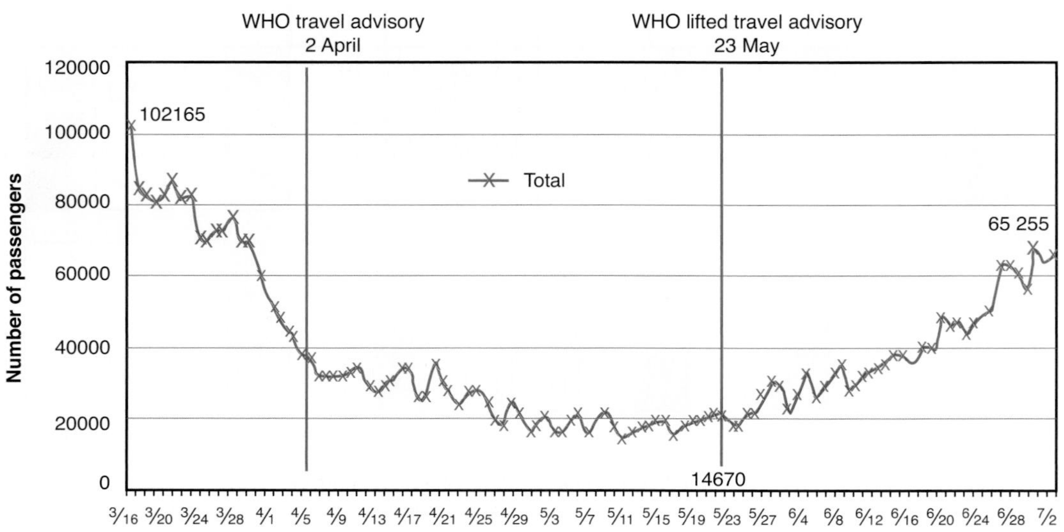

FIG. 11-16 Airport passenger movements, Hong Kong International Airport, 2003.

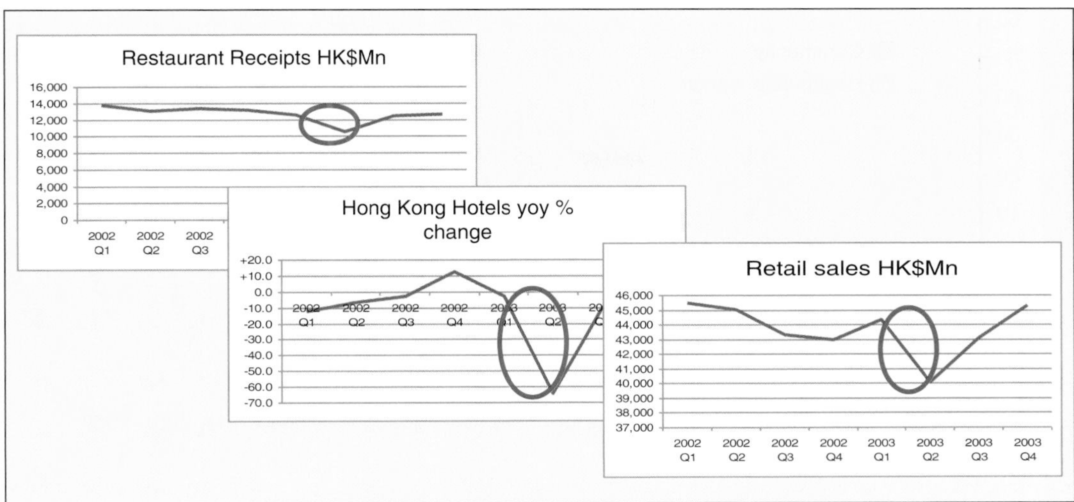

FIG. 11-17 Economic impact, SARS, Hong Kong 2003.

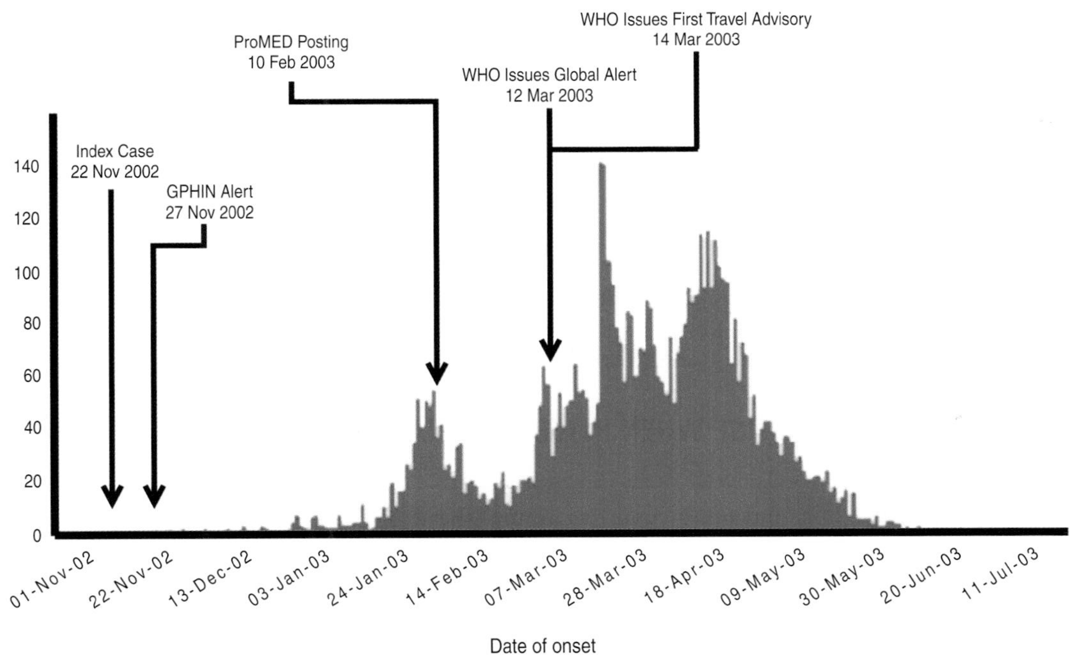

FIG. 11-18 SARS, probable cases by date of onset, worldwide, 2002–2003.

The Asian Development Bank estimated the economic impact of SARS at approximately US$18 billion in East Asia, or approximately 0.6% of gross domestic product. Fortunately, economic recovery was rapid once international spread had stopped.

The SARS outbreak of 2003 provides a clear example of how an infectious disease that originates in one part of the world can cause a public health security threat to the entire planet. From its origins—probably as a simple coronavirus that had a reservoir in wild animals and gained human-to-human transmissibility through a one-time

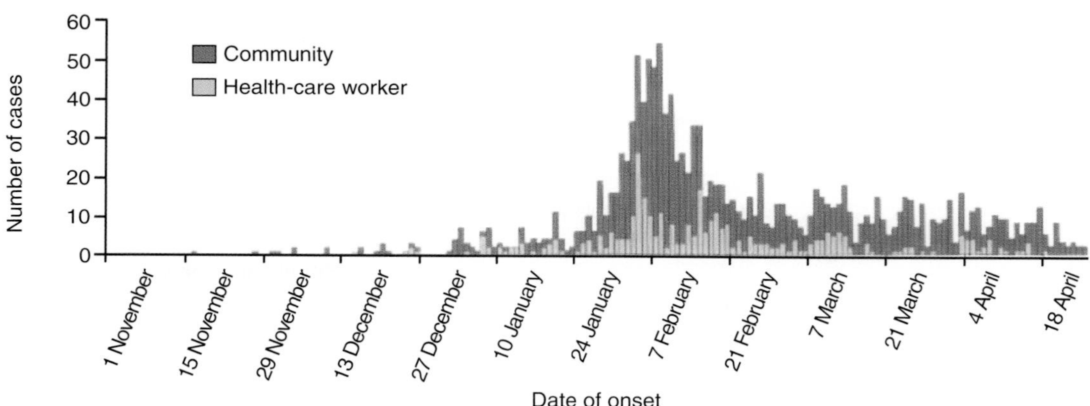

FIG. 11-19 SARS, probable cases by date of onset, Guangdong Province China, 2001–2003.

mutation as it replicated in either a human or an animal host in China—the SARS coronavirus caused an outbreak of global dimension as it crossed international borders. The SARS coronavirus caused an outbreak that demonstrated not only the risk of emerging infections to human health, but also to the world's interlinked economy—an example of the full potential of infections that breach the animal/human species barrier anywhere in a globalized and interconnected world.

Detection and Response where and when the Outbreak Occurred

Based on retrospective analysis, hospital workers in China became infected with the SARS coronavirus early in the outbreak and amplified transmission within hospitals and through close contacts and family members to the community (Fig. 11-19).

It was at this time—in November 2002—that PMM and GPHIN began to detect the outbreak and notified the international community. Had the outbreak been detected and responded to in China, when and where it was occurring, it might not have spread to Hong Kong and then internationally. If that had been the case, the morbidity and mortality, not to mention the severe economic disruption, might have been avoided or mitigated.

PREPAREDNESS AND RESPONSE WHEN INTERNATIONAL BORDERS CANNOT PROTECT POPULATIONS

Since the SARS outbreak, China and other countries around the world have begun to strengthen national alert, preparedness, and response systems and processes for emerging infections and other naturally occurring public health events. Several new national institutes of public health have been established, including the Public Health Agency of Canada, the Health Protection Agency in the UK (recently transformed into Public Health England), and the Hong Kong Centre for Health Protection. Many more countries strengthened their preparedness and capacity to detect and respond to public health events that threaten national populations, and a majority of countries in the world have developed pandemic plans for influenza and other pandemic diseases.

At the same time, the IHR were revised and today place great emphasis on the legally binding requirement of countries to develop eight core capacities in public health. These core capacities include preparedness, surveillance, laboratory, response mechanisms, and risk communication, so that public health events can be better detected and managed nationally, decreasing their potential for international spread.

Emphasis on national core capacity in public health moves actions for public health security from a global to a national perspective. There is, however, still a need for global surveillance systems to ensure public health security and preparedness, and for global alert and response systems to provide a safety net when national capacity fails to detect and/or report a public health event of international concern and international spread occurs.

Biological Weapons, Bioterrorism, and Public Health

Global alert and response systems are also considered important for identifying the deliberate use of biological agents or toxins to cause harm. The same systems that have been developed for the detections and response to naturally occurring emerging infections described in this chapter are also useful for detecting and responding to those that are deliberately caused.

Biological weapons, or harmful biological agents used as a weapon of mass destruction,[46] became a major concern during the Cold War period when countries around the world were known to have programs on the research and development of biological weapons. In 1972, a multilateral disarmament treaty banning the development, production, and stockpiling of biological weapons was opened, and over 170 countries have now become signatories and ratified the treaty. This treaty, the Biological Weapons Convention (BWC), has developed agreement among signatories to provide annual reports, in standard format, on specific activities related to the BWC, including research; vaccine production; national biological defense research and development; past activities in offensive and/or defensive biological research and development if not previously reported; outbreaks of infectious diseases and/or toxins; publications; and legislation/regulation.

In 1991, a group of experts was established under the BWC to identify and examine potential scientific and technical verification measures, but this group was unable to develop consensus on a draft inspection protocol, and the process was ended in 2001, just after the deliberate use of anthrax spores to cause harm in the USA. The absence of any formal verification regime to monitor compliance is thought by some countries to limit the effectiveness of the BWC, but consensus has been developed gradually on measures that would contribute to security from deliberately used agents. These measures include the following:

- national mechanisms to establish and maintain the security and oversight of pathogenic microorganisms and toxins;
- enhanced international capabilities for detecting, responding to, investigating, and mitigating the effects of deliberate use of biological or toxin weapons;
- strengthening and broadening the capabilities for international institutions to detect and respond to the outbreak of infectious diseases (including diseases affecting plants and animals); and
- codes of conduct for scientists.

Many systems that address these measures are already in place for naturally occurring public health events, and are described in this chapter. It has been understood over time in discussions surrounding the BWC that these surveillance, alert, preparedness, and response activities aimed at naturally occurring public health emergencies—mechanisms such as PMM, GPHIN, GOARN, and the IHR—also serve to provide the same support for any events that might be deliberately caused.

The same is true for pandemic planning for surge capacity and resilience. Preparedness for naturally occurring events such as pandemic influenza is now also considered vital for deliberately caused public health events.

CONCLUSION

Though international borders cannot protect against the international spread of infectious diseases, as was thought until the late twentieth century; increased understanding of the potential of emerging infections, electronic communications, digital data sharing platforms, and concerted global action have led to many recently developed mechanisms that have led to stronger public health security.

In addition, animal and human health agencies are beginning to work more closely together to assess the risks of emerging infections and to prevent or mitigate their emergence internationally, regionally, and nationally in a One Health movement that continues to gain momentum.

Innovations in surveillance and detection that use hand-held digital devices have opened the way for participatory, real-time surveillance among entire populations. And finally, the understanding that mechanisms in place for preparing for, detecting, and responding to naturally occurring emerging disease events are the same as required for those that are deliberately caused have created the potential for closer collaboration among sectors dealing with public health and defense.

With increased understanding about the risks caused by infectious disease, and the fact that they can cross international borders with relative ease, public health surveillance and risk assessment have come a long way since the pandemics of the fourteenth century, making the future of global health security bright.

KEY SUMMARY POINTS

- While there have been many successes in global disease surveillance, some challenges remain. Transparency, trust and sharing of data are key governance issues that need to continue to be addressed, as they are essential elements of success.
- The spread of disease has always been a major concern, and public health security measures have become a part of national defense.
- International collaboration began as a collective defense mechanism, resulting in many international treaties, conventions, and regulations, to control the spread of disease through international borders.
- Disease spread cannot be stopped at international borders, as demonstrated by EIDs. EIDs are threats to public health security that have high human and economic costs, as demonstrated by H1N1, vCJD, and SARS.
- Global surveillance and sharing of the benefits of surveillance is a public good. Influenza surveillance in humans and animals demonstrate the network of global laboratories and surveillance networks that work to detect clusters and outbreaks of potential public health importance.
- Global alert and response systems are an important way to ensure public health security.
- The SARS outbreak demonstrates the spread of disease across international borders and the importance of early detection and alert, as well as outbreak mitigation strategies.
- The IHR (2005) emphasize core public health capacities to better detect and manage public health events.
- Preparedness and global alert and response systems for naturally occurring infectious diseases are important in identifying potential use of biological weapons or bioterrorism.

DISCUSSION QUESTIONS

1. Give some examples of public health security risk caused by infectious diseases.
2. What are the key characteristics of emerging infectious diseases? List some examples.
3. Which recent events demonstrate that stopping the international spread of emerging infectious diseases requires more than action at international borders?
4. Give some other examples of the human and economic costs of emerging infectious diseases in addition to those listed in the chapter.
5. Do you agree that global surveillance is necessary for global health security? Why or why not? Is it a global public good?
6. How do the laboratory networks, surveillance systems, and alert systems help ensure global security?
7. What are the underlying characteristics of the innovative alert and response described in the chapter? Use these characteristics to describe a potential future innovative system—what would it do? How would it provide an alert for public health action? How would it use more traditional systems or information sources?
8. How can the IHR (2005) core capacities be described in relation to global security?
9. Describe how the lessons learned from the examples provided throughout the chapter could enhance a country's ability to detect a deliberately caused outbreak and protect its population against a biological weapon.

REFERENCES

1. Rodier G, Greenspan AL, Hughes JM, Heymann DL. Global public health security. Emerg Infect Dis 2007;13(10):1447–52.
2. Kilwein JH. Some historical comments on quarantine: part one. J Clin Pharm Ther 1995;20(4):185–7.
3. Stuard SM. A state of deference: Ragusa/Dubrovnik in the Medieval Centuries: University of Pennsylvania Press; 1992. p. 269.
4. Harvard University Library Open Collection. Cholera epidemics in the 19th century, <http://ocp.hul.harvard.edu/contagion/cholera.html/>; [cited June 06, 2014].
5. Lloyd BJ. The Pan American Sanitary Bureau. Am J Public Health Nations Health 1930;20(9):925–9.
6. Stowman K. International sanitary regulations. Public Health Rep 1952;67(10):972–6.
7. INTERNATIONAL sanitary regulations. World Health Organization regulations No. 2. World Health Organ Tech Rep Ser 1951;41:1–100.
8. Hahn BH, Shaw GM, De Cock KM, Sharp PM. AIDS as a zoonosis: scientific and public health implications. Science 2000;287(5453):607–14.
9. Health CoEMTt, Medicine Io. Emerging infections: microbial threats to health in the United States. In: Lederberg J, Shope RE, Oaks Jr SC, editors. National Academies Press; 1992. p. 312.
10. Morse SS. Factors in the emergence of infectious diseases. Emerg Infect Dis 1995;1(1):7–15.
11. Jones KE, Patel NG, Levy MA, Storeygard A, Balk D, Gittleman JL, et al. Global trends in emerging infectious diseases. Nature 2008;451(7181):990–3.
12. Sharp PM, Hahn BH. Origins of HIV and the AIDS pandemic. Cold Spring Harb Perspect Med 2011;1(1):a006841.
13. Kruse H, Kirkemo AM, Handeland K. Wildlife as source of zoonotic infections. Emerg Infect Dis 2004;10(12):2067–72.
14. Thorns CJ. Bacterial food-borne zoonoses. Rev Sci Tech 2000;19(1):226–39.
15. Reusken CB, Haagmans BL, Muller MA, Gutierrez C, Godeke GJ, Meyer B, et al. Middle East respiratory syndrome coronavirus neutralising serum antibodies in dromedary camels: a comparative serological study. Lancet Infect Dis 2013;13(10):859–66.
16. Han J, Jin M, Zhang P, Liu J, Wang L, Wen D, et al. Epidemiological link between exposure to poultry and all influenza A(H7N9) confirmed cases in Huzhou city, China, March to May 2013. Euro Surveill 2013;18(20).
17. Ostroff S. Perspectives: the role of the traveler in translocation of disease. The yellow book: CDC health information for international travel 2014. U.S. Centers for Disease Control and Prevention; 2014.
18. Heymann DL, Dar OA. Prevention is better than cure for emerging infectious diseases. BMJ 2014;348:g1499.
19. Bank TW. People, pathogens, and our planet. Washington, DC: The World Bank; 2012.
20. Heymann DL, Reinhardt K. Emerging infections, the international health regulations, and macro-economy. In: Culyer AJ, editor. Encyclopedia of health economics. San Diego: Elsevier; 2014. p. 272–6.
21. Vargas-Parada L. H1N1: a Mexican perspective. Cell 2009;139(7):1203–5.
22. Organization WHO. Pandemic (H1N1) 2009 - update 82: World Health Organization, <http://www.who.int/csr/don/2010_01_08/en/>; [updated December 2, 2010; cited June 6, 2014].
23. Prevention USCfDCa. Seasonal influenza (Flu): information on swine influenza/variant influenza viruses, <http://www.cdc.gov/flu/swineflu/>; [cited June 6, 2014].
24. Rassy D, Smith RD. The economic impact of H1N1 on Mexico's tourist and pork sectors. Health Econ 2013;22(7):824–34.
25. Organization WHO. Joint FAO/WHO/OIE statement on influenza A(H1N1) and the safety of pork: World Health Organization, <http://www.who.int/mediacentre/news/statements/2009/h1n1_20090430/en/>; 2009 [updated December 10, 2010; cited June 6, 2014].
26. Galante M, Garin O, Sicuri E, Cots F, Garcia-Altes A, Ferrer M, et al. Health services utilization, work absenteeism and costs of pandemic influenza A (H1N1) 2009 in Spain: a multicenter-longitudinal study. PLoS One 2012;7(2):e31696.
27. The Impact of the H1N1 Pandemic on Canadian Hospitals. 2010.
28. Hill AF, Desbruslais M, Joiner S, Sidle KC, Gowland I, Collinge J, et al. The same prion strain causes vCJD and BSE. Nature 1997;389(6650):448–50, 526.
29. Collee JG, Bradley R, Liberski PP. Variant CJD (vCJD) and bovine spongiform encephalopathy (BSE): 10 and 20 years on: part 2. Folia Neuropathol 2006;44(2):102–10.
30. Brown P, Will RG, Bradley R, Asher DM, Detwiler L. Bovine spongiform encephalopathy and variant Creutzfeldt-Jakob disease: background, evolution, and current concerns. Emerg Infect Dis 2001;7(1):6–16.
31. Atkinson N. The impact of BSE on the UK economy, <http://www.veterinaria.org/revistas/vetenfinf/bse/14Atkinson.html/>. [cited June 06, 2014].
32. Organization WH. Global Influenza Surveillance and Response System (GISRS): World Health Organization, <http://www.who.int/influenza/gisrs_laboratory/en/>; 2014. [updated May 23, 2014; cited June 06, 2014].
33. FluNet: World Health Organization, <http://gamapserver.who.int/GlobalAtlas/home.asp/>; [cited 2014].
34. OFFLU OIE/FAO Network of expertise on animal influenza, <http://www.offlu.net/>; [cited June 06, 2014].
35. Public Health England. Human animal infections and risk surveillance group London: Health Protection Agency, <http://www.hpa.org.uk/Topics/InfectiousDiseases/InfectionsAZ/EmergingInfections/HAIRS/>; [updated February 11, 2014; cited June 6, 2014].
36. World Health Organization. Poliovirus detected from environmental samples in Israel - update, <http://www.who.int/csr/don/2013_07_15/en/>; 2013. [updated August 26, 2013; cited June 6, 2014].
37. World Health Organization. Surveillance of drug resistance in tuberculosis, <http://www.who.int/tb/challenges/mdr/surveillance/en/>; 2014. [updated March 14, 2014; cited 2014].
38. Heymann DL, Aylward RB. Poliomyelitis eradication and pandemic influenza. Lancet 2006;367(9521):1462–4.
39. ProMED-mail. About ProMED-mail, <http://www.promedmail.org/aboutus/>; [cited 2015].
40. ProMED-mail. <http://www.promedmail.org/>; [cited June 6, 2014].
41. Healthmap, Boston Children's H, American Public Health A, Skoll Global Threats F. About - flu near you, <https://flunearyou.org/>; 2013.
42. HealthMap. <http://healthmap.org/>; [cited June 6, 2014].
43. Mykhalovskiy E, Weir L. The Global Public Health Intelligence Network and early warning outbreak detection: a Canadian contribution to global public health. Can J Public Health 2006;97(1):42–4.
44. Heymann DL, Rodier GR. Hot spots in a wired world: WHO surveillance of emerging and re-emerging infectious diseases. Lancet Infect Dis 2001;1(5):345–53.
45. Heymann DL. SARS and emerging infectious diseases: a challenge to place global solidarity above national sovereignty. Ann Acad Med Singapore 2006;35(5):350–3.
46. Merriam-Webster, <http://www.merriam-webster.com/>.

CHAPTER

12

Smart Governance of Public Health Surveillance

Affan T Shaikh, Scott JN McNabb

Of all the forms of inequality, injustice in health care is the most shocking and inhuman.

Martin Luther King Jr

KEY WORDS

Governance
Statist
Globalist
Human security
Global public health security
Viral sovereignty
Universal Declaration of Human right
Smart governance

PERSPECTIVES ON GLOBAL HEALTH GOVERNANCE

Ethical considerations in public health governance are critical for the success and sustainability of public health surveillance initiatives across the world. Yet, despite remarkable achievements in both public health and medicine over the past century, for those left behind, the status quo remains one sided and a further "indictment of our collective failure to ensure the equitable sharing of health progress."[1] Global health governance—a potential equalizing force—is the "collective forms of governance, from the subnational to the global level, which address health issues with a global dimension."[2] But despite US$30 billion per year in funding for global health initiatives, global health suffers from poor governance, in part due to lack of coordination and competing visions.[3,4] However, "no country can protect the health of its citizens alone,"[5] and therefore global health governance is informed by several multidisciplinary paradigms to approach these difficult issues.[6]

Chief among these various global health governance models, two diverging attitudes permeate governance discussions, as depicted in the global health governance compass (Fig. 12-1). On this compass, threats can exist on two axes. The x-axis runs between statist and globalist. The **statist** perspective is concerned primarily with the security and stability of the state, while the **globalist** perspective focuses primarily on the well-being of individuals and communities.[7] The y-axis runs between global health security and human security. **Global health security** focuses on securitization, containment, and the inside/outside dynamic. **Human security** focuses on stability, health equity, sustainable development, moral obligation, and root causes of disease.[8] While proponents for each perspective may not always exclusively favor one approach over the other, public health governance issues are heavily influenced by the actions, inactions, and prioritization based on each perspective. Both perspectives are criticized, yet both hold an important place in global discourse.[4,7] Global health security arguments use the rationale that an action is justified if it ultimately benefits the state, while human security arguments use the rationale that an action is justified if it ultimately benefits humanity.

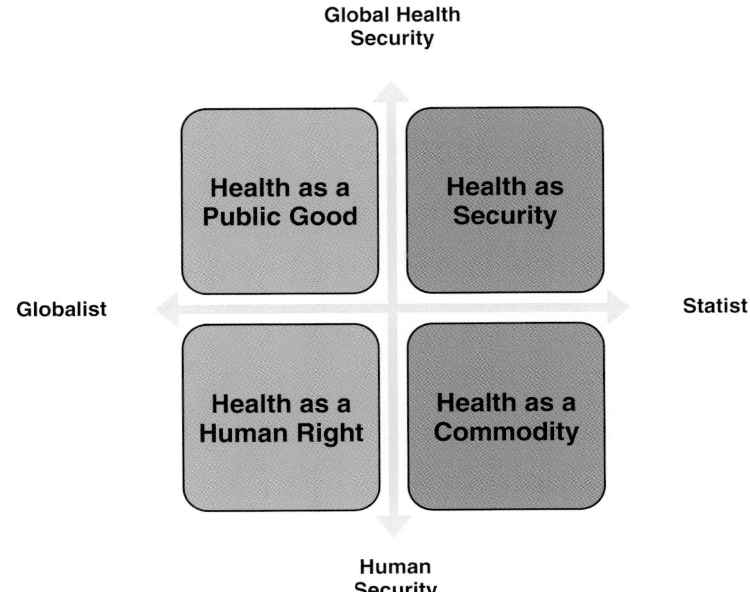

FIG. 12-1 Global health governance compass.

The global health governance compass is a useful tool for organizing and understanding various approaches to governance. It is by no means an absolute or static measure. Determining one's position on the compass requires two questions. Firstly, is the intervention under consideration motivated by a desire to ultimately secure the state (statism) or by more altruistic persuasions to protect vulnerable populations regardless of their nationality (globalism)? This will determine who will ultimately benefit from the intervention. Secondly, is the proposed action using language in support of state interests (global health security) or of vulnerable populations (human security)? Using this framework, health concerns are consequently framed as security issues (upper right quadrant), commodity issues (lower right quadrant), human right issues (lower left quadrant), or public good issues (upper right quadrant). The quadrants of this compass will be used to organize our discussion throughout this chapter.

Considering emerging and re-emerging infectious diseases (EIDs) and noncommunicable diseases (NCDs), let's explore the global health compass further. A statist perspective is interested in ultimately protecting the state and may adopt a global health security or human security position to do so. Framed as a global health security issue, a statist, for example, would enact policies that directly support system strengthening of state interests. These actions may include building national epidemic response capacities. On the other hand, statism framed as a human security issue would enact policies that support vulnerable populations in only so far that they would ultimately benefit state interests. These policies may include supporting vaccine research and biomedical interventions targeting EIDs heavily present in foreign states. On the other side of the spectrum, a globalist perspective is less concerned with protecting individual states, but more focused on securing the health of all, especially the most vulnerable, regardless of nationality. As with statism, a globalist can adopt a global health security or human security approach. Framed as a global health security issue, a globalist would enact policies that directly support system strengthening of foreign institutions according to the needs of the foreign state. These actions may include supporting foreign workforce capacities. On the other hand, globalism framed as a human security issue would support policies that support the greatest challenges facing vulnerable populations. These actions may include eradication efforts targeting neglected tropical diseases or supporting foreign efforts to combat NCDs. These variations in approach are summarized in Table 12-1.

In public health surveillance, organizations supporting one of the perspectives in this compass utilize different missions and agendas that affect their attitude toward ethical concerns. Between individual actors, these issues may

TABLE 12-1 Public Health Governance Perspectives

		STATIST	GLOBALIST
Referent		State	Individual
Threat		Does the disease threaten the well-being of the state?	Who is the most vulnerable to disease?
Response		Strengthen institutions protecting the state system	Alleviate the impact of disease on individuals
Ethical stance		Self-protection	Common humanity
Value framework			
	Values	Securitization, preparedness, containment, inside and outside dynamic, and prioritization and collective action against ongoing or future acute threats	
Global health security	*Health as*	Security	Public Good
	Examples	Develop global disease surveillance systems, **national** response capacities, and biomedical interventions targeting **EIDs** threatening **wealthy** countries	Develop global disease surveillance systems, **foreign** response capacities, and biomedical interventions targeting **EIDs** threatening **all** countries, especially **most vulnerable**
	Values	Security, stability, health equity, apolitical, long-term investments, sustainable development, root cause of disease, moral obligation	
Human security	*Health as*	Human right/development	Commodity
	Examples	Provide access to vaccines, drug and vaccine research and development targeting **EIDs** threatening **wealthy** countries in **vulnerable** countries	Provide access to essential medicines, drug, and vaccine research and development targeting **EIDs or NCDs** threatening **most vulnerable**

include privacy, consent, disclosure, and moral obligations to prevent the spread of disease. Between populations, national and international governments, nongovernmental organizations, and private corporations, these issues may include ownership of biological materials and intellectual property, data sharing, and moral obligations to prevent the spread of disease (Fig. 12-2).

This chapter will focus on issues at this broader level, including the statist and globalist perspectives and the values of global health security and human security that are used to frame arguments and mobilize action between populations. We will describe the frames of security, commodity, human rights, development, and the global public good. The implications of these issues for global public health surveillance will be discussed. Two examples will be presented, the first about the recent claims of viral sovereignty and the ongoing debate over ownership and patenting of biological material and its consequences for public health surveillance. The second example is about the emergence of antimicrobial resistance and the ongoing need to strengthen health systems. However, as we will demonstrate, a new holistic approach to the governance of public health surveillance or what we will coin as smart public health governance that balances the statist and globalist views is needed.

Interoganizational

- Ownership of biological materials and intellectual property
- Data sharing
- Access to benefits
- Moral obligations

Interpersonal

- Privacy
- Consent
- Dosclosure
- Moral obligations

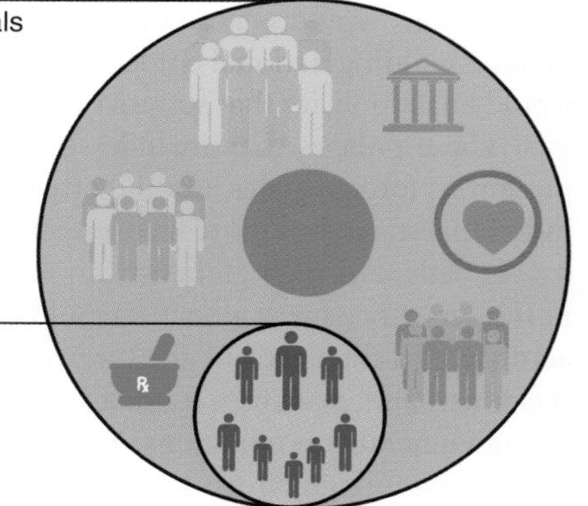

FIG. 12-2 Ethical considerations of public health surveillance at the micro- and macro-levels.

STATISM IN THE GOVERNANCE OF PUBLIC HEALTH SURVEILLANCE

With the emergence of a globalized world, we now readily acknowledge that microbes know no boundaries—in today's interconnected world, public health threats in one part of the world can affect the entire global population very easily.[10]

In 1851, a group of delegates from 12 countries met in France to standardize international quarantine measures against the spread of cholera, plague, and yellow fever,[11,12] the first of 14 International Sanitary Conferences spanning 87 years. These conferences formed the foundation on which the World Health Organization (WHO) was built in 1948,[11] and illustrate one of the first coordinated efforts to protect the state by limiting the spread of epidemic diseases—a hallmark of the statist perspective.

History is filled with records of epidemics; before the more widespread movement and exchange of people and goods these outbreaks remained localized incidents.[13] With increased interaction, however, microbes spread more quickly than ever, and new populations with little past exposure were exposed to new pathogens. Spurred by fears of the rapid spread of disease, states devised elaborate precautions to prevent the spread of pestilence, despite knowing little about the diseases' etiology and epidemiology.[11,14,15] Their primary concern was to protect the booming economic networks that marked the beginning of the globalized world. Yet, early quarantine precautions often resulted in delays, costs to merchants and business owners, sequestration of crewmembers and passengers, and destroyed cargo.[15,16] These mounting costs led European nations to request lifting undue restrictions.

In order to ease difficulties for international trade and commerce, the first International Sanitary Conference took place in 1851 in Paris.[11] A debate over proper quarantine procedures of cholera at this first meeting indicates the developing statist sentiment. The Spanish medical delegate said cholera was not "constantly, essentially, and universally contagious" and that quarantine caused a loss of time, to which an English delegate retorted, "time is money [but] public health is gold."[11] This short exchange demonstrates the early understanding that public health actions were linked inextricably to economic consequences and it was therefore necessary to protect the state from external microbial threats.[17] The International Sanitary Conference was the first major event to establish health protection for international consultation through cooperation[11] and set a global precedent for the statist perspective. The conferences sought to deal with both hypothetical and actual dangers to economic, military, and political interests through scientific debate and coordinated responses.[11,15]

The golden age of microbiology ushered in a new era of public health and medicinal advances improving our understanding of the etiology and epidemiology of infectious diseases. While this decreased the incidence of new disease and greatly improved sanitation standards, it did little to help already infected patients until after World War II, when antibiotics were discovered. After successfully defeating smallpox, polio, and other infectious diseases, most western nations felt the threat of infectious diseases was waning.

Over the past two decades this sentiment has all but changed again, as the threat of emerging and re-emerging infectious diseases returns.[19] As one expert puts it, "despite [...] enormous technological and economic power, [many policy experts have failed to realize] it is extremely unlikely that developed countries will be able to remain an island of health in a global sea of disease."[20] The statist perspective uses the language of security to reprioritize health issues from "low politics" to "high politics,"[21] in order to capture the attention of decision-makers.[21]

The statist rationale begins and ends with the state. Statists are focused on determining the role health plays in economic, military, and political interests in order to better prepare the state to respond to threats of disease.[7] They ask whether a particular disease threatens the state, and, if so, what actions can be taken to strengthen institutions protecting the state.

This perspective is illustrated by health policy development in the USA. The USA hosted an International Sanitary Conference to promote international acceptance of the first US Federal Quarantine Act.[11,22] This act aimed to create a national notification system of the sanitary conditions of ports and vessels outside and destined for the USA. This proposal called for the right to inspect foreign ships not only on their arrival but also on their departure,[11] which many saw as a breech of sovereignty. More recently, US officials have underscored the fundamental need to protect the state from emerging threats from not only traditional security threats such as nuclear incidents and terrorism but also public health threats such as avian influenza pandemics.

Statism and Global Health Security

Health security is the recognition that "infectious diseases constitute a verifiable threat to national security and state power"[20] and require the government's engagement.[24] For example, HIV/AIDS brought the recognition of an emerging threat to the state that could—and did—disrupt global health. A number of scientists have argued the need for international relations and health experts to address the security implications of emerging diseases.[20,24–27] The statist perspective, in the language of global health security, was further endorsed by a 2007 WHO report that stated the importance of global public health security:

Global public health security is defined as the activities required, both proactive and reactive, to minimize vulnerability to acute public health events that endanger the collective health of populations living across geographical regions and international boundaries [...] Global health security, or the lack of it, may also have an impact on economic or political stability, trade, tourism, access to goods and services and, if they occur repeatedly, on demographic stability.[28]

In the US, the Obama administration oversaw the creation of the Global Health Security Agenda[29] with the principal aim of strengthening capacitates in low- and middle-income countries to prevent, detect, and respond to outbreaks of infectious diseases, epidemics, and bioterrorism.[5] This agenda represents the US shift in thinking of health threats as security threats as well as the need to address such threats across sectors.[30] The agenda streamlines the state's security needs into three simple goals (prevent, detect, and respond) and nine key operational objectives and creates clear actionable priorities for global public health security that make sense to diplomats and security officials. The agenda uses the language of security, preparedness, and containment—the language of global health security—to broaden the statist health perspective out of the traditional technical realm.[31]

Health as Security

After the Cold War ended, academics and policy experts began to explore nonmilitary threats. While this new area received guidance (e.g., from the United Nations Development Program's 1994 report *New Dimensions of Human Security*, a foundational globalist and human security document discussed later in the chapter) there was still a need to identify how health challenges become identifiable security threats.[32]

The Copenhagen School of Security Studies demonstrated how a perceived threat could be securitized in order to "takes politics beyond the established rules [...] and frame the issue as a special kind of politics or above politics"[33] along a spectrum of issue types. Depending on the circumstances, issues can be located anywhere on the spectrum, which will differ from state to state and across time. On one end of the spectrum, issues are nonpoliticized, meaning that the state does not deal with the issue, and it is not vital to the state's survival. On the other end, issues are securitized, or characterized as existential threats that require emergency measures. In the middle, politicized issues are part of public policy and require government decisions and resource allocation (Fig. 12-3).

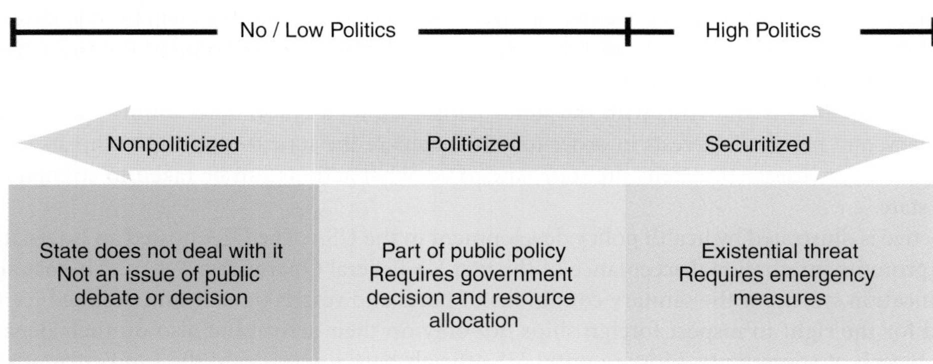

FIG. 12-3 Securitization spectrum.

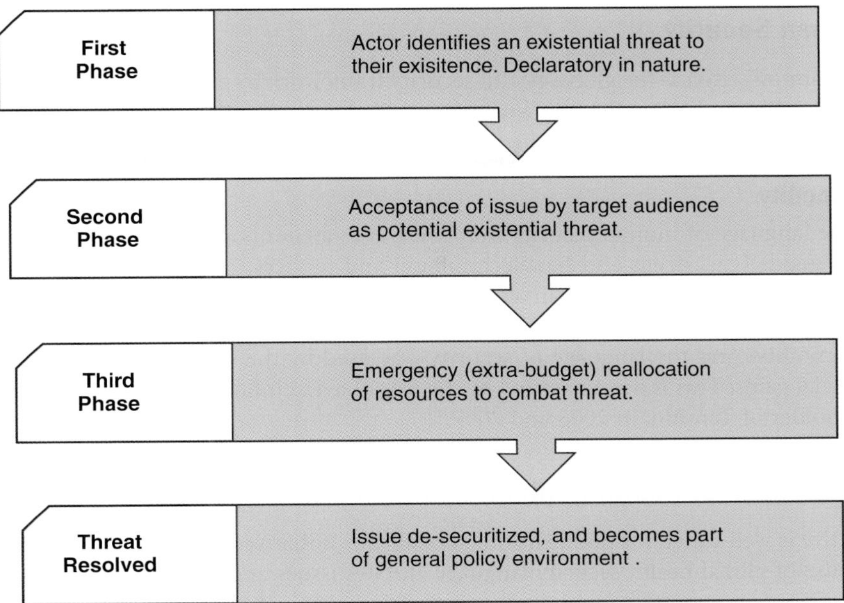

FIG. 12-4 Copenhagen School's phases of threat identification.

This spectrum identifies how health challenges become identifiable security threats, which occurs in several phases (Fig. 12-4).[33] However, this model does not address the politics of existential threats, where policy makers may chose to deliberately ignore or misallocate resources to existential threats or even securitize nonexistential threats.[34]

Health security draws recognition to emerging infectious diseases that pose grave threats to state security and that could cripple populations and economies.[20,24] Securitizing the threat attracts greater political attention and resources for protecting health and lives in the face of specific threats, and thus EIDs are grouped with other national security threats such global terrorism and nuclear proliferation.[35] Securitization requires that states identify the threat's source,[33] making acute threats like infectious diseases[36,37] the primary targets for securitization. Typically the best candidates for securitization are infectious disease threats that "inspire particular human dread, and which therefore often generate a level of societal disruption disproportionate to the mortality and morbidity they pose."[35] EIDs, as opposed to NCDs, have been more readily securitized for a number of reasons[33]:

- They evoke human anxiety and fear of the unknown and of silent, invisible, and lethal threats.
- They pose a threat to economic, military, political, or social domestic and foreign policies and the state itself.
- Their source can be identified.
- They require intensive short-term interventions by states.

Securitization creates an inside-outside dynamic; the state on the inside must protect itself and its citizenry from outside threats.[38] While this is a useful strategy for prioritizing health, the idea that a serious pathogenic threat from the outside can be vanquished or contained is an oversimplification.[7,39] The best strategies states develop involve implementing health security policies and capacity. It is clear that public health surveillance is critical for detecting and preventing epidemics. In particular, surveillance that detects known communicable diseases, especially those with high epidemic potential, early recognition of new infections, and monitoring the growing resistance to antimicrobial drugs.[40]

The premise of the health securitization argument rests on the argument that states and international organizations are more likely to take health risks seriously if they are presented as security threats to the states well-being.[7] This is well demonstrated in the rapid acceleration of biosecurity and pandemic preparedness policies in security agendas.[37,41–46]

Statism and Human Security

Although not as commonly used as the global health security framework by statists, the use of human security values evokes the values of health as a commodity and business-minded investments to help the most vulnerable of populations. Ultimately, this benefits the security of the state.

Health as a Commodity

Statists invoking the language of human security frame health as a commodity to be sold to populations. Health is thereby reduced to goods (e.g., drugs and new technology) and services.[9] The commodification of health is most apparent in the pharmaceutical sector and can also be seen in efforts to privatize health systems, workforce movements, health tourism, and the export–import of addictive substances.[7] Economic interests often underlie the use of health as a commodity. And the language of security—as used by the statist perspective—evokes fear that can translate into financial gains. This is demonstrated by the fear of avian influenza and subsequent windfall profits for Roche, the patent holder of Tamiflu, in 2006 and 2007.[47]

Implications of Statism for Public Health Surveillance

The statist perspective is well suited for public health surveillance initiatives aimed to protect the state from external threats. While the use of global health security language elevates issues and catches the attention of major governmental actors, securitization may fail to address the underlying causes that allow infectious diseases to perpetuate. As another global health expert states, "Global health security is essentially a defensive, reactive strategy because it seeks to ensure that [s] tates are prepared to detect and respond to public health threats and emergencies of international concern."[48]

Governments will support and set thresholds for surveillance systems according to their own perceived threats to sovereignty.[49] Indicative of statism, "There is no escaping for the conclusion that the harvest of outbreak intelligence overseas is essentially geared to benefit wealthy nations."[49] The factors that contribute to the spread of infectious diseases—poverty, poor nutrition, and inadequate health infrastructure—are not easily securitized and therefore secondary concerns, if considered at all.[37] While calls for statist global health security are rooted in a justifiable need for self-protection, failure to address the underlying causes of disease may also affect state security. Securitization absolves state actors from any moral obligation to respond to health crises beyond their needs.[39] Furthermore, an exclusive focus on economic and military interests may further perpetuate colonial models of health.[50] Securitization of health issues targets the diseases most likely to hinder global trade, finance, or travel to developed nations.[51] Preying on emotions of helplessness without checks and balances, securitization uses fear to transform the possible into the probable.[52] Unfortunately, this implementation of securitization sanctions actions that may unreasonably circumvent human rights.[53]

Health as a commodity has important implications as well, particularly with regard to patent issues and access to essential medicines. As the mantra of public health surveillance is detect, analyze, and respond, access to essential medicines is critical to utilizing public health surveillance for disease management. However, the Trade-Related Aspects of Intellectual Property Rights (TRIPS) agreement of 1994 establishes a comprehensive standard for many forms of intellectual property applicable to members of the World Trade Organization. While the intent is to ensure products developed would be protected from cheaper copies, TRIPS has been criticized for curtailing access to affordable generics.[54] TRIPS protects the high initial investment costs of pharmaceutical companies—estimated to be US$26.4 billion annually for R&D,[55] from major generic pharmaceutical industries in Brazil and India. But much of the world's population—as much as 80%—do not have access to essential medicines due to nonavailability and high costs and may rely on such sources.[56]

The recent calls for microbial sovereignty demonstrate the limitations of the statist perspective through over securitization of health issues and curtailing access to drugs.

MICROBIAL SOVEREIGNTY AS AN EXAMPLE OF STATISM

The WHO revised International Health Regulations (IHR [2005])—the modern day application of the International Sanitary Conferences—provide a global framework to prevent, protect against, control, and facilitate public health response to the international spread of disease. Its success firmly rests on mutual trust and transparency among parties. Claims of viral sovereignty indicate the worst-case scenario of the statist perspective, where individual state actors act in their own self-interest often conflicting with shared goals.

Issues of sovereignty have long existed in the realm of governance of public health surveillance, since the early years of the International Sanitary Conferences when the British Empire was sensitive of claims of cholera originating in British-controlled India.[11] Conference delegates defeated a proposal to send an international scientific commission to India to study cholera at its source; the rejection contended that this would "constitute an infringement of the sovereignty of governments with possessions in India."[11] Delicate issues of sovereignty were discussed regularly at the conferences, where decisions were often interpreted as a means of intervention in states' domestic affairs.[12]

Today, **viral sovereignty** refers to a sovereign state's ownership rights over pathogens found within its borders.[57] The term was used to describe tensions rising from the Indonesian government's decision to conditionally withhold samples of H5N1 avian influenza (commonly known as bird flu) in 2007.[58] Drawing from past experiences with the SARS epidemic, experts argued that "globally shared health risk demands absolute global transparency."[58] However, the Indonesian health minister's decision to withhold samples was not baseless; she argued that sharing virus samples is a country's sovereign right for several reasons.[59,60] First, there was concern that WHO would share virus samples with big pharmaceutical companies without their authorization, contrary to WHO guidelines. There was no guarantee that the pharmaceutical companies would develop drugs that could respond to strains circulating in developing countries. Developing countries have limited access even to reasonably priced vaccines because developed nations tend to buy out stock. Indonesian authorities were also alarmed about reports that samples of the Indonesia strain were sent to a US laboratory famous for weapon development. Finally, Indonesia's claims were supported by international law, including the Convention on Biological Diversity and the Nagoya Protocol on Access and Benefit-sharing.

While many found Indonesia's decision a major setback for public health,[61-63] others, such as the editor of *The Lancet*, were sympathetic with Indonesia's position.

"To protect the global population, 6.2 billion doses of pandemic vaccine will be needed, but under current manufacturing capacity the world can only produce 500 million doses. And, in a pandemic, it is industrialized countries that will have access to available vaccines, whereas developing countries—where a pandemic is likely to emerge—will be left wanting. In November 2004, a WHO consultation reached the depressing conclusion that most developing countries would have no access to vaccine during the first wave of a pandemic and possibly throughout its duration."[64]

Securitization of this case led to two consequences. First, the surge in demand to procure pharmaceutical countermeasures favored developed countries with vaccine manufacturing capacity.[65,66] Second, the high level of concern over this emerging threat and the need for samples to sustain countermeasures with virus mutation substantially increased the value of the viruses circulating in Indonesia, essentially creating a diplomatic bargaining chip.[66] While the IHR (2005) were not prepared to address this situation, three years later the World Health Assembly adopted the Pandemic Influenza Preparedness Framework that would support the equitable sharing of vaccines in a pandemic scenario.[67] However the framework, legally nonbiding, avoided issues of intellectual property and merely reinforced a global norm rather than altering the status quo.[68]

Issues of viral ownership were renewed in 2012 when a former microbiologist in Saudi Arabia shared samples of the Middle East Respiratory Coronavirus with an external institution, and the virus genome was subsequently sequenced and patented.[69] As some argued, patenting the genome prevented access to necessary materials[70,71] and eventually prompted WHO to take a strong stance against this action. As the WHO Director General stated, "Making deals between scientists because they want to take intellectual property, because they want to be the world's first to publish in scientific journals, these are issues [that need to be addressed]. No IP will stand in the way of public health actions".[72]

Continuing claims of viral sovereignty bring up unresolved controversies that challenge ethical public health governance and add unnecessary risk of global pandemics. They exemplify a statist perspective framed as a global health security issue being used by both developed and developing countries. Indonesia and Saudi Arabia were both faced with situations where they were required to act in their own self-interest to ensure the well-being of their state, and ultimately citizen. Although this caught many developed countries supporting disease surveillance under the auspices of global health security off guard, the same statist perspective justified the actions of developing countries.

GLOBALISM IN THE GOVERNANCE OF PUBLIC HEALTH SURVEILLANCE

Although, health as a fundamental human right, the primary driver in the globalist perspective, has evolved over the years, this basic tenet has been reinforced in a number of governance documents. Some of these documents obligate states to ensure that all people enjoy the same access to goods and services essential to enjoyment of this right. The recent International Covenant on Economic, Social and Cultural Rights (ICESCR) obligates states to ensure provision of a number of health care and public health services, as well as equitable and affordable access to underlying health determinants such as water and sanitation, adequate and safe food, nutrition and housing, healthy occupational and environmental conditions, and health-related education and information, including on sexual and reproductive health.[73] The ICESCR obligates states to respect the right to health in other countries, often contradictory to trade and intellectual property agreements.[74]

Primary Health Care for All

As discussed above, the supposed conquest of microbes was attributed primarily to revolutionary advances in public health and medicine as well as vast improvements in sanitation. In the midst of this, a reevaluation of the traditional, strong biomedical and curative health care paradigm was well under way in the mid-twentieth century. British professor of social medicine, Thomas McKewon, controversially argued that England's gains in population health and decreased mortality rates were due to better standards of living and nutrition.[75,76] Canada was the first official western government to recognize that our "emphasis upon biomedical healthcare system is wrong, and that we need to look beyond the traditional healthcare (sick care) system if we wish to improve the health of the public."[77,78] This shift, coined as the "epidemiological transition" by Abdel Omran, accounts for the vast decrease in infectious diseases over time due to expanded public health and sanitation.[79] This transition helped support early globalists in arguing for the right to health in global public health governance documents, such as the 1946 preamble to the WHO constitution that calls for "the enjoyment of the highest attainable standard of health."[80]

A Shifting Global Health Agenda

While WHO first focused on technical projects such as reducing morbidity and mortality through massive vertical programs, such as smallpox eradication or nutrition initiatives, in 1973, the new Director General, Halfan Mahler, took a decisively different and idealistic approach to health, one that emphasized strengthening health systems.[81] Mahler sought to use WHO and its newfound credibility to advocate for primary health care and health equity across the world.[7,81]

WHO and the United Nations Children's Fund supported a 1975 joint report, "Alternative Approaches to Meeting Basic Health Needs in Developing Countries." The report highlighted WHO increases in "basic health services" projects (from 85 in 1965 to 156 in 1971) and criticized vertical programming and the application of western approaches to developing countries for meeting the needs of the common people.[82,83] Vertical programs advocated for disease surveillance and eradication for western perceived threats, but the report identified leading causes of morbidity and mortality in developing countries to be malnutrition, vector-borne respiratory disease, and diarrheal disease, which themselves are "the results of poverty, squalor, and ignorance."[83] Furthermore, vertical programming risks duplicative efforts due to lack of coordination, "recipient fatigue" in health ministries forced to administer multiple programs, disruptions in local resource allocation, and crowding out of local needs.[84] The report sparked a worldwide debate and prompted WHO to restructure.[82]

In his 1976 World Health Assembly Speech, Mahler controversially told the assembly, "many social evolutions and revolutions have taken place because the social structures were crumbling [...] There are signs that the scientific and technological structures of public health are crumbling," going on to argue for increased attention for the social determinants of health.[85] He also used this platform to announce the "Health for All by the Year 2000" goal, which would become an integral part of primary health care.[82]

Opposite of the statist perspective, the globalist perspective addresses the insecurities of the individual and considers the state as one of a number of actors able to provide security to the most vulnerable populations. Two driving characteristics define this position. First, the primary referent is the individual, no matter his or her socioeconomic or geographic position. Second, the purpose of bringing health into the realm of international relations serves to promote health equity, that is, everyone should enjoy similar health resources and access to care.[7] The globalist approach seeks to understand which populations are the most vulnerable to disease, what the roles of various actors in global health governance are, who the best actors to deliver health are, and what the best way to alleviate the impact of disease is.[7,86]

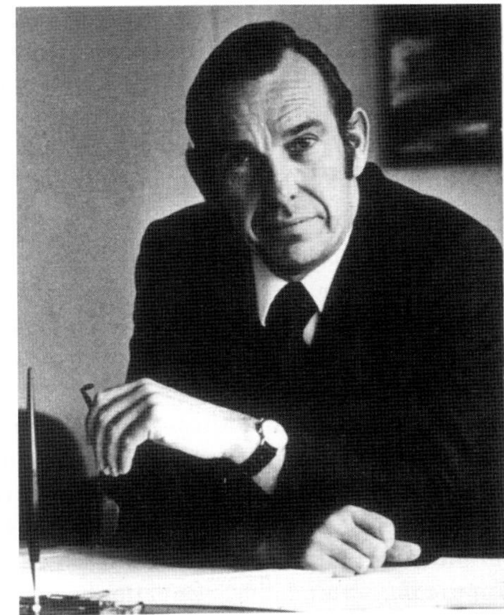

FIG. 12-5 Halfdan T. Mahler, Director General of the World Health Organization, 1973–1988. (Source: https://en.wikipedia.org/wiki/Halfdan_T._Mahler#/media/File:Halfdan_Mahler_by_Erling_Mandelmann.jpg).

Declaration of Alma-Ata

The globalist perspective is illustrated by the Declaration of Alma-Ata of 1978, led in many ways by WHO director Mahler. The International Conference on Primary Health care took place in Alma-Ata, Kazakhstan, in 1978 and involved over 3000 delegates from 134 governments and 67 multilaterals and nongovernmental organizations. At the end of the 1960s and 1970s counterculture revolution, this conference was biggest convergence of world leaders in history. Mahler opened the conference by asking questions calling for immediate action, including the following[82]: Are you ready to introduce, if necessary, radical changes in the existing health delivery system so that it properly supports [primary health care] as the overriding health priority? Are you ready to fight the political and technical battles required to overcome any social and economic obstacles and professional resistance to the universal introduction of [primary health care]? The conference's main document, the Declaration of Alma-Ata, called for health for all people by 2000.

The declaration advocated for three key ideas.[87] First, it stated a preference for nontechnological interventions such as nutrition and sanitation. Second, it opposed medical elitism in favor of genuine community involvement in health care strategies. Finally, it introduced the idea that health care is inseparable from socioeconomic development. A landmark event for primary health care, the Declaration of Alma-Ata had very strong sociopolitical implications, addressing underlying social, economic, and political causes of poor health and justifying health as a major driver and vehicle for social justice issues. "Primary healthcare is essential healthcare based on practical, scientifically sound, and socially acceptable methods and technology made universally accessible to individuals and families in the community through their full participation and at a cost that the community and the country can afford to maintain at every stage of their development in the spirit of self-reliance and self-determination [...] It is the first level of contact of individuals, the family, and community with the national health system bringing healthcare as close as possible to where people live and work."[87]

Addressing the 61st World Health Assembly, Dr Halfdan Mahler quoted from the Declaration of Alma-Ata saying that "primary healthcare includes at least education about prevailing health problems and the methods of preventing and controlling them; promotion of food supply and proper nutrition; an adequate supply of safe water and basic sanitation; maternal and child healthcare, including family planning; immunization against major infectious diseases; prevention and control of locally endemic diseases; appropriate treatment of common diseases and injuries; and provision of essential drugs."[88]

Selective Primary Health Care

A major limitation of the Declaration of Alma-Ata was that it was too broad and set unrealistic expectations. Opponents advocated to instead enact Selective Primary Healthcare, an interim strategy through which basic health services could be developed to target the most common diseases in developing countries.[89] Selective primary health care was seen as a balance between scarcity and choice and attracted the support of some donors, scholars, and agencies. The debate over the effectiveness of each approach inevitably followed.[82,90] Supporters of the original model believed this was just a repackaging of the vertical programs that focused on specific diseases and lacked the holistic approach needed to address underlying issues.[91] Each side debated issues such as the meaning of primary health care, how it would be financed and implemented, and whether primary health care is cheaper than traditional health interventions or demands a greater investment of resources.[92]

Although Mahler never took part in the debate, he recognized the risk of national and international donor biases in the selective primary health care model and continued to push for a holistic anthropocentric agenda that focused on the most vulnerable, even after he left WHO in 1988.[81] Primary health care continues to be advocated and practiced by a number of nonstate actors and has contributed to the Beijing Declaration[93] and Holistic Primary Health Care,[94] both taking shape in 2008. These documents have shaped the globalist perspective seeking to alleviate the burden of disease.

Globalism and Human Security

In the post-Cold War era, the concept of "human security" emerged to describe global vulnerabilities outside of the traditional framework of "national security" and advocate for a person-centered view of security as a necessity for stability. The United Nations Development Program's 1994 Human Development Report helped shape the principles of human security. The report argued for sustainable human development that responds to crises of underdevelopment, global poverty, population pressures, and environmental degradation. For too long, the report argues, our idea of security has focused on conflict between states and threats to international borders, but that "for most people today, a feeling of insecurity arises more from worries about daily life than from the dread of a cataclysmic world event" and that "human security [...] is a concern with human life and dignity."[32] Human security focuses on two aspects: safety from chronic threats, such as hunger, disease, and repression, and protection from sudden and hurtful disruptions in the patterns of daily life. The report argues that human security should include threats in seven areas, including health (Fig. 12-6):

1. Community
2. Economy
3. Environment
4. Food
5. Health
6. Personal
7. Politics

Human security as it relates to health involves addressing the major causes of death linked with poor nutrition and unsafe environments or lifestyles. Human security seeks to maximize protection from diseases and unhealthy lifestyles. As such, many issues outside of the purview of infectious diseases are considered, including violence and injury prevention, climate change, and man-made disasters.[95-100] Furthermore, an index of human security as it relates to life expectancy, access to sanitation, and access to health services—albeit with its limitations—demonstrates the wide range of health inequity across the world (Fig. 12-7).[101]

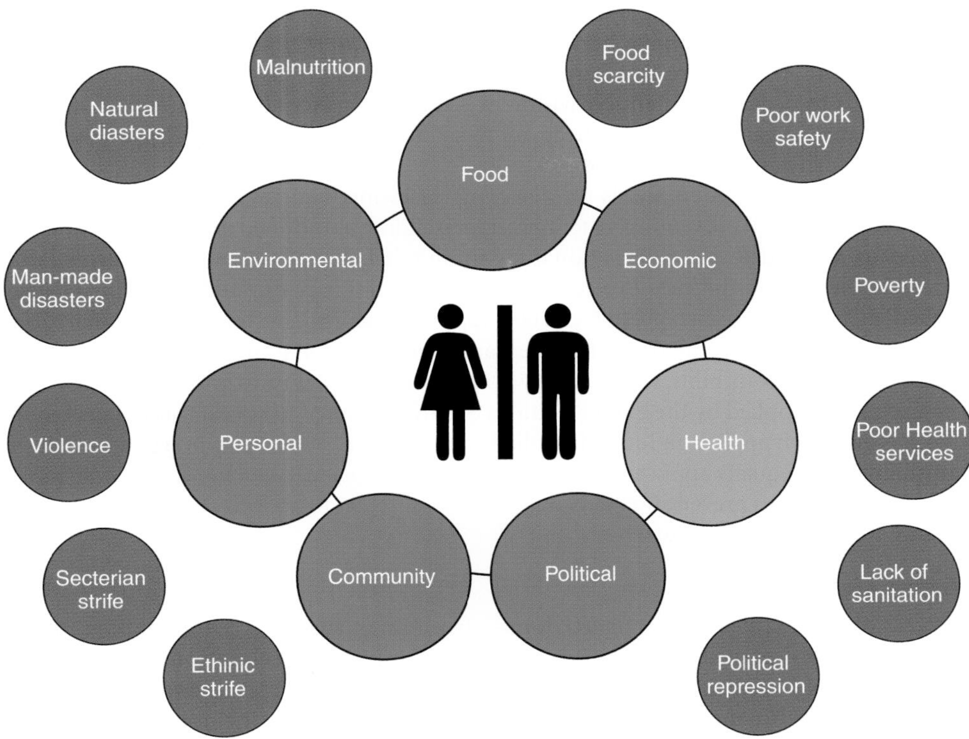

FIG. 12-6 Seven areas contributing to human security.

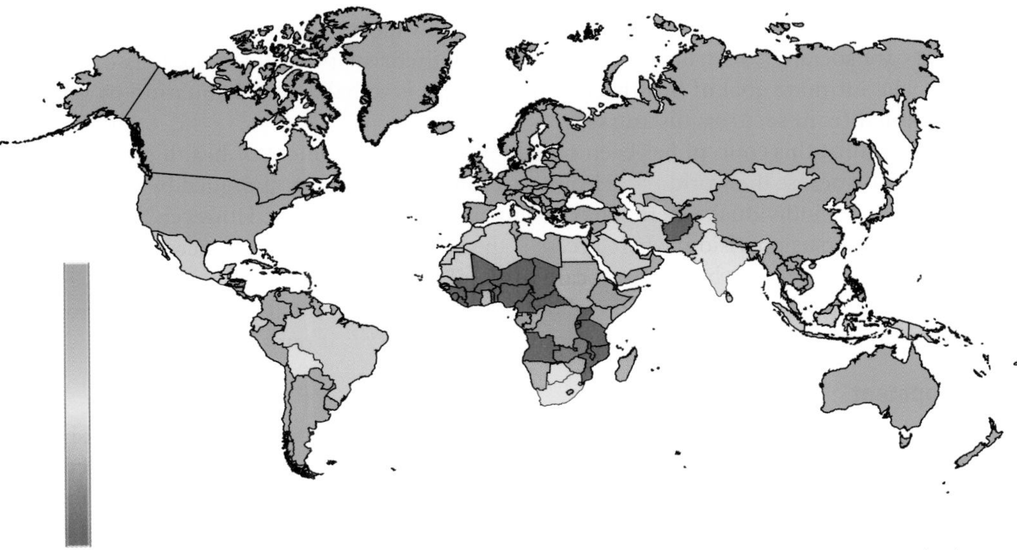

FIG. 12-7 Human security index measure of health based on life expectancy, access to sanitation, equality of access to health services, 2010. (http://www.humansecurityindex.org)

Its been argued that the state-based governance of global health, valuing health security, needs to radically change to incorporate a globalist perspective valuing human security.[10] As such, many globalists adopting human security values are critical of existing governance structures. Because this radical reshaping is unlikely,[7] many proponents believe that change needs to occur incrementally within existing governance structures, including the state.[102] This strategy must find a balance to galvanize the political will to act in the name of the voiceless and vulnerable without succumbing to health securitization.[7]

Similar to global health security's emphasis on detecting, assessing, and responding, human security seeks to address underlying causes through preventing, reacting, and rebuilding as outlined in the Responsibility to Protect.[103] Although developed to respond to the international community's failure to respond the Rwandan and Serbian genocides in the 1990s, the Responsibility to Protect acts as a reformulation of our understanding of state sovereignty and can be applied to health circumstances.[104] A 2001 report developed by the International Commission on Intervention and State Sovereignty at the request of the Canadian government further outlines that sovereignty not only entail rights but also responsibilities, specifically a state's responsibility to protect its people.[103] While this concept has been exclusively applied by the United Nations Security Council to conflict situations requiring military interventions[103] it has also been applied in limited public health contexts of violence prevention.[105] Sovereign states' rights and responsibilities can equally apply to health crises outside genocide scenarios when a state refuses to address health threats, requiring action to prevent further spread of disease, react to address causes of disease, or rebuild the health infrastructure to be prevent reoccurrences.

Health as a Human Right

Amidst World War II, the principle of the four freedoms—freedom of speech, freedom of religion, freedom from fear, and freedom from want—served as the foundation for the **Universal Declaration of Human Rights** in 1948 and further endorsement of health as a human right. The declaration states, "everyone has the right to standard of living adequate for the health and well-being of himself and of his family, including food, clothing, housing, and medical care and necessary social services."[107] It establishes that health and social determinants of health have equal responsibility.[108] Endorsement of this rights-based approach to health care ensures that those with the greatest need can access the health care services they need, shifting the emphasis from disease to individual and community health.

Following the Cold War era, there was a great hope that the hard-won peace could be channeled into improving human security for millions across the world, allowing for new ideas of security to be explored.[106] Recognizing that security threats are socially constructed, critical security theorists prioritized the bias of perceived threats over other voices.[7] The ultimate goal of health as a human right is to balance the equation by giving a platform to voices often excluded from security discourse.

Arguing for health equity, this concept has been called for in the development of health programs to address the root causes of poor health across the world.[10,109] Health as a fundamental right, as argued by many globalists, would reprioritize the health of the individual, where states downplay this responsibility. However, health as a human right entails a debate of access versus provision, where access is the obligation not to deny access to basic health care and provision is the obligation to provide basic health care to all.[7] This debate rests on two questions. First, what is the scope of right and responsibility? And second, on whom does this obligation fall? While many have argued this is a shared responsibility between the state and nongovernmental actors,[110,111] it remains unclear.[7]

Health as Development

One of the best measures of a health system's performance is its impact on health outcomes, but health outcomes remain dismal across much of the developing world. Globalists using the language of human security may frame health as an indicator of development to advocate for strengthening health systems. Although linked, this concept is different than human development, which aims to widen the range of people's choices; human security ensures that people can exercise their choices safely and freely.[112] Health is a desired outcome of development, and a number of global initiatives have been established to improve health and further economic development. The Millennium

Development Goals have been hailed as the "world's biggest promise"[113] and commit world leaders to specific, measurable, attainable, reasonable, and time-bound improvements in global poverty, health, education, and other key areas (see Chapter 29).

However, as a 2013 United Nations report notes, "more than 40 developing countries lack sufficient data to track progress [for the Millennium Development Goals],"[114] leading to calls for a "data revolution" to better measure progress. "Better data and statistics will help governments track progress and make sure their decisions are evidence-based; they can also strengthen accountability."[115] Contributing to better data and statistics for measurement of Millennium Development Goals progress, or any public health surveillance activities, require strengthening public health surveillance and surveillance systems.

Globalism and Global Health Security

The use of global health security language by globalists attempts to prioritize the health issues of vulnerable populations. Globalists use the global health security framework to justify addressing threats to vulnerable populations by demonstrating that there is a threat to the stability of the state if no action is taken. Under this argument, health is typically framed as a global public good. With this perspective, this is done for the security of the individual, but it is framed to appeal to statists because "the massive amount of disease burden in the world's poorest nations poses a huge threat to global health and security."[116] Furthermore, "the security of the most affluent state can be held hostage to the ability of the poorest state to contain an emerging disease."[114]

Health as a Global Public Good

Public goods encompass a range of physical commodities and services, and once provided, no one can be excluded from their benefit. Thus, global public goods, like reducing infectious diseases, are goods whose benefit cross borders and are global in scope.[117] Globalists framing health as a global public good using global health security seek to galvanize global action by emphasizing the consequences of failing to act against threats in the developing world.[20] Rather than appealing to the support of developed countries under humanitarian pretenses, health as a global public good encourages the globalist perspective as a state investment in self-protection.[118] There is no commercial incentive for producing global public goods, however, since they do not result in any direct financial gains. Furthermore, as a public good, free riding may lead to an underprovision of goods or services, overusage and degradation of common resources, or lack of initiative. Therefore, a global public good is to be pursued by the collective[119] and demonstrates the benefit of the rich helping the poor. It provides a rationale for developed countries to complement traditional aid.[117]

Implications of Globalism

The globalist model is well suited to address the root causes of public health issues that affect populations' most vulnerable citizens. The model argues that the security of the state depends on the security of its citizens.[120] Globalists tend to frame health as a human right or a development issue supported by the human security framework; however, there is not clarity about what a right entails and who is responsible for delivering it.[121] There are also ongoing debates about the benefits of existing development aid programs.[122-124] Furthermore, while economic development raises living standards,[6] most international agencies remain interested in short-term technical programs with clear budgets rather than longer term broad programs that address the social determinants of health.[125]

Health as a global public good has impacted public health surveillance. The term itself has been overused, diminishing its effect and devaluing the term when it is used appropriately.[119] The concept of global public good has been most usefully applied to two aspects of health, research and development and disease control.[126] However, contrary to the primary health care movement, health as a global public good is often used to justify increased disease-specific systems. While scaling up some disease-specific programs such as HIV/AIDS, malaria, and tuberculosis has led to substantial reductions in morbidity and mortality, this also highlights the relative biases in targeting some diseases over others and failing to strengthen the overall health system.[127] In particular, vertical programs for immunizations, malaria, and tuberculosis demonstrate sector-wide shortcomings including lack of cold chain, shortages in a skilled workforce, insufficient resources, and poor health infrastructure.[119,128] Furthermore, many countries risk failing to meet the IHR (2005) without renewed commitments to build capacities.

Antimicrobial Resistance

The limitations of the globalist perspective include a lack of clarity of scope and a failure to prioritize investments to strengthen health systems. These limitations are illustrated by the emergence of antimicrobial resistance. Common and treatable diseases pose a grave threat to developed and developing countries in the form of antimicrobial resistance. Seen across the world, new and evolving resistant pathogens continue to challenge the health and public health systems. In 2012, there were approximately 450,000 new cases of multidrug-resistant tuberculosis (MDR TB), and extensively drug-resistant tuberculosis (XDR TB) has been identified in 92 countries by September 2013. Yet, despite growing concerns, MDR TB is largely underreported. Surveillance for antimicrobial resistance is neither coordinated nor harmonized due to vertical siloed programming. Patients infected with drug-resistant microbes are generally at an increased risk of worse clinical outcomes and death, and they consume more health care resources than patients infected with nonresistant strains of the same bacteria. Recognizing this growing issue and knowledge gap, WHO published the first "Antimicrobial Resistance: Global Report on Surveillance" in 2014 to bring attention to the issue, were they state:

"Without urgent, coordinated action by many stakeholders, the world is headed for a post-antibiotic era, in which common infections and minor injuries which have been treatable for decades can once again kill [...] Effective antibiotics have been one of the pillars allowing us to live longer, live healthier, and benefit from modern medicine. Unless we take significant actions to improve efforts to prevent infections and also change how we produce, prescribe and use antibiotics, the world will lose more and more of these global public health goods and the implications will be devastating."[129]

The overuse of antibiotics in people and animals, often unnecessarily, contributes to growing antimicrobial resistance.[130] The failure of health systems to effectively mitigate antimicrobial resistance, whether through maintaining surveillance or through response capacities and hygienic environments, also contributes to the problem.[131] Ultimately, the problem is the result of poverty, ignorance, poor sanitation, hunger and malnutrition, inadequate access to drugs, poor and inadequate health care systems, civil conflicts, and bad governance in developing countries.[40]

The WHO report makes recommendations for individual citizens, for health workers and pharmacists, policy makers, and industry on how to tackle antimicrobial resistance.[132] We need to strengthen global surveillance systems and build national capacities, both of which are critical to tackling this challenge. Prevention activities are also important, such as improving hygiene and infection prevention and control measures, improving sanitation and access to clean water, and encouraging more widespread use of vaccines. The development of new antibiotics through research and development activities can also contribute to long-term progress.

Finally, we need to rebuild our thinking of health to acknowledge the shared threat of antimicrobial resistance. However, many countries suffer from short-term orientation and lack of coordination. Greater local ownership and participation in global health initiatives about antimicrobial resistance are critical for development and sustainability.[133] The globalist perspective has failed to effectively prioritize and utilize resources or to raise awareness of the growing antimicrobial resistance challenge.

As antimicrobial resistance brings to light the shortcoming of existing public health surveillance capacities, the globalist perspective, protecting the most vulnerable, will become increasingly critical. Framed with human security and as a human right issue, diseases associated with poverty are increasingly affected by antimicrobial resistance and represent a significant obstacle to achieving health gains worldwide. Framed within global health security and seen as a global public good, all countries share in the benefit of fighting antimicrobial resistance, yet little focus has been given to surveillance and response capacity building.

THE PROMISE OF SMART GOVERNANCE OF PUBLIC HEALTH SURVEILLANCE

At the intersection of global health and international relations, statism and globalism are two major drivers for political and humanitarian engagement in global public health surveillance. Both perspectives are framed with values of global health security or human security to achieve different visions. While it is common for statists to develop and implement initiatives primarily through a global health security lens, they can invoke language from the human security perspective, and vice versa for globalists. Health concerns are consequently framed as security, development, global public good, commodity, and/or human right issues depending on the perspective and framework utilized.[9] Ultimately, statists or globalists are interested in pursuing actions that address the state or vulnerable populations, respectively, but diverging views risk discord in governance and the ability to effectively and efficiently address health issues.

There are several epidemiologic, economical, and political challenges to global health governance. Among them is antimicrobial resistance, access to health care, counterfeit drugs, growing burden of NCDs, emerging and re-emerging infectious diseases, and shortcomings in the public health workforce. Our current practice of global health governance falls short in preparing us for these challenges. "The current regime complex for global health governance suffers [from] failures to prevent health problems from becoming global dangers, to produce effective responses to global health threats, to implement important treaties on global health, to develop stronger health systems in developing countries, and to stimulate sufficient progress on social determinants of health"[128] However, our interest and understanding of the institutions, rules, regulations, and processes are rapidly evolving and becoming more visible to policy makers. While the approaches of statist and globalist perspectives towards public health governance differ, a balanced approach between the two is optimal for the public's health.

Drawing from political theory, Joseph Nye's concept of "smart power"[134] can be applied to the governance of public health surveillance, in what can be called "smart public health governance." **Smart public health governance**, the combination of hard and soft governance strategies, holds the promise of balancing statism and globalism. By acknowledging that strengthening foreign capacities is ultimately a benefit to state interests in our globalized world, applying smart governance can achieve a safer world through utilizing the global health security and human security concepts. This idea is captured in the shared health governance model, based on the moral concept of global health justice known as provincial globalism.

This approach could be a balancing force that melds values among different actors into a shared vision of health and health provision.[133,136] A consensus of goals and strategies can foster agreements on program design, implementation, evaluation, and coordination. Shared global governance focuses on norms as shared authoritative standards; ethical commitments, shared goals, and role allocation; shared sovereignty and constitutional commitments; legitimacy and accountability; and country-level attention to international health relations.[136] In the face of growing public health challenges, a balanced approach to global health governance—one that accounts for statism and globalism—holds the promise to a more equitable sharing of our health progress, ultimately securing the state as well as the individual.

KEY SUMMARY POINTS

- The global health governance compass is used to discuss global public health governance today. The compass has two axes balancing the statist and globalist perspectives and the human security and the global health security perspectives.
- Health challenges are framed as security, commodity, human right, development, or global public good issues.
- Ethical considerations of public health surveillance include privacy, consent, disclosure, and moral obligations at an individual level and include ownership of biological materials and intellectual property, data sharing, access to benefits, and moral obligations at a population level.
- The statist perspective, strongly shaped by the rise, fall, and return of the microbial threat, is primarily interested in the security of the state.
- The globalist perspective, strongly shaped by the primary health care movement, is primarily interested in the security of individuals and communities.

DISCUSSION QUESTIONS

1. Give a public health example for each of the four quadrants of the global health governance compass. Which is the hardest to think of? Why do you think this is?
2. Is there one quadrant or perspective that is more prevalent in public health or public health surveillance? Why?
3. How did International Sanitary Conferences influence public health governance?
4. Are there any current public health issues that have recently been, or may be in the future, securitized? Is this good or bad?
5. Do you agree with Indonesia's decision about its case of viral sovereignty? Why or why not?
6. To prioritize primary health care for all, what issues would governments need to emphasize? Which would need to be de-emphasized?
7. Is there more than one way to implement primary health care for all? Give some examples of both advantages and disadvantages.
8. Do you agree that health is a human right? Why or why not?
9. How is governance important in tackling antimicrobial resistance?
10. Do you think balancing statism and globalism is feasible? Why?

REFERENCES

1. Frenk J, Chen L, Bhutta ZA, Cohen J, Crisp N, Evans T, et al. Health professionals for a new century: transforming education to strengthen health systems in an interdependent world. Lancet 2010;376(9756):1923–58.
2. Lee K, Goodman H. Global policy networks: the propagation of health care financing reform since the 1980s. Health policy in a globalising world. Cambridge University Press; Cambridge, UK, 2002.
3. Murray CJL, Anderson B, Burstein R, Leach-Kemon K, Schneider M, Tardif A, et al. Development assistance for health: trends and prospects. Lancet 2011;378(9785):8–10.
4. Lakoff A. Two regimes of global health. Humanity 2010;1(1):59–79.
5. US Department of Health and Human Services. Global health security agenda: toward a world safe and secure from infectious disease threats. <http://www.globalhealth.gov/global-health-topics/global-health-security/GHS%20Agenda.pdf>; February, 2014, Accessed 01 April 2015.
6. De Cock KM, Simone PM, Davison V, Slutsker L. The new global health. Emerg Infect Dis 2013;19(8):1192–7.
7. Davies S. Global Politics of Health. 1st ed. Cambridge, UK: Polity; 2010. p. 224.
8. Programme UND. Human development report: United Nations Development Programme, <http://hdr.undp.org/en/content/human-development-report-1994/>; 1994 [cited 2015].
9. Labonte R. Global health in public policy: finding the right frame? Crit Public Health 2008;18(4):467–82.
10. Aginam O. Global health governance: international law and public health in a divided world. Toronto, Buffalo: University of Toronto Press, Scholarly Publishing Division; 2005. p. 240.
11. Howard-Jones N, World Health Organization. The scientific background of the International Sanitary Conferences, 1851-1938/Norman Howard-Jones. Geneva: World Health Organization; 1975.
12. Ersoy Nermin GY. International sanitary conferences from the Ottoman perspective (1851–1938). Hygiea Internationalis 2011:10(1);53–79.
13. Sherman IW. Twelve diseases that changed our world. 1st ed. Washington, DC: ASM Press; 2007. p. 219.
14. Chiffoleau S. [Pilgrims to Mecca, germs and the international community]. Med Sci (Paris) 2011;27(12):1121–5.
15. Liverani M, Coker R. Protecting Europe from diseases: from the international sanitary conferences to the ECDC. J Health Polit Policy Law 2012; 37(6):915–34.
16. Bynum WF. Policing hearts of darkness: aspects of the international sanitary conferences. Hist Philos Life Sci 1993;15(3):421–34.
17. Huber V. The unification of the globe by disease? The international sanitary conferences on cholera, 1851–1894. Hist J 2006;49(02):453–76.
18. Spellberg B, Taylor-Blake B. On the exoneration of Dr. William H. Stewart: debunking an urban legend. Infect Dis Poverty 2013;2(1):3.
19. Garrett L. The coming plague: newly emerging diseases in a world out of balance. Reprint ed. New York: Penguin Books; 1995. p. 768.
20. Price-Smith AT. The health of nations: infectious disease, environmental change, and their effects on national security and development. Cambridge, Mass: The MIT Press; 2001. p. 232.
21. Beitz CR. Political theory and international relations. Revised ed. Princeton, N.J: Princeton University Press; 1999. p. 224.
22. Act to prevent the introduction of contagious or infectious diseases into the United States 1878, 20 Stat. L. 37. 1878.
23. Obama B, Lugar R. Grounding a Pandemic. The New York Times. 2005. 2005/06/06/; [Sect. Opinion].
24. Fidler DP. International law and infectious diseases. Oxford: Clarendon Press; 1999.
25. Elbe S. Should HIV/AIDS Be Securitized? The ethical dilemmas of linking HIV/AIDS and security. Int Stud Quart 2006;50(1):119–44.
26. Ostergard Jr RL. Politics in the hot zone: AIDS and national security in Africa. Third World Q 2002;23(2):333–50.
27. Singer PW. AIDS and international security. Survival 2002;44(1):145–58.
28. World Health Organization. The world health report 2007: a safer future: global public health security in the 21st century. 2007.
29. Frieden T. Why global health security matters to U.S., <http://globalpublicsquare.blogs.cnn.com/2014/05/05/why-global-health-security-matters-to-u-s/>; 2014.
30. John Kerry KS, Lisa M. Why global health security is a national priority, <http://www.cnn.com/2014/02/12/opinion/kerry-sebelius-health-security/index.html/>. <http://www.cnn.com/2014/02/12/opinion/kerry-sebelius-health-security/>; 2014 [updated June 19, 2014].
31. Morrison JS. The global health security agenda: a snowy promising start | The CSIS Global Health Policy Center, <http://www.smartglobalhealth.org/blog/entry/the-global-health-security-agenda-a-snowy-promising-start/>; 2014 [updated June 19, 2014].
32. Human Development Report 1994, <http://hdr.undp.org/en/content/human-development-report-1994/> [updated June 26, 2014].

33. Buzan B, Wæver O, Wilde Jd. Security: a new framework for analysis. Boulder, Colorado: Lynne Rienner Publishers; 1998. p. 252.
34. Lo Yuk-ping C, Thomas N. How is health a security issue? Politics, responses and issues. Health Policy Plan 2010;25(6):447–53.
35. Enemark C. Disease and security: natural plagues and biological weapons in East Asia. Abingdon, Oxon: Routledge; 2007.
36. Collier SJ, Lakoff A. The problem of securing health. In Biosecurity interventions: global health and security in question. Columbia University Press, New York, 2008. p. 7–32.
37. McInnes C, Lee K. Health, security and foreign policy. Rev Int Stud 2006;32(01):523.
38. Walker RBJ. Inside/outside: international relations as political theory: Cambridge University Press; Cambridge, UK, 1993.
39. Peterson S. Epidemic disease and national security. Secur Stud 2002;12(2): 43–81.
40. Byarugaba DK. Antimicrobial resistance in developing countries and responsible risk factors. Int J Antimicrob Agents 2004;24(2):105–10.
41. Cooper M. Life as surplus: biotechnology and capitalism in the neoliberal era. University of Washington Press; Seattle, Washington, 2008.
42. Elbe S. Security and global health. Polity; Cambridge, UK, 2010.
43. Enemark C. Is pandemic flu a security threat? Survival 2009;51(1):191–214.
44. Koblentz GD. From biodefence to biosecurity: the Obama administration's strategy for countering biological threats. Int Aff 2012;88(1):131–48.
45. Lakoff A, Collier SJ. Biosecurity interventions: global health & security in question. Columbia University Press; New York City, New York, 2008.
46. Rushton S, Youde J. Routledge Handbook of Global Health Security, Milton Park, Abingdon, Oxon; New York, NY: Routledge; 2014. p. 376.
47. Anon. Roche says Tamiflu capacity outstrips demand. Reuters; 2007. [UTC].
48. Fidler DP. From international sanitary conventions to global health security: the new International Health Regulations. Chinese J Int Law 2005;4(2):325–92.
49. Calain P. From the field side of the binoculars: a different view on global public health surveillance. Health Policy Plan 2007;22(1):13–20.
50. King NB. Security, disease, commerce ideologies of postcolonial global health. Soc Stud Sci 2002;32(5–6):763–89.
51. Thieren M. Health and foreign policy in question: the case of humanitarian action. B World Health Organ 2007;85(3):218–24.
52. Durodié B. Inclusion versus experimentation. Crit Rev Int Soc Pol Philos 2005;8(3):359–62.
53. Szreter S. Health and security in historical perspective. In: Lincoln C. Chen JL, Vasant N, Charles DA, editors. Global health challenges for human security. Global Equity Initiative, Harvard University; Boston, Massachusetts, 2003.
54. Kumaranayake L. Global governance of international public health: the role of international regulatory cooperation. In: Roberts JA, editor. The economics of infectious disease. Oxford: Oxford University Press; 2006.
55. Resnik DB. Developing drugs for the developing world: an economic, legal, moral, and political dilemma. Dev World Bioeth 2001;1(1):11–32.
56. Leach B, Paluzzi JE, Munderi P. Prescription for healthy development: increasing access to medicines. London, UK: Earthscan; 2005.
57. Mullis K. Playing Chicken with Bird Flu: "Viral Sovereignty," the right to exploit natural genetic resources, and the potential human rights ramifications. Am Univ Int Law Review 2009;24(5):943–67.
58. Holbrooke R, Garrett L. 'Sovereignty' That Risks Global Health. The Washington Post; August 10, 2008 [Sect. Opinions].
59. Supari SF. It's Time for the World to Change in the Spirit of Dignity, Equity and Transparency. 2nd ed. Jakarta: Penerbit Lentera; 2008. p. 287.
60. Yu PK. Virotech Patents, Viropiracy, and Viral Sovereignty. SSRN Scholarly Paper. Rochester, NY: Social Science Research Network; 2003. Report No.: ID 451640.
61. Mike L. Secretary Mike Leavitt's Blog: Pandemic Influenza 2008, <http://archive.hhs.gov/secretarysblog/my_weblog/pandemic_planning/index.html/>; 2008 [updated June 26, 2014].
62. Mullis K. Playing chicken with bird flu: "Viral sovereignty," the right to exploit natural genetic resources, and the potential human rights ramifications. American University International Law Review 2009;24(5):943–967.
63. Scoones I. Avian Influenza: science, policy and politics. London, Washington, DC: Routledge; 2010. p. 288.
64. Global solidarity needed in preparing for pandemic influenza. Lancet 2007;369(9561):532.
65. WHO. Avian influenza: assessing the pandemic threat, <http://www.who.int/influenza/resources/documents/h5n1_assessing_pandemic_threat/en/>; 2005 [updated June 26, 2014].
66. Elbe S. Haggling over viruses: the downside risks of securitizing infectious disease. Health Policy Plan 2010;25(6):476–85.
67. WHO. Pandemic influenza preparedness Framework, <http://www.who.int/influenza/resources/pip_framework/en/>; 2011 [updated June 26, 2014].
68. Fidler DP, Gostin LO. The WHO pandemic influenza preparedness framework: a milestone in global governance for health. JAMA 2011;306(2):200–1.
69. Butler D. Tensions linger over discovery of coronavirus. Nature. 14 January 2013. <http://www.nature.com/news/tensions-linger-over-discovery-of-coronavirus-1.12108>; 26 June 2014.
70. Anon. Saudi coronavirus work stymied at Canadian lab, <http://www.cbc.ca/1.1322426/>. <http://www.cbc.ca/news/health/saudi-coronavirus-work-stymied-at-canadian-lab-1.1322426/>; [updated June 23, 2014].
71. Associated Press. World Health Organisation calls for greater cooperation in fight against deadly coronavirus. 2013.
72. Miles T, Nebehay S. WHO warns countries not to hoard secrets of coronavirus. Geneva: Reuters; 2013 [UTC].
73. United Nations (UN) ECOSOC. The Right to the Highest Attainable Standard of Health. In: Comments ECG, editor. 2000.
74. Hunt P, Khosla R. Are drug companies living up to their human rights responsibilities? The perspective of the former United Nations Special Rapporteur (2002-2008). PLoS Med 2010;7(9): e1000330.
75. McKeown T, Brown RG. Medical evidence related to English population changes in the eighteenth century. Pop Stud 1955;9(2):119–41.
76. Colgrove J. The McKeown thesis: a historical controversy and its enduring influence. Am J Public Health 2002;92(5):725–9.
77. Lalonde M. A new perspective on the health of Canadians. 1974.
78. Lemco J. National Health Care: Lessons for the United States and Canada. University of Michigan Press; Ann Arbor, Michigan, 1994. p. 304.
79. Omran AR. The epidemiologic transition: a theory of the epidemiology of population change. Milbank Mem Fund Q 1971;49(4):509–38.
80. Constitution of the World Health Organization as adopted by the International Health Conference, New York, 19-22 June, 1946; signed on 22 July 1946 by the representatives of 61 States (Official Records of the World Health Organization, no. 2, p. 100) and entered into force on 7 April 1948.
81. Tine H. Biographical Dictionary of Secretaries-General of International Organizations: Mahler, Halfdan Theodor, World Health Organization, 1973-1988, <http://www.ru.nl/politicologie/koppeling/reinalda/io-bio-biographical/>; 2013 [updated June 26, 2014].
82. Cueto M. The origins of primary health care and selective primary health care. Am J Public Health 2004;94(11):1864–74.
83. Djukanovic V, Mach EP, World Health Organization, UNICEF. Alternative approaches to meeting basic health needs in developing countries: a joint UNICEF/WHO study /. World Health Organization. 1975.
84. Waddington C. Does earmarked donor funding make it more or less likely that developing countries will allocate their resources towards programmes that yield the greatest health benefits? Bull World Health Organ 2004;82(9):703–8.
85. Mahler HT. Social perspectives in health: address in presenting his report for 1975 to the twenty-ninth world health assembly. Geneva: WHO Library; 1976.
86. Woodward D, Drager N, Beaglehole R, Lipson D. Globalization and health: a framework for analysis and action. Bull World Health Organ 2001;79(9): 875–81.
87. World Health Organization. Declaration of Alma-Ata, 1978. World Health Organization; 2005.
88. Halfdan M. WHO | Address to the 61st World Health Assembly. <http://www.who.int/mediacentre/events/2008/wha61/hafdan_mahler_speech/en/>; 2008 [updated June 26, 2014].

89. Walsh JA, Warren KS. Selective primary health care: an interim strategy for disease control in developing countries. N Engl J Med 1979;301(18): 967–74.
90. Evans JR, Hall KL, Warford J. Shattuck lecture—health care in the developing world: problems of scarcity and choice. N Engl J Med 1981;305(19): 1117–27.
91. Gish O. Selective primary health care: old wine in new bottles. Soc Sci Med 1982;16(10):1049–54.
92. Breilh J. Community medicine under imperialism: a new medical police? Int J Health Serv 1979;9(1):5–24.
93. WHO. "Beijing declaration," <http://www.who.int/medicines/areas/traditional/congress/beijing_declaration/en/>; [updated June 23, 2014].
94. Cueto M. The ORIGINS of primary health care and SELECTIVE primary health care. American Journal of Public Health. 2004;94(11):1864–1874.
95. Cerqueira MT. Health and human security in border regions. Rev Panam Salud Publica 2012;31(5):359–64.
96. Onuoha FC. Why the poor pay with their lives: oil pipeline vandalisation, fires and human security in Nigeria. Disasters 2009;33(3):369–89.
97. Parmar PK, Agrawal P, Goyal R, Scott J, Greenough PG. Need for a gender-sensitive human security framework: results of a quantitative study of human security and sexual violence in Djohong District, Cameroon. Confl Health 2014;8:6.
98. Rabaia Y, Giacaman R, Nguyen-Gillham V. Violence and adolescent mental health in the occupied Palestinian territory: a contextual approach. Asia Pac J Public Health 2010;22(Suppl. 3):216S–21S.
99. Verhoeven H. Climate change, conflict and development in Sudan: global neo-Malthusian narratives and local power struggles. Dev Change 2011;42(3):679–707.
100. Ziadni M, Hammoudeh W, Rmeileh NMEA, Hogan D, Shannon H, Giacaman R. Sources of human insecurity in post-war situations: The case of Gaza. Journal of Human Security. 2011;7(3):10.3316/JHS0703023. doi:10.3316/JHS0703023.
101. Hastings DA. The Human Security Index: pursuing enriched characterization of development. Development 2013;56(1):6678.
102. Pogge T. World poverty and human rights. Ethics Int Affairs 2005;19(01): 1–7.
103. Intervention ICo, Sovereignty S, Evans GJ, Sahnoun M. The responsibility to protect: report of the International Commission on Intervention and State Sovereignty. Canada: International Development Research Centre; 2001.
104. Annan KA. We, the peoples of United Nations in the 21st Century. New York: United Nations; 2000.
105. Adler RN, Smith J, Fishman P, Larson EB. To prevent, react, and rebuild: health research and the prevention of genocide. Health Serv Res 2004; 39(6 Pt 2):2027–51.
106. Booth K. Theory of World Security. 1st ed. Cambridge, New York: Cambridge University Press; 2008. p. 516.
107. UN General Assembly, Universal Declaration of Human Rights, 10 December 1948, 217 A (III). <http://www.refworld.org/docid/3ae6b3712c.html>; 17 October 2015.
108. Gruskin S, Mills EJ, Tarantola D. History, principles, and practice of health and human rights. Lancet 2007;370(9585):449–55.
109. Sen A, Farmer P. Pathologies of power: health, human rights, and the new war on the poor. [With a New Preface by the Author]. Berkeley: University of California Press; 2004. p. 438.
110. Gruskin S, Grodin MA, Marks SP, Annas GJ. Perspectives on health and human rights. Taylor & Francis; London, UK, 2004. p. 643.
111. Hunt P. Neglected diseases, social justice and human rights: some preliminary observations. Geneva: WHO. Health and Human Rights Working Paper Series; 2003;(4).
112. Thomas C, Wilkin P. Globalization, Human Security, and the African Experience. Boulder, Colo: Lynne Rienner Pub; 1998. p. 211.
113. Hulme D. The millennium development goals (MDGs): a short history of the world's biggest promise. Manchester: University of Manchester Brooks World Poverty Institute; 2009.
114. Panel UNHL. A new global partnership: Eradicate poverty and transform economies through sustainable development. Final Report of the UN High-Level Panel of Eminent Persons on the Post-2015 Development Agenda. New York: United Nations Publications; 2013.
115. Pande V, Elgin-Cossart M. Africa: fight poverty - with data. New York: High Level Panel of Eminent Persons on the Post-2015 Development Agenda; 2013.
116. Organization WH. Macroeconomics and health: Investing in Health for Economic Development: Report of the Commission on Macroeconomics and Health. 1st ed. Geneva: World Health Organization; 2001. p. 210.
117. Smith RD. Global public goods and health. Bull World Health Organ 2003;81(7):475.
118. Kaul I, Faust M. Global public goods and health: taking the agenda forward. Bull World Health Organ 2001;79(9):869–74.
119. Smith RD, MacKellar L. Global public goods and the global health agenda: problems, priorities and potential. Global Health 2007;3(1):9.
120. Curley M, Thomas N. Human security and public health in Southeast Asia: the SARS outbreak. Aust J Int Aff 2004;58(1):17–32.
121. Paris R. Human Security: Paradigm shift or hot air? Int Secur 2001;26(2): 87–102.
122. Bond P. The dispossession of African wealth at the cost of Africa's health. Int J Health Serv 2007;37(1):171–92.
123. Easterly W. The white man's burden: why the west's efforts to aid the rest have done so much ill and so little good. Reprint ed. New York: Penguin Books; 2007. p. 448.
124. Moyo D, Ferguson N. Dead aid: why aid is not working and how there is a better way for Africa. 1st Reprint ed. New York: Farrar, Straus and Giroux; 2010. p. 208.
125. Rifkin SB, Muller F, Bichmann W. Primary health care: on measuring participation. Soc Sci Med 1988;26(9):931–40.
126. Smith R, Beaglehole R, Woodward D, Drager N. Global Public Goods for Health: Health economic and public health perspective. Oxford; New York: Oxford University Press; 2003. p. 312.
127. El-Sadr WM, De Cock KM. Health systems exist for real people. Introduction. J Acquir Immune Defic Syndr 2009;52(Suppl. 1):S1–2.
128. Garret L. The Challenge of Global Health, <http://www.cfr.org/world/challenge-global-health/p12361/>; 2007 [updated June 26, 2014].
129. WHO. WHO's first global report on antibiotic resistance reveals serious, worldwide threat to public health, <http://www.who.int/mediacentre/news/releases/2014/amr-report/en/>; 2014 [updated June 26, 2014].
130. Davies SC, Fowler T, Watson J, Livermore DM, Walker D. Annual report of the chief medical officer: infection and the rise of antimicrobial resistance. Lancet 2013;381(9878):1606–9.
131. Girou E, Legrand P, Soing-Altrach S, Lemire A, Poulain C, Allaire A, et al. Association between hand hygiene compliance and methicillin-resistant Staphylococcus aureus prevalence in a French rehabilitation hospital. Infect Control Hosp Epidemiol 2006;27(10):1128–30.
132. WHO. Antimicrobial resistance, <http://www.who.int/mediacentre/factsheets/fs194/en/>; 2014 [updated June 26, 2014].
133. Ng NY, Ruger JP. Global health governance at a crossroads. Glob Health Gov 2011;3(2):1–37.
134. Nye Jr JS. Smart power. Great leaders know when hard power is not enough. Harv Bus Rev 2008;86(11):55–9, 135.
135. Definition provided by the chapter author.
136. Ruger JP. Global health justice and governance. Am J Bioeth 2012;12(12):35–54.

CHAPTER 13

Achieving the Right Balance in Governance of Public Health Surveillance

Jennifer B Nuzzo, Gigi Kwik Gronvall

Let both sides seek to invoke the wonders of science instead of its terrors. Together let us explore the stars, conquer the deserts, eradicate disease, tap the ocean depths and encourage the arts and commerce.

John F Kennedy (1961 Inaugural Address)

KEY WORDS

Cooperation | Multicountry disease surveillance networks | PIP

INTRODUCTION

In 2011, a toxin-producing strain of *Escherichia coli* bacteria infected thousands of people in Germany and France and killed dozens.[1] Shortly after the outbreak was first recognized, health officials in Germany launched an investigation to identify the cause in hopes of preventing additional illnesses and deaths. Initially they suspected, based on available epidemiologic data, that cucumbers from Spain might be to blame and cautioned the public not to consume raw produce.[2] In response, many countries around the world announced bans on produce from Germany and Spain.[3] Some countries, like Russia and Lebanon, opted to ban all produce from the EU, citing ongoing uncertainty about the true cause of the outbreak.[4] German retail sales in May fell by 2.8%, the fastest decline in 4 years.[5] But these moves were called into question when shortly thereafter Germany's health authorities retracted their conclusion that the outbreak was caused by Spanish cucumbers and began scrutinizing other possible sources.[6] Many weeks later, after the outbreak seemed to be on the decline, an analysis of import and supply chain data identified the more likely cause: sprouts made from seeds imported to Europe in 2010.[7]

The 2011 *E. coli* outbreak was one of the most deadly and expensive outbreaks in Europe's recent history. It also serves as an important example of how infectious diseases pose threats to global health and security and why there is need for improved information sharing and global cooperation to combat these threats. The contaminated seeds from one part of the world managed to sicken thousands and caused economic repercussions throughout Europe illustrates how the health, political, and economic consequences of infectious disease outbreaks can be severe and can extend well beyond those areas where human infections are actively occurring. It demonstrates that the toll outbreaks take can be exacerbated in the absence of timely and accurate information. Uncertainty about the cause of the outbreak and questions about whether it would spread made it difficult to isolate affected produce and issue cautionary guidance to the public and, as a result, multiple countries issued bans on broad categories of produce, with deleterious effects on whole sectors of their economies.

In the last 15 years, events like the *E. coli* outbreak in Europe, the anthrax attacks of 2001, the rapid global spread of severe acute respiratory syndrome (SARS) in 2003, the 2009 influenza A (H1N1) pandemic, and the emergence and international spread of the Middle East respiratory syndrome coronavirus (MERS-CoV) have all increased global political concerns about emerging infectious disease threats and deliberate epidemics and have demonstrated both the important connection between global public health and security.[8]

Yet, while global health and security rely on timely sharing among international partners of disease surveillance information, a balanced approach is required to ensure full participation by the nations involved. When countries see tangible benefits from participating in global surveillance programs, great strides can be made toward achieving global health and security. A good example of this can be found in seasonal influenza surveillance. Each year, institutions in more than 100 countries around the world collaborate to identify and share information about which influenza strains are in circulation with the goal of informing global production of a seasonal influenza vaccine that is well matched to the dominant influenza threat. In the USA, the estimated 40% of Americans who avail themselves of the seasonal influenza vaccine are among some of the direct beneficiaries of this global surveillance collaboration.[9]

However, despite strong reasons for countries to take collective action to improve the detection and response to infectious disease outbreaks, there are clear disincentives to information sharing, which inhibit nations from fully engaging. Strong disagreements between countries as to whether and how to share data have hindered the response to several high-profile global outbreaks, including SARS, H5N1, and MERS-CoV. In each of these outbreaks, there have been tensions between the global community's need for shared information to ensure global security and individual nations' needs to protect the health of their citizenry, as well as their economies.

This chapter will discuss the importance of maintaining global surveillance for infectious diseases and why a balanced approach to the conduct of surveillance is needed to ensure full participation by countries. Specifically, it will discuss the current challenges facing global surveillance, why enhanced global governance is required, and what actions the global community can take to achieve a balanced governance system.

PROGRESS MADE TOWARD ENHANCED GLOBAL COOPERATION FOR GLOBAL SURVEILLANCE

Revision of the International Health Regulations

In 2005, the IHR were significantly revised, in part due to experience during the 2003 SARS outbreak. Global perception that SARS was worsened by China's lack of communication about the outbreak called into question the effectiveness of the existing IHR and led many to call for the regulations to be updated and strengthened.[10] A key provision of the revised IHR is that the short list of reportable diseases contained in previous IHR was abandoned in favor of a broad definition of what constitutes a reportable event. The IHR now require that State Parties build and maintain the capacity to detect and respond to any public health event of international concern (PHEIC). The World Health Organization (WHO) has developed an algorithm that countries can use to assess whether an event constitutes a likely PHEIC, but generally speaking, any health event that has the potential to spread internationally and cause harm to other countries is a likely candidate for designation as a PHEIC. Under the revised IHR, countries must report potential PHEIC to WHO within 24 h of their recognition. The IHR also require signatories to provide assistance to countries with fewer resources to help improve their capacity to achieve these new IHR requirements. Many have interpreted this requirement to mean that countries must help others improve their capacity to conduct surveillance.

Formation of Multicountry Disease Surveillance Networks: A Promising Sign of Increased Interest in Global Cooperation for Surveillance

The formation of **multicountry surveillance networks**[11] shows promise for enhanced global cooperation for detecting and responding to infectious disease outbreaks. In response to the increasing frequency of disease outbreaks that have spread across national borders, some countries have formed agreements and partnerships with their geographic neighbors for the purpose of improving their individual and collective abilities to detect, investigate, and respond to disease outbreaks and epidemics.[12] Countries that participate in surveillance networks typically agree to share disease outbreak information and to collaborate in efforts to control disease spread.[12] Some also agree to share technical methods, tools, and other resources that can enhance the disease surveillance practices of each country within the network. In some cases, the sharing and joint analysis of surveillance data across a network has contributed to a more complete understanding of scientific evidence about the nature of the outbreaks.[13,14] For example, health officials from Israel, Jordan, and the Palestinian authority formed a surveillance network to improve their collective response to food-borne outbreaks. The resulting Middle East Consortium on Infectious Disease Surveillance (MECIDS) network has shared data, laboratory capacities and protocols, and conducted joint training and data analysis to improve detection and response to food-borne outbreaks, as well as to other regional outbreaks, such as the 2009 H1N1 influenza pandemic and H5N1 avian influenza.[11,13,14] Multicountry disease surveillance networks now exist in many other parts of the world, such as Southeast Asia, Southern Africa, southeastern Europe, and East Africa.[15]

Global Health Security Agenda

The opportunities for collective action to counter infectious disease threats took another step forward on February 13, 2014, when the White House announced the Global Health Security (GHS) Agenda. The GHS Agenda is intended to signal a new commitment to prevent, detect, and rapidly respond to infectious disease threats. The White House along with more than 30 partner nations, WHO, the World Organization for Animal Health, and the Food and Agriculture Organization of the United Nations stated that they will commit to a 5-year effort to significantly accelerate activities to address biological threats, whether they are naturally occurring, deliberate, or accidental.[16] In an editorial, Secretary of State John Kerry, Secretary of Health and Human Services Kathleen Sebelius, and Assistant to the President for Homeland Security and Counterterrorism Lisa Monaco[17] wrote that with today's technology, nations "can put in place a safe, secure, globally linked, interoperable system to prevent disease threats, detect outbreaks in real time, and share information and expertise to respond effectively." At the time of writing it is early to project what the GHS Agenda will mean for enhanced PHS, but it underscores the necessity of these issues, and that disease surveillance is a priority across multiple sectors and government agencies.

REMAINING CHALLENGES TO DATA SHARING

Economic Disincentives to Report Outbreaks

Though countries are required by the IHR to report in a timely manner any public health events of international concern that have occurred, the penalties for countries that fail to do so are unclear. From the perspective of a nation, there may be few direct incentives to report the presence of a disease to the international community. Historically, countries that have reported major outbreaks have endured significant drops in tourism and trade, closings of borders, and other economically damaging measures. Such was the case during the 2009 influenza A/H1N1 pandemic. At the onset of the pandemic, WHO issued clear recommendations that countries should not ban imports, close borders, or restrict travelers to contain the outbreak at national borders.[18] Despite these recommendations, however, a number of countries pursued these measures, which caused undue economic harm to other nations.[10,18] A more detailed discussion of the 2009 influenza pandemic can be found in the pandemic influenza case study (Box 13.1).

Many Health Priorities, Not Enough Resources

Another challenge for global surveillance is that many countries across the globe lack the capabilities necessary for detecting and responding to infectious disease threats.[30] Though the revised IHR call upon countries to improve

BOX 13-1 Case Study: 2009 Influenza Pandemic

The 2009 H1N1 influenza pandemic, which represented one of the first global tests of the revised IHR, serves as an unfortunate cautionary tale for countries that might consider whether and when to report an outbreak. Most countries generally adhered to the requirements of the IHR during the pandemic by sharing information and enacting policies consistent with WHO, but there were some notable exceptions.[10,19] Shortly after the pandemic was recognized, WHO made it clear that, based on the rapid spread of influenza cases that was occurring, no practical measures existed that would prevent the disease from being spread from country to country. Consequently, WHO recommended that countries not ban imports, close borders, or restrict travelers in attempts to contain the outbreak at national borders, as these would do more harm than good. The WHO recommendations were well informed by science and global experience during previous pandemics. Historically, closing airports and detaining travelers at borders has not been effective in preventing disease importation. For example, in reviewing evidence from multiple countries' experiences with SARS, a WHO expert group concluded that screening and detaining travelers at international borders had "little documented effect on detecting SARS cases."[20] Furthermore, a historical analysis of previous influenza pandemics conducted by WHO concluded that "screening and quarantining entering travelers at international borders did not substantially delay virus introduction in past pandemics … and will likely be even less effective in the modern era."[21]

However, during the 2009 H1N1 pandemic, a number of countries pursued control measures in defiance of WHO recommendations and efficacy, which caused economic damage and great inconvenience to affected groups and individuals. Around the world, many countries restricted flights to or from North America in defiance of WHO guidance.[22] China[23] and Singapore[24] quarantined Mexicans and other North Americans traveling to those countries regardless of H1N1 exposure. Fever screens were also employed in 2009 for H1N1 at 22 international airports in countries such as China and India despite WHO judgment that such measures would hinder trade and travel without compensatory public health benefit[25–27] and on evidence that suggested they would not work well to control influenza.[21,27] In addition, some countries banned pork from the affected countries in spite of a joint statement by WHO, United Nations Food and Agriculture Organization (FAO), the World Organization for Animal Health (OIE), and the World Trade Organization (WTO), which stated that pork and pork products could not transmit H1N1 influenza.[28,29]

their surveillance capabilities, progress toward full implementation of these requirements has been slow. Fewer than 20% of countries reported having met the 2012 deadline for IHR implementation.[31,32] However, even with additional time, gaps in countries' surveillance capacities are likely to persist for some time.

A key challenge is that in areas of the world where surveillance needs are greatest, there are few resources available to make needed improvements. While all countries require information about infectious disease events that occur across the globe, they do not equally share the burden of having to conduct surveillance for such outbreaks. The geographic distribution of most infectious disease outbreaks suggests that much of the burden of global surveillance falls on the developing world—countries where there is already a high burden of infectious diseases (such as HIV, TB, and malaria) and where trained personnel, diagnostic laboratories, and funding required to support surveillance are in short supply. For example, though there have been great advances in the technologies available to diagnose or detect infectious diseases, WHO has reported that more than 60% of laboratory equipment in developing countries is outdated or not functioning.[33]

The current outbreak of Ebola virus disease (EVD) in West Africa illustrates both the importance of having in place throughout the world adequate surveillance capabilities for the early detection outbreaks that threaten global health and security, as well as the severe resource shortages that exist in some countries to combat deadly outbreaks. The Ebola crisis in West Africa, which WHO declared on August 8, 2014, to be a PHEIC, likely began in Guinea as early as December 2013—close to 3 months before WHO was notified. Since its emergence, the absence of a strong diagnostic and treatment facilities have contributed to the exponential spread of the disease in several countries.

For such countries, it may be difficult to prioritize allocation of a nation's scarce health resources to improve surveillance for rare events, like PHEIC, when there are insufficient resources available to address endemic disease threats. The funding required to implement the central requirements of the IHR are significant. Katz and Fischer[34] have estimated the total costs of implementing the core capacities in a representative southeast Asian country may require US$230–280 million. Though the IHR call upon member states to help others implement the requirements by sharing technical and financial support, as Katz and Fischer[35] have pointed out, countries have been "slow to roll out comprehensive assistance packages to help resource-constrained countries."

Insufficient Governance for Global Surveillance

Though the revised IHR have helped to improve the frequency with which countries share information about outbreaks and other public health events of international concern, there continue to be disagreements among countries over what level of data sharing is necessary. Fueling these tensions is the absence of specific international frameworks to govern when and how countries should share information in the midst of an outbreak. Though the IHR set the expectation that countries will report the occurrence of a PHEIC in a timely manner, the IHR do not contain specific provisions as how and when countries should share clinical and environmental specimens obtained from outbreaks of international concern and other data that are critical components of effective surveillance. Two case studies—Indonesia's refusal to share H5N1 specimens and Saudi Arabia's response to MERS-CoV—illustrate how the absence of comprehensive governance frameworks for international surveillance has complicated the response to outbreaks.

H5N1 and Indonesia

In 2006, Indonesia announced that it would no longer cooperate with the WHO-led international surveillance efforts by sharing its H5N1 influenza specimens. As the country hardest hit by avian influenza, Indonesia's announcement worried international health authorities who feared that lack of access to virus samples from Indonesia would compromise global efforts to keep tabs on the evolving H5N1 threat. Indonesia justified its sudden refusal to share this critical surveillance information on having learned that an Australian pharmaceutical company had developed an H5N1 vaccine based on a specimen that was originally isolated in Indonesia.[36,37] Indonesia's health officials worried that in sharing samples from its H5N1 outbreaks, it would be increasing the probability that the country's clinical specimens would either be developed into vaccines that Indonesia could not afford or be patented by vaccine companies, which would complicate Indonesia's or other countries' efforts to develop their own vaccines. Invoking the 1992 United Nations Convention on Biological Diversity (CBD), Indonesia further claimed that it was an act of "biopiracy" for pharmaceutical companies to profit from the Indonesian avian samples.[38] Indonesia argued that viruses obtained within a country are the sovereign property of that nation.

The standoff over H5N1 specimens lasted for several years until WHO announced that it had brokered an agreement with Indonesia and other countries regarding sharing and access to influenza specimens.[39,40] The WHO's **Pandemic Influenza Preparedness Framework (PIP Framework)** for the Sharing of Influenza Viruses and Access to Vaccines and Other Benefits, which was adopted in 2011, encourages countries to share influenza samples by addressing some of the concerns about who has access to specimens and any commercial products (such as vaccines) that may be developed from specimens shared by countries.[41] The PIP Framework contained two key provisions. First, it aims to address vaccine inequities by increasing resource limited countries' access to medicines and vaccines derived from shared virus samples through monetary support and in-kind contributions from the pharmaceutical industry. Second, it tries to control the transfer of specimens that countries share through the adoption and use of material transfer agreements (MTAs). The agreements discourage treating virus samples as intellectual property.[42]

MERS-CoV and the Kingdom of Saudi Arabia

In June 2012, Dr Ali Mohamed Zaki, a physician in Jeddah, Saudi Arabia, isolated and cultured an unknown, potentially dangerous virus. The sample had come from a man who died from severe pneumonia and acute renal failure, and the viral cause of death was not identified through routine diagnostic tests. The physician sent the sample to Dr Ron Fouchier, a virologist at Erasmus Medical Center (EMC) in Rotterdam, the Netherlands, for identification (see case studies).[43]

Fouchier sequenced the virus and discovered that it was a previously unknown coronavirus, which is the same family of viruses to which SARS belongs. Dr Zaki announced the news of the new virus, provisionally named human betacoronavirus 2c EMC after the research center in Rotterdam, on ProMED-mail, a free, infectious diseases reporting system. Saudi health officials learned of the new virus through the ProMED-mail announcement.[43] Dr Zaki, dismissed from his position, has since moved to Egypt. Saudi health authorities were not pleased that the virus was not reported through the Ministry of Health (MoH), and that although the virus was first isolated in Saudi Arabia, the action of sending a sample to Fouchier handed over the sovereign and intellectual property rights on diagnostic tests or treatments.

After the ProMED announcement, the Erasmus researchers required laboratories to sign an MTA in order to gain access to samples of the virus. An MTA typically governs what the receiving laboratories can do with the virus and is now a customary part of sharing samples; in the MERS-CoV case, the agreement stipulates that the samples belong to Erasmus MC and that the receiving laboratory cannot share or give the samples to other laboratories.[44] Erasmus also filed for a patent based on the gene sequence of MERS-CoV, with the hope of one day being able to commercialize a diagnostic test, vaccine, or other medicine to combat the new virus. The Jeddah physician was listed as the first name on the patent, and Erasmus claims that it intended to share all along.[44] Nonetheless, the patent and MTA moves angered Saudi health officials who felt that their own ability to use the virus to protect citizens from the lethal virus was limited. The Saudi MoH contested Erasmus' right to control a virus that was isolated from the Kingdom.[45]

Though the Kingdom of Saudi Arabia (KSA) health officials have yet to cite "viral sovereignty" in their arguments against Erasmus University, the dispute bears similarity to concerns raised by Indonesia in 2006. These examples illustrate how a country's officials may decide that in sharing with the international community there may also be loss of full control or access to specimens needed to protect the citizenry from an infectious disease threat within the country's borders. These concerns were echoed by the WHO Director General Margaret Chan. Addressing the MERS-CoV disagreement between KSA and Erasmus, Director General Chan asked why "scientists would send specimens out to other laboratories on a bilateral manner and allow other people to take intellectual property rights on a new disease … No [intellectual property] should stand in the way of you, the countries of the world, to protect your people."[45]

The MERS-CoV situation also demonstrates the inadequacy of existing international agreements for global surveillance. Though international agreements like the IHR and the PIP Framework exist, neither has been shown to fully address the countries' concerns about sharing surveillance information. Though the PIP Framework mitigated Indonesia's concerns about sharing H5N1 specimens, the agreement applies to influenza viruses only; other viruses, like MERS-CoV, are not covered by any existing specimen-sharing framework.

International Disagreements over Data Necessary to Maintain Adequate Surveillance

In addition to the problems of coordinating sharing of physical samples between nations, there have been problems coordinating how much information is required for adequate public health surveillance, and therefore what studies are required to assess the emerging threat. This is particularly the case for influenza surveillance, where there is always the potential that a pandemic strain may emerge, and where there is a great deal of evolutionary change in the viral strains from season to season. Though there have been many outbreaks of seasonal influenza, and handfuls of pandemics, there is still a great deal of uncertainty about why a particular strain of influenza would spark a pandemic over another strain, and a general lack of information about how pandemic strains evolve. This complicates surveillance, as it makes it difficult to adequately interpret the information that is received. In particular, scientific uncertainty has complicated the surveillance for H5N1 avian influenza.

H5N1 is currently an avian disease but occasionally crosses over to infect people. WHO reported last year that since 2003, there have been 622 laboratory-confirmed cases of H5N1, of which 371 resulted in death, an approximately 60% mortality rate.[46] Considering that the most devastating influenza pandemic in history, the 1918 influenza pandemic, had a 2.5% fatality rate and still killed at least 50 million people, the potential consequences if H5N1 could evolve to transmit between people without losing much of its mortality rate would be immense.[47] It is unclear why H5N1 has not yet emerged as a pandemic strain, or whether it will.

The great uncertainty about whether this potentially devastating disease should be prepared for has led some scientists to pursue studies to validate whether H5N1 is indeed a public health threat. In 2000, the Centers for Disease

Control and Prevention (CDC) started experiments with H5N1 strains isolated from Hong Kong from the first human H5N1 outbreak in 1997. They performed "reassortment" studies to determine whether one of those influenza mixing vessels was likely to produce a human pandemic strain.[48]

Research continued in this area for years, but did not attract much attention outside of the influenza research community. That changed after a scientific presentation by Ron Fouchier from Erasmus Medical Center at the European Scientific Working Group on Influenza's conference in Malta in 2011. Fouchier described how his laboratory pushed the virus to evolve under controlled circumstances so that it was contagious among ferrets, the preferred animal model for studying influenza.[49] When the transmissible strain was isolated from the ferrets and genetically sequenced, it was found to differ from the starting strain in only five areas.[50] All of the mutations that had been laboratory-evolved were already seen in samples isolated from sick birds in nature, though not all together in one strain.[50,51] This suggested that H5N1 might have been incrementally evolving to become a mammalian pathogen. Yoshihiro Kawaoka, a scientist who runs virology laboratories at both the University of Wisconsin–Madison and University of Tokyo, performed a different type of experiment that produced the same general conclusion: H5N1 could be transmissible among humans.[50] Both scientists submitted their work to major scientific journals; Fouchier submitted his work to *Science*, and Kawaoka submitted his work to *Nature*.

Prior to publication, the papers were considered by the National Science Advisory Board for Biosecurity (NSABB), which, along with the US government, recommended redaction of methodological details. The disagreement about what to do with these articles, and the line of inquiry for influenza research, provoked 6 months of public discussion, a self-imposed moratorium on this type of work by the influenza research community, a series of high-profile international meetings, a reversal of the US government stance, and ultimately the publication of the articles in leading scientific journals. Disagreement remains, however, about whether the research—which has been termed "gain-of-function research"—should be pursued or funded. US policy for research governance has added additional oversight for gain-of-function research using 15 biological pathogens, including highly pathogenic avian influenza and botulinum toxin, all of which are already regulated as select agents. The United States Department of Health and Human Services has also introduced a set of rules for how they will fund research projects anticipated to generate highly pathogenic H5N1 viruses, which are transmissible among mammals by respiratory droplets.[52] It is possible that the US government may take further actions to govern dual-use research of concern (DURC), which they define as "life sciences research that … could be directly misapplied to pose a significant threat with broad potential consequences to public health and safety, agricultural crops and other plants, animals, the environment, materiel or national security."[52] In the end, there is no clear international agreement about how much research is required for adequate disease surveillance. It is, however, clear that if research were to be curtailed in the US on these studies, it will be pursued elsewhere.[53]

Keeping Pace with Technological Changes

The challenges of sample sharing and information sharing are not likely to diminish in the future, though technological changes may change the nature of the debate. For years, it has been routine for new pathogen samples to be genetically sequenced in their entirety, and the information published in scientific journals and databases. More recently, however, the synthesis of genetic material has become more reliable and less expensive. While the technological feats accomplished by Craig Venter and colleagues at the J. Craig Venter Institute in synthesizing an entire bacterial genome and "booting" it up to create a synthetic cell are beyond the capacities of most laboratories, it is certainly possible for many scientists around the world to synthesize small viruses, including influenza.[54] If it is beyond the capacity of an individual laboratory, there are companies that can supply synthesized strands of genetic material for an increasingly reasonable price.

The ability to synthesize a virus strain for research purposes, without having to wait for or apply for an MTA or to have to deal with viral sovereignty issues, is a relatively new development that could affect how virus samples are shared. If the sequence is published, it certainly inhibits the ability of a nation to claim viral sovereignty. If worries about loss of viral sovereignty lead to sequences not being analyzed, that could be a detriment to disease surveillance.

The Nagoya Protocol on Access and Benefit Sharing (NP), part of the CBD, touches on this possibility, but the actual effect it will have on disease surveillance is now unclear. Treaty experts have recommended that scientific researchers try to determine the origin of the viral strain, even if they are only examining digital sequences, because provider countries "may assert that such information falls within the scope of the CBD/NP."[55] This information may change, however, because the Nagoya Protocol is not in effect (it will go into effect 90 days after 50 countries ratify the agreement, but so far only 6 countries and the EU have even taken initial steps of submitting implementing legislation to the convention).[55] Though the USA is not a party to the CBD and there are no apparent plans to become one, the convention and protocol still affects US researchers, particularly if they try to obtain genetic resources from other nations, or seek to commercialize or acquire intellectual property from a nation that is party to the treaty.

VISION FOR THE FUTURE

Though the global community has recognized the need for international cooperation to detect and respond to outbreaks, experience in recent outbreaks, such as the 2009 H1N1 influenza pandemic, H5N1 avian influenza outbreaks, and MERS-CoV, shows that progress toward this goal is lacking. Economic consequences that befall countries that report outbreaks and disagreements on data ownership serve as powerful disincentives to global information sharing. If the international community desires full cooperation and engagement of nations in global surveillance initiatives, it will have to find ways to address these issues. Going forward, the goal for global surveillance efforts should be to pursue approaches that balance both the need for global information sharing and countries' individual obligation to protect their own citizens.

A necessary first step is to recognize that countries will only cooperate with global surveillance initiatives if they feel it is in their best interest to do so. Though the IHR require countries to report PHEIC, in the absence of enforceable penalties for failing to share information, countries' participation in global surveillance is largely voluntary and dependent on their perception of the value of sharing with other nations. Compliance is possible in a voluntary system. In the USA, the primary legal responsibility for conducting surveillance for and responding to outbreaks rests not with the federal government but with individual states. The USA maintains national surveillance for important diseases because states voluntarily share this information with the CDC's National Notifiable Diseases Surveillance System (NNDSS). States participate in this program because they see value for their own programs in having aggregated information—that is, national statistics about the occurrence and trends of important diseases. A similar dynamic governs nations' willingness to participate in global surveillance programs.

It is also important that the global community take steps to reduce the economic disincentives to report infectious disease outbreaks. Countries that impose travel restrictions and trade barriers on countries that report disease outbreaks could face consequences if those measures are not supported by WHO guidance. Mechanisms within the IHR to do so, such as the possibility of revoking World Health Assembly membership, have not been used to date and are unlikely to be used in the future. But countries that violate WHO guidance could be strongly condemned by other IHR treaty members, and diplomatic and other channels can be used to prevent unnecessary restriction of trade and travel.[18] Providing incentives to countries to report infectious disease outbreaks tying the willingness to report to the access and benefit sharing of medical countermeasures and public health assistance may also be merit consideration.

The international community will also need to develop a consensus framework that governs how countries share critical surveillance information, such as virus samples and specimens. This governance framework must establish a process by which data and specimens are shared between countries, international health authorities (including WHO), and scientists. It must also establish international consensus regarding the "rights" of countries from where the specimen is isolated and outline a process for developing derivative products (e.g., vaccines and diagnostics) and expectations about countries' access to those products.

KEY SUMMARY POINTS

- Over the last decade there have been significant efforts to improve surveillance for global infectious diseases, including recent revisions of IHR to expand reportable events, formation of multicountry disease surveillance and laboratory networks to increase sharing of capacities and data with neighboring countries, and the launch of the Global Health Security Agenda to increase political will for surveillance.
- Despite recent progress, there still remains insufficient funding to assist nations to improve surveillance capacity for global infectious disease threats, particularly in countries with limited health resources and a high burden of endemic diseases.
- There is currently a lack of international agreements and a corresponding governance structure to guide the sharing surveillance data and specimens among countries and between researchers and public health practitioners.
- The international community must ensure to reduce and minimize the economic disincentives, such as interfering with travel and trade, to ensure willingness of countries to report all PHEIC to WHO.

DISCUSSION QUESTIONS

1. What are some of the ways in which infectious disease outbreaks can undermine global health and security?
2. How do the revised (2005) International Health Regulations aim to improve global response to infectious disease outbreaks?
3. Give some reasons why implementation of the revised IHR has been slow.
4. Give some reasons why countries may not want to report outbreaks.
5. Is it possible to maintain effective global surveillance if participation is voluntary?
6. Discuss some of the ways in which a country's duty to its citizens conflicts with international need for information about outbreaks?
7. What do countries mean when they use the term "viral sovereignty?" How has this concept affected global response to past outbreaks?
8. In what ways has the absence of global agreement over what surveillance information is necessary to control outbreaks led to international disagreements?
9. In what ways may future scientific advances affect the sharing of surveillance information between countries?
10. What are some ways to encourage countries to share data with each other?

REFERENCES

1. Frank C, Faber MS, Askar M, et al. HUS investigation team. Large and ongoing outbreak of haemolytic uraemic syndrome, Germany. Eurosurveillance 2011;16(21):1–3.
2. Kupferschmidt K. Cucumbers may be culprit in massive *E. coli* outbreak in Germany. Science Insider, <http:// news.sciencemag.org/scienceinsider/2011/05/cucumbers-may-be-culprit-in-mass.html/>; May 26, 2011.
3. Goodman A. Warning lifted against Spanish cucumbers suspected in *E. coli* outbreak. CNN, <http://www.cnn.com/2011/WORLD/europe/06/01/spain.germany.e.coli/ index.html/>; June 1, 2011.
4. Norman L. *E.coli* row could overshadow EU-Russia summit. Wall Street Journal, <http://www.wsj.com/articles/SB1000142405270230439270457637372003094005 8>; June 9, 2011.
5. *E. coli* outbreak hits German retail sales in May. Reuters, <http://in.reuters.com/article/2011/06/30/ idINIndia-58006420110630/>; June 30, 2011. [accessed July 28, 2011].
6. Tremlett G, Pidd H. Germany admits Spanish cucumbers are not to blame for *E. coli* outbreak. Guardian.co.uk, <http://www.guardian.co.uk/uk/2011/may/31/e-coli-deaths-16- germany-sweden/>; May 31, 2011. [accessed July 28, 2011].
7. European Food Safety Authority. Tracing seeds, in particular fenugreek (Trigonella foenum-graecum) seeds, in relation to the Shiga toxin-producing *E. coli* (STEC) O104:H4 2011 outbreaks in Germany and France. EFSA/ECDC Joint Rapid Risk Assessment, <http://ecdc.europa.eu/en/publications/Publications/2011June29_RA_JOINT_EFSA_STEC_France.pdf/>; June 29, 2011.
8. Rodier G, Greenspan AL, Hughes JM, Heymann DL. Global public health security. Emerg Infect Dis 2007;13(10):1447–52.
9. McIntyre AF, Gonzalez-Feliciano AG, Bryan LN, Santibanez TA, Williams WW, Singleton JA, et al. Seasonal influenza vaccination coverage – United States, 2009-10 and 2010-11. MMWR Surveill Summ 2013;62(Suppl. 3):65–8.
10. Katz R, Fischer J. The revised international health regulations: A framework for global pandemic response. Global Health Governance 2010;III(2), <http://ghgj.org/Katz%20and%20Fischer_The%20Revised%20International%20Health%20Regulations.pdf/>.
11. Leventhal A, Ramlawi A, Belbiesi A, et al. Enhanced surveillance for detection and management of infectious diseases. Regional collaboration in the Middle East to deal with H5N1 avian flu. BMJ 2006;333(7573):856–8.
12. Gresham L, Ramlawi A, Briski J, Richardson M, Taylor T. Trust across borders: responding to 2009 H1N1 influenza in the Middle East. Biosecur Bioterror 2009;7(4):399–404.
13. Cohen D, Gargouri N, Ramlawi A, Abdeen Z, Belbesi A, Al Hijawi B, et al. A Middle East subregional laboratory-based surveillance network on foodborne diseases established by Jordan, Israel, and the Palestinian Authority. Epidemiol Infect 2010;138(10):1443–8.
14. M'ikanatha NM, Iskander J, editors. Concepts and methods in infectious disease surveillance. Oxford, UK: John Wiley & Sons Ltd; 2015.
15. CORDS. Connecting organizations for regional disease surveillance: strategic plan. 2011.

16. US Department of Health and Human Services. Office of Global Affairs. The global health security agenda, <http://www.globalhealth.gov/global-health-topics/global-health-security/ghsagenda.html/>; 2014.
17. John K, Kathleen S, Monaco L. Why global health security is a national priority. CNN; November 12, 2014.
18. Nuzzo JB, Gronvall GK. Global health security: closing the gaps in responding to infectious disease emergencies. Glob Health Govern 2011;4(2):1–15.
19. Katz R. Use of Revised International Health Regulations During Influenza A (H1N1) Epidemic, 2009. Emerging Infectious Diseases 2009;15(8):1165–1170.
20. Bell DM and World Health Organization Working Group on Prevention of International and Community Transmission of SARS. Public Health Interventions and SARS Spread, 2003. Emerg Infect Dis 2004;10(11):1900–1906.
21. World Health Organization Writing Group. Nonpharmaceutical Interventions for Pandemic Influenza, International Measures. Emerg Infect Dis 2006;12(1):81–87.
22. World Health Organization. Statement by Director. Global Alert and Response (GAR): No rationale for travel restrictions, <http://www.who.int/csr/disease/swineflu/guidance/public_health/travel_advice/en/index.html#/>; May 1, 2009. [accessed June 1, 2011].
23. Jackson K. U.S. Warns Travelers about China's 7-day Flu Quarantine. The Seattle Times, <http://seattletimes.nwsource.com/html/travel/2009368666_webchinaflu22.html/>; 2009. [accessed March 22, 2011].
24. Singapore Ministry of Health. Press Release: Update on Influenza A (H1N1-2009), <http://www.news.gov.sg/public/sgpc/en/media_releases/agencies/mica-nrd/press_release/P- 20090504-1.html/>; May 3, 2009. [June 1, 2011].
25. Stolberg S, Robinson O. Swine Flu Diary: Caught in a Beijing Dragnet. New York Times, <http://www.nytimes.com/2009/07/28/health/28flu.html/>; July 27, 2009.
26. Sinha K. American & European visitors to be screened for swine flu. The Economic Times, <http://articles.economictimes.indiatimes.com/2009-04-28/news/27649958_1_health-secretary-naresh-dayal-influenza-symptoms-swine-flu/>; April 28, 2009.
27. Anon. Stop screening for H1N1 at airports: WHO. Deccan Herald <http://www.deccanherald.com/content/20406/stop-screening-h1n1-airports-who.html/>; August 18, 2009.
28. Doering C. USDA may help ailing pork industry hit by H1N1. Reuters, <http://www.reuters.com/article/2009/05/07/us-flu-usa-vilsack-idUSTRE5466J420090507/>; March 7, 2009.
29. Joint FAO/WHO/OIE/WTO Statement. Joint FAO/WHO/OIE Statement on influenza A (H1N1) and the Safety of Pork. Media Centre, World Health Organization, <http://www.who.int/mediacentre/news/statements/2009/h1n1_20090502/en/index.html/>; 2009, [accessed March 22, 2011].
30. Wilson K, von Tigerstrom B, McDougall C. Protecting global health security through the international health regulations: requirements and challenges. CMAJ 2008;179(1):44–8.
31. Ijaz K, Kasowski E, Arthur RR, Angulo FJ, Dowell SF. International health regulations—what gets measured gets done. Emerg Infect Dis 2012;18(7):1054–7.
32. Frieden TR. Why global health security is imperative, <http://www.theatlantic.com/health/archive/2014/02/why-global-health-security-isimperative/283765/>; 25 February 2014.
33. U.S. Government Accountability Office. Challenges in improving infectious disease surveillance systems (GAO-01-722). 2001.
34. Katz R, Hate V, Kornblet S, Fischer JE. Costing framework for international health regulations (2005). Emerg Infect Dis 2012;18(7):1121–7.
35. Fischer JEKS, Katz R. The international health regulations (2005): surveillance and response in an era of globalization, <http://www.stimson.org/images/uploads/The_International_Health_Regulations_White_Paper_Final.pdf/>; 2011. [accessed February 18, 2014].
36. Aglionby J. Indonesia agrees to share bird flu samples. Financial Times. February 16, 2007. <http://www.ft.com/intl/cms/s/0/4d1995ae-bdf1-11db-bd86-0000779e2340.html#axzz3rCtO6klq>.
37. Irwin R. H5N1 and global diplomacy. Indonesia, <http://eprints.lse.ac.uk/28272/1/Irwin_Indonesia_and_Global_Health_Diplomacy.pdf>; 2010. [accessed March 3, 2014].
38. Irwin R. Indonesia, H5N1, and global health diplomacy, <http://ghgj.org/Irwin_Indonesia H5N1 and Global Health Diplomacy.pdf/>; 2010.
39. World Health Organization. Pandemic influenza preparedness framework for the sharing of influenza viruses and access to vaccines and other benefits ("PIP Framework") questions and answers, <http://www.who.int/influenza/pip/PIP_FQA_Nov_2011.pdf/>; 2011.
40. World Health Organization. Sixty-fourth World Health Assembly. Pandemic influenza preparedness: sharing of influenza viruses and access to vaccines and other benefits (Report by the Open-Ended Working Group of Member States). 2011.
41. WHO. Pandemic influenza framework, <http://apps.who.int/iris/bitstream/10665/44796/1/9789241503082_eng.pdf/>.
42. Fidler DP, Gostin LO. The WHO pandemic influenza preparedness framework: a milestone in global governance for health. JAMA 2011;306(2):200–1.
43. Butler D. Tensions linger over discovery of coronavirus. Nature News, <http://www.nature.com/news/tensions-linger-over-discovery-of-coronavirus-1.12108/>; 2013.
44. Kupferschmidt K. As outbreak continues, confusion reigns over virus patents. Science Insider, <http://news.sciencemag.org/people-events/2013/05/outbreak-continues-confusion-reigns-over-virus-patents/>; 2013.
45. Fidler DP. Who owns MERS? The intellectual property controversy surrounding the latest pandemic, <https://www.foreignaffairs.com/articles/saudi-arabia/2013-06-06/who-owns-mers>; 2013.
46. World Health Organization. H5N1 avian influenza: timeline of major events. 2012.
47. Taubenberger JK, Morens DM. 1918 influenza: the mother of all pandemics. Emerg infect dis 2006;12(1):15–22.
48. Enserink M. Virology. Tiptoeing around Pandora's Box. Science 2004;305(5684):594–5.
49. Katz R, Fischer J. The revised international health regulations: a framework for global pandemic response. Glob Health Govern 2010;3(2):1–18.
50. Gronvall G. H5N1: a case study for dual-use research. New York: Council on Foreign Relations Press, <http://www.cfr.org/public-health-threats-and-pandemics/h5n1-case-study-dual-use-research/p30711/>; 2013.
51. Kawaoka Y. H5N1: flu transmission work is urgent. Nature 2012;482(7384):155.
52. Office of Science and Technology Policy. United States Government Policy for institutional oversight of life sciences dual use research of concern. Federal Register, <https://federalregister.gov/a/2013-04127/>; 2013. p. 12369–72.
53. Zhang Y, Zhang Q, Kong H, Jiang Y, Gao Y, Deng G, et al. H5N1 hybrid viruses bearing 2009/H1N1 virus genes transmit in guinea pigs by respiratory droplet. Science 2013;340(6139):1459–63.
54. Wade N. Synthetic bacterial genome takes over a cell, researchers report. New York Times; May 20, 2010.
55. Bagley MA, Rai AK. The Nagoya Protocol and Synthetic Biology Research: a look at the potential impacts. Synthetic Biology Project at the Wilson Center. Wilson Center, <http://www.synbioproject.org/process/assets/files/6672/_draft/nagoya_final.pdf/>; 2013.

3 SECTION

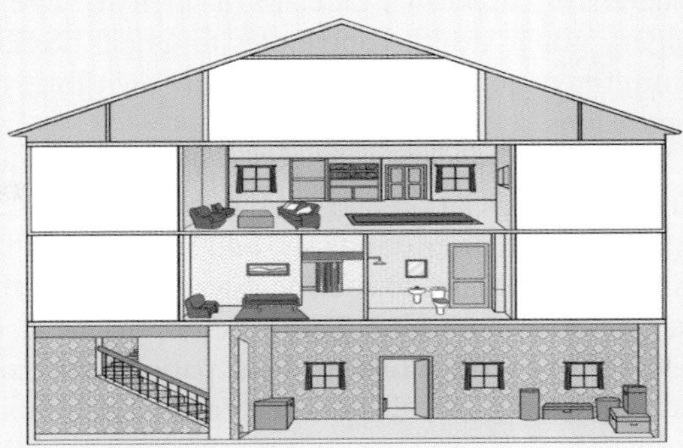

Collaboration Fuels Transformation

Stacy Okutani

Section Outline

Collaboration is integral to twenty-first century Public Health Surveillance Strengthening (PHSS) as new technologies and data sources enable new insights and knowledge about disease emergence and transmission. These collaborations can transform global PHS. Partnerships and networks provide contextual knowledge and expertise, sustain interest, and support the rapid sharing of information and best practices. Much of what public health requires to develop into a dynamic and forward-leaning practice depends on engaging with new groups and deepening established relationships. Understanding how these enriched collaborations are beginning to enhance PHS is a first step toward making new types of collaborations standard practice for PHS.

Developing new collaborations with the military, clinical practice, societies, communities, and experts outside the traditional realm of human and public health will contribute to a revitalized and strengthened system for PHS. This section explores collaborations within each of these areas. The first chapter explores the concept of One Health, describing the importance of a sustained investment in understanding the human–animal–environment interfaces. The authors are deeply engaged in implementing this approach and discuss both the challenges to achieving this vision and opportunities to build upon developing efforts. The next chapter provides a vision for how biosurveillance can be achieved through global collaborations. The lead author was the Assistant Secretary of Defense for Nuclear, Chemical, and Biological Defense. This theme of military contributions is further explored in

Chapter 16. The former Director of the Armed Forces Health Surveillance Center describes the many ways in which military public health contributes to global health security. The US Department of Defense has a long history of commitment to the health of both its own forces and improvements in the health and capabilities of the world's populations.

The chapter on nonprofit associations directly addresses the essential role that associations play in the PHS enterprise. Associations serve as important advocates for PHS both within countries and globally while building capacity, developing standards, and improving the public health workforce. Next, the focus of the section moves from the global level to specific ways that the public health and clinical medicine sectors can mutually benefit from increased collaborations. There are important factors that make collaboration difficult, but more important ones yield improved outcomes for both patients and communities. The final chapter in this section explores the variety and importance of collaborations at the community level. The authors describe the significant benefits to public health from reaching out to both new and established communities at the local level to address both routine and novel outbreaks.

The types of engagements described in this section contribute to the transformation of PHS just as collaboration enhances the renovation of a home in a historic district. Many communities must be engaged in order to achieve an outcome that is in harmony with all stakeholders and serves their needs. Through collaborations, the home acquires welcoming spaces, such as a porch, and doors and windows to allow for movement and greater transparency.

LEARNING OBJECTIVES

- Define the One Health approach and its importance to the future of PHS.
- Identify the current efforts and systems that are using the One Health approach.
- List examples demonstrating the intersection between human health, animal health, and environmental health.
- Define biosurveillance and how it supports and differs from PHS.
- Describe the DOD's future vision for biosurveillance and how they plan to achieve this vision.
- Describe the role that military can and has played in public health.
- Identify the US DoD's current initiatives to improve collaboration and information sharing
- Explain the role and importance of associations in PHS.
- List different types of associations.
- Describe the importance of clinicians and clinical facilities to PHS.
- Define the differing priorities that often exist between clinicians or clinical facilities and public health units, and how these differing priorities can present challenges to achieving optimum PHS data.
- Describe possible actions that can be used to enhance the relationship between clinical medicine and public health practitioners to strengthen PHS.
- Recognize the importance and benefits of engaging communities in public health surveillance.

CHAPTER 14

One Health in the Twenty-first Century

Jonna AK Mazet, Haley McDermott, Tracey Goldstein

Limit your life to concentration on the self and your world will only be small. Embrace interconnectedness and unity and the world becomes endlessly full of possibilities.

AC Ping

KEY WORDS

One Health
Interspecies transmission
Field sampling
Diagnostic testing
Information management
MBDS (Mekong Basin Diseases Surveillance)
Emerging Pandemic Threats Program
OFFLU (OIE/FAO Network of Expertise on Animal Influenza)
FoodNet Canada (formerly, C-EnterNet)
CIPARS (The Canadian Integrated Program for Antimicrobial Resistance Surveillance)
Canary Database

THE ONE HEALTH PERSPECTIVE ON GLOBAL PROBLEM SOLVING AND PUBLIC HEALTH SURVEILLANCE

Though the threat of zoonoses to human health has long been understood, the call to action for public health practitioners has never been more imperative. Over 60% of human infectious diseases are shared with animals,[1] and most global pandemics including HIV/AIDS, severe acute respiratory syndrome (SARS), and pandemic influenzas are triggered by viral pathogens originating from wildlife.[1,2] The costs of these pandemic pathogens are often catastrophic, involving not only treatment and control costs but also detriments to trade and travel.[1] As public health practitioners, it is therefore crucial that we recognize the threat of zoonotic pathogens to public health and work to understand the drivers that influence their global emergence and resurgence.

In light of recent scientific discoveries highlighting the human–animal–environment interface and its role in pandemics, the need for adequate disease surveillance, prevention strategies, and outbreak protocols that incorporate these ideas are as pressing as ever. In just the past 2 years, both avian influenza strain H7N9[3] and the suspected zoonosis Middle East Respiratory Syndrome Coronavirus (MERS-CoV)[4] (see case studies*) have been identified as novel pathogens posing a serious threat to human health. Simultaneously, researchers have provided evidence for cross species transmission and movement of the 2009 pandemic influenza virus H1N1[5] in wildlife, and have identified the Chinese horseshoe bat as a likely reservoir of the 2002–2003 pandemic virus SARS-CoV.[6] While animals are an important component of the transmission pathway, a zoonosis' pandemic potential is equally impacted by its surrounding environment.[7] Ecological changes related to anthropogenic practices, social conditions, and human behaviors are often the primary reasons that pathogens undergo changes in transmission patterns that alter pathogenicity. Additionally, while studies have shown that a primary driver of pathogen introduction is an accelerating

*Available at http://booksite.elsevier.com/9780702063374/

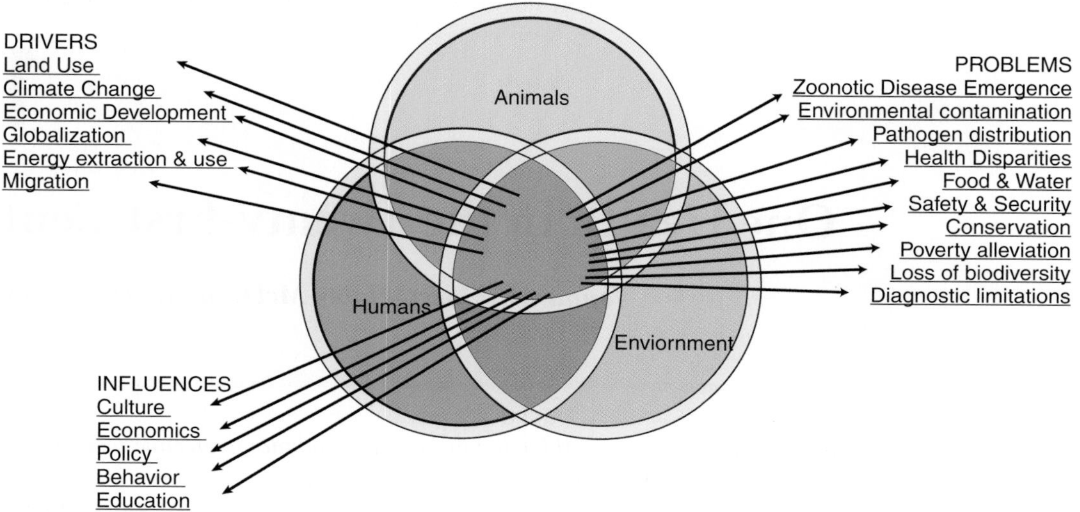

FIG. 14-1 Utilizing the One Health approach to address drivers, influences, and problems arising at the human–animal–environment interface. One Health is not a new discipline, but rather an approach recognizing the inextricable connection between human, animal, and environmental health and its role in the prevention, detection, and response to important problems of global health concern. As shown here, these problems occur at the human–animal–environment interface and are influenced and driven by anthropogenic practices, social conditions, and human behaviors that are likely only to be exacerbated as the human population continues to increase. The success of the One Health approach hinges on its central tenet that we must work in interdisciplinary teams—breaking silos and joining sectors for improved knowledge, understanding, and innovation. Illustration credit: M. Blake

increase in trade and travel, other drivers including intensive agricultural practices, antimicrobial drug resistance, land use change, and extraction industries are equally important for pathogen alteration or emergence.[7] Alarmingly, with a human population predicted at 9 billion by 2050, these conditions driving pathogen emergence or outbreaks are likely to be exacerbated.[1]

The message is clear. The health of the organisms around us and that of our supporting environment are directly connected to the health of people worldwide. We must consider these axioms in order to improve the surveillance, detection, control, and prevention of emerging and re-emerging global pathogens. The concept of One Health represents the application of these ideas put into the context of public health practice. As depicted in Fig. 14-1, One Health is not a unique discipline, but rather an approach recognizing the inextricable connection between human, animal, and environmental health to prevent the emergence and spread of both novel and re-emerging global pathogens. The success of the One Health approach hinges on its central tenet that we must work in interdisciplinary teams—breaking silos and joining sectors for improved knowledge, understanding, and innovation. In combination with scientific and technological advances, the concept of One Health represents an important opportunity to improve public health surveillance worldwide.

ONE HEALTH IN PRACTICE: GOALS, BENEFITS, AND CHALLENGES

The overarching goals of One Health in the public health surveillance arena are to bring together knowledgeable and empowered stakeholders to utilize necessary information and technology, fill gaps in established surveillance systems (human and animal), make information accessible for all users, and provide ground-truthed data to jurisdictional authorities for improved health surveillance and implementable policy development. Unfortunately, despite growing acknowledgement of the utility of the approach and the ample areas that could be improved through effective collaborations and inclusion of additional disciplines, the acceptance of One Health by policy makers at the highest levels of international governance is not often translating to on the ground implementation. Successful One Health application requires the cooperation of experts from numerous disciplines, including but not limited to human medicine, veterinary medicine, public health, environmental science, ecology, conservation biology, nursing, social sciences, the humanities, engineering, economics, education, and public policy, all of which are active forces in the ministries and other essential elements of civil society, also represented by NGOs, academic institutions, and communities. Unfortunately, these disciplines and sectors seldom act in cooperation, a strategy that is essential to improving surveillance and global problem solving through One Health.

When applied successfully, the One Health approach can be used most effectively to bring essential stakeholders together to solve complex health problems, especially those that involve multisectoral influences or that require input and acceptance from those invested on different sides of social, political, economic, or disciplinary boundaries, such as zoonoses. The key to modern health problem solving is the fostering of effective partnerships and collaborations at these local, national, regional, and global levels, especially considering the challenges of infectious disease surveillance. A historical lack of collaboration among ministries and across jurisdictional authorities has severely limited the identification of solutions to global health problems, like emerging infectious coronaviruses, including those responsible for SARS and MERS, as well as the implementation of effective surveillance and interventions. However, with energized international policy support for One Health and with the World Health Organization (WHO), the Food and Agriculture Organization (FAO), and the World Organization for Animal Health's (OIE) commitment to multilateral engagement and joint programs for surveillance and public health solution development, an integrated approach to human, animal, and ecosystem health has begun to be implemented and is driving a rational approach to global health that will likely improve the prediction, prevention, recognition, and response to diseases.

Though replete with opportunity, the One Health approach is not without its challenges and limitations. Still lacking is awareness of the role that environmental influences play in the transmission and propagation of diseases. Unfortunately, this lack of awareness is compounded by the fact that critical natural resource management agencies are often underfunded and slow to be invited to or to join surveillance activities due to perceived mission conflicts and competing priorities. Additionally, One Health research and surveillance projects and interventions are limited because of unwillingness of traditional funders to redirect resources across sectors and expand out of siloed missions. Other challenges are poor coordination among stakeholders; lack of policy and legal framework for One Health; unwillingness to share data; inadequate human resources and laboratory capacity; and continuing weak representation and engagement of stakeholders from the ecosystem/environment sector.[8]

ONE HEALTH IN ACTION: REGIONAL AND GLOBAL UTILIZATION OF THE CONCEPT

Despite the aforementioned challenges, excellent examples of One Health-oriented surveillance efforts highlight the perspective and its use in public health. For example, the 12-year-old **Mekong Basin Diseases Surveillance** (MBDS) network is a cross-border collaboration including Cambodia, China, Myanmar, Lao PDR, Thailand, and Vietnam, that has been attempting to combat and control outbreaks of disease through collaborative regional surveillance, reporting, joint outbreak investigation, and capacity building since 2001(through initial support from the Rockefeller Foundation).[9, 10] Similarly, there are focal disease surveillance projects, such as the Health for Animals and Livelihood Improvement (HALI) Project exploring disease transmission and control, especially tuberculosis and brucellosis, at the human–animal–environment interface in rural Tanzania.[11] Additional examples, including The United States Agency for International Development's (USAID) **Emerging Pandemic Threats Program**[12] (EPT) and the WHO, OIE, and FAO's collaborative global early warning system for animal diseases transmissible to humans (GLEWS) clearly exemplify the One Health approach and how it is being utilized to strengthen disease detection and preparedness programs both regionally and internationally.

USAID's EPT was created in 2009 in an effort to respond to the growing need for improved detection, identification, and response for emerging zoonoses.[12,13] The EPT 1 program consists of four overall projects: PREDICT, RESPOND,

IDENTIFY, and PREVENT, and also includes the Center for Disease Control (CDC), all working in concert to build local, regional, and national One Health capacity for disease detection, diagnosis, risk reduction, and response.[12-14] Utilizing a true One Health approach to public health surveillance, PREDICT partners University of California Davis, EcoHealth Alliance, Metabiota, Smithsonian Institution, and Wildlife Conservation Society with support from Columbia and Harvard Universities,[15] focus on the discovery and detection of zoonoses at the wildlife–human interface, strengthening laboratory and surveillance capacity, and monitoring human–wildlife interactions for emerging, re-emerging, or novel pathogens posing a substantial public health threat.[14,15] PREDICT partners also work to define ecological drivers of disease spillover to humans and to improve models for predicting global zoonotic disease emergence. Through coordination with 59 ministries in 20 countries, PREDICT has built capacity for diagnostic testing in 33 laboratories and is working toward sustainable improvements in a total of 35 laboratories. They have optimized surveillance and response by standardizing animal sampling protocols, improving cold chain access, responding to deadly outbreaks with animal and environmental best practices, and identifying an efficient diagnostic paradigm for diseases of unknown origin. In total, PREDICT has trained over 2500 people worldwide, sampled over 50,000 animals, and discovered almost 1000 viruses in genera or families known to cause epidemics.[15,16]

On a global level, the need for increased understanding of disease ecology and epidemiology among animals and people motivated the creation of a One Health surveillance partnership among the WHO, OIE, and FAO. Together, the group has been working since 2006 on the One Health inspired early warning system, GLEWS.[17] The overall objective of GLEWS is to improve early warning capacity for animal disease threats for the benefit of the international community.[18] This aim is accomplished by combining and coordinating the intelligence mechanisms of the three organizations through sharing of information, risk assessment strategy, and epidemiological analysis.[18] Among many shared activities, agencies participate in thematic and working group meetings, collaborate on normally exclusive research and regulatory work, and coordinate disease alert and response mechanisms, avoiding duplication and enhancing verification of pathogen threats.[18] Largely due to the One Health approach taken by GLEWS, each of the tripartite organizations has been able to participate in the building of newly developed programs and systems that support the prevention and prediction of zoonotic and other high impact diseases originating at the human–animal–environment interface. The World Animal Health Information System and Database (WAHIS and WAHID) created by the OIE, the global food safety and alert system (INFOSAN) created by WHO and FAO, and the network of expertise on animal influenza (OFFLU) developed by FAO and OIE are just a few of the examples of programs that now benefit from free-flowing information exchange and collaboration within GLEWS.[19] **OFFLU** is the OIE-FAO global network of expertise on animal influenza that works to reduce the negative impacts of animal influenza viruses by promoting effective collaboration between animal health and human health experts.[20] Moving forward, GLEWS aims for better coordination of fragmented surveillance efforts and more connections between expert institutions and organizations for improved diagnostics, data analysis, risk assessment, epidemiology, social science, and communication.[19]

The above uses of the One Health approach in public health surveillance are just a portion of those in existence. As the recognition of animals and the environment as significant contributors to human health continues to grow, numerous surveillance tools modeled on One Health have been created, including the International society for Infectious Diseases' ProMED-mail (PMM), the Public Health Agency and Government of Canada's FoodNet Canada (formerly known as C-EnterNet) and CIPARS programs, Boston Children's Hospital's HealthMap, and the Yale University's Canary Database to name a few.[17] **Foodnet** (formerly known as C-EnterNet) is a program developed to improve Canada's food safety surveillance. It is composed of three food safety surveillance sites that collects detailed information about food-borne illness in Canadians and traces those illnesses back to their sources in food, water, or animals.[21] **CIPARS** is the Canadian Integrated Program for Antimicrobial Resistance Surveillance. It monitors trends in antimicrobial use and antimicrobial resistance in selected bacterial organisms from human, animal, and food sources across Canada.[22] The **Canary Database** was developed by Yale University (Occupational and Environmental Medicine, School of Medicine) that selects, curates, and indexes thousands of scientific studies from MEDLINE, CAB Abstracts, and Agricola to collate the evidence for animals as "early warning" sentinels of human health hazards.[23]

To exemplify the opportunity that these One Health surveillance tools present for the detection, identification, and response to emerging zoonoses, we may turn to a pathogen with both zoonotic significance and pandemic potential, influenza A.

UNDERSTANDING THE ONE HEALTH PERSPECTIVE: THE RISK OF INTERSPECIES TRANSMISSION OF INFLUENZA A (H1N1, H3N8) AMONG SEALS, BIRDS, AND HUMANS

Interspecies transmission of influenza A is an important factor in the evolution and ecology of influenza viruses. **Interspecies transmission** is the transmission occurring between species.[24] Marine mammals are in contact with a number of influenza reservoirs, including aquatic birds and humans, and this may facilitate transmission among avian and mammalian hosts.[5] The emergence of new strains of influenza virus is always of great public concern, especially when the infection of a new mammalian host has the potential to result in a widespread outbreak of disease.[25] Thus, multiple host species must be considered when evaluating the risks for viral transmission and potential for viral recombination.

Previously, there has been documentation of interspecies transmission of influenza A between birds and marine mammals, as well as between seals and people. Avian origin isolates H4N5 and H3N8 have been found in harbor seals dying with pneumonia, and H7N7 transmission has been documented in humans following exposure to infected seals dying of respiratory disease.[26-28] When at sea, seals spend much of their time feeding off the coast or concentrated in regions off the continental shelf, which are highly productive areas where many marine species and fisheries converge.[29,30] Thus, there is ample opportunity for exposure to and transmission of viruses through contact with other marine species thought to be reservoirs for influenza viruses such as aquatic birds, and through environmental exposures such as feces discharged from shipping vessels at sea.[31,32] Recently, two new examples have highlighted the continued occurrence of such events and the critical need for holistic approaches that incorporate the risk factors and mechanisms at play leading to them. In 2009, a new strain of H1N1 re-emerged in people resulting in the first influenza pandemic of the twenty-first century, as declared by the WHO. This virus was thought to be a mutation of four known strains of influenza A subtype H1N1; one endemic in humans, one endemic in birds, and two endemic in pigs.[33]

In 2010, exposure to pandemic H1N1 influenza virus (pH1N1) occurred among free-ranging Northern Elephant Seals after the animals had returned to the central Californian coast from their short postbreeding migration in the northeast Pacific.[5] Sequencing revealed greater than 99% homology with influenza strain A/California/04/2009 (H1N1) that emerged in humans and swine in 2009, and serology indicated that exposure was widespread in elephant seals along the Californian coast. Furthermore, mutations indicated that the virus had only recently become a seal-adapted virus; thus, in a short time the virus acquired adaptive mutations that allowed for replication and transmission in the elephant seal population while reducing replication fitness in human epithelial respiratory cells, illustrating the readily adaptive ability of these viruses. Then, more recently in 2011, more than 150 harbor seals off the US Coast in New England died during an outbreak of pneumonia. Analysis revealed the presence of an avian H3N8 influenza A virus similar to the one that had been circulating in North American waterfowl since 2002.[25] The virus not only had mutations that indicated recent adaption to mammalian hosts but also had the potential ability to replicate in multiple mammalian hosts, including in humans. Thus, as indicated in Fig. 14-2, the virus was able to increase its spread not only geographically between land and sea but also between species.

In 2010, exposure to pH1N1 was found to have occurred among free-ranging northern elephant seals after the animals had returned to the central Californian coast from their short postbreeding migration in the northeast Pacific. As shown in Fig. 14-2, subsequent analysis and sequencing revealed that the virus was able to adapt for replication and transmission in a new mammalian host. Given that direct contact between humans and elephant seals is unlikely in the remote region while at sea, it may be possible that exposure occurred through contact with aquatic avian hosts, thus expanding its geographical pathogenicity by cycling among mammalian, avian, and human hosts both at sea and on land.

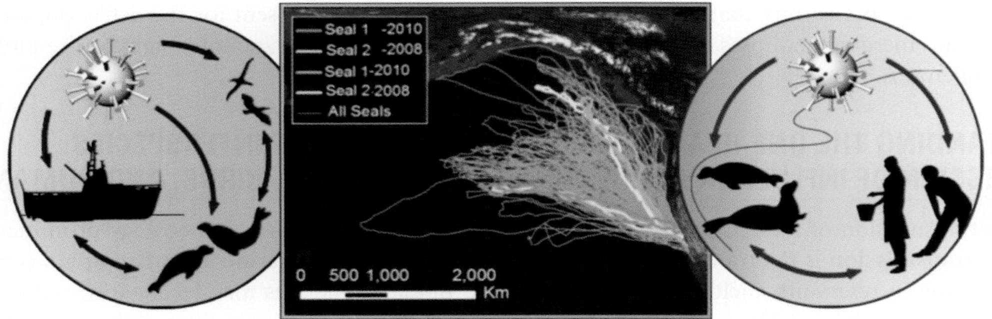

FIG. 14-2 A visual representation of the geographical and interspecies spread of the pathogen influenza A. In 2010, exposure to pandemic H1N1 influenza virus (pH1N1) was found to have occurred among free-ranging Northern Elephant Seals after the animals had returned to the central Californian coast from their short postbreeding migration in the northeast Pacific. Subsequent analysis and sequencing revealed that the virus was able to adapt for replication and transmission in a new mammalian host. Given that direct contact between humans and elephant seals is unlikely in the remote region while at sea, it may be possible that exposure occurred through contact with aquatic avian hosts, thus expanding its host species range by cycling among mammalian, avian, and human hosts both at sea and on land. *Source:* Mazet J, H McDermott, T Goldstein. In Press. One Health in the 21st century. In: Transforming Public Health Surveillance. Elsevier.

Both the documented outbreak of H3N8 in harbor seals and infection with pH1N1 in elephant seals are particularly significant because in both examples the viruses had naturally acquired mutations that are known to increase transmissibility and virulence in mammals. Additionally, in the case of the pH1N1 in elephant seals, none of the animals that were handled on the beach or that died in the rehabilitation hospital appeared to be ill, instead it seemed that the infection was asymptomatic and the disease self-limiting. Therefore, although seals may be infected with zoonotic pathogens that provide no clinical signs of illness, the risk to people cannot be ignored. This work highlights the need for additional surveillance and biosafety measures, not only to monitor and prevent disease exposure for people working with and around animals but also to prevent those very people from transmitting diseases to susceptible animals. Only with the One Health approach can we utilize these factors at the human–animal–environment interface to facilitate our understanding of both epizootic and zoonotic global disease emergence and respond accordingly with appropriate public health surveillance and response protocols.

PRACTICAL CONSIDERATIONS IN ONE HEALTH: BUILDING A SUCCESSFUL PROGRAM

Thus far, we have discussed the benefits and challenges of the One Health approach, and have shown examples of how it is being utilized to strengthen public health surveillance worldwide. However, in order to build a successful One Health program, there are several practical components that one must first consider. Among others, this includes how to build a functional team; how to construct an appropriate response; and how to design protocols for sampling, testing, and information management appropriate for the surveillance situation at hand. It is the careful consideration of these factors, along with a constant focus on collaboration that moves the One Health concept from an important philosophy to a useful approach.

Building a Functional Team

The first step in addressing the obstacles blocking the implementation of One Health surveillance is to become less focused on these challenges and more concerned with bringing together a team for active problem solving, in other words, getting the job done. Clearly, identifying the problem or issue for which you need a more effective surveillance approach is the key; for example, how to identify an unknown host for an emerging pathogen such as MERS-CoV. Developing an effective team in this context includes identifying the stakeholders who have the mandate to get the work initiated and to engage the disciplines that will be required to efficiently design and successfully implement the activity. Also important at this early stage is the structure of the collaborative framework through which those involved will engage. During an epidemic emergency response that structure will likely be more top-down driven with a well-defined chain of command. This phase is generally organized and led by a government agency or task force or is delegated to an international authority. However, once the initial emergency has been abated, this operational framework may change and become more flexible, allowing the inclusion of additional expert inputs as needed. Excellent communications and clear expectations on the frequency and content of information sharing are essential at all stages. In the MERS-CoV example, the critical emergency response would likely be led by a Ministry of Health, as the presenting cases have been in people, but that Ministry would also likely engage the other important ministries, for example, tourism, trade, agriculture, and the environment, as well as international response organizations and experts from multiple intersecting disciplines, including epidemiology, medicine, public health, veterinary medicine, molecular biology, virology, ecology, economics, and social science.

Constructing an Appropriate Response

Once the team has been constructed and the modes and frequency of communication and oversight have been put into place, the approach must be designed based on the best available data. In some circumstances, there are adequate statistics on which to base choices for the number and types of surveillance targets and the distribution of sampling, such as for seasonal human influenza surveillance. In other scenarios, such as identifying and monitoring for pandemic pathogen emergence, the data are limited and speculative. In this case, forecasting with mathematical models is necessary, using the best available historical data on pathogen emergence, as well as current information on demographic, commercial, and environmental factors that could be evolving and influencing emergence. These models can be used to initially target surveillance geographically and demographically, and for high-risk groups that may practice specific behaviors increasing their contact with potential pathogens.

The surveillance program then should be tailored most specifically to the job at hand, while considering the human–animal–environment connections relevant for disease transmission. Sample size targets may be difficult to establish, given the uncertainty inherent in problems that lend themselves to the One Health approach. However, estimates of pathogen diversity and prevalence should be used to make the most scientifically rigorous sampling plan.[25] Targeting of sampling at interfaces where people and animals come together in environments conducive for pathogen transmission may be the most efficient.[2] For example, the HALI Project mentioned above focuses sampling at locations where livestock, wildlife, and people come together to share dwindling water sources and the pathogens present therein.[11] Once targeted with the best available data, sampling should then proceed, optimally with results fueling improved forecasting models to direct the ongoing surveillance. Of course, excellent laboratory capacity is required for quality data and may not be available in all areas where sampling will occur. Therefore, successful surveillance programs often must invest in laboratory improvements and effective networking to assure consistency of methods for comparable data. Data analysis plans must also be anticipated in advance to allow for the most appropriate design. Good preparation in the design of the surveillance approach will allow the best development of data management and the most successful outcomes.

Designing One Health Protocols: Field Sampling

Field sampling is the collection of human, animal, and ecologic samples and data at predetermined times.[24] Coordination of data and sample collection for all aspects of the project jointly is key, including human, animal, and ecologic variables and samples collected at the same site and at the same time. Targeted sampling locations should be based on on-the-ground knowledge and the ability to do tandem sampling at critical places where contact between humans and animals is the most intimate and environmental factors facilitate transmission in order to best obtain comparable data across the groups. Depending on the question at hand, the animals to be included in the study may be domestic species, wildlife species, or both. It is important to perform a site characterization or assessment to collect data on environmental variables at the same time when collecting the human and animal samples. Ideally the sampling design will include longitudinal sampling, repeated at each site during each season (fall, winter, spring, and summer or wet and dry depending on location of study and what is appropriate). The field team should include animal health and medical professionals, as well as field biologists to ensure the needed expertise is available to collect samples for all aspects (e.g., appropriate personnel to capture, anesthetize, and sample animals; clearance and experience to collect samples from humans; and the ability to accurately collect environmental data). The sampling design should be adaptive to be able to address problems that may arise such as the number of days spent at each site if not enough animals are captured (wildlife, domestic animals) or humans are not available for testing (when enrolling patients into a study at a clinic or hospital). The sampling process should also be iterative. Whereas the project may start with field studies and surveillance, it should be flexible enough to change once laboratory testing and diagnostic feedback to better target and inform surveillance.

Designing One Health Protocol: Diagnostic Testing

Diagnostic testing is any type of laboratory test that is performed to aid in the diagnosis or detection of disease.[24] An additional component that is key to the One Health strategy is testing of targeted, clinically relevant samples based on the close contact between the human and animal groups, the potential route(s) of exposure of the pathogen, and the environmental circumstances that may promote disease. The challenge in such a One Health project is to develop and implement a framework for diagnostics that can be used across host species to detect known, new, and emerging pathogens or health threats. Currently, most projects focus on traditional testing, which generally incorporates the detection of one or more specific pathogen that is/are often specific to a certain host. Thus, it is often difficult to obtain data that can be comparable across host species, as different testing methods and assays are used to test samples from each. Because One Health projects include examining samples from varied species, often for which there are a lack of reagents or established diagnostic tests, a shift in the diagnostic methodology is needed to incorporate a more widely applicable strategy. Broadly reactive consensus polymerase chain reaction (cPCR) assays that target a family of pathogens, rather than a specific species or strain, have been used extensively in research laboratories to detect and characterize novel pathogens.[34,35] This type of tactic represents a potentially powerful change in the approach with the ability to produce specific, high-resolution data when casting a wide net for potential pathogens. More general tools, like family-level PCR, could allow for quicker detection of both known and new pathogens for all host species, as the strategy depends on focusing on detecting a pathogen group and is not dependent on the sample type virus or host. Employing these types of methods in both human and animal health laboratories on samples from all host species could lead to a more sustainable approach to discovery of new and shared pathogens and diagnosis of mystery illnesses affecting multiple hosts.

Designing One Health Protocols: Information Management

Information management is the entry of data and management of information from one or more sources and the distribution of that information to one or more audiences.[24] The ability to store and access accurate and comprehensive data is critical for a One Health project, and the key to success is the need to use or develop a searchable and queryable database that holds information for all human, animal, and environmental project data in a single platform. Thus, the information management platform must be able to store and integrate field, surveillance, and diagnostic data. Levels of security must be assigned to all project personnel so that data accessibility can be managed and limited as needed, and keep human identifying information separate and secure to comply with Health Information Privacy (HIPAA) rules.[36] The system must also facilitate timely sharing of data and results as appropriate. Information needs to flow from and between the field and the laboratory with standard fields linking data, individuals, and sites used by all team members. The importance of a strong database development team with expertise in database structure and familiarity with the data that are collected is essential. This team must be able to rapidly address data needs, changes, reorganizations, and problems as they arise and on an ongoing basis for the success of the project. Additionally, identifying a data quality manager with knowledge of health, biology, and diagnostic data is an important component of the information management team. Frequent communication is necessary between database managers and users to ensure accurate entry and extraction of data if possible. Finally, a platform should be chosen that allows for efficient online data entry and updates with a feature to temporarily "hold" data until the quality and completeness can be assessed. The platform should also be presented in a user-friendly interface, with the ability to expand function and size (memory, server size, software) to address projects needs and expansion over time, and it should be able to interface with statistical software packages so that frequent data queries and extracts are possible for analyses.

CREATING A ONE HEALTH WORKFORCE: NEEDS AND OPPORTUNITIES

It is indisputable that no single discipline, organization, or sector has the knowledge, expertise, or resources to combat the emergence or resurgence of global zoonotic pathogens in the manner outlined above. In the twenty-first century, just as we have learned that disease does not distinguish between the boundaries of nations or species, we have also learned that it does not adhere to the artificial boundaries that exist between disciplines or sectors.[37] Still, working across these long-standing partitions requires a great breadth of skill that is often not inherent nor taught in traditional educational programs. Thus, the need for this type of approach in surveillance also underscores the need for a public health workforce trained in One Health ideals and practices.

For these reasons, it is imperative that we begin to build capacity for One Health skill sets in the form of new workshops, curricular content, and educational programs. Simultaneously, we must provide built-in incentives that reward multidisciplinary and collaborative work. Having such systems in place would pave the way for truly paradigm shifting One Health approaches, like the appointment of novel "One Health practitioners" with the training and capacity to see through disciplinary confines and facilitate global health problem solving. Though important, this vision will require the time, effort, and resources of many. During the current interval, individuals can obtain further training in One Health specific job functions that will facilitate their ability to become an integral member of a One Health team. Though the approach may be limited by difficult system-wide constraints, a commitment to collaboration and a willingness to strengthen competencies[38-40] will provide the public health professional with the means to utilize the One Health approach within public health surveillance worldwide.

KEY SUMMARY POINTS

- In light of recent scientific discoveries and intensifying environmental drivers, it is crucial that public health practitioners recognize the threat of zoonotic pathogens to public health and work to understand the drivers and dynamics that influence their global emergence and resurgence.
- The concept of One Health represents an approach to zoonotic pathogen detection, prevention, and control, utilizing the interconnectivity of animals, humans, and their surrounding environment alongside interdisciplinary and intersectoral collaboration to improve public health surveillance worldwide.
- When successful, the One Health approach can bring stakeholders together to solve complex health problems, but these benefits are challenged by a deficiency in environmental expertise, an unwillingness of funders to reallocate resources across sectors, inadequate human resources and laboratory capacity, and poor coordination across stakeholders.
- Despite its challenges, USAID's EPT program and the WHO, FAO, and OIE collaborative early warning system GLEWS represent excellent examples of the One Health approach and its utilization in surveillance, both regionally and internationally.
- The relevance of One Health surveillance is clearly demonstrated by recent discoveries of interspecies transmission of Influenza A (H1N1, H3N8) among seals, birds, and humans along the Californian coast.
- In order to move the One Health concept from an important philosophy to a useful approach, careful consideration should be given to team selection; appropriate response design; and development of sampling, testing, and information management protocols.
- The One Health concept requires a breadth of skill that is often not inherent nor taught in traditional education programs. Thus, the increasing utilization of the approach in surveillance underscores the need for educational capacity building, paradigm shifting job creation, and individual training that support a competent One Health workforce.

DISCUSSION QUESTIONS

1. In light of recent scientific discoveries and intensifying environmental drivers, it is crucial that public health practitioners recognize the threat of zoonotic pathogens to public health and work to understand the drivers and dynamics that influence their global emergence and resurgence.
   a. Given the gravity of the threat of zoonotic pathogens to human health, list some ways that we might significantly increase the understanding and skill set of One Health among public health practitioners. Can you think of an example outside of those detailed in this chapter when a new idea and/or skillset needed to be distributed both quickly and comprehensively within a field or workforce? How did they do it?
2. The concept of One Health represents an approach to zoonotic pathogen detection, prevention, and control, utilizing the interconnectivity of animals, humans, and their surrounding environment alongside interdisciplinary and intersectoral collaboration to improve public health surveillance worldwide.
   a. Both interdisciplinary and intersectoral collaboration are widely recognized as vital for innovation and successful application of ideas, but are often met with opposition. What are some reasons for the opposition faced at both the discipline and sector levels, and how might these barriers be addressed?
3. When successful, the One Health approach can bring stakeholders together to solve complex health problems, but these benefits are challenged by a deficiency in environmental expertise, an unwillingness of funders to reallocate resources across sectors, inadequate human resources and laboratory capacity, and poor coordination across stakeholders.
   a. Given its fundamental place in the One Health approach, why do you think that environmental expertise is consistently deficient from the discussion? Aside from the One Health approach, is this deficiency found in other areas of public health? If so, how has this been addressed?
4. Despite its challenges, USAID's EPT program and the WHO, FAO, and OIE collaborative early warning system GLEWS represent excellent examples of the One Health approach and its utilization in surveillance both regionally and internationally.
   a. While it may seem inherent that collaboration is imperative to comprehensive surveillance, what can we measure to show meaningful impact? What can't we measure? How can we define the costs and benefits of a One Health approach?
5. The relevance of One Health surveillance is clearly demonstrated by recent discoveries of interspecies transmission of Influenza A (H1N1, H3N8) among seals, birds, and humans along the Californian coast.
   a. What type of additional surveillance and biosafety measures are needed, not only to monitor and prevent disease exposure for people working with and around animals, but also to prevent those very people from transmitting diseases to susceptible animals? What stakeholders would support these types of reforms? Who might oppose them?
6. In order to move the One Health concept from an important philosophy to a useful approach, careful consideration should be given to team selection; appropriate response design; and development of sampling, testing, and information management protocols.
   a. Identify a public health issue that might benefit from a One Health approach. How would you develop a team to address it?
   b. What other considerations are relevant to moving the One Health concept from philosophy to approach? How does the perception of One Health by the general public factor into this movement? How should One Health be presented to the general public? What unintended consequences may arise from a poorly crafted message?
7. The One Health concept requires a breadth of skill that is often not inherent nor taught in traditional education programs. Thus, the increasing utilization of the approach in surveillance underscores the need for educational capacity building, paradigm shifting job creation, and individual training that support a competent One Health workforce.
   a. When building education capacity for a new approach to global health issues, how do you go about defining a set of universally agreed upon competencies? How do you promote marketability for this skill set?

b. In rural communities both in the USA and abroad, a lack of financial resources for multiple specialized health providers has highlighted the potential of paraprofessionals who are trained in the One Health approach to provide health deliver support in human, environmental, and animal medicine. How would you define the scope of work for this type of professional? How might this type professional best be trained? What are the potential limitations of this approach?

REFERENCES

1. Karesh WB, Dobson A, Lloyd-Smith JO, Lubroth J, Dixon MA, Bennett M, et al. Ecology of zoonoses: natural and unnatural histories. Lancet 2012;380(9857):1936–45.
2. Morse SS, Mazet JA, Woolhouse M, Parrish CR, Carroll D, Karesh WB, et al. Prediction and prevention of the next pandemic zoonosis. Lancet 2012;380(9857):1956–65.
3. Investigation E. Emergence of avian influenza A (H7N9) virus causing severe human illness—China, February–April 2013. Am J Transplant 2013;13:2216–21.
4. World Health Organization. Middle East respiratory syndrome coronavirus Joint Kingdom of Saudi Arabia/WHO mission Riyadh, 4–9 June 2013. Geneva: WHO; 2013.
5. Goldstein T, Mena I, Anthony SJ, Medina R, Robinson PW, Greig DJ, et al. Pandemic H1N1 Influenza Isolated from free-ranging Northern Elephant Seals in 2010 off the central California coast. PloS one 2013;8(5):e62259.
6. Ge XY, Li JL, Yang XL, Chmura AA, Zhu G, Epstein JH, et al. Isolation and characterization of a bat SARS-like coronavirus that uses the ACE2 receptor. Nature 2013;503:535–8.
7. Kilpatrick AM, Randolph SE. Drivers, dynamics, and control of emerging vector-borne zoonotic diseases. Lancet 2012;380(9857):1946–55.
8. Murray JG, Aviso SM, Karesh W, Machalaba C. Policy opportunities for linking animal and human health. Animal health and biodiversity: preparing for the future. Compendium of the OIE Global Conference on Wildlife, Paris, France, February 23–25, 2011; 2012.
9. Secretariat PMAC. A World United Against Infectious Disease: Cross-sectoral Solutions. Bangkok, Thailand: Prince Mahidol Award Conference 2013; 28 Jan–2 Feb, 2013.
10. Phommasack B, Jiraphongsa C, Ko Oo M, Bond KC, Phaholyothin N, Suphanchaimat R, et al. Mekong Basin Disease Surveillance (MBDS): a trust-based network. Emerg Health Threats J 2013;6. doi.10.3402/ehtj.v3406i3400.19944.
11. Mazet JA, Clifford DL, Coppolillo PB, Deolalikar AB, Erickson JD, Kazwala RR. A "one health" approach to address emerging zoonoses: the HALI project in Tanzania. PLoS Med 2009;6(12):e1000190.
12. Bogich TL, Chunara R, Scales D, Chan E, Pinheiro LC, Chmura AA, et al. Preventing pandemics via international development: a systems approach. PLoS Med 2012;9(12):e1001354.
13. U.S. Agency for International Development. Development UAfI. Emerging Pandemic threats Program Overview. Washington, DC: 2010. www.usaid.gov.
14. Development USAfI. Emerging pandemic threats program: Fact Sheet, <http://www.usaid.gov/news-information/fact-sheets/emerging-pandemic-threats-program/>; 2013.
15. University of California Davis OHI. PREDICT, <http://www.vetmed.ucdavis.edu/ohi/predict/>; 2013. [accessed 2013].
16. Partnership: UP. A briefing on PREDICT: Update on progress through year 3 in building global surveillance to detect and prevent spillover of pathogens of pandemic potential that can move between wildlife and people. Washington, DC: United States Agency for International Development; 2013.
17. Zinsstag J, Schelling E, Bonfoh B, Fooks AR, Kasymbekov J, Waltner-Toews D, et al. Towards a 'One Health' research and application tool box. Vet Ital 2009;45(1):121–33.
18. The FAO OIE WHO. 2011 GLEWS: global early warning and response system for major animal diseases, including zoonoses, <http://www.glews.net/>; January 5, 2011.
19. Collaboration F-O-W. Sharing responsibilities and coordinating global activities to address health risks at the animal-human-ecosystems interfaces. 2010.
20. OFFLU OIE/FAO Network of expertise on animal influenza, <http://www.offlu.net/>; June 6, 2014.
21. FoodNet Canada (formerly known as C-EnterNet): Reducing the burden of gastrointestinal disease in Canada, <http://www.phac-aspc.gc.ca/foodnet-canada/overview-apercu-eng.php/>; 2006. [accessed 2015].
22. Canadian Integrated Program for Antimicrobial Resistance Surveillance (CIPARS), <http://www.phac-aspc.gc.ca/cipars-picra/index-eng.php/>; 2007. [accessed 2015].
23. Canary Database | Animals as Sentinels of Human Environmental Health Hazards, <http://canarydatabase.org/about/description/>. 2015.
24. Definition provided by the chapter author.
25. Anthony SJ, St Leger JA, Pugliares K, Ip HS, Chan JM, Carpenter ZW, et al. Emergence of fatal avian influenza in New England harbor seals. MBio 2012;3(4):e00166–12.
26. Hinshaw VS, Bean WJ, Webster RG, Rehg JE, Fiorelli P, Early G, et al. Are seals frequently infected with avian influenza viruses? J Virol 1984;51(3):863–5.
27. Mandler J, Gorman OT, Ludwig S, Schroeder E, Fitch WM, Webster RG, et al. Derivation of the nucleoproteins (NP) of influenza A viruses isolated from marine mammals. Virology 1990;176(1):255–61.
28. Webster RG, Geraci J, Petursson G, Skirnisson K. Conjunctivitis in human beings caused by influenza A virus of seals. N Engl J Med 1981;304(15):911.
29. Ayers JM, Lozier MS. Physical controls on the seasonal migration of the North Pacific transition zone chlorophyll front. J Geophys Res: Oceans (1978–2012) 2010;115(C5).
30. Polovina JJ, Howell E, Kobayashi DR, Seki MP. The transition zone chlorophyll front, a dynamic global feature defining migration and forage habitat for marine resources. Prog Oceanogr 2001;49(1):469–83.
31. Hinshaw VS, Webster RG, Turner B. The perpetuation of orthomyxoviruses and paramyxoviruses in Canadian waterfowl. Can J Microbiol 1980;26(5):622–9.
32. Hinshaw VS, Wood JM, Webster RG, Deibel R, Turner B. Circulation of influenza viruses and paramyxoviruses in waterfowl originating from two different areas of North America. Bull World Health Organ 1985;63(4):711–9.
33. Enserink M. WHO Declares Official End to H1N1 'Swine Flu' Pandemic. Science Insider, Health, <http://news.sciencemag.org/2010/08/who-declares-official-end-h1n1-swine-flu-pandemic/>; 2010. [accessed 2013].
34. Marchesi JR, Sato T, Weightman AJ, Martin TA, Fry JC, Hiom SJ, et al. Design and evaluation of useful bacterium-specific PCR primers that amplify genes coding for bacterial 16S rRNA. Appl Environ Microbiol 1998;64(2):795–9.
35. VanDevanter DR, Warrener P, Bennett L, Schultz ER, Coulter S, Garber RL, et al. Detection and analysis of diverse herpesviral species by consensus primer PCR. J Clin Microbiol 1996;34(7):1666–71.
36. United States. Health insurance portability and accountability act of 1996. Public Law 104–191. US Statut Large 1996;110:1936–2103.
37. McMichael AJ. Planetary overload: global environmental change and the health of the human species. Cambridge University Press; Cambridge, 1993.
38. Kunkel R, Hueston W, Christian K, et al. One Health Core Competency Workshop. Rome, Italy: March 12–13, 2012. USAID/RESPOND.
39. Mountain S. One Health (OH) Core Competencies by Proficiency Level. 2011.
40. RESPOND U. Global One Health Core Competencies. 2012.

CHAPTER

15

Collaboration for Biosurveillance

Andy Weber, Julia Dooher

. . . we must come together to prevent, and detect, and fight every kind of biological danger—whether it's a pandemic like H1N1, or a terrorist threat, or a treatable disease.

President Barack Obama, 2011

KEY WORDS

Biosurveillance
National Strategy for Biosurveillance
Emerging pathogens
Information communication technology (ICT)
Information sharing
Transparency
Collaboration

INTRODUCTION

Over the past half century, advances in biological research, increased access to basic hygiene, improved medical interventions and public health practice, and the **information and communication technology**[1] (ICT*) revolution have dramatically enhanced the delivery of health care. However, both recurring and **emerging pathogens** continue to threaten human health worldwide (see Chapter 11 for further discussion). Emerging pathogens are the causative agents of an infectious disease whose incidence increases following appearance in a new host population or whose incidence increases in an existing population as a result of long-term changes in the underlying epidemiology.[2] There is a broad expert consensus that these threats will grow in number and magnitude as a result of increased globalization and the resulting ability of infectious microbes to move and proliferate more efficiently (see Chapter 11).[3] Pathogens' ability to be carried by animal and insect hosts and jump to humans further expand this threat.[4] Also troubling is the sharp rise in antimicrobial resistance due to overuse of antibiotics in humans and in livestock, which is expected to lead to the spread of diseases for which we lack effective therapeutic countermeasures.[5] Finally, in addition to the spread of naturally occurring infectious diseases, the ever-increasing expansion of biological know-how and easier access to technology and laboratory methods increases the risk that rogue nations or terrorists will be able to obtain, develop, weaponize, and use biological weapons. Further complicating the picture, many human, animal, and plant pathogens identified as posing potential intentional security risks (termed "select agents") are in fact present in nature and distributed globally.[6] Together, it is clear that the global community faces a complex and expanding landscape of risks to health as well as to economic well-being and national stability (see Chapter 11).

Our shared vision is that health threats, no matter what their cause, are detected in real time so that governments, international organizations, and individuals are properly informed and can take appropriate action to minimize negative impacts and the spread of infectious agents as early as possible. One of the most important means to

*ICT: Refers to all the technology used to handle telecommunications, broadcast media, intelligent building management systems, audiovisual processing and transmission systems, and network-based control and monitoring functions.[1]

accomplish this is to improve and connect national and global public health surveillance systems. Health surveillance is the major input to the broader concept of **biosurveillance.** Biosurveillance, discussed throughout this chapter, is defined as the process of gathering, integrating, interpreting, and communicating essential information related to all-hazards threats or disease activity affecting human, animal, or plant health to achieve early detection and warning, contribute to overall situational awareness of the health aspects of an incident, and to enable better decision-making at all levels.[7] Biosurveillance includes the analysis and interpretation of biosphere data that might relate to disease activity and threats to human or animal health – whether infectious, toxic, metabolic, or otherwise, and regardless of intentional or natural origin – in order to achieve early warning of health threats, early detection of health events, and overall situational awareness of disease activity.[8] In today's globalized world of rapid travel, expanding commerce, increasing urbanization, and consequently pathogen spread, optimizing public health surveillance and integrating other environmental information at the source of an outbreak is increasingly important for the safety of all (see Chapters 3 and 11). Effective public health surveillance and biosurveillance (which can include monitoring of environmental samples, food, or wildlife for microbes, chemical threats or other toxins affecting health, for example) for improved decision-making involves the convergence of multiple elements, including:

- raw data (e.g., symptoms, diagnoses, and microbial genomic sequences);
- basic data collection processes (e.g., epidemiology and social media);
- cutting-edge information technologies that help manage large data sets;
- mechanisms for data analysis;
- sharing of information with stakeholders and partners (e.g., public health, scientific and medical communities, authorities, international governing bodies, and individual citizens) in a smooth, networked fashion;
- professionals trained and equipped to conduct the above activities.

Smart enhancements to the system elements listed above and, importantly, the linkages between these elements will help us reach our shared vision. This complex endeavor requires global leadership and prioritization of activities such as technical innovation, program planning, coordination, and implementation. Given the complexity inherent in each of these elements and their integration into a broader system, the fundamental keystone to achieving this shared vision is a culture of **collaboration**[9] across multiple sectors. These sectors include both health and security professionals of governmental entities, nongovernmental organizations, academia, and industry. Through bringing talents and resources together collaboratively we will strengthen, link, and amplify current surveillance activities and bring to bear novel solutions and innovative approaches.

Thus, this chapter focuses on the central role of collaboration in building and using effective biosurveillance systems. After a brief background and description of where we stand today and selected elements of the biosurveillance system we envision for the future, we identify important steps needed to develop the next generation of collaboration that will lead to success in using biosurveillance to mitigate threats to global health and security.

HISTORICAL BACKGROUND

Our understanding continues to evolve about current and possible future infectious diseases and deliberate biological threats as well as how best to counter them and minimize their effects. Rapid technological advances and our ever-deeper scientific understanding facilitate a more comprehensive view of biological risks; however, challenges remain in multidisciplinary collaboration and leveraging technology to its full potential. A historical backdrop is useful to better understand man-made and emerging natural biological threats over the past 40 years in order to appreciate the need for innovative surveillance approaches and partnerships to fuel effective **information sharing** for the future. We refer to information sharing as the ability to conduct multijurisdictional, multidisciplinary exchange of health-related information and situational awareness data among federal, state, local, territorial, and tribal levels of government, and the private sector.[10]

A substantial factor motivating us to recognize how important it is to be aware of biological risks comes from experiences with man-made security threats. Looking back to the Cold War era, the Soviet Union's massive offensive biological weapons program provides a chilling example of the threat of biological weapons of mass destruction. Just one Soviet era biological weapons plant in Stepnogorsk, Kazakhstan, once was able to produce 300 metrics tons of anthrax agent during a single burst of mobilization for wartime.[11] Countering this biological warfare threat required the USA to undertake the meticulous work of piecing together bits of information about Soviet biological weapons programs, which had always been shrouded in secrecy. This required earning the trust of ex-Soviet researchers and apparatchiks who for years conducted this deadly program, partly coerced by a totalitarian system, which taught them to hate the West, and partly to put food on the table for their families. One important step forward came after the Soviet Union disintegrated, when President Nursultan Nazarbayev of the newly independent Kazakhstan led the elimination of the biological weapons infrastructure through a partnership with the Department of Defense Nunn–Lugar Cooperative Threat Reduction Program (CTR). The CTR approach during that time proved successful through trusted relationships built with scientists previously engaged in Soviet biowarfare efforts. These scientists were equipped with the support that enabled them to channel their expertise into health-promoting activities instead. The experience with managing the Soviet biothreat through CTR in the 1990s provides (i) a real-life case study of the threat of engineered biological weapons as well as (ii) the transformative effect of international partnership and exchange of scientific expertise across borders. Over the years, and as discussed later in this chapter and in Chapter 16, the biological component of the CTR program, implemented through the Defense Threat Reduction Agency (DTRA), has evolved to address ways to reduce a diverse array of global biological threats—still working hand-in-hand with trusted partners.

During the 1990s, visionary scientists in the USA also advanced our scientific knowledge of human health risks by describing the types of systems and approaches needed to help address both natural and intentional biological threats.[12] Dr Joshua Lederberg, a professor of genetics who received the 1958 Nobel Prize for his work elucidating the genetic recombination mechanisms of bacteria, was one such leader in modernizing the world's understanding of biological threats. A scientific advisor to nine US presidents, Lederberg was a pioneering scientist and humanitarian who focused on the nexus of microbiology, health, and security, as well as the risks that infectious agents pose to functioning of societies. In 1992, Dr Lederberg coedited the groundbreaking Institute of Medicine (IOM) report "Emerging Infections: Microbial Threats to Health in the United States."[13] The report served as a call to action for government and other sectors to address concerns of microbial spread. The report used "examples to illustrate fundamental principles involved in [the] emergence of contemporary infectious diseases and the resurgence of old diseases."[13] This report was one of the first to direct multisectoral attention to the impending threat of pathogenic and newly emerging, naturally occurring microorganisms and the importance of developing techniques to detect such organisms. The report conveyed the importance of developing surveillance mechanisms to identify and communicate the presence of these organisms at population-based levels. In 2003 (coincidentally at the same time as the severe acute respiratory syndrome [SARS] outbreak in China), Dr Lederberg cochaired another IOM committee that updated information from the 1992 report and approached infectious disease risks from an even more global vantage point. This report highlighted additional risks and considerations for pathogen spread including those stemming from animal–human interactions. Importantly, the report called upon the human, veterinary, and agricultural communities to work together more closely.[14] This concept—which recognizes that the health of humans is connected to the health of animals and the environment—is now termed "One Health" (see Chapter 14).[15]

Whether a biological incident results from natural causes, an accidental incident, or a deliberate attack, our ultimate collective goal is to save lives and promote global well-being. Advances have been made in pursuing this goal, but many challenges exist. In terms of progress, the US Department of Defense has been thoroughly engaged in developing tools for detecting naturally occurring pathogens and infections and also as a means to detect engineered biothreats. The continued development of advanced technologies and systems for identifying pathogens, diagnosing infections, monitoring disease spread, and sharing information in real time by the USA and others will allow the public health and security sectors to make better decisions to protect civilians and service members from infectious disease and minimize the potential for deliberate biological attacks. However, a major impediment to the promise of regional and global biosurveillance remains the existence of numerous individual, stove-piped surveillance systems that house small subsets of data (e.g., disease specific, subpopulation specific, or country specific) that may not always be up-to-date and that cannot (or will not) share data with each other. Unable to fully use the available data and information sources about health risks, and unable to share information rapidly, we are all getting only a partial picture, a fuzzy and delayed snapshot, of biological threats to the public's health.

VISION FOR THE FUTURE

Moving beyond the status quo, we must create a broadly distributed public health surveillance network that delivers accurate, early information to government bodies, international organizations, and citizens. Our vision is a world in which health workers, government agencies, and private citizens are equipped with an integrated biosurveillance system that rapidly communicates accurate information about potential health threats (whether infectious or noninfectious), providing early warning and facilitating action that limits negative consequences. This future can be created only by improving understanding, cooperation, and coordination among all communities of interest. A web of supportive policies that set achievable goals with clear guidance for attaining them, and an intent to foster, share, and adopt advances in technology and practice, will enable effective collaboration and progress.

All Communities of Interest are United

No single organization or sector of society (e.g., government, industry, or academia, and health and security communities) can provide or operate a comprehensive biosurveillance system without a range of partners contributing information and expertise. For example, information uncovered by medical and public health practitioners and first responders on the front lines is critical to decision-makers at all levels; this was experienced during the Ebola epidemic in West Africa. Government agencies should track and leverage promising technological advances from the private sector and academia on a routine basis. We must continually forge strong partnerships among global leaders in science, public health, technology innovation, public policy, program implementation, academia, and private industry.

Embracing the overlaps between the health, agricultural, and security communities will lead to a more effective system to prevent, protect against, and respond to natural infectious diseases, accidental releases, and intentional biological threats. However, institutional and historical challenges exist. The size, structure, and subcultures of some of the organizations involved can, at times, impede progress. Despite this, the fact that people work in different disciplines or offices should not block the exchange of ideas, the opportunity to solve problems together in a new way, or the chance to develop technologies that address the needs of multiple groups. To transform our collective efforts to minimize health threats, whether natural or deliberate, it is imperative to strengthen discourse and partnerships between the biodefense and public health communities, both within the USA and with international partners. And although the security and health communities bring critical knowledge, competencies, technologies, and resources to the table, they have been isolated from each other for too long.

The US Department of Defense has taken steps to address the challenge of the "health-security divide". In 2009, the Office of the Assistant Secretary of Defense for Nuclear, Chemical, and Biological Defense Programs issued a memorandum specifically stating that the Department of Defense's chemical and biological defense mission would encompass emerging infectious diseases; this served as formal notice that the Department must consider all threats—not just traditional biological warfare agents—in order to better protect our soldiers and citizens. The US military also contributes to public health through a worldwide network of laboratories and health surveillance activities that are linked to other governments and international organizations, as described in Chapter 16. As will be discussed later in the current chapter, it is encouraging that strong White House leadership, in concert with the US Departments of Health and Human Services, State, Defense, Homeland Security, and Agriculture and other US government departments and agencies, in tandem with numerous international counterparts, has demonstrated a commitment to collaboration and action to confront global health risks in transformative ways through the Global Health Security Agenda. Thus, important strides have been made to bridge health and security sectors, but improvements are still needed.

Comprehensive Policy in Place

The right technologies and effective collaboration across sectors and disciplines could theoretically help us meet various biosurveillance subgoals, but the glue that will bind these elements together in an enduring manner that responds to changing circumstances is a comprehensive body of local, national, and international policies. For the USA, a few high-level building blocks are already in place. A series of national US strategies and directives have set policy priorities that describe the range of hazards we must confront and high-level approaches toward tackling these complex problems. These policy documents note the strategic need for enhanced approaches for biosecurity, biosurveillance, and emergency preparedness for both public health and security purposes. For instance, the 2009 *National Strategy for Countering Biological Threats* stated that "the rapid detection and containment of, and response to, serious infectious disease outbreaks—whether of natural, accidental, or deliberate origin—advances both the health of populations and the security interests of States."[16] Building on such foundations, the 2012 ***National Strategy for Biosurveillance*** sets forth the US Government's approach to strengthening the national biosurveillance enterprise.[7] The strategy builds on existing biosurveillance concepts and capabilities to enable more rapid detection, knowledge, and characterization of human, animal, or plant disease activity to improve incident situational awareness.[7] The strategy presented a set of guiding principles, core functions, and enabling activities that organized a national-level effort to advance biosurveillance that is also tied to state and local efforts.[7] Importantly, this US policy document also specifically highlighted the need for an approach that takes into account the broad range of potential health threats, the "all-hazards approach," by stating that we must "[embrace] the need to engage in surveillance for [weapons of mass destruction] threats and a broader range of human, animal, and plant health challenges, including emerging infectious diseases, pandemics, agricultural threats, and food-borne illnesses." Together these strategic-level policy documents support a shared understanding and elevate concerns to the level of national priorities. These documents and their associated fora provide a common touchstone and compass from which US government entities obtain guidance and share expertise. Importantly, other sectors (e.g., academic, nonprofit, industry) and partners (e.g., those outside the USA) may draw from and build upon these documents as well.

A key example of policy supporting collaborative action is the Global Health Security Agenda, initiated by the Obama Administration and joined by international governments and organizations.[17] This agenda, formally released in February 2014, highlights a set of nine core objectives that would substantially improve global health security—a world safe and secure from infectious disease threats. By articulating these objectives, efforts and resources from numerous US government departments and agencies are being aligned for maximal benefit in partnership with nations and international organizations around the globe. The agenda has thus provided energy for an effort that would otherwise be pursued by different communities in smaller and disconnected ways. The ultimate goal of this global effort is to energize meaningful, measureable progress along three main trajectories: prevent avoidable epidemics, detect threats early, and respond rapidly and effectively. Numerous countries and international organizations are enthusiastically participating and have rallied to assist in addressing these core objectives in a powerful, collaborative fashion; in September 2014, 44 countries came together to announce 100 new commitments including ways to build, measure, and maintain improved activities and systems. Results from individual projects initiated in one country or region (e.g., emergency operation centers, laboratory practices, or ICT projects) will be shared more broadly, offering the opportunity for fine-tuning and expansion to other locales.[18, 19] Working with international partners to bolster all regions' resilience can be thought of as preventive medicine—we mitigate or "buy down" risk when the global community is equipped to detect threats earlier and has a shared understanding of a common desired "end state" and ways to get there. From a policy standpoint, the development and communication of priority goals, outcomes, and overarching measures through the Global Health Security Agenda encourages leaders throughout the global community to contribute and leverage ideas, expertise, capabilities, and resources while minimizing redundancies. We expect that these objectives will grow deep roots that support the development, planning, coordination, implementation of an array of activities that will make measureable differences in improving our collective ability to prevent, identify, and contain the spread of infectious diseases in the future.

Cutting-Edge Technology Embraced

Modernized Diagnostic and Detection

In order to provide public health surveillance and biosurveillance practitioners with a comprehensive and dynamic picture of a population's current health status and any indicators for alarm, we must embrace the opportunities offered by technological advances in science and engineering. Tools for accessing and interpreting data will equip our workforces, and must be designed for a range of workers trained and capable of using them. These are core areas requiring our attention, leadership, and investment.

One critical area for improvement is in approaches to detect the "unknown"—the newest, emerging, heretofore unseen threats for which we may not yet have specific diagnostic tests or detectors. As Lederberg's 1992 IOM report notes, "current U.S. and international surveillance efforts are certainly of great value in detecting known infectious and noninfectious diseases. They fall short, however, in their ability to detect emerging infectious diseases. There has been no effort to develop and implement a global program of surveillance for emerging diseases or disease agents."[12] While many scientific and technological advances have come to fruition since publication of this seminal report, its stark conclusion captures one of the biggest public health surveillance challenges: the unknown biological threats that loom over the horizon. Middle East Respiratory Syndrome Coronavirus (MERS-CoV), avian influenza A (H7N9), and Ebola in West Africa are recent examples from 2012, 2013, and 2014. We must continue to focus on the continued development of technical capabilities and trained workforces required for identifying and assessing such emerging diseases.

Our vision for a future of effective applied ("operational") biosurveillance requires investment in advanced laboratory, detection, and diagnostic technologies. Novel emerging pathogens, especially those that result from animal-to-human leaps (also known as "zoonotic jumps"), can be major blind spots. In addition, the increase in antimicrobial resistance and the consequent reduced strength of our arsenal of antibiotics pose critical challenges. We must expand the repertoire of tools that equip primary care providers, public health personnel, and scientists to collect information required for an accurate and informed regional and global picture of the presence and spread of new pathogens or toxic agents. Addressing the call of Lederberg and colleagues, the availability of less expensive and more accurate next-generation sequencing and other identification and characterization methodologies and analysis tools will speed surveillance. Metagenomics, advanced proteomics, sample preparation methodologies, and bioinformatics will aid the accurate and rapid analysis of complex environmental and clinical samples, including the assessment of antimicrobial resistance markers or virulence factors. The development and use of diagnostic and detection technologies that do not require culturing of pathogens, where possible, will ensure a safer environment for laboratory workers and reduce opportunities for spread of dangerous pathogens through accidental release or malevolent theft.

A key area that will transform our approach to health surveillance, make timely clinical treatment decisions, and limit outbreak spread is the ability to diagnose infections on the spot, outside of clinic walls and laboratory infrastructure—termed the "point-of-care." To reduce turnaround times for diagnosis or surveillance, the Department of Defense is investing in the development and testing of reliable point-of-care diagnostics that can be used in remote locations. Such technologies are urgently needed in austere locations for civilian care as well, for quick and appropriate treatment of the individual and containment of an outbreak.[20] Point-of-care diagnostics or pathogen detection platforms that tie directly into electronic surveillance systems would allow us to rapidly identify infectious agents or an outbreak, and thus enable faster containment or intervention measures. Additionally, devices or assays that instantly distinguish between bacterial and viral infections would also dramatically cut down on unnecessary antibiotic use, resulting in improved patient care, a preserved medical countermeasure arsenal, and decreased rate of antimicrobial resistance spread.

Information Technology Advances

Ultimately the goal of disease surveillance activities and our emphasis on the development of rapid clinical and detection methodologies is to provide the earliest indications and warnings of health threats, no matter the cause. The biosurveillance user community of interest is varied and includes public health subject matter experts, clinical and laboratory staff, military health planners, emergency operations staff, public safety personnel, government decision-makers, researchers, and the general public. In addition to improvements in laboratory technologies, advancements in ICT and improved data management are necessary to realize real-time biosurveillance for different types of users. Computational methods for handling big data and the algorithms for making sense of it are required to help us ingest and find meaning in the vast amount of information available now and in the future. Mathematics and bioinformatics are needed to define baselines and the threshold above which we determine a situation is abnormal. To accomplish these goals, we must foster collaborations between technical disciplines (e.g., microbiology, medicine, and computer science) and support the science and technology (S&T) and research and development activities that meet these challenges in innovative ways.

One technological approach is to explore the use of nontraditional information sources for early warning. Informal sources of information such as media reports, early syndromic data, event-based surveillance (including social trends or market information), and social media represent a relatively untapped data resource (see Chapters 3 and 11). By pulling together all of the available data that hint at a potential problem, experts and decision-makers gain valuable time to intervene before a situation increases in magnitude or complexity. In a concept borrowed from national security called "tip and cue," early indicators of an event or circumstances out of the ordinary can focus attention on that area and increase directed monitoring activities. Because informal information sources may be of varying confidence levels, it will be critical to avoid issuing alarms without appropriate follow-up. Nontraditional, early reports would provide a "tip," which would then "cue" more traditional methods to substantiate, validate, or correct the initial signal using high confidence, vetted activities such as formal disease reporting or detailed, targeted health surveillance and epidemiological analysis. Such an approach may enable fast and effective actions to confirm, communicate, contain, and respond to an incident or outbreak.

Additional approaches to improving biosurveillance-driven decision-making include the development of capabilities for prediction and forecasting. Prediction refers to the capability to anticipate the emergence of infectious disease outbreak given factors that promote a pathogen's appearance or re-emergence in the human population and its ability to spread. Forecasting refers to the means to project the likely progression of an infectious disease outbreak or incident, including the impact of specific mitigation measures on the event's trajectory. These efforts will require the development of advanced modeling and simulation methods that incorporate information on pathogen characteristics, climate, human or animal population dynamics, and possible interventions. Ecologists, veterinarians, microbiologists, computational biologists, health informaticians, physicians, public health practitioners, and mathematicians will need to collaborate to develop and refine prediction and forecasting models using data from past and present events. Ultimately these teams will need to develop practical applications to inform preparedness and alert and response activities for both military and civilian use.

Members of the varied biosurveillance user community of interest will benefit from improved tools for real-time data presentation and information sharing among and between communities, organizations, and varying levels of expertise. Advanced data fusion, visualization, and mapping tools will provide a dynamic and intuitive view of events such as a flu pandemic or food-borne outbreak. Such capabilities will better equip users to interpret and convey evolving situations in temporal and geospatial ways to expedite trend determination and the monitoring of outbreak or incident progression, guiding and speeding our ability to respond.

ICT is the technology of the production, manipulation, storage, and communication of information using computers and microelectronics.[1] The examples of ICT advances noted above reflect technologies highlighted by the 2013 *National Biosurveillance S&T Roadmap* developed by the US Office of Science and Technology Policy in conjunction with the US interagency.[21] The development and improvement of such innovative computational tools are being supported by the Department of Defense as it continues its long-standing commitment to supporting a robust and forward-thinking science and technology infrastructure and its practice of converting technological advances into operational tools.

As we invest in, develop, and employ new information technologies, we must do so smartly. Ultimately we seek to maximize collaboration, promoting the exchange of data, reports, hypotheses, interpretations, potential interventions, practical insight, and best practices. To do this, ICT systems must be configured to provide fast and straightforward ways of communicating between colleagues across multiple organizations and country boundaries. Software applications and platforms must be compatible and interoperable. To ensure the unimpeded flow of information, developers will need to utilize established, common data standards for electronic health records and electronic health surveillance as well as software architectures that allow systems and analytic tools to tie into each other. Software should be simple to use, adaptable, scalable, and widely available. Systems should be designed to be flexible so that they can accommodate the addition of future pioneering advances, including new software applications to revolutionize approaches for data analysis and fusion, visualization, prediction, forecasting, language interpretation, and unstructured data processing.

The role of ICT in public health surveillance and biosurveillance is to link people and information to achieve distributed "situational awareness." Through working across sectors and utilizing the appropriate software features, we should strive to share innovations and develop technologies that are flexible, applicable to, and practical for a wide range of international users. As we design a solution for one purpose or user group, we should keep in mind other potential applications. We should look for opportunities to equip other user groups with capabilities to improve information sharing and thus readiness. The Department of Defense has fostered this approach through the science and technology and advanced development efforts of the Nuclear, Chemical, and Biological Defense Program. One example of this is the codevelopment of an ICT platform for information sharing for public health and biological incident preparedness with counterparts in the Republic of Korea. In the future, IT efforts should increasingly consider international government partners, nongovernmental organizations, international organizations, and decision-makers at all levels, from senior level decision-makers to operational staff across disciplines (e.g., public health, emergency operations, and academia). Going forward, it will be very important focus to consider ICT applications for individual citizen users who may access relevant biosurveillance information through a mobile phone or tablet device—this represents the "democratization" of health surveillance and biosurveillance information.

HOW TO ACHIEVE THE VISION

Based on our experiences implementing the vision of modern biosurveillance systems within the US government, we believe the next generation of collaboration will require five core actions. First, our partners and we must leverage existing expertise from our stakeholders. Second, we need to promote deeper and broader information sharing. Third, we should identify and build on successful models of collaboration and programs that demonstrate high impact within and among disciplines, and apply lessons learned from them. Fourth, we need to prove that health surveillance is a crucial component of effective emergency response. Finally, we must invest in future generations of experts who will both ensure that our current vision is met and conceive even better biosurveillance systems for the future.

Leveraging Existing Expertise through Innovative and Enduring Partnerships

When we consider how to harness expertise to achieve our shared vision for a healthier, safer world, it is important to recognize some of the key ways that the US Department of Defense can and does contribute. The US military routinely shares its know-how and capabilities with global partners in support of global health security; understanding better how it does so would allow for improved collaboration and problem solving. There is great potential in applying the military's scientific, public health, and medical expertise to improve global health in the course of ensuring troop health and conducting the military mission. The US military's workforce includes experts in an array of fields including laboratory medicine and research, development and acquisition of diagnostic and other laboratory equipment and ICT tools, and practitioners in public health, occupational health, preventative medicine, veterinary medicine, and operational emergency response. These capabilities are shared with global partners both in the case of acute emergencies (e.g., humanitarian assistance) and long-term relationships with host countries, as noted below and in Chapter 16.[22] Despite this potential, we still have work to do in challenging myths and stereotypes. The US military's activities that benefit public health globally are often not well understood beyond extensive, but episodic, humanitarian assistance activities. It is important to correct misunderstandings and appropriately leverage the military's expertise both by improving the military's own ways of operating and collaborating across disciplines, and by communicating the military's commitment to global well-being through the sharing of technology and expertise with global partners.

A major source of expertise that is channeled for public health on a long-standing, ongoing basis is the globally distributed network of overseas laboratories operated by the US Navy, Army, and other partners that are part of the Armed Forces Health Surveillance Center (AFHSC) Global Emerging Infections Surveillance and Response System

(GEIS) network, as discussed in Chapter 16. These laboratories work closely with host nation partners and local workers to conduct research on diseases of local importance. These facilities and their workers function as nodes for health surveillance in support of the host country and deployed US service members. The Department of Defense also contributes to partner capabilities through the CTR program's biological component, the Cooperative Biological Engagement Program (CBEP). CBEP partners with host nations around the globe and offers specialized support on an array of laboratory, research, health surveillance, and biosecurity activities. These activities are both material based and nonmaterial based. Workforce training reduces the worldwide biological threat through laboratory and health provider training, for example, in order to bolster partner capabilities and capacities in sustainable ways for the long term. Implementation efforts are designed in concert with the partner and focus on strengthening capabilities to prevent, detect, and respond to a variety of health threats within their borders and to facilitate reporting of disease outbreaks to the World Health Organization (WHO) through International Health Regulations (2005) procedures. Many of these activities are coordinated with and implemented by the US Centers for Disease Control and Prevention (CDC), providing a vital, responsive link to civilian health communities abroad. The Department of Defense's Chemical and Biological Defense Program (CBDP) also collaborates with the CDC. The CBDP conducts the early research and development and the advanced development of diagnostics, medical countermeasures, and biosurveillance information system technologies. CDC enhances and complements these efforts through specialized laboratory capabilities and subject matter expertise in public health, pathogen biology, field epidemiology and health surveillance, informatics, ICT, and emergency operations for accurate public health surveillance and biosurveillance. Such collaborative efforts between the leading US security and health sectors support the national security mission of protecting US citizens and those of US friends and allies, and contribute to regional and global public health, resiliency, and stability.

Improving Information Sharing

Our collective ability to leverage knowledge and expertise depends upon systems and norms that support effective and efficient health information sharing at a variety of levels. Individual collaboration among subject matter experts, communication within national borders and between international counterparts, technical collaboration, and promoting overall **transparency** among stakeholders all contribute to the interconnected biosurveillance system we envision. When discussing transparency, we are referring to the release of information by institutions, which is relevant to evaluating those institutions and allows citizens and markets to hold institutions accountable for their policies and performance.[23]

Building personal relationships is essential if various communities are to understand and learn from one another's capabilities and experiences. We must prioritize strengthening partnerships between biodefense and public health. Interaction between biodefense and public health communities at both leadership levels and program implementation levels is foundational to building long-lived relationships that will enable information sharing under both steady-state and emergency circumstances. Such dialogue and exchange should be encouraged within and between government departments and other entities, and through efforts to strengthen international global health security.

Transparency and an established culture of trust and responsibility are needed for communities and governments to be willing to share information on public health threats across organizational boundaries or national borders. Insight on how to effectively combat potential threats should be shared readily, including initial clinical warning signs, pathogen attributes, and risk factors influencing an outbreak. The willing sharing of data, analysis, and contextual information is required for a truly functional and integrated global biosurveillance system. One important exemplar comes from the remarkable strides the Chinese government made improving transparency over the past decade.[24, 25] In 2003, China suppressed information on the appearance and spread of the deadly SARS virus. In 2013, however, the Chinese government and academic institutions rapidly identified and swiftly communicated the presence of the novel H7N9 influenza virus to other nations and WHO. This example illustrates how information sharing and transparency in sharing virus samples, scientific data, and surveillance results led to effective biosurveillance and outbreak response.

Moving beyond the outmoded protectiveness about health threats within a country's borders to more openness and transparency can be challenging, but this shift is critical. While we recognize the potential economic and political ramifications of sharing health and agricultural information and considerations of sovereignty, countries and international bodies must promote information sharing as the standard in today's interconnected world. Anything less is reckless. It is the responsibility of leaders and international organizations, both governmental and nongovernmental, to set the example of transparency and to stand together in establishing the expectations and goals of heath information and sample sharing.

Building on Successful Models and Programs

Identifying lessons from past successes in countering health and biosecurity threats will allow us to build on successful programs and the expertise resident in public and private organizations. As noted earlier, the Department of Defense expanded the Nunn–Lugar CTR program from its beginnings in deterring nuclear and biological weapon threats following collapse of the Soviet Union to now include a focus on enhancing the abilities of partner countries to counter a range of biological threats. This is because of the scientific understanding that dangerous pathogens are endemic in many parts of the world, and that the core public health surveillance, biosurveillance, and preparedness activities necessary to detect, characterize, and counter biological threats are common whether a threat is natural, deliberately made, or accidentally released (see Chapter 11). (Notably, the cause of a health incident or outbreak is not often known for some time.) Through its more than 20-year history, scientific engagement and trusted relationships remained core to CTR efforts and success, and this same approach is used to drive efforts on biological threats to health. Today's biology-focused efforts involve collaborative strengthening of biosecurity, research, and health surveillance capabilities, primarily through engagement with the civilian sector of partner nations. The global reach of these partnerships is broad, with collaborators in science, health, security, and emergency response in the Middle East, South and Southeast Asia, and Africa, as well as nations of the former Soviet Union.

Recognizing and flexibly addressing new threats is vitally important for both the security and health sectors. A key way to counter an emerging and complex threat landscape is for communities and disciplines to collaborate creatively and effectively. For example, it is now widely accepted that approximately 75% of recently emerging infectious diseases affecting humans are diseases of animal origin and that approximately 60% of all human pathogens are zoonotic.[4] Responding to this evolving and expanding threat, and recognizing the fact that zoonotic pathogens represent significant biosecurity threats, CTR efforts now include a substantial focus on One Health activities. This involves training and support of surveillance and research activities involving the partner's veterinary sector. Continued progress will rely on maintaining a focus on enduring, trusted relationships; identifying partner needs; providing capabilities that fit with existing partner processes and which can be sustained independently; reacting and adapting to an evolving biological risk landscape; and working effectively with internationally recognized leaders such as CDC and international governmental and nongovernmental organizations.

Proving the Importance of Health Surveillance for Emergency Response

Effective public health surveillance depends upon the establishment of routine, day-to-day information uptake in order to provide trusted and actionable guidance upon recognition of an apparent incident or an outbreak. Some of the most important pieces of essential information that inform our initial understanding that an event has occurred is early health surveillance data and related analyses. Sick people go to clinics and hospitals generally before anyone knows the cause of the problem. Effective technologies and protocols for health surveillance must be in place for handling and processing health data under normal circumstances as well as under conditions of a rapidly filling emergency department. Understanding and improving the role that health surveillance plays within the broader biosurveillance construct (which also includes environmental surveillance and communication measures, for example) is needed to optimally guide sound contingency planning and emergency operations management.

Conducting collaborative international exercises is a very effective means to integrate and optimize the functional elements of health surveillance, biosurveillance, and emergency response. Exercises can test what we think we know about how information flows and how decisions are made. From there we can identify how to speed up slower steps, determine technological requirements, make workflow or protocol improvements, or focus on areas requiring policy improvements. The annual Republic of Korea Able Response exercise series, initiated in partnership with the USA in 2011, is an outstanding example of the value of strengthening a whole-of-government biological crisis response capacity that incorporates biosurveillance. Able Response is a biopreparedness exercise that examines and refines procedures by the USA and the Republic of Korea to prepare for and handle a biological threat event on the Korean Peninsula. The key innovation is bringing together the interagency of both countries, including defense, health, and law enforcement communities. Through this model, colleagues who previously focused on roles and responsibilities within their own organization become skilled at coordinating with others. This helps develop a more holistic, well-informed, efficient, and resilient biosurveillance and response capability. While held in the Republic of Korea, US interagency colleagues who participate in the event often report that the exercise also strengthens US government linkages and procedures. Together, Able Response actively supports global health security objectives through fostering strategic and practical whole-of-government actions.

Investing in the Next Generations

While policy and technological advances provide key foundations for the biosurveillance enterprise, there is nothing more critical than our people and workforce. In order to realize the vision of reliable, real-time, and distributed detection and awareness of disease threats globally, we must cultivate the next generation of biosurveillance leaders and practitioners. Let us ignite the minds and channel the talents of those workers with skills in biological and chemical research, computer science, engineering, primary health care, veterinary health, public health, and international relations. Fostering these diverse skill sets is critical to ensuring continued growth, flexibility, and innovation in the multidisciplinary field of biosurveillance.

Building workforce capacity with international partners is at the core of fostering a network of trained colleagues and enduring global partnerships. The objective should be to build from the ground up, ensuring communication and trust, so that programs and solutions are selected and implemented, and are practical, scalable, and sustainable by the partner country. Health workers at local, district, and national levels should have training and proficiency in the tasks needed for effective health surveillance and biosurveillance, including diagnostic testing, data collection and analysis, and trend identification. The goal is that health surveillance and biosurveillance activities become part of the fabric of every day work, and that these practices are shared among colleagues and with the coming generations. Technologies to facilitate information sharing will complement a country's trained workforce, and they must be matched with the user and the current local processes in mind. One particularly notable regional model for enhancing workforce capabilities is the African Field Epidemiology Network (AFENET), which supports African nations through workforce training in building sustainable capacity in field epidemiology, public health laboratory management, health surveillance, outbreak prevention, investigation, and response. Other key examples are the Field Epidemiology Training Program (FETP) and associated Field Epidemiology and Lab Training Program (FELTP) that are coordinated and operated by the CDC in dozens of countries, with support from the Department of Defense. These programs are designed to build sustainable capacity for detecting and responding to health threats so that disease outbreaks can be detected locally and prevented from spreading.

Ensuring and expanding workforce capacity also involves cultivating future national biosurveillance leaders. One way we can do this is by encouraging the best scientists and other professionals to pursue fellowships and internships in public service, including the Emerging Leaders in Biosecurity Initiative and the American Association for the Advancement of Science (AAAS) Science and Technology Policy Fellowship. Senior leadership should encourage colleagues in their organizations to recruit and inspire talented young people. We should embrace mentoring and cultivate opportunities to pioneer new directions and share ideas across sectors. We benefit not only from the experience of seasoned experts but also from others' fresh perspectives. New voices should be encouraged to participate and contribute to this civic mission. The key to fostering the next generation of collaboration will be establishing a culture that naturally values bold thinking, transparency, communication, teamwork, and an unflinching commitment to tackle the tough problems head-on.

CONCLUSION

Today we benefit from the accumulated knowledge and expertise in science, health, and information technology developed over the past several decades. However, there is work to be done. Civilian and military populations, both in the USA and around the world, are still at risk from health threats that can cause severe economic damage and, in certain cases, destabilizing crisis conditions. Technological advances in pathogen, toxin and disease detection and ICT would allow us to react more quickly, ultimately improving national security and saving lives. It is critical to strengthen our ability to collect and communicate information accurately and quickly through technological enhancements, workforce development, and improvements in the norms of information sharing across borders. Together these activities will allow the global community to be informed about the appearance of potential health threats whether they are naturally occurring, intentionally created, or as a result of accidental release. Such vigilance will position leaders, practitioners, and individuals to make appropriate and educated decisions to protect health and limit disease spread and minimize disruption to society. Our shared vision is one of preparedness, rooted in science. As we strive to prevent, detect, and respond to health threats posed by microbial evolution, globalization, accidents, and malicious actors, we must draw together forward-thinking subject matter experts, innovators, and policy makers to enhance our situational awareness and access to reliable, actionable information. Expertise in microbiology, chemistry, medicine, epidemiology, public health, computer science, engineering, and other disciplines will be in high demand. Professionals with competency in these areas will be called upon to collaborate in order to expand and refine biosurveillance solution sets, and to communicate opportunities and challenges to senior leaders and policy makers for support and advocacy. As a society, we need government leaders who understand the potential impacts of natural and other threats to health and how public health and security should be strengthened through interagency and multisectoral activities. Effective policy and supporting programs must continue to be shaped, articulated, and championed across communities to foster linkages between organizations and disciplines and to align complementary problem-solving efforts. In order to reach the promise of the next generation of public health surveillance, biosurveillance, and global health security, all must embrace a culture of bold innovation and collaborative partnership.

RELEVANT JOB FUNCTIONS FOR BIOSURVEILLANCE

This chapter calls for participation and collaboration by professionals from many disciplines. Biosurveillance efforts are conducted at multiple levels of government and involve interactions between government, industry, and academia. There are opportunities to work at technical and operational levels, as well as at strategic and policy-oriented positions. We have grouped some of these professions and list key professional skills and attributes, and selected examples of ways to gain applicable training or experience.

- Information technology professionals
  - Currency on the latest programming and agile software development approaches
  - Ability to communicate effectively with non-ICT professionals and translate their needs into applied tools
  - Systems engineering training and experience
  - Computer scientists, informaticians, and computational biologists who can integrate computational approaches with biological principles
  - Training conducted at Bachelor's, Master's, and PhD levels
  - Industry experience in software development and computer science
- Scientific, medical, and public health subject matter experts
  - Disciplines in high demand include epidemiologists and other public health professionals, microbiologists, chemists, laboratorians, biomedical engineers, clinicians, veterinarians, and ecologists
  - Practical experience treating patience and conducting epidemiological analysis and outbreak investigation in military or civilian settings; field experience highly desirable
  - Ability to critically evaluate emerging technologies and conduct "technology watches"

  - Exposure to government through employment or fellowships
  - Interest in contributing subject matter expertise to government decision-makers
  - Interest and skill in translating between strategic-level policy priorities and programmatic initiatives
  - Medical school or graduate-level training, often with additional career experience
- Policy and international relations
  - Excellent writing and oral communication skills
  - Understanding of geopolitical dynamics and diplomacy
  - Formal training (e.g., Master's level) obtained in public policy, international relations, or analogous training acquired through fellowships or internships
  - Experience in international and government settings
- Program management and implementation
  - Management of technical research and development efforts, obtained in the commercial sector or government
  - Practical experience in planning, contracting, or implementing training activities, either domestically or internationally
- Emergency operations and planning
  - Ability to communicate effectively with subject matter experts and decision-makers at various levels of government
  - Ability to utilize information communication technologies and to develop practical response protocols
  - Experience gained from military service or law enforcement
  - Formal training from undergraduate or graduate training
  - On-the-job training from state/district or municipal/city government

KEY SUMMARY POINTS

- By improving national and global public health surveillance systems, one reduces the risks and effects of infectious disease outbreaks and biological or chemical weapons.
- While great efforts have been made in detection of infectious and noninfectious diseases, it is the unknown or emerging diseases that need additional attention since the current technologies are not as strong in detection or identification of such emerging pathogens.
- For biosurveillance, investments in workforce capacities and advanced laboratory detection and diagnostic technologies are essential for combating and detecting emerging pathogens.
- While many of the necessary tools to better address global health security through surveillance exist, a major impediment to regional and global biosurveillance remains: the existence of vertical surveillance systems that focus on subsets of data (e.g., disease specific, subpopulation specific, country specific).
- Information sharing and interdisciplinary collaboration are critical to a comprehensive biosurveillance system.
- Although many technical tools exist, ICT and other technological tools must be enhanced, particularly to detect new and emerging threats.
- The USA prioritizes biosurveillance and US departments and agencies are guided by national and international policies including the 2009 US National Strategy for Countering Biological Threats, the 2012 US National Strategy for Biosurveillance, 2013 National Biosurveillance Science and Technology Roadmap, and the Global Health Security Agenda. These policies aim to enhance collaboration and information sharing, and support the establishment of a more comprehensive biosurveillance system to quickly identify and minimize the effects of health threats whether natural, intentional, or accidental.

DISCUSSION QUESTIONS

1. Discuss several examples of public health threats, including potential biological or chemical weapons, drawing from this chapter and other experiences. Are these threats increasing, decreasing, or remaining stable? Why?
2. How has the US experience during the last 50 years influenced our understanding of biosurveillance and public health surveillance?
3. Partnerships and information sharing are discussed throughout the chapter. Which partnerships are most important for biosurveillance and global health security? Why?

4. How can public health agencies at all levels balance detecting emerging new threats with addressing known threats? Consider risk size, human resources, financial resources, and security in your response.
5. What kinds of data can media reports and event-based surveillance provide for public health use?
6. What are the ways in which the health and security communities can contribute to each other, and to health surveillance, biosurveillance, and global health security?
7. What is the role for policy in promoting biosurveillance initiatives and global health security objectives?

REFERENCES

1. Information and communication technology, <https://www.techopedia.com/definition/24152/information-and-communications-technology-ict>; September 25, 2015.
2. Woolhouse ME. Population biology of emerging and re-emerging pathogens. Trends Microbiol 2002;10(Suppl. 10):S3–7.
3. Institute of Medicine Forum on Microbial T. The National Academies collection: reports funded by National Institutes of Health. Infectious disease movement in a borderless world: workshop summary. Washington, DC: National Academies Press, National Academy of Sciences; 2010.
4. Taylor LH, Latham SM, Woolhouse ME. Risk factors for human disease emergence. Philos Trans R Soc Lond B Biol Sci 2001;356(1411):983–9.
5. U.S. Centers for Disease Control and Prevention. Antibiotic resistance threats in the United States, 2013, <http://www.cdc.gov/drugresistance/threat-report-2013/>; September 30, 2015.
6. Rambhia KJ, Ribner AS, Gronvall GK. Everywhere you look: select agent pathogens. Biosecur Bioterror 2011;9(1):69–71.
7. National Strategy for Biosurveillance. Washington, DC: The White House; 2012.
8. Homeland Security Presidential Directive/HSPD-21 National Strategy for Public Health Preparedness [news release]. Washington, DC: The White House; October 18, 2007. <http://www.whitehouse.gov/news/releases/2007/10/20071018-10.html>; 19 October, 2007.
9. Collins English Dictionary. Collaboration, <http://www.collinsdictionary.com/>; September 30, 2015.
10. U.S. Centers for Disease Control and Prevention. Public health preparedness capabilities: capability 6: information sharing. U.S. Centers for Disease Control and Prevention; 2011.
11. Bozheyeva G, Kunakbayev Y, Yeleukenov D. Former Soviet biological weapons facilities in Kazakhstan: past, present, and future. Monterey, CA: Monterey Institute of International Studies; 1999.
12. (IOM) IoM. Microbial evolution and co-adaptation: a tribute to the life and scientific legacies of Joshua Lederberg. Washington, DC: National Academies Press; 2009.
13. National Research Council. Emerging infections: microbial threats to health in the United States. Washington, DC: National Academy Press; 1992.
14. National Research Council. Microbial threats to health: emergence, detection, and response. Washington, DC: National Academic Press; 2003.
15. Rabinowitz PM, Kock R, Kachani M, Kunkel R, Thomas J, Gilbert J, et al. Toward proof of concept of a one health approach to disease prediction and control. Emerg Infect Dis 2013;19(12).
16. National Security Council. National Strategy for Countering Biological Threats. Washington, DC: The White House; 2009. p. 4.
17. U.S. Department of Health and Human Services. The Global Health Security Agenda, <http://www.globalhealth.gov/global-health-topics/global-health-security/ghsagenda.html/>; September 25, 2015.
18. Statement by the Chair of Global Health Security Agenda White House Event, September 26, 2014 [press release]. Washington, DC: The White House; 2014.
19. U.S. Centers for Disease Control and Prevention. CDC Global Health - Global Health Security Agenda, <http://www.cdc.gov/globalhealth/security/>; September 25, 2015.
20. Nuzzo JB, Rambhia K, Morhard R, Watson M, Adalja A, Toner E, et al. Diagnosing infection at the point of care. UPMC Center for Health Security; Baltimore, Maryland. 2013.
21. Executive Office of the President National Science and Technology Council. National biosurveillance science and technology roadmap. Washington, DC: The White House; 2013.
22. Michaud J, Moss K, Kates J. U.S. Global Health Policy. The U.S. Department of Defense and Global Health; Menlo Park, California, 2012.
23. The World Bank. Anti-corruption and transparency, <http://web.worldbank.org/WEBSITE/EXTERNAL/COUNTRIES/LACEXT/EXTLACREGTOPPUBSECGOV/0, content MDK:20830474~pagePK:34004173~piPK:34003707~theSitePK:832592,00.html/>; [cited 2015].
24. Wang Y. The H7N9 influenza virus in China—changes since SARS. N Engl J Med 2013;368(25):2348–9.
25. Liu Q, Cao L, Zhu XQ. Major emerging and re-emerging zoonoses in China: a matter of global health and socioeconomic development for 1.3 billion. Int J Infect Dis 2014;25:65–72.

CHAPTER

16

Contributions of the United States' Military Public Health Surveillance to Global Public Health Security

Kevin L Russell

The prayer that has been mine for twenty or more years, that I might be permitted in some way or some time to do something to alleviate human suffering, has been answered.

Walter Reed

KEY WORDS

Health care encounter monitoring
Reportable medical events
Field activities
Deployment surveillance
Environmental and occupational monitoring
Force Health Protection
GEIS
CBEP
CBD
Reference laboratory

INTRODUCTION

The engagement of the United States Department of Defense (DoD) in health surveillance activities might not be intuitive to the lay public at first glance, but disease and nonbattle injuries (as opposed to battle injuries) have been the major cause of troop morbidity throughout the history.[1] The DoD has an obligation to keep its men and women in uniform as healthy as possible; this obligation is not only to the men and women who choose to serve their country but also to the leadership and the country as a whole, ensuring there is a fit force to "deter war and protect the security of the United States."[2] To do this, the DoD must monitor the health of its men and women in uniform and continually assess health risks in the regions throughout the world where they are asked to operate.

Many surveillance programs in the DoD are established to monitor and mitigate health risks. Research and development initiatives are informed by this surveillance, producing countless disease countermeasures including vaccines, antimicrobials, antimalarials, diagnostic tests, and vector surveillance tools to maintain and improve the health of service members at home and abroad. These countermeasures have frequently found applications outside of the military and are used in other countries to keep their citizens healthy and productive. The current Ebola crisis in West Africa is a timely example of DoD's contributions. From diagnostics to medical countermeasure developments in both antivirals and vaccines, the DoD's contributions have been substantial, but sadly and clearly, not sufficient to prevent this catastrophe.

The DoD operates throughout the world and thus has disease exposures throughout the world. Collaboration and transparent communication are crucial for the DoD to prepare for those exposures. Collaboration allows the DoD to learn from others' experiences as well as to share its own information and products.

This chapter will explore the history and current landscape of the US DoD's public health surveillance—both inside and outside of active-duty uniformed populations—and resulting contributions that have impacted global public health security. In the context of collaborations, past and current examples of successes will be outlined and a future vision will be discussed with some ideas of how that vision can be attained. Combat situations might draw a line in the sand at times, but at the end of the day, we all share one world, and our vision is, more often than not, a shared one: a safe, healthy world free of preventable diseases.

THE HISTORY OF MILITARY CONTRIBUTIONS TO GLOBAL PUBLIC HEALTH

From a historical perspective, public health surveillance in the DoD and medical countermeasure development and research are intimately intertwined. One cannot determine the medical countermeasures to develop without an understanding of health risks, and, likewise, one cannot determine the effectiveness of medical countermeasures without monitoring outcomes. Combining these closely related processes is as important today as it was decades ago; public health measures developed for service members very often have benefits for other populations.[1,3,4]

The DoD's historical contributions to global public health include, but are not limited to, infectious disease epidemiology,[5] advances in vaccines,[4,6,7] antimicrobial development,[8] diagnostic tests, health informatics that assist host countries or foreign militaries in monitoring disease distributions and outbreaks,[9] and predictive technologies. Table 16-1 outlines many of these contributions to give the reader an appreciation of the breadth and diversity of contributions, as a comprehensive list would be near impossible to construct. Three disease areas deserve special attention and are discussed as examples in subsequent sections: malaria and vector-borne diseases, diarrheal diseases, and influenza and respiratory diseases.

Malaria and Vector-Borne Diseases

Malaria, both historically and currently, has devastating global public health ramifications, and the DoD has had important contributions to this and other vector-borne infectious diseases. Since the early 1800s, the Army Medical Department struggled with control of "intermittent fevers" in the Americas. Avoidance of marshes was commonly advised, but control remained poor. French researchers Pelletier and Caventau[10] successfully isolated the active ingredient, quinine, from the cinchona tree bark that had been used for centuries as a "remedy" for these fevers, and Army physicians refined the dosing regimen throughout the mid- to late 1800s.[8] In the late 1800s and into the 1900s, enormous strides were made by Major Walter Reed and Col William Crawford Gorgas and others in markedly decreasing the transmission of yellow fever in Cuba and then in Panama. Malaria was more difficult; the tactics employed by Col Gorgas in Panama to finally achieve success required a multifaceted approach: (1) eliminating vector breeding grounds by draining swamps and spraying oil, (2) using mosquito "swatters," (3) using screens on living quarters, and (4) administering quinine for prophylaxis. Malaria rates dropped from 800 cases to 16 cases per 1000 workers.[11] "The result was staggering; perhaps the greatest single achievement in public health prevention in the 20th century."[8,12]

In the pre-World War II era, efforts within the US Army shifted to the development of chemical prophylaxis, partly because the Japanese and Germans controlled many of the quinine plantations in the Philippine islands. Since that time, the DoD malaria drug program has been involved with the development of nearly all antimalaria medications available, many of which are now used throughout the world for malaria chemoprophylaxis and treatment. Efforts to develop new antimalaria drugs and vaccines continue to this day. Also notable, recent surveillance efforts were instrumental in discovering the first evidence of artemisinin resistance in Southeast Asia,[13,14] a major public health concern as artemisinin is the key ingredient in many antimalaria drugs in the region. In the realm of malaria and other vector-borne pathogens, the DoD has had monumental contributions within environmental control, vector control, personal protective measures, chemical chemoprophylaxis, and vaccine development that have benefitted the entire world, although further progress is needed.

TABLE 16-1 Selected DoD Contributions to Public Health

	VACCINE DEVELOPED	VACCINE RESEARCH	EPIDEMIOLOGY AND PATHOGENESIS	TREATMENT REGIMENS	DIAGNOSTIC TESTING	ANTIMICROBIAL DEVELOPMENT	TRAINING AND CAPACITY BUILDING	PUBLIC HEALTH AND VECTOR-CONTROL MEASURES	DISCOVERY
Adenovirus	✓	✓	✓						✓
Amoebiasis			✓		✓				
Angiostrongyliasis			✓		✓				
Anthrax		✓	✓	✓					
Arenaviruses		✓	✓	✓					
Bartonellosis		✓	✓	✓					
Brucellosis		✓	✓	✓					
Campylobacter		✓	✓	✓					
Chikungunya		✓	✓						
Cholera	✓	✓	✓	✓			✓		
Cyclosporiasis				✓					
Dengue	✓	✓	✓	✓	✓		✓	✓	
Diarrheal diseases		✓	✓	✓			✓		
Ebola-Reston									✓
Ehrlichioses			✓	✓	✓			✓	
Epidemic typhus (*Rickettsia prowazekii*)	✓	✓	✓	✓	✓			✓	
ETEC		✓	✓	✓					
Filariasis			✓		✓			✓	
Filoviruses		✓	✓	✓					
Gastrointestinal parasites			✓						
Gonorrhea	✓	✓	✓	✓			✓		
Guanarito virus									✓
Hantaviruses		✓	✓	✓					
Hepatitis A	✓	✓	✓	✓					
Hepatitis B	✓		✓	✓					
Hepatitis E	✓	✓	✓						
HIV		✓	✓	✓			✓		
Hookworm (*A. duodenale*)			✓	✓					✓

TABLE 16-1 Selected DoD Contributions to Public Health—cont'd

	VACCINE DEVELOPED	VACCINE RESEARCH	EPIDEMIOLOGY AND PATHOGENESIS	TREATMENT REGIMENS	DIAGNOSTIC TESTING	ANTIMICROBIAL DEVELOPMENT	TRAINING AND CAPACITY BUILDING	PUBLIC HEALTH AND VECTOR-CONTROL MEASURES	DISCOVERY
IHR (2005) compliance							✓		
Influenza	✓						✓		
Intestinal capillariasis			✓	✓					
Intestinal trematodes			✓						
Japanese encephalitis	✓	✓	✓		✓				
Leishmaniasis			✓	✓	✓	✓			
Leptospirosis			✓	✓	✓				
Malaria	✓	✓			✓	✓	✓		
Meningococcal disease	✓	✓							
Murine typhus (*Rickettsia typhi*)				✓	✓			✓	
New nematode (*A. malaysiensis*)									✓
Oliveros virus									✓
Plague		✓	✓	✓					
Pneumococcus	✓								
Q fever *(Coxiella burnetii)*		✓	✓		✓				
Rabies								✓	
Rift Valley fever			✓		✓				
Rubella	✓								
scrub typhus (*Orientia tsutsugamushi*)		✓	✓	✓	✓			✓	
Shigella		✓	✓	✓					
Schistosomiasis			✓	✓	✓			✓	
Smallpox	✓								
Spotted fevers	✓		✓		✓				
Syphilis			✓	✓					
Tick-borne encephalitis	✓	✓							
Traveler's diarrhea		✓		✓					

Continued

TABLE 16-1 Selected DoD Contributions to Public Health—cont'd

	VACCINE DEVELOPED	VACCINE RESEARCH	EPIDEMIOLOGY AND PATHOGENESIS	TREATMENT REGIMENS	DIAGNOSTIC TESTING	ANTIMICROBIAL DEVELOPMENT	TRAINING AND CAPACITY BUILDING	PUBLIC HEALTH AND VECTOR-CONTROL MEASURES	DISCOVERY
Trypanosomiasis			✓	✓		✓			
Tularemia		✓							
Typhoid	✓			✓					
VEE, WEE		✓							
West Nile virus		✓	✓						
Yellow fever	✓	✓	✓					✓	

Sources:

1. Endy TP, Thomas SJ, Lawler JV. History of U.S. military contributions to the study of viral hemorrhagic fevers. Mil Med 2005;170(4 Suppl):77–91.
2. Dooley DP. History of U.S. military contributions to the study of viral hepatitis. Mil Med 2005;170(4 Suppl):71–6.
3. Artenstein AW, Opal JM, Opal SM, Tramont EC, Peter G, Russell PK. History of U.S. military contributions to the study of vaccines against infectious diseases. Mil Med 2005;170(4 Suppl):3–11.
4. Bavaro MF, Kelly DJ, Dasch GA, Hale BR, Olson P. History of U.S. military contributions to the study of rickettsial diseases. Mil Med 2005; 170(4 Suppl):49–60.
5. Ockenhouse CF, Magill A, Smith D, Milhous W. History of U.S. military contributions to the study of malaria. Mil Med 2005;170(4 Suppl):12–6.
6. Lim ML, Murphy GS, Calloway M, Tribble D. History of U.S. military contributions to the study of diarrheal diseases. Mil Med 2005;170(4 Suppl): 30–8.
7. Christopher GW, Agan MB, Cieslak TJ, Olson PE. History of U.S. military contributions to the study of bacterial zoonoses. Mil Med 2005;170(4 Suppl):39–48.
8. Rasnake MS, Conger NG, McAllister K, Holmes KK, Tramont EC. History of U.S. military contributions to the study of sexually transmitted diseases. Mil Med 2005;170(4 Suppl):61–5.
9. Hoke Jr CH. History of U.S. military contributions to the study of viral encephalitis. Mil Med 2005;170(4 Suppl):92–105.
10. Crum NF, Aronson NE, Lederman ER, Rusnak JM, Cross JH. History of U.S. military contributions to the study of parasitic diseases. Mil Med 2005;170(4 Suppl):17–29.
11. Peake JB, Morrison JS, Ledgerwood MM, Gannon SE. The Defense Department's enduring contributions to global health: the future of the U.S. Army and Navy overseas medical research laboratories. Washington, DC: Center for Strategic and International Studies; 2011.
12. Russell KL Johns M, Lipnick R, Sessions C. Global militaries unite. Discussion of responsibilities under the International Health regulations (2005): Saint Petersburg 2010. JHSH 2011;Spring 1(1):131–40.

Gastrointestinal Diseases

Diarrheal diseases have long taken a grim toll on mankind. Military operations have been particularly hard hit, given difficulties with sanitation and food safety practices. The US military's engagement with cholera is an impressive example of its impact on public health. This work eventually benefited public health's understanding of all causes of human diarrheal illness.

Dr Robert Phillips's role in cholera started in 1947 at the Naval Medical Research Unit 3 (NAMRU-3) in Cairo, Egypt. Cholera was a devastating disease with mortality in excess of 20% at times. Phillips' research,[15] first in Egypt and later in Taiwan and Thailand, demonstrated that cholera caused an isotonic fluid loss with excess sodium; that an intravenous, slightly hypertonic saline solution could reduce mortality from cholera; and that cholera is a non-invasive disease. By the late 1950s, it was discovered that glucose in oral rehydration solutions facilitated sodium absorption and decreased fatality rates to less than 1%. Oral rehydration solutions became affordable and available throughout the world.[15] *The Lancet* reported in an editorial that this work was "potentially the most important medical advance of this century."[16]

Dr Walter Reed's work on typhoid led to the observation that asymptomatic carriers could spread typhoid. It was more than a decade later that Typhoid Mary's (the first person in the USA identified as an asymptomatic carrier of typhoid) role in sustaining an outbreak of typhoid was recognized.[15] The lessons learned from this work and expertise gained by the US military eventually extended to many other bacterial gastrointestinal pathogens such as dysentery caused by *Shigella*,[17] as well as enteroinvasive *Salmonella*, pathogenic *Escherichia coli*,[18] and *Campylobacter jejuni*.[19]

Influenza and Respiratory Diseases

Respiratory illnesses have also been among the major contributors to morbidity and mortality throughout the history of military forces. The 1918–1919 global influenza pandemic is a prime example, where military forces not only suffered a catastrophic impact but also, unfortunately, contributed to the global spread.[20]

Close living conditions, physical stress, potential poor sanitation and hygiene, and extensive environmental exposures all contribute to the rapid spread of respiratory pathogens in a military setting. For these reasons, the DoD was instrumental in early influenza vaccine development efforts. The DoD initiated a global respiratory surveillance network using the DoD OCONUS (outside the continental United States) Navy and Army laboratories and this network continue to provide critical information on strain circulation (Fig. 16-1). Partners in this network monitor for emerging strains globally. This information is collected and shared in close communication with the US Centers for Disease Control and Prevention (CDC) and the World Health Organization (WHO).[21] Research on other respiratory viruses has been conducted by the DoD, including development of unique oral adenovirus vaccines in the 1960s that provide near 100% protective effectiveness against serotypes 4 and 7 adenovirus infections.[22,23] DoD researchers also substantively contributed to the understanding of Group A *Streptococcus*, *Pneumococcus*, rhinovirus, pertussis, respiratory syncytial virus, human Middle East respiratory syndrome coronavirus (MERS-CoV), and many other respiratory diseases.[21,24]

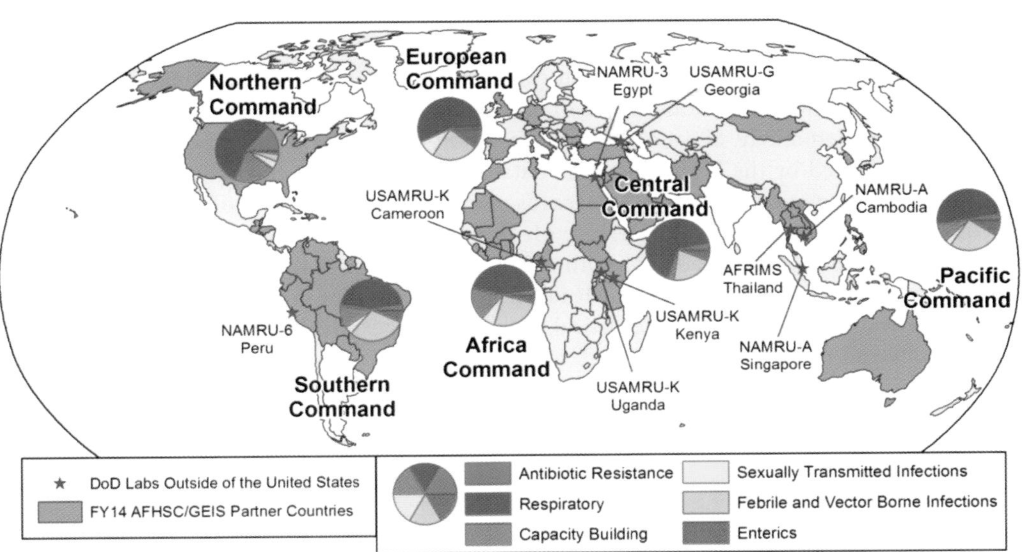

FIG. 16-1 DoD OCONUS laboratory network.

Other Infectious Agents

Given the military's role, it is not surprising that considerable work has also been done throughout history to understand the epidemiology, clinical manifestations, and virulence mechanisms for a variety of bacterial zoonoses and other infectious agents that could be used against its troops and citizens through biological warfare. Chemoprophylaxis, antimicrobial treatments, and vaccines were developed for many of these pathogens. Table 16-1 lists DoD's work on many of these agents, including plague, Q fever, anthrax, brucellosis, and tularemia.[25] These agents are robust examples of how the DoD public health programs, from surveillance to development of diagnostics and medical countermeasures, have benefitted global public health.

THE CURRENT ENVIRONMENT

Health surveillance conducted in the US military today is multifaceted and complex. It is conducted in different ways by each Service and with different central or DoD-level components. The ultimate purpose of health surveillance in the DoD, as described above, is "Force Health Protection." **Force Health Protection** is defined as all measures taken by commanders, supervisors, individual Service members, and the military health system (MHS) to promote, protect, improve, conserve, and restore the mental and physical well-being of Service members across the range of military activities and operations. These measures enable the fielding of a healthy and fit force, prevention of injuries and illness and protection of the force from health hazards, and provision of medical and rehabilitative care to those who become sick or injured anywhere in the world.[26] For the purposes of this chapter, these activities can be summarized as (1) health care encounter monitoring, (2) DoD reportable medical events, (3) field activities, (4) deployment surveillance, (5) environmental and occupational monitoring, (6) the OCONUS laboratory surveillance efforts, (7) threat-reduction activities, and (8) other activities.

Health Care Encounter Monitoring

Health care encounter monitoring is electronic monitoring of any care for active duty or beneficiaries (defined as those that have access to benefits such as retirees and family members) paid for by the DoD.[26] The DoD is uniquely capable of robust health care encounter monitoring, which is accomplished through administrative databases that include International Classification of Diseases, 9th revision (ICD-9) diagnostic codes. Briefly, any care for active duty or beneficiaries (defined as those that have access to benefits, such as retirees and family members) paid for by the DoD creates an electronic file in the DoD monitoring system. Knowing the denominator, or how many active-duty personnel there are, allows generation of rates of encounters for any number of health-related issues. Rates are the gold standard for epidemiology, and no other organization in the world can do this to the same extent and breadth as that accomplished by the DoD. The DoD database of health care encounters includes both outpatient and inpatient visits, resulting in over 185,000,000 records per year. One of several DoD systems that captures health information for surveillance purposes is the Defense Medical Surveillance System (Fig. 16-2).

All military Services and DoD-level public health organizations produce various analytic reports from available medical databases for DoD and US government leaders. Recent examples include trends of traumatic brain and hearing injuries and health outcomes after theoretical environmental exposures. Additionally, reports can be generated for organizations and health care providers about specific issues or concerns, such as low back pain in pilots, vaccine coverage, or Lyme disease. The reports vary widely and cover several broad categories of reports: disease, injury, deployment, vaccine, and special reports.

DoD Reportable Medical Events

Reportable medical events are health conditions that must be monitored and reported according to DoD guidance. This list is influenced by CDC's notifiable events list and includes events identified as representing significant military

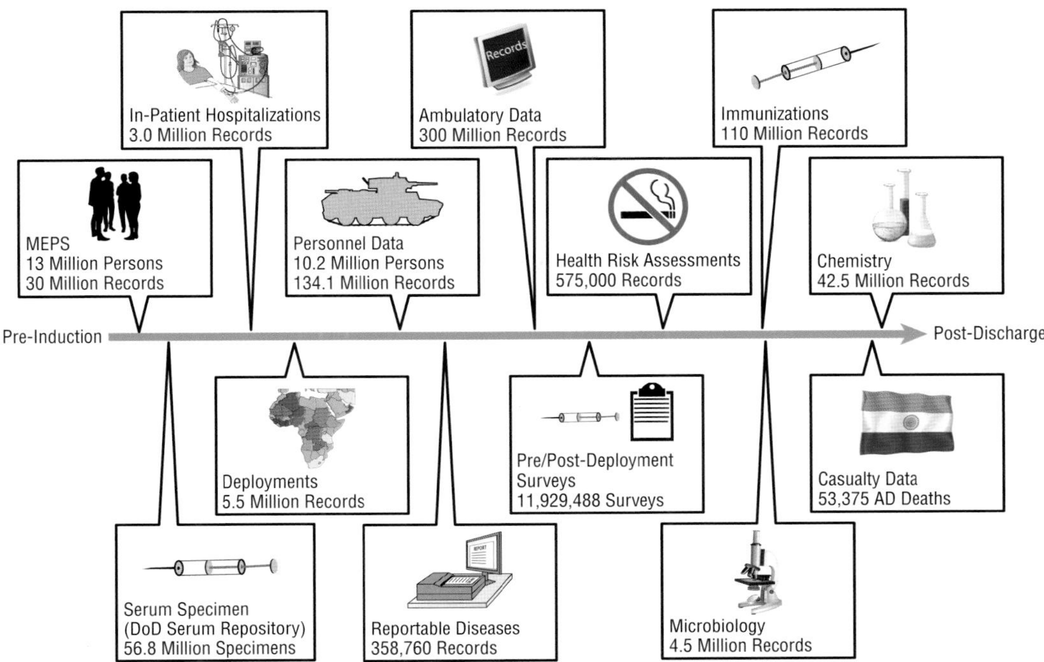

FIG. 16-2 Defense Medical Surveillance System. A comprehensive system which aggregates various health information on active duty and beneficiaries at the individual level. It is utilized to monitor trends and answer queries on any number of health-related conditions.

threats. Much as the CDC and states must monitor reportable medical events, so too does the DoD. Sixty-six health conditions are monitored closely by the DoD based on the most recent guidance from March 2012.[27] This guidance is influenced by the list of notifiable diseases from the CDC and the Council of State and Territorial Epidemiologists (CSTE) and by events that the "military public health experts have identified as representing significant military threats that deserve additional emphasis for surveillance"[27] such as heat and cold injuries. Each of the Services monitor submitted events, validating the information and providing needed follow-up. There is also a program for monitoring electronic laboratory data for diseases that should be reported.[28] The public health assets within each Service then reach out to the associated clinic or hospital to facilitate more comprehensive reporting. Health care providers and local military hospitals also have a responsibility to report notifiable diseases to the appropriate federal and state agencies.

Field Activities

Field activities require attention to health surveillance initiatives. Indeed, it has been noted how infectious diseases "are the true beneficiaries of war."[29] The conditions found in these settings often require special attention to health protection measures, both before arrival and during operations. Field activities range from food and water monitoring, sewage treatment, waste management activities, vector and rodent surveillance and control, disease and battle injury monitoring, determination of occupational and environmental exposures, and monitoring of psychological health status.[26] Guidelines for these programs are abundant, both Service-specific[30] and DoD-wide.[31]

Deployment Surveillance

Deployment surveillance is required by the US Congress in response to concerns from veterans. Extensive questionnaires are now collected before deployment, within 30 days after deployment, and 90–180 days after return.[32] The primary purpose of these questionnaires is to identify conditions that may need further clinical support or intervention, but they are used for analytic and health trend analysis surveillance purposes as well.

Environmental and Occupational Monitoring

Environmental and occupational monitoring here refers to DoD efforts to document the extent and short-/long-term consequences of military environmental and occupational exposures. Military environmental and occupational exposures have been an issue of considerable concern and attention in recent years, such as concern over lead exposure on military firing ranges or "burn pit" exposures in the Middle East. Documenting the extent and long-term consequences of such exposures has been a focus both within the DoD and by external groups such as the Institute of Medicine and the National Research Council.[33]

The DoD maintains extensive databases to archive much of this information, including the Defense Occupational and Environmental Health Readiness System—Industrial Hygiene and Military Exposure Surveillance Library. However, much of the data contained in these modules are area-based measurements, and they lack a robust collection of individual-level or service member-specific exposure information. There are differences among the Services in the amount of data they collect as well; the Air Force conducts more individual exposure sampling than the Navy or Army and catalogs it in the database.[33] The Future Vision section of this chapter elaborates on future efforts.

US DoD OCONUS Laboratory Surveillance Efforts

As briefly alluded to at the beginning of this chapter, the US DoD has long maintained and utilized laboratories in strategic locations throughout the world, primarily for researching and developing medical countermeasures. These laboratories enabled much of the countermeasure development also outlined in the section, "History of Military Contributions to Global Public Health". At present, the DoD maintains six laboratories as seen in Fig. 16-1. Laboratories in Kenya, Thailand, and the Republic of Georgia are supported by the Army and those in Egypt, Asia, and Peru are supported by the Navy.

Before 1997, infectious disease surveillance through the OCONUS laboratories was largely limited to specific disease countermeasure development programs. In 1997, the Presidential Decision Directive, National Science and Technology Council—#7, was released, specifically stating that "the mission of DoD will be expanded to include support of global surveillance, training, research and response to emerging infectious disease threats."[34] The **Global Emerging Infections Surveillance and Response System (GEIS)** was established in part to help fulfill this mandate. Now a division of the Armed Forces Health Surveillance Center (AFHSC), GEIS funding in support of this mission has expanded, with a majority of the support provided to the DoD OCONUS Navy and Army laboratories. This has enabled DoD laboratories throughout the world to engage more fully with local organizations such as Ministries of Health, Ministries of Defense, regional academic institutions, and other government and nongovernmental organizations in mutually beneficial ways. Through the building of these strategic partnerships, relevance to local host countries has been sustained and mission capabilities retained.

The GEIS network and its partners support a wide range of global surveillance efforts through a holistic approach that includes surveillance activities to prevent, detect, and respond to infectious diseases; training; surveillance innovation and integration; and coordination, communication, and collaboration among GEIS partners to facilitate responsive information sharing.[26] In 2014, GEIS network surveillance and training efforts reach 71 countries (Fig. 16-1). Outbreak assistance efforts are highlighted in Table 16-2. AFHSC effectively communicates information from the GEIS portfolio to support increased public awareness and understanding of important global issues and shaping of public health decisions. Surveillance findings are routinely shared with the defense and health ministries in host partner countries. GEIS encourages its partners to present and publish their findings in medical journals and at scientific meetings and to be compliant with the WHO International Health Regulations (IHR) (2005).[35,36]

Threat-Reduction Efforts

A chapter on DoD contributions to global public health would not be complete without highlighting the many contributions of the DoD's Cooperative Biological Engagement (CBEP) and Chemical Biological Defense (CBD) Programs. **CBEP** is a DoD program that works with partner countries to dismantle, destroy, and prevent the sale, theft, diversion, or use of biological weapons and to enhance the partner country's capability to survey, detect, diagnose, identify, secure, and report pathogens, diseases, or events of security concern.[26] CBEP is the biological threat-reduction component of the DoD's Cooperative Threat Reduction Program that has historically addressed the offensive biological weapons program and the scientific expertise left vulnerable after the collapse of the Soviet Union. CBEP has since expanded its cooperative threat-reduction efforts to the Middle East, Africa, and Southeast Asia.

The **CBD** program was established by the DoD to provide state-of-the-art defense capabilities to allow military forces of the USA to operate and successfully complete missions in chemical and biological warfare environments.[37] The CBD programs are working toward improved diagnostic capabilities that can be used in the field, and have several medical countermeasures in the pipeline that, if cleared by the Food and Drug Administration, will enable vaccination against or treatment of various infectious diseases. CBD is also funding the development of improved electronic surveillance tools that will assist in detection of and situational awareness for infectious disease outbreaks. Metrics are being developed to determine the outcome of these efforts, which will provide enormous benefits for global public health through prevention, early detection, and adequate recovery from any number of natural or intentional exposure events.[38]

It is critical to note that the public health programs in the DoD are working more closely than ever with the programs and products being developed by the CBEP and CBD programs. Many of the medical countermeasures and electronic surveillance tools will facilitate the integration that is badly needed in the DoD as well as information sharing with non-DoD partners and stakeholders throughout the world.

SUPPORT AND COLLABORATION WITH OTHER US GOVERNMENT AND INTERNATIONAL ENTITIES

Thus far, a basic understanding of the history of DoD public health surveillance and contributions to global public health has been outlined, followed by a glimpse of the breadth of activities that are currently underway. With this background, a few ongoing collaborations that the DoD has with other US government and international organizations will be highlighted, although many other examples could be provided.

Global presence brings global responsibilities, which means that the DoD must not work in a vacuum. Rather, the DoD has an obligation to share its knowledge and achievements. The DoD recognizes its responsibilities for "core competencies" and reporting under the IHR (2005). Article 9 of IHR (2005) states that parties have a responsibility to inform WHO within 24 h of receipt of evidence of a public health risk identified outside their territory that may cause international disease spread.[35,36] However, it is DoD policy to defer to the host country or country of identification if at all possible for decision to report. The DoD also attempts to defer to the host country or country of identification when diseases are detected during routine infectious disease surveillance or when health care is provided to local nationals or to US active-duty personnel. Indeed, with the 2009 influenza A H1N1 pandemic, the DoD found itself in this situation. When the emerging influenza strain was found within service members in various locations abroad, the DoD's first reporting responsibility was to the country where they were located, deferring to those countries to report through their regional WHO alerting avenues. Although this process is not always seamless, the intent strengthened collaborations and lines of communication with local health officials.[35]

TABLE 16-2 Fiscal Year 2013 Global Outbreaks with DoD Assistance

PILLAR	DISEASES	DATES	COUNTRY	USG PARTNERS AND OTHER COLLABORATORS	NO. OF CASES	IMPACT/CONTRIBUTION TO HOST COUNTRY HEALTH OFFICIALS
AMR	Nosocomial pseudomonas infection	April 2013	Peru	Ministry of Health	4	Diagnostic support
Enterics	*Vibrio parahaemolyticus*	September 2013	Thailand	Ministry of Defense	40	Epi and labs support
	Typhoid fever	October 2012	Peru	Ministry of Defense	3	Epi support through advisory
	Gastroenteritis	June 2013	Peru	Ministry of Defense	16	Epi support through advisory
	Acute gastroenteritis	October 2012-May 2013	USA	NRTC Great Lakes; MCRD-San Diego	2216	
FVBI	Brucellosis	January 2013	Nepal	Ministry of Health	9	Provided tube agglutination testing following initial slide agglutination screening performed at NPHL
	Dengue	June 2013	Cambodia	CDC; Ministry of Health	29	NAMRU-2 intensified surveillance in the area and provided expert advice on vector control
	Malaria	March 2013	Djibouti	Ministry of Health, Djibouti; National Institute of Public Health, Djibouti; Combine Task Force- Horn of Africa (CJTF-HOA)	1250+	Identification of malarial flambeau, assisted in identification of antimalarial resistance and parasite lineage, as well as id'd it was in fact endemic transmission
	Probable Mayaro fever	September 2012	Peru	Ministry of Health	1	Diagnosis advice
	Chickenpox	March 2013	Peru	Ministry of Defense	3	Epi support through advisory
	Nonspecific febrile illness	March 2013	Peru	Ministry of Defense	9	Epidemiologic, diagnostic and logistic support to Peruvian Navy, access to a fast diagnosis that allows early implementation of control measures
	Leptospirosis (probable)	June 2013	Peru	Ministry of Defense	1	Diagnostic support
Respiratory	Respiratory	November 2012–August 2013	Thailand	Ministry of Defense	187	Possible infection control and vaccination policy changes
	Influenza A/H5N1	August 2013	Nepal	Ministry of Health	No human cases	Provided surge diagnostic capacity to test samples of humans in contact with birds infected with H5N1 (e.g., cullers) for H5N1

TABLE 16-2 **Fiscal Year 2013 Global Outbreaks with DoD Assistance—cont'd**

PILLAR	DISEASES	DATES	COUNTRY	USG PARTNERS AND OTHER COLLABORATORS	NO. OF CASES	IMPACT/CONTRIBUTION TO HOST COUNTRY HEALTH OFFICIALS
	Influenza A/H5N1	January, July 2013	Cambodia	CDC; Ministry of Health; Ministry of Agriculture; Institute Pasteur, Cambodia	2	Infected child recovered; Ministry of Health investigation did not determine additional human cases; recent poultry die offs evident
	Convulsive cough	September 2012	Peru	Ministry of Defense	1	Epi support through advisory
	Viral meningitis	April 2013	Peru	Ministry of Defense	5	Epi support through advisory
	Conjunctivitis	January 2013	Peru	Ministry of Defense	29	Epi support through advisory
	Hyperendemics: Influenza A H1N1	June 2013	Peru	Ministry of Defense		Epidemiologic, diagnostic, and logistic support to Peruvian Navy, access to a fast diagnosis that allows early implementation of control measures
	Influenza A/H1N1	October 2012; June 2013	USA; US Deployed (Persian Gulf)	MCRD Parris Island, USAFSAM, USN 3rd Fleet	17	Among the earliest 2012–2013 season influenza isolates
	RSV	October 2012	USA	Tripler AMC, NEPMU-6	12	
	Respiratory illness	October 2012	USA	MCRD Parris Island	11	
	Pneumonia	June 2013	USA	Naval Air Facility, DC; AFHSC-GEIS	2	Ruled out potential 1st US case of MERS-CoV
	Influenza A and B	July 2013	US Deployed (Persian Gulf)	USN 3rd Fleet	19	
	MERS-CoV	April 2012–June 2013	USA	AFHSC-GEIS; CDC; State Health Departments; base-level public health/preventive medicine staff	4 PUI	Diagnostic support of hospital-based outbreak in Jordan in April 2012; two of the four investigations involved MERS-CoV testing at USAFSAM; both specimens tested negative for MERS-CoV, allowing for a more rapid stand-down of investigations that were utilizing numerous resources
	Chlamydia pneumonia	June 2013	USA	WRNMMC	1	Support to WRNMMC utilizing new capabilities

Another example of DoD's responsibilities under IHR (2005) also focuses on collaboration. The DoD sponsored a forum in St. Petersburg, Russia, in September of 2010, at which military medical department representatives from 41 countries discussed their responsibilities for reporting to and supporting their civilian counterparts. It was recognized that in many countries the military has the strongest medical infrastructure and capability that should be leveraged. Participants were encouraged to identify their local civilian focal point for reporting to WHO and establish open communication and information sharing.[39]

The DoD's global laboratories, discussed above, are guests within their respective countries, and as such each laboratory is sponsored by either the local Ministry of Health or Ministry of Defense. Although each laboratory has a cadre of active-duty researchers, the vast majority of support comes from locally hired staff. Each laboratory maintains close collaborations with not only its host organization but also with many other governmental and academic groups in strategic partnerships. These partnerships must provide added value to the local government with complete transparency. Although this could be viewed as health diplomacy, in reality it is using DoD assets for both force protection and global public health benefits.[40]

Through these collaborations and support to regional surveillance and research assets, the DoD global laboratories also hold various WHO designations. The laboratory in Bangkok, Thailand, for example, is a collaborating center for diagnostics and training. This designation defines its role in supporting member states to coordinate and harmonize disease outbreak diagnostics and response activities to strengthen the Global Outbreak Alert and Response Network; to disseminate findings of emerging and re-emerging disease research and laboratory diagnostics for the benefit of regional health surveillance activities; and to encourage greater mobilization of country-level diagnostics and prevention activities through innovative global, regional, and local partnerships. The laboratory in Kenya is a WHO regional reference laboratory for yellow fever and a member of the African Regional Office Emerging Dangerous Pathogen Laboratory Network. A **reference laboratory** is a laboratory that provides authoritative test results.[26] WHO has a network of reference laboratories, for example. The laboratory in Cairo, Egypt, also has WHO collaborating center responsibilities for emerging and re-emerging infectious diseases with three reference laboratory designations that fall under this umbrella: (1) malaria microscopy and antimalarial drug resistance; (2) influenza, including H5N1 and H1N1; and (3) genotyping rotavirus for the Eastern Mediterranean Regional Office. Additionally, the CDC's Global Disease Detection center is co-located within the Cairo laboratory. In a true "whole of government" approach, Naval researchers are able to benefit from the expertise that CDC brings while limiting redundancy and expense by sharing facilities and administrative infrastructure. Depending upon the collaboration that is needed, the laboratory can play a military, CDC, or WHO role in facilitating outreach efforts and minimizing sensitivities.

The DoD effort in influenza surveillance is another example of collaboration with CDC and WHO to benefit global public health. Although some aspects of this program were covered previously, the extensive collaborations deserve mention here. Since the creation of the AFHSC in early 2008, centralized DoD influenza and other respiratory disease surveillance efforts have been in place, spanning over 400 sites in over 70 countries, including active-duty US military as well as host-country civilian and military personnel at health facilities, research laboratories and field locations worldwide.[41] Priority is given to rapid molecular processing of influenza samples to determine strain type and monitoring for new strain emergence. Relevant portions of the sequenced genome are forwarded to CDC for integration with their influenza genome databases. Unique samples may then be requested by the CDC for further testing and investigation. Original samples from sequences that exhibit evidence of strain variation are often requested by CDC for culturing and inclusion in reference panels or vaccine seed preparations.[42] At the beginning of the 2009 influenza A H1N1 pandemic, the military's laboratory-based, respiratory disease surveillance efforts were responsible for the initial detection of this virus, which occurred among four military dependents who presented with ILI symptoms at DoD military medical treatment facilities and US–Mexico border clinics in San Diego, California, and San Antonio, Texas. Through rapid sequencing and communication with CDC, investigations demonstrated that the viruses were identical but lacked evidence of an epidemiologic link. This was the beginning of the 2009 influenza A H1N1 pandemic, during which DoD–CDC collaboration helped facilitate global public health responses.[43-46]

Another example of collaboration is with the US Department of Health & Human Services (HHS) Office of the Assistant Secretary for Preparedness and Response (ASPR). HHS-ASPR oversees US government (USG) International Capacity Building under the IHR (2005). Many USG departments and agencies partner with other countries and WHO to support the development and strengthening of IHR core capacities. However, to know exactly who is doing what and where, a tool to improve coordination and provide a comprehensive picture of USG IHR capacity-building efforts internationally is needed. This effort, with partial support from GEIS, is to develop and provide a USG collaboration web-accessible tool that comprehensively captures and illustrates IHR capacity-building efforts internationally as performed by different USG agencies. It is being developed in the form of a common operating picture, facilitating visualization and strategic assessment of current and future USG international engagements to build IHR core capacities, thereby promoting interagency coordination of IHR core capacity-building efforts internationally.

Many other collaborative efforts with the US DoD exist but cannot be expanded upon in this venue. They include, but are not limited to (1) US DoD "Secondees" to the WHO Headquarters in Geneva and European regional office in Copenhagen to facilitate bilateral and transparent information sharing; (2) support to and collaborations with the International Committee of Military Medicine, in partnership with WHO, to train and provide public health tools to militaries throughout the world, in keeping with the IHR (2005);[39] (3) collaborations with information sharing on a common information technology internet-accessible tool within the Republic of Korea—including the Korean Armed Forces, Korean Center for Disease Control, and US Forces Korea; (4) development, in conjunction with the Johns Hopkins University Applied Physics Laboratory, and sharing of a tool called Suite for Automated Global Electronic bioSurveillance to enhance open-source and adaptable electronic disease surveillance ideally adapted for resource-poor settings, now being leveraged by 12 countries; and (5) support for the multidrug-resistant organism Repository and Surveillance Network that comprises a public health diagnostic laboratory within the military enterprise, with extensive testing for existing and emerging antimicrobial resistance, and sharing of findings with national and international communities.

FUTURE VISION FOR HEALTH SURVEILLANCE IN THE DOD

The primary purpose of DoD health surveillance is to provide a fit and healthy military. However, as outlined in the introduction and further illustrated in the historical contributions and collaborations sections, there are secondary effects that can offer significant advantages and benefits to the USA and other populations. Despite robust surveillance on many levels, there is still much room for improvement.

First and foremost, integration needs to be improved within the DoD to increase the visibility of all activities and the sharing of such information. Many of the Services in the DoD continue to run activities independent of each other. One effort currently underway to help integrate the Services is the ambitious and wide scale "Defense Health Agency," the intent of which is to consolidate redundant Service-specific capabilities into DoD-wide capabilities to serve the entire DoD. The impetus of this consolidation is not only cost savings but also improving communication and coordination and eliminating redundancy. This effort will help DoD achieve better visibility and integration of information.

Another example of DoD future vision initiatives is the collection of individual-level environmental and occupational exposure data. This can be in the form of a database that takes institutional or community-wide data, identifies all individuals in that community, and applies those data to individually linked databases. This information could also be collected from personal exposure monitors, much like the radiation exposure that individual dosimeters track for service members with potential radiation exposure. The "Individual-Level Exposure Records" initiative is attempting to address part of this gap in health surveillance within the DoD. Technological advances might facilitate the identification of exposures that utilize biological material collected from service members and test them for metabolic products that can signify exposures that could have health consequences. These exposure determinations could then be linked to health outcomes in order to identify risky practices or exposures that can be mitigated.

Next, the DoD has a unique opportunity to contribute to global public health through enhanced interactions with other countries' military forces. No other organization in the USA currently emphasizes working with militaries in other countries. Military forces around the world can work together to demonstrate their support to civilian authorities with primary responsibility for responding to global infectious disease or public health emergencies. Militaries have unique logistical and transportation infrastructures that can and should be leveraged.[39,47] At the time of publication of this book, this is being demonstrated robustly within Liberia in response to the West Africa Ebola crisis. The US DoD has been asked to engage with logistics, construction of vital infrastructure, training, and Command Center coordination.

Finally, DoD and USG integration and collaboration would mean nothing if the USA, as part of the global community, does not share transparently with the global community. A collaborative, online sharing tool, open to all countries and allowing integration within and across governments, would be one way to accomplish this. An international organization is likely to be more globally accepted in championing and driving this type of vision than the USA or DoD. Although some countries might be reluctant to share this type of information, given potential economic ramifications or social isolation, this mentality seems to be much less prominent than it once was. This shift may be due to the paradigm-breaking IHR (2005), which minimizes the importance of national borders for disease surveillance. Using H5N1 influenza as an example, Davies[48] and colleagues report "strong support to the claim that East Asian states have come to accept and comply with the duty to report infectious disease outbreaks and that the assertions of sovereignty in response to global health governance frameworks have not systematically inhibited reporting compliance."

The US DoD's efforts to improve force health protection has yielded important medical benefits to people throughout the world. Lives have been saved through active surveillance, improved public health and medical countermeasure practices, diagnostic assays development and other studies leading to a better understanding of endemic and emerging diseases. DoD's assistance to the international community's efforts to respond to the unprecedented outbreak of Ebola in West Africa is just one example of how unique DoD capabilities contribute to life-saving missions globally. Through active engagement and collaborative efforts among militaries, among organizations, and among countries, global health surveillance and response capabilities can be improved for the benefit of all.

KEY SUMMARY POINTS

- The engagement of the DoD in health surveillance activities might not be intuitive to the lay public at first glance, but disease and nonbattle injuries (as opposed to battle injuries) have been the major cause of troop morbidity throughout the history.
- The DoD's historical contributions to global public health have included malaria and vector-borne diseases, diarrheal diseases, and influenza and respiratory diseases.
- DoD health surveillance activities include health care encounter monitoring, reportable medical events, field activities, deployment surveillance, environmental and occupational monitoring, the OCONUS laboratory surveillance efforts, threat-reduction activities, and others.
- The DoD has an obligation to share its knowledge and achievements and to collaborate with other US agencies and international organizations.
- DoD has several initiatives and efforts underway to improve collaboration, increase information sharing, and enhance integration with other entities.

DISCUSSION QUESTIONS

1. How are the military and the DoD uniquely positioned to improve public health for malaria, gastrointestinal diseases, and respiratory diseases or other conditions, based on the historical examples included in the chapter and outside information?
2. What emerging public health threats would the DoD likely be involved with? Why?
3. How are the DoD's seven surveillance activities described above (health care encounter monitoring, reportable medical events, field activities, etc.) similar to or different from how a local, state, or federal public health agency might conduct surveillance?

4. In what ways do the IHR (2005) facilitate the DoD's efforts to improve integration, collaboration, and coordination? How might they hinder these efforts?
5. Based on the information in the chapter and outside information, evaluate the DoD's initiatives to increase integration and transparency.
6. How can technology and IT solutions help DoD achieve its surveillance goals?

Acknowledgments

A sincere thanks to Jennifer Rubenstein for her extensive assistance with research for this chapter. Many thanks to Joel Gaydos, Julie Pavlin, and Jose "Toti" Sanchez for their suggestions and edits. Penny Masuoka was extremely helpful for the maps used in the chapter, and finally, thanks to Ramzy Azar, Kelly Vest, William Meyer, and Kevin Haines for their specific contributions.

Disclaimer

The opinions and views expressed in this chapter are those of the author and do not necessarily represent the official opinion of the US Department of Defense. The author has no financial disclosures to report.

REFERENCES

1. Beaumier CM, Gomez-Rubio AM, Hotez PJ, Weina PJ. United States military tropical medicine: extraordinary legacy, uncertain future. PLoS Negl Trop Dis 2013;7(12):e2448.
2. About the DoD: Department of Defense, <http://www.defense.gov/about/%5D/>.
3. Bayne-Jones S. The evolution of preventive medicine in the United States Army, 1607-1939. In: Anderson RS, editor. Washington, DC: U.S. Government Printing Office; 2009.
4. Wintermute BA. Public health and the US Military: a history of the Army Medical Department, 1818-1917. New York: Routledge; 2011. p. 284.
5. Hoke Jr CH. History of U.S. military contributions to the study of viral encephalitis. Mil Med 2005;170(Suppl. 4):92–105.
6. Artenstein AW, Opal JM, Opal SM, Tramont EC, Peter G, Russell PK. History of U.S. military contributions to the study of vaccines against infectious diseases. Mil Med 2005;170(Suppl. 4):3–11.
7. Grabenstein JD, Pittman PR, Greenwood JT, Engler RJ. Immunization to protect the US Armed Forces: heritage, current practice, and prospects. Epidemiol Rev 2006;28:3–26.
8. Ockenhouse CF, Magill A, Smith D, Milhous W. History of U.S. military contributions to the study of malaria. Mil Med 2005;170(Suppl. 4):12–6.
9. Hitchcock P, Chamberlain A, Van Wagoner M, Inglesby TV, O'Toole T. Challenges to global surveillance and response to infectious disease outbreaks of international importance. Biosecur Bioterror 2007;5(3):206–27.
10. Rocco F. The miraculous fever-tree. New York: HarperCollins; 2003.
11. Russell PF. Man's mastery of malaria. London: Oxford University Press; 1955.
12. Harrison G. Mosquitoes, malaria, and man. New York, NYC: E.P. Dutton; 19878.
13. Noedl H, Se Y, Schaecher K, Smith BL, Socheat D, Fukuda MM. Evidence of artemisinin-resistant malaria in western Cambodia. N Engl J Med 2008;359(24):2619–20.
14. Saunders D, Duplessis C, Lescano A, Andagalu B, Thomas A, Fukuda M, et al. US Department of Defense contributions to malaria surveillance. Lancet Infect Dis 2013;13(4):293–4.
15. Lim ML, Murphy GS, Calloway M, Tribble D. History of U.S. military contributions to the study of diarrheal diseases. Mil Med 2005;170 (Suppl. 4):30–8.
16. Water with sugar and salt (editorial). Lancet 1978;2(8084):300–1.
17. DuPont HL, Levine MM, Hornick RB, Formal SB. Inoculum size in shigellosis and implications for expected mode of transmission. J Infect Dis 1989;159(6):1126–8.
18. O'Brien AO, Lively TA, Chen ME, Rothman SW, Formal SB. Escherichia coli O157:H7 strains associated with haemorrhagic colitis in the United States produce a Shigella dysenteriae 1 (SHIGA) like cytotoxin. Lancet 1983;1(8326 Pt 1):702.
19. Hoge CW, Gambel JM, Srijan A, Pitarangsi C, Echeverria P. Trends in antibiotic resistance among diarrheal pathogens isolated in Thailand over 15 years. Clin Infect Dis 1998;26(2):341–5.
20. Patterson KD, Pyle GF. The geography and mortality of the 1918 influenza pandemic. Bull Hist Med 1991;65(1):4–21.
21. Ottolini MG, Burnett MW. History of U.S. military contributions to the study of respiratory infections. Mil Med 2005;170(Suppl. 4):66–70.
22. Takafuji ET, Gaydos JC, Allen RG, Top Jr FH. Simultaneous administration of live, enteric-coated adenovirus types 4, 7 and 21 vaccines: safety and immunogenicity. J Infect Dis 1979;140(1):48–53.
23. Kuschner RA, Russell KL, Abuja M, Bauer KM, Faix DJ, Hait H, et al. A phase 3, randomized, double-blind, placebo-controlled study of the safety and efficacy of the live, oral adenovirus type 4 and type 7 vaccine, in U.S. military recruits. Vaccine 2013;31(28):2963–71.
24. Russell K. Respiratory infections in military recruits. In: Lenhart MK, Lounsbury DE, North Jr, RB, editors. Textbooks of military medicine: recruit medicine. Washington, DC: Borden Institute; 2006.
25. Christopher GW, Agan MB, Cieslak TJ, Olson PE. History of U.S. military contributions to the study of bacterial zoonoses. Mil Med 2005;170 (Suppl. 4):39–48.
26. Definition provided by the chapter author.
27. Armed Forces Reportable Medical Events Guidelines and Case Definitions. Armed Forces Health Surveillance Center, <http://www.afhsc.mil/Home/ReportableEvents>; September 30, 2015.
28. Medical Surveillance and Medical Event Reporting Technical Manual. Portsmouth, VA: Navy and Marine Corps Public Health Center; 2011.
29. Ball J. Infections are the true beneficiaries of war. BBC News; 2013.
30. Field hygiene and sanitation. US: Department of the Army and Commandant. Marine Corps 2000; FM 21-10 <https://archive.org/details/FM21-10_2000>.
31. Deployment Health. Under Secretary of Defense for Personnel and Readiness. 2011.

32. Comprehensive Health Surveillance. In: Department of Defense Directive, editor; 2013.
33. DeFraites RF, Richards EE. Assessing potentially hazardous environmental exposures among military populations: 2010 symposium and workshop summary and conclusions. Mil Med 2011;176(Suppl. 7):1–112.
34. Clinton W. Presidential decision directive NSTC-7 emerging infectious diseases. Washington, DC: The White House; 1997.
35. Johns M, Blazes DL, Fernandez J, Russell K, Chen DW, Loftis R. The United States Department of Defense and the International Health Regulations (2005): perceptions, pitfalls and progress towards implementation. Bull World Health Organ 2011;89(3):234–5.
36. Johns MC, Blazes DL. International Health Regulations (2005) and the U.S. Department of Defense: building core capacities on a foundation of partnership and trust. BMC public health 2010;10(Suppl. 1):S4.
37. Chemical and biological defense small business innovation research, <http://www.cbdsbir.net/>; September 30, 2015.
38. 2013 Department of Defense Chemical and Biological Defense annual report to Congress. In: Program CaBD, editor. U.S. Department of Defense; 2013. <http://www.acq.osd.mil/cp/docs/2013%20DoD%20CBDP%20ARC_FINAL_13%20May%202013.pdf>.
39. Russell K, Johns M, Lipnick R, Sessions C. Global militaries unite. Discussion of responsibilities under the International Health regulations (2005): Saint Petersburg 2010. JHSH 2011;1(1):131–40. Spring.
40. Russell KL, Rubenstein J, Burke RL, Vest KG, Johns MC, Sanchez JL, et al. The Global Emerging Infection Surveillance and Response System (GEIS), a U.S. government tool for improved global biosurveillance: a review of 2009. BMC public health 2011;11(Suppl. 2):S2.
41. Sueker J, Blazes D, Johns M, Blair P, Sjoberg P, Tjaden J, et al. Influenza and respiratory disease surveillance: the US military's global laboratory-based network. Influenza Other Respir Viruses 2010;4(3):155–61.
42. Canas LC, Lohman K, Pavlin JA, Endy T, Singh DL, Pandey P, et al. The Department of Defense laboratory-based global influenza surveillance system. Mil Med 2000;165(7 Suppl. 2):52–6.
43. Swine influenza A (H1N1) infection in two children—Southern California, March-April 2009. MMWR Morb Mortal Wkly Rep 2009;58(15):400–2.
44. Dawood FS, Jain S, Finelli L, Shaw MW, Lindstrom S, Garten RJ, et al. Emergence of a novel swine-origin influenza A (H1N1) virus in humans. N Engl J Med 2009;360(25):2605–15.
45. Petruccelli B, Otto JL, Johns MC, Lipnick RJ. U.S. military public health surveillance and response to pandemic influenza A (H1N1). Am J Prev Med 2010;39(5):483–6.
46. Johns MC, Burke RL, Vest KG, Fukuda M, Pavlin JA, Shrestha SK, et al. A growing global network's role in outbreak response: AFHSC-GEIS 2008-2009. BMC Public Health 2011;11(Suppl. 2):S3.
47. Blazes DL, Russell KL. Medicine in war and peace: joining forces. Nature 2011;477(7365):395–6.
48. Davies S. The International Politics of Disease Reporting: towards Post-Westphalianis. Int Polit 2012;49(5):591–613.

CHAPTER

17

Nonprofit Associations and Cultivating Collaboration to Advance Public Health Surveillance

Laura C Streichert, Paula Soper, Ian Watson

In the long history of humankind (and animal kind, too) those who learned to collaborate and improvise most effectively have prevailed.

Charles Darwin

KEY WORDS

Association
Partnership
Nongovernmental organization (NGO)
Capacity building assistance (CBA)
Technical assistance

INTRODUCTION

More than a decade into the twenty-first century, it is still difficult to effectively forecast, detect, and respond to disease outbreaks and other events of public health significance in the rapid timeframe that the public expects. Nonprofit associations serve a vital role in helping governmental public health agencies by providing the collaboration, information exchange, workforce development, knowledge management, system improvements, and advocacy needed to tackle challenges in disease surveillance in new ways.[1] An **association** is any organization of people who share similar interests, professions, or other commonality.[2]

Innovations in public health surveillance often stem from the convergence of ideas provided when people with different perspectives take coordinated action. While technological tools assist the innovation process, building trust and aligning priorities among stakeholders with similar interests is key to adapting to a rapidly evolving surveillance landscape. Among other roles, nonprofit membership-based associations (hereafter Associations) tap into the collective experience and energies of their networks to identify how to improve public health programs, services, and policies. Associations focused on public health surveillance serve as champions for positive change in this arena.

Nonprofit organizations provide the sustained support needed for public health agencies to get data in the right hands at the right time. Current reports of the cross-border spread of Middle Eastern Respiratory Syndrome (MERS), caused by a novel virus, are reminders of the need for public health agencies to be ever vigilant and have systems in place for public health response.[3] Associations are well positioned to help public agencies maintain readiness to detect and respond to the growing risk of emerging infectious diseases, the rising burden of chronic conditions, increase in the number and severity of natural events, and other known and unforeseen events. They achieve this by bringing ideas to action—by harmonizing efforts, creating linkages between jurisdictions and program areas, advocating for funding and policy changes, and maintaining the momentum needed to implement new practices and policies.

The strategic vision for an integrated surveillance enterprise expressed by national and international leaders calls for efficient, flexible, and comprehensive systems that will require partnerships to attain these goals.[4] A **partnership** is an association of two or more persons or entities typically involving close cooperation to achieve common goals.[2] When formalized into legal and incorporated nonprofit associations or professional societies, these partnerships create an organizational home and a structure for coordinated action on short- and long-term goals.

This chapter will highlight examples of nongovernmental, independent membership-based associations with a strong focus on disease surveillance in the USA and abroad. A professional association is just one of the many ways in which **nongovernmental organizations (NGOs)** are structured throughout the world. An NGO is any nonprofit, voluntary group of citizens organized on a local, national, or international level that performs service, educational, or humanitarian functions, advocates or monitors policies, and/or encourages informed decision-making.[2] Some are organized as a quasi-autonomous nongovernmental organization (quango), defined as a government-funded body working in the private sector.[5] Others are organizations with organizational members, as described later in the chapter.

ASSOCIATIONS AND THE PUBLIC HEALTH SURVEILLANCE ENTERPRISE

The effective functioning of the public health system relies on the individual and coordinated efforts of its different components (Fig. 17-1). In the realm of public health surveillance, nonprofit associations play an important role by working directly with the front line of surveillance: local and state health departments. Associations provide the cross-jurisdiction perspective and support practitioners need in order to keep up-to-date with new perspectives, best practices, and resources needed to improve their public health surveillance practices.

Professional associations typically originate when a group of colleagues identify an unfilled need that could be best addressed with coordinated action. For example, the Council of State and Territorial Epidemiologists (CSTE) grew out of a need identified in the 1950s for collective input into national disease reporting.[7] The Association of State and Territorial Health Officials (ASTHO) was officially incorporated in 1942, but its roots date back to a Sanitary Council of the Mississippi Valley discussion in 1879 about strategies for controlling cholera outbreaks.[8] The International Epidemiological Association (IEA) began in 1954 as the International Corresponding Club to foster communication between physicians working in academics and research institutions. After hosting a number of conferences throughout the world, they incorporated as IEA to focus on the scholarly exchange of research in epidemiology, especially among academic researchers.

There are three primary types of membership associations that address public health surveillance issues. The first type supports a range of activities in a particular domain of public health. The Safe States Alliance, for example, is an association that focuses on a wide range of injury and violence prevention issues, including surveillance. The second type of association represents executive leaders of governmental public health agencies while supporting programmatic functions within those agencies. The two primary US associations in this category are ASTHO and the National Association of County and City Health Officials (NACCHO), which represent state and local public health officials, respectively. Both associations are deeply involved in workforce development, advocacy, and programmatic support across a wide range or areas of public health surveillance.

The third type of association focuses primarily on public health surveillance and epidemiology through interdisciplinary partnerships. CSTE, for example, supports a wide range of program areas within surveillance, including infectious disease, chronic disease, environmental health and injury. The International Union for Health Promotion and Education (IUHPE; http://www.iuhpe.org/) is similarly working to build professional public health networks with projects to advance public health, although they are not focused strictly on disease surveillance.

The International Society for Disease Surveillance (ISDS) is another example of this third type of association. ISDS began as a grassroots initiative, partly in response to the need for real-time situational awareness after the terrorist events of 9/11 and the mailing of anthrax letters in the USA.[9] The first National Syndromic Surveillance Conference was held in New York City in 2002 to advance knowledge and create innovative approaches for collecting and sharing real-time data for public health surveillance. Successive annual conferences established the scientific foundations of the field and helped define a new community of surveillance professionals drawn from public health practice, academia, and the private sector with expertise in epidemiology, informatics, and statistics. In response to the need for an institutional home for this interdisciplinary community, ISDS was launched in 2005 as a national independent nonprofit professional society.

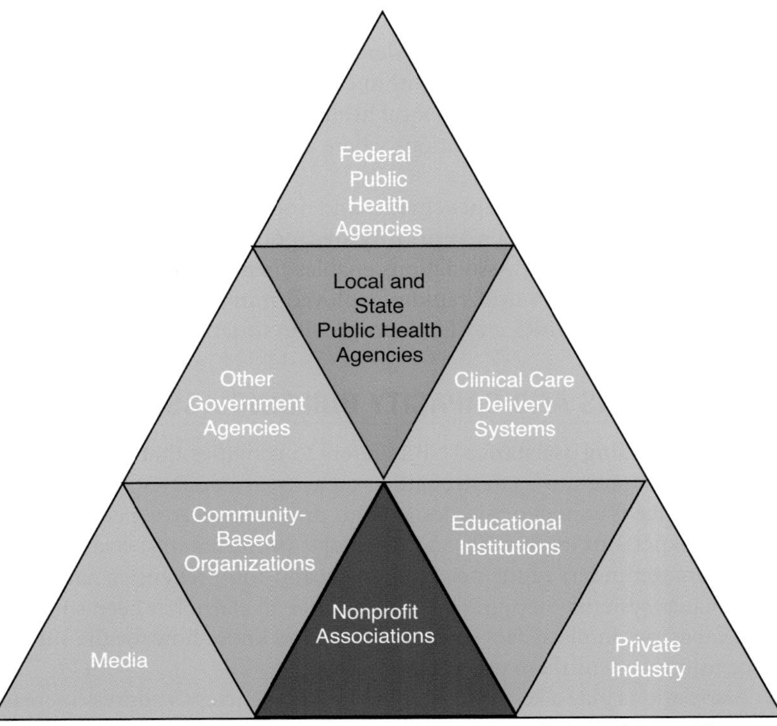

FIG. 17-1 Components of the public health system. *(Adapted from Chapman K, 2013[6])*

Associations represent a discrete component of the public health system primarily because of their designation as nongovernmental entities with a public-oriented mission. In the USA, nonprofit associations are legal entities recognized by the Internal Revenue Service (IRS) as tax-exempt, charitable organizations that must meet certain requirements as "charitable, educational, medical, religious, or scientific organizations" that provide some type of public good. [10] Internationally, nonprofit organizations are typically required to register in the countries in which they operate.

People join a society or association to be part of a community of professionals addressing similar topics and challenges. Membership is based on a relationship with the scope, mission, and activities of those organizations. The "communities of practice" that Associations establish through volunteer committees and workgroups provide a means for channeling the collective knowledge and experience of a group of professionals toward a common goal through regular interaction.[11] They also provide opportunities to engage public health practitioners in leadership roles as, for example, committee chairs and representatives in national advisory groups.

Ongoing collaboration builds trust and leverages previous investments in money, time, and energy that are then compounded as activities build on one another. The networking and intellectual excitement at conferences and meetings often spark ideas for new collaborations that lead to other joint activities. For example, at a recent Regional Data Sharing workshop organized by ISDS and ASTHO, workshop participants continued to work together after the workshop on data sharing issues. They submitted an abstract for further discussion at the next ISDS conference[12] that subsequently led to a paper and recommendations for strategies to facilitate data sharing. The final steps are now underway to work with associations to implement and disseminate the work to a broader audience. This example illustrates how Associations can take a logic-model approach to coordinating a project from new idea to objectives, outputs, outcomes, and impact.

Unlike government or corporate organizations, nonprofit associations take a nonpartisan approach to problems and solutions. As private organizations, Associations have established relationships with their members and the agility to support public health agencies through activities that may be prohibited or outside the scope of work of other organization types, notably federal agencies. As politically neutral third-party entities, they can bridge government sectors, both between and within countries—such as between the federal US Centers for Disease Control and Prevention (CDC) and state and local health departments. This enables collaborations that may not otherwise occur, especially in international situations where affiliation with a governmental entity can raise political sensitivities and questions of authority.

Associations also can adapt activities and resources to address new concerns, such as emergency events or outbreak situations, recognition of a new priority area, policy changes, and funding opportunities. The leaner and less bureaucratic structure of many Associations enables them to mobilize resources as needed. For example, in 2014, associations throughout the world rapidly deployed initiatives for public health jurisdictions to collect and report any suspected cases of MERS and Ebola to provide situational awareness on a global scale.

ASSOCIATIONS AND CAPACITY BUILDING ASSISTANCE

Capacity building assistance (CBA) refers to activities that provide guidance, support, and technical assistance to people and organizations to strengthen capacity in a designated area (e.g., to deliver public health services).[2] **Technical assistance** is a form of aid designed to provide expertise needed to promote surveillance practice. It can include sending experts to teach skills and help solve problems in specialized areas.[2] Throughout the world, emergent outbreaks are reminders of the need for strong and comprehensive national preparedness programs that rely on robust surveillance systems. Stepping up systems after an alarm has been sounded is ineffective. Public health agencies must have capacities in place. However, resources and know-how for the surveillance practices needed and a skilled workforce to implement them are often lacking.

Associations play a key role in aiding health agencies to address increasing pressure to provide more public health services with fewer resources, while increasing adoption of evidence-based practices. In the USA, CDC has recognized the role of national nonprofit associations to provide CBA as a means "to optimize the quality and performance of public health systems, the public health workforce, public health data and information systems, public health practice and services, public health partnerships, and public health resources."[13]

By assessing the priorities and capacities of their sector of the public health community, Associations identify where CBA is most needed through activities that include technical consultations and assistance, information transfer, training, and funding. While the interaction between an Association and its members is ongoing, Associations will step up to address new concerns that arise in times of outbreak or policy change, as described above.

Associations help public health surveillance professionals stay abreast of the latest methodologies, models, business processes, policies, roles, and procedures.[14] Public health authorities do not have extra time, energy, or financial resources to "reinvent the wheel"—and they do not need to when resources are available from Associations. Furthermore, surveillance responsibilities within health departments are often siloed such that different components—such as those addressing infectious disease and chronic diseases or injury—do not interact as effectively as possible. Associations contribute by providing opportunities for colleagues who work specifically in surveillance, such as epidemiologists and analysts, to collaborate and share information across agencies and sectors. This includes a number of ways to collaborate, including webinars, committees, workgroups, and online trainings.

For example, ASTHO, with initial funding and support from CDC, has brought together a steering committee of members from more than 10 associations and 3 federal agencies to collaboratively plan the Public Health Community Platform (PHCP). **ASTHO** is the national nonprofit organization representing public health agencies in the USA, the US territories, and the District of Columbia and over 100,000 public health professionals these agencies employ.[8]

The PHCP is a public health community-owned asset to support data sharing and data exchange; sharing of technical services and applications; sharing of analytic and visualization tools, surveillance methodologies and data sets; and the sharing of other resources to support the state, territorial, local, and tribal governmental public health enterprise. The PHCP represents a significant change in public health business practices around data collections, sharing, and analysis. The vision for this platform is driven by many of the Associations most actively engaged in public health surveillance activities.

Associations are also hubs for rapidly disseminating information to their members through multiple communication mechanisms, including websites, forums, blogs, and social media to keep the dialogue going within a community. A challenge for the Associations themselves is to be aware of the latest communication modalities and tools to improve reach and impact.

Although public health agencies are strongly encouraged to implement evidence-based measures and procedures, there is a lack of rigorously reviewed information on which to base action. Associations help overcome this challenge by building bridges between the public health and academic research communities through journal publications, conference proceedings, manuscripts, and other resources in the published and gray literature. New results are disseminated through presentations, webinars, and workshops to introduce and share best practices, new tools, and other recommendations.

Many associations routinely poll their members to ensure that programmatic, policy, and research initiatives are aligned with the needs of their constituencies and to tailor their work more effectively. These assessments range from informal surveys from a convenience sample of respondents to more structured surveys subject to qualitative and quantitative analysis. ISDS, in association with ASTHO, for example, has twice conducted a nationwide survey of syndromic surveillance practice to identify areas for technical assistance, standards development, and targeted knowledge and skill-building training. CSTE regularly conducts assessments to determine epidemiology workforce capacity and needs, which can lead to new policy priorities or activities that reflect changing needs among the current workforce.

There is wide variability in surveillance systems' capability and workforce capacity. By providing CBA in the form of technical consultations, information transfers, fellowships, funding for pilot projects, and training opportunities, such as workshops, to identify and implement standards of practice, associations can help bring health departments to a minimum level of surveillance capability. Associations also facilitate peer-learning networks to help public health professionals learn from and assist one another. For instance, CSTE has a peer-to-peer technical assistance program where HIV-surveillance coordinators go to another jurisdiction to help newer surveillance coordinator learn how to conduct HIV surveillance activities.

One area of future development for Associations is promotion of more rigorous and outcome-based evaluations for information exchange, training, and technical support. There is a growing body of evidence from the emerging field of dissemination and implementation research that applies elements of translational science relevant to public health in order to "accrue the most public health benefit from scientific discoveries."[15] By using education and communication principles, such as the diffusion of innovations theory,[16] associations can hone their communications, marketing, and community-building activities to be even more effective.

The Distribute Project as an Example of Association Capacity Building Assistance

The importance of associations in helping jurisdictions provide data for situational awareness became evident on June 11, 2009, when the World Health Organization (WHO) declared a global pandemic of novel influenza A (H1N1).[17] In the USA, H1N1 cases were appearing throughout the nation, and health departments wanted to confirm the data anomalies they were seeing. Public health agencies across the country ramped up surveillance for influenza-like illness (ILI). Many jurisdictions activated their automated syndromic surveillance system (some for the first time), which was a relatively new addition to the arsenal of surveillance tools used by public health practitioners.

Earlier, in 2006, colleagues from state and large metropolitan area health jurisdictions, with support from ISDS, initiated the Distributed Surveillance Taskforce for Real-time Influenza Burden Tracking and Evaluation (hereafter Distribute) project as a pilot to demonstrate how the surveillance community could voluntarily share summarized, de-identified ILI data for the purpose of situational awareness.[18] As the pandemic unfolded, ISDS, with CDC funding, stepped in to provide the coordination and fiscal management required to expand the project. Working with the

University of Washington, ISDS set up a collection point for jurisdictions to send syndromic surveillance system data that classified hospital emergency department medical records and other data into a collection of symptoms that define "syndromes." Comparisons of de-identified aggregate data provided the most near real-time (usually every 24 h) data available on a potential outbreak. At the height of the pandemic, Distribute grew to become a nationwide system that received data from 43 state and local health jurisdictions, representing over 50% of the US population and more than 35% of all emergency department visits nationwide.[19] Many of the principles of Distribute have been integrated into BioSense 2.0, a nationwide syndromic surveillance system.

Key to Distribute's success was the enthusiastic and engaged community of practice created to tap into the expertise of those using a syndromic surveillance system for ILI surveillance. The learning community started by Distribute continues today with ISDS support for ongoing collaboration among surveillance colleagues from jurisdictions and partner organizations from the academic, government, and private sectors.

ASSOCIATIONS AND STANDARDS DEVELOPMENT

The surveillance systems used by health departments are traditionally based on local priorities and available funding. Consequently, public health jurisdictions worldwide vary greatly in their surveillance capacity and the components of their systems. This variability can be seen in the National Profile of Local Health Departments published annually by NACCHO.[20] This report documents differences in epidemiology and surveillance services and provides baseline information for goal setting, measuring progress, and targeting education and training activities.

The era in which every health department can develop its own surveillance processes, policies, and practices is no longer viable given human and financial resource constraints and increasing drives to standardize the collection, analysis, and sharing of data. In the USA, the health care sector has increasingly adopted electronic health record (EHR) technology and programs to put data to "meaningful use" by exchanging it with public health agencies. Meaningful use has fueled a drive toward enhanced systems and greater standards for what data are collected, how they are exchanged, and their application for different public health purposes, including electronic laboratory reporting, syndromic surveillance, and cancer and immunization registries.[21]

As national organizations that cover public practitioners across jurisdictions and sectors, Associations provide critical services at every stage of standards development, from the identification of the need for a standard and in creating a demand for it, to development, implementation, evaluation, and, in some cases, ongoing stewardship. Specifically, Associations can help to develop case definitions, usage of new technologies, data collection tools, evaluation platforms, algorithms, data transport mechanisms, and syndromic surveillance syndrome definitions, to name a few. Some associations, such as the American Health Information Management Association (AHIMA), which recently merged with the Public Health Data Standards Consortium, are specifically focused on standards for integrating health information technology (IT) into public health practice.

Acting as neutral facilitators, Associations have played a key role in the adoption of new standards by addressing needs for interoperability yet allowing flexibility for local practices. One example is ISDS's role in developing recommendations for standards for the use of EHR data from hospital settings for the purpose of syndromic surveillance. Standards were developed with active input from a multidisciplinary workgroup of public health practitioners, health care professionals, and academic researchers with sustained implementation support through regular teleconference calls open to the surveillance community.[22, 23] By engaging stakeholders in the standards development, ISDS helped to ensure that the standards resonated with actual data availability and surveillance practice for applicable public health purposes.

At the global surveillance level, greater population mobility and the subsequent need to cross borders to gather surveillance data are triggering a need for standards to promote "apples-to-apples" data aggregation and exchange for situational awareness and public health response. While there are currently multiple evaluation frameworks for surveillance, they do not allow comparisons or aggregation. As difficult as it is to establish standards within a nation, it is especially challenging across autonomous nations. To address this, WHO, as the primary global regulatory body, has created the International Health Regulations (2005), which delineate core competencies in surveillance as well as other public health functions. While all countries have buy-in for reaching the goals, many fall short. Associations working to expand global standards in surveillance, therefore, more generally address strategies for complying with IHR (2005) goals rather than developing standards.

By bringing their broad constituencies to the table, Associations help ensure that systems and standards are aligned with real-world constraints and priorities. Without engaging end users and considering both the processes and the products of change, even well-intentioned efforts can be doomed for failure. This is where the strength of Associations are often evident: by building consensus within the community and providing subject matter expertise, Associations can address the variables that underlie successful standards implementation, such as cost in human and financial resources, scalability, time to implement, training needs, and adaptability to context changes. The pace of implementation is also critical, since it has been demonstrated (and logic follows) that it is generally more feasible to move stepwise toward standards-based interoperable systems rather than to attempt any comprehensive surveillance integration project all at once.[24]

ASSOCIATIONS AND PUBLIC HEALTH WORKFORCE DEVELOPMENT[2]

All health departments seek to maintain a skilled public health workforce using the best available technologies working on the most significant issues. Associations have long played an important role in providing professional development and training in surveillance outside of the traditional academic environment.

As surveillance changes, so too do the knowledge and skills public health practitioners need to perform their work effectively. Surveillance professionals at all stages of their career need help to keep abreast of the latest methodologies, policies, roles, and procedures.[14] Building the competencies of the surveillance workforce through training and the dissemination of information that is aligned with the stated needs of surveillance professionals are key ways that Associations build the competencies of the public health workforce.

With recent advances in the automated exchange of a growing volume and variety of health and health-related data, surveillance professionals must be proficient in public health informatics to fully understand and trust data quality, as it flows from clinical records to information for policy makers.

Public health informatics, which combines principles and methods from epidemiology, statistics, and computer science, is increasingly part of the core curriculum at schools of public health, but the field is new to many practitioners who were trained as epidemiologists or data analysts. There is a growing portfolio of learning opportunities, including workshops, webinars, and online resources, developed by associations to address this need. For example, ASTHO, NACCHO, and CSTE collaboratively sponsor fellowships, such as the Applied Public Health Informatics Fellowship, that place trainees in local and state health departments where they gain practice-based experience.

In addition to working with individuals as units of change, efforts are also underway to create system-level changes in the public health surveillance workforce. Currently, hiring can be constrained such that, for example, epidemiology departments can only hire an epidemiologist. CDC worked with the US Department of Labor to establish an informatics fellowship as an official apprenticeship program—the first step in getting new position classifications recognized. The nonprofit Public Health Informatics Institute (PHII) then collaborated with CDC and ASTHO and NACCHO members and staff to create job description templates for four levels of informatics positions. The Associations provided the critical subject matter expertise to modify the classifications to be applicable and feasible for local and state health departments.[25]

Areas for future advancement in CBA include more rigorous evaluations of the true impact of training on changes in individual behavior and organizational capacity in surveillance, as determined by the identification and tracking of metrics for surveillance performance. In addition, associations may increase the connection between process and outcome evaluation. For example, training evaluations could determine how improving statistical skills result in improvements in the technical and more objective attributes of the surveillance systems—such as system sensitivity—as well as more subjective attributes such as acceptability of new methodologies. Principles of the emerging field of change management, which have traditionally been applied to corporate situations, have increasing relevance in the public health environment, as well.

Demonstrating the impact of workforce development initiatives will demonstrate the rationale for investing time and money in education and training activities. This benefits not only the Associations developing the trainings to demonstrate the return on investment to funders but also the public health agencies that support such activities. Ultimately, surveillance professionals at all career levels should have access to a portfolio of opportunities with different levels of engagement, using a variety of mechanisms on different topics of relevance.[26] Associations must also revisit whether some partnerships are as productive as they can be or, alternatively, undeveloped, while others may need to be created.

ASSOCIATIONS AND ADVOCACY FOR PUBLIC HEALTH SURVEILLANCE

Associations give voice to their constituencies at multiple levels of decision-making. Whether identifying changes in business practice, impacting policy through education, or testifying on community priorities, Associations help ensure that input from the community is heard. Associations can facilitate the early and ongoing engagement that is often instrumental to successfully implementing new processes, tools, or approaches.

Associations often create policy analysis documents that help with decision-making. For example, CSTE annually develops and disseminates a collection of position statements on topics chosen by their membership. The responses by decision-makers to the statements are then also shared back with the community for further discussion to help extend the information flow and feedback. Other methods for soliciting input on policy issues include workgroups, committees, testimonies at high-level committee meetings, and other forums that provide opportunities for public health practitioners to contribute to the dialogue.

The legal and funding status of Associations limits their ability to perform certain advocacy activities. Nonprofit organizations in the USA that qualify for 501(c)[3] status, for example, are subject to specific allowances with regard to the type and proportion of their activities that are considered "influencing legislation" or lobbying, as determined by the time devoted by both compensated and volunteer workers and the expenditures for the activity.[27] However, nonprofits are allowed to play an educational role, so long as they do not issue an overt call to action for the adoption or rejection of any specific legislative action, such as a bill.[28, 29] Some organizations, such as ASTHO, CSTE, and NACCHO, nonetheless, have dedicated lobbying staff paid with nongovernmental dollars as part of their advocacy efforts.

Associations can also utilize the power of coalitions to amplify their messages and to reach greater audiences. One example is the Joint Public Health Informatics Taskforce (JPHIT), founded in 2008 as a consortium of public health membership associations to coordinate advocacy efforts. JPHIT is committed to improving population health surveillance and outcomes through informatics, health IT, and information exchange. JPHIT is unique within the field of public health, as it provides a forum that enables coordinated and collaborative development and implementation of public health informatics priorities, a unified voice on national informatics policy issues, and a focus on improving performance of the public health system through informatics.[30] Since its creation, JPHIT has developed and communicated unified positions on issues such as proposed meaningful use requirements, public health representatives on national health IT advisory committees, the organization of informatics within CDC, and other issues.[30] The JPHIT member organizations routinely develop unified responses to federal notices of proposed rulemaking and provide testimony before national advisory committees on public health informatics and surveillance issues. JPHIT continues to successfully advocate for the inclusion of public health in the larger national health IT conversation.

A vision for the future role of Associations in advocacy includes a system whereby lines of communication and access to data and information are available to all stakeholders in the public health system. Public health agencies, policy makers, and others should be aware of where to go for the information they need for informed decision-making. Associations can play a role by working with public health agencies to develop, disseminate, and implement best practices in creating communication resources and reports that are targeted to decision-makers at different levels of authority.

ASSOCIATIONS AND THE GLOBAL PUBLIC HEALTH SURVEILLANCE ENTERPRISE

The global surveillance landscape can be summarized as daunting and fragmented, with great disparities that challenge traditional and regimented methodologies and approaches. Though there are clearly individual standouts and regions with high-surveillance competency (e.g., Europe), approaches to public health surveillance capacity building has failed to create a surveillance infrastructure capable of detecting and responding to emerging threats consistently across individual countries and regions in compliance with IHR (2005) requirements and most other expectations. Varying resource environments, security realities, transboundary monitoring deficiencies, and a lack of sufficient public health training, among many other factors, contribute to what would already be considered a monumental undertaking. In this environment, the role of Associations is paramount, both for the problems to which they may unintentionally contribute and the benefit that can be realized if coordinated and galvanized under a common ideal.

As is mostly recognized, enhancements to global surveillance should result in measured improvement in time-to-detection, time-to-response, data fidelity, and readily disseminating disease and condition information considered important for public health purposes. With this in mind, Associations committed to the global surveillance mission must focus resources and efforts toward impacting key functions in the surveillance chain, ensuring that these efforts are not only coordinated, but synergizing and enhancing investments throughout the chain, whether ongoing or planned.

In this way, Associations can make a difference in regions where a public health framework is needed and where vertically implemented projects and programs conceived and executed in isolation to address a particular public health need can fall short. Associations' longer term and inherently collaborative projects can, thereby, improve the public health landscape and contribute toward increased sustainability.

Associations can take action to shape the current global public health surveillance situation into something that addresses existing gaps and deficiencies and, more importantly, presents alternative strategies for achieving global surveillance in response to ever-evolving public health threats.

Progress toward disease surveillance capability deployment pivots on defined public health system requirements and program-level standards and specifications, supported by methods specific to each country's needs, sustained through reliable information infrastructure, and appropriately addressing deficiencies within a trained workforce, supporting the required skill sets necessary to use and develop information solutions for public and population health needs. Above all else, leadership is the foundation by which all expectations, investments, and objectives fail or prosper. Association programs should identify an end-state upfront in order to maximize the host country's or region's benefit. Program objectives should be well defined with a clear strategy in place to transition capability and capacity directly to the partner with which the association is working.

A leader or champion must be identified to advocate for a particular approach, to advise on regulatory and legislative modifications needed, to recommend standards and consistent systems, and more. The leader can set commonly accepted requirements that meet measurable objectives and end states and promote curricula and training approaches to increase the throughput for public health individuals being trained and assure competency to operate in the field. This championing body or bodies is made up of Associations, and in particular, those that understand that the common goal can only be reached through dedicated coordination, cooperation, communication, shared principles, and most importantly, ability to compromise on overarching end states. This model can be constructed by many means and hold various philosophical characteristics, but ultimately, the established entity must have credibility and legitimacy in the country or region it operates.

Regardless of whether a champion is led by a larger international organization with many smaller Associations involved or defined by a coalition of like-minded Associations geared toward surveillance challenges described above, a champion must be able to generate its own sustainable propulsion.

One example of a coalition of associations is the World Federation of Public Health Associations (WFPHA), whose members represent national public health associations, and schools of public health. While not focused exclusively on surveillance, WFPHA activities include international conferences to bring international professionals together to share best practices, advocacy through position statements, and training fellowships.[31] Similarly, Connecting Organizations for Regional Disease Surveillance (CORDS), a nonprofit organization based in Lyon, France, was established "to improve global capacity to respond to infectious disease" through activities that leverage the assets of the individual member organizations.

Associations and organizations come and go, resources and financial investments rise and fall, political priorities and public health initiatives ebb and flow. Through it all a championing body must persist and stay true to the set requirements, objectives, and end states of achieving global public health surveillance. No one party's importance can define success for such an entity, and thus, the imperative for maintaining an even keel throughout change is growth, incorporation, and advocacy. This champion must become an institution. This is neither easy nor novel, but it is essential to overcoming surveillance challenges with any degree of continuity and effectiveness.

To orchestrate action in a given country or region, there must exist incentives for partners to trust Associations and/or a championing body. The obvious answer is to make certain that they are not only involved but also invested in the planning, process, and implementation. Integrated disease and public health surveillance has a common purpose of helping all—the country improves its reporting and response, the region benefits from early warning and shared resource approaches, and the international community gets more time to prepare and respond to health-related threats, no matter where they might present.

It is an easy endeavor to work toward, but instead of Associations deploying molecular diagnostic capabilities into resource-constrained and/or remote areas, for example, it is far better to work with that country in a more methodical manner. Organizations should focus on country representatives and experts while advising and working with them to implement surveillance to achieve their goals, integrate and synchronize with regional systems, and influence international behavior toward partnership.

ASSOCIATIONS AND SUSTAINABLE BUSINESS MODELS

Associations need sustainable business models that can adapt to the changing public health landscape in order to remain a foundational component of the public health system. Passion for improving population health is necessary but not sufficient when bills need to be paid. As business enterprises, public health associations share the same challenges and uncertainties as all nonprofits to maintain a financially healthy organizational structure, especially in times of economic downturn.[32] To fully understand this concept, it is necessary to consider Associations' organizational structure and funding.

Associations working in public health surveillance vary in size, reach, influence, and capacity as measured by membership, annual budget, history, and level of influence with decision-makers. Most are governed by an elected or appointed board of directors with roles and responsibilities articulated in the organization's bylaws. Financial and other information, including the "greater-good" purpose that demonstrates compliance with the tax-exempt qualifications for nonprofit organizations can be found on the IRS 990 form, which organizations are required to make publicly available.

Grants and contracts are the major source of revenue for Associations working in public health surveillance. A financial benefit of retaining a tax-exempt status is eligibility for funding from private, foundation, and governmental sources that cannot give funds to individuals or private entities.

In the USA, CDC is a major funder of the CBA work of Associations. A primary funding mechanism is a 5-year cooperative agreement under a funding opportunity called, "Building Capacity of the Public Health System to Improve Population Health through National, Nonprofit Organizations."[6] With shifting priorities and siloed funding, however, Associations can no longer rely on dependable funding sources and amounts from year to year. In the global arena, CBA activities for public health have traditionally been funded by major foundations with program areas in public health generally or surveillance, more specifically. Examples include the Bill & Melinda Gates Foundation, the Rockefeller Foundation, the Clinton Foundation, and the Skoll Global Threats Fund.

Increase in the number and focus of funding mechanisms, such as grants and contracts, targeted to advancing public health surveillance specifically, would ensure that CBA activities aimed at building surveillance capabilities are funded. However, in a political climate that seeks to reduce government spending, regardless of need, public health is, unfortunately, in a difficult position to get increased funding for its activities. Associations recognize that diverse funding sources—to include a variety of public, private, and governmental sources—reduces the vulnerability that results from dependence on one primary funder. In the global arena, contracted work to Associations is supported by CDC and other federal agencies, including the Defense Threat Reduction Agency (DTRA) and the US State Department. Foundations working in global health, such as the Bill & Melinda Gates Foundation, the Skoll Emerging Threats Fund, and the Rockefeller Foundation are just a few major supporters of capacity-building activities in global health surveillance.

Even member-based Associations working in public health surveillance do not receive much revenue from individual donations or membership dues. APHA, the oldest and largest public health Association, receives less than 20% of its revenue from membership dues.[33] Cuts have also been made in employer payment of professional dues and membership fees, further reducing membership renewals. This can be detrimental to Associations that rely on their membership for volunteers to supplement staff and thereby increase organizational capacity.

Conventions and annual events are a major source of unrestricted revenue for many public health associations. Although in-person meetings are the lifeblood of a strong community of practice, they are often considered expendable for budget-cutting purposes. Recently, new policies and tightened restrictions on governmental spending (especially for travel and food) have negatively affected conference attendance, making this a less reliable revenue source for Associations. Furthermore, students and those early in their careers, who depend on showing their work and networking at conferences, may be unable to do so.[34] Associations are addressing this by working together to co-host or co-locate meetings, holding fewer meetings (e.g., hosting biannual instead of annual events), or using more interactive virtual event technologies, such as those used by CDC to host the 2013 Public Health Informatics Virtual Event.[35] A benefit is the ability to provide access to the presentations after the event.

Looking ahead, Associations must take a more corporate perspective to strategic planning and business development to remain financially viable. Strategic planning and reevaluating the mission and vision of an organization is a fundamental task, usually undertaken by the board of directors of the organization. This will require increased focus by individual associations on the value they add and by the network of public health surveillance associations working on how they can work together more effectively and efficiently.

Through improved communications and transparency, Associations can work more synergistically to promote collaborative and complementary initiatives without redundancy. Furthermore, with increased emphasis on funders to demonstrate outcomes, it is imperative that Associations develop performance measures that demonstrate the impact of their work on advancing surveillance goals. While the market for the work of associations is growing, the realities of financial and political climates will continue to shape their position in the overall public health system.

KEY SUMMARY POINTS

- Associations work directly with governmental public health agencies to enable them to prevent and respond to events of public health concern.
- Associations cultivate collaboration and engage members with other stakeholders across disciplines and sectors to create communities of practice and opportunities for sharing experience and expertise.
- Associations provide the CBA needed to develop and maintain a skilled public health workforce using the best available technologies working on the most significant issues.
- A unified voice is presented for the surveillance community through associations and it is through this unified voice that advocacy occurs to create system-level change across jurisdictions.
- Associations face challenges common to nonprofit organizations for maintaining sustainable business plans during changes in political, economic, and social landscapes.
- Throughout the world, associations that work to advance public health have been founded to serve similar core functions.

DISCUSSION QUESTIONS

1. Compare and contrast the ways by which different components of the public health system can work to advance public health surveillance.
2. Describe three ways by which the implementation of surveillance data standards promotes situational awareness.
3. List some of the issues to consider when Associations work in an international environment. Describe the consequences of poor planning.
4. A new bill is before Congress to increase funding for a nationwide syndromic surveillance system and you are meeting with a local legislator. What are three key messages you will be discussing? What topics will you be avoiding?
5. Choose a nonprofit organization and create a logic model (resources, objectives, outputs, outcomes, impact) that describes its work to advance public health surveillance.

REFERENCES

1. The White House. National Strategy for Biosurveillance. July 2012. <https://www.whitehouse.gov/sites/default/files/National_Strategy_for_Biosurveillance_July_2012.pdf>; September 25, 2015.
2. Definition provided by the chapter author.
3. US Centers for Disease Control and Prevention. Middle East Respiratory Syndrome (MERS) Home Page. <http://www.cdc.gov/coronavirus/mers/>; September 30, 2015.
4. Perry HN, McDonnell SM, Alemu W, Nsubuga P, Chungong S, Otten Jr MW, et al. Planning an integrated disease surveillance and response system: a matrix of skills and activities. BMC Med 2007;5:24.
5. Pifer A. Letter: on quasi-public organizations; whence came the quango, and why. The New York Times. New York. September 5, 1987. <http://www.nytimes.com/1987/09/05/opinion/l-letter-on-quasi-public-organizations-whence-came-the-quango-and-why-969587.html>; September 30, 2015.
6. Chapman K, Weaver G, Taveras S. US Centers for Disease Control and Prevention. Building capacity of the public health system to improve population health through national, non-profit organizations. 2013. <http://www.cdc.gov/stltpublichealth/funding/rfaot13.html>; September 30, 2015.
7. Council of State and Territorial Epidemiologists. About CSTE. <http://www.cste.org/?page=About_CSTE&hhSearchTerms=%22history%22>; September 30, 2015.
8. Association of State and Territorial Health Officials. History of ASTHO. <http://www.astho.org/About/History/>; September 30, 2015.
9. International Society for Disease Surveillance. <http://www.syndromic.org/about-isds>; September 30, 2015.
10. U.S. Internal Revenue Service. Exemption requirements - 501(c)(3) organizations. <http://www.irs.gov/Charities-&-Non-Profits/Charitable-Organizations/Exemption-Requirements-Section-501(c)(3)-Organizations>; September 30, 2015.
11. Wenger E, McDermott R, Snyder WM. Cultivating communities of practice: a guide to managing knowledge. Boston, MA: Harvard Business Review Press; 2002. p. 284.
12. Rennick M, Swenson DJ, Hoferka S, Ishikawa C, Zwickl R. Check! explore barriers and solutions to data sharing on BioSense 2.0. Online J Publ Health Inform 2014;6(1):e83.
13. US Centers for Disease Control and Prevention. Overview of CDC-RFA-OT13-1302: building capacity of the public health system to improve population health through national, nonprofit organizations. 2013.
14. Syndromic surveillance. Reports from a national conference, 2003. MMWR Morb Mortal Wkly Rep 2004;53(Suppl.):1–264.
15. Brownson RC, Colditz GA, Proctor EK, editors. Dissemination and implementation research in health: translating science to practice. New York, NY: Oxford University Press; 2012. p. 560.
16. Greenhalgh T, Robert G, Macfarlane F, Bate P, Kyriakidou O. Diffusion of innovations in service organizations: systematic review and recommendations. Milbank Q 2004;82(4):581–629.
17. World Health Organization. Pandemic (H1N1) 2009, <http://www.who.int/csr/disease/swineflu/en/>; September 30, 2015.
18. Olson DR, Paladini M, Lober WB, Buckeridge DL. Applying a new model for sharing population health data to national syndromic influenza surveillance: DiSTRIBuTE Project proof of concept, 2006 to 2009. PLoS Curr 2011;3:RRN1251.
19. Lober WB, Reeder B, Painter I, Revere D, Goldov K, Bugni PF, et al. Technical description of the Distribute Project: a community-based syndromic surveillance SYSTEM implementation. Online J Public Health Inform 2014;5(3):224.
20. National Association of County and City Health Officials. National profile of local health departments, 2013. 2014.
21. Blumenthal D, Tavenner M. The "meaningful use" regulation for electronic health records. N Engl J Med 2010;363(6):501–4.
22. International Society for Disease Surveillance. Final recommendation: core processes and EHR requirements for public health syndromic surveillance. 2011.
23. International Society for Disease Surveillance. Electronic syndromic surveillance using hospital inpatient and ambulatory clinical care electronic health record data: recommendations from the ISDS meaningful use workgroup. 2012.
24. Samb B, Evans T, Dybul M, Atun R, Moatti JP, Nishtar S, et al. An assessment of interactions between global health initiatives and country health systems. Lancet 2009;373(9681):2137–69.
25. Public Health Informatics Institute. Resources. <http://www.phii.org/resources/browse/topics>; September 30, 2015.
26. Drehobl PA, Roush SW, Stover BH, Koo D. Public health surveillance workforce of the future. MMWR Surveill Summ 2012;61(Suppl.):25–9.
27. Internal Revenue Service. Measuring lobbying activity: expenditure test. <http://www.irs.gov/Charities-&-Non-Profits/Measuring-Lobbying-Activity:-Expenditure-Test>; September 30, 2015.
28. Internal Revenue Service. Lobbying. <http://www.irs.gov/Charities-&-Non-Profits/Lobbying>; September 30, 2015.
29. US Centers for Disease Control and Prevention. Anti-lobbying restrictions for CDC grantees. 2012. p. 6.
30. Public Health Data Standards Consortium. Health information technology standards. <http://www.phdsc.org/standards/health-information/D_Standards.asp/>; September 30, 2015.
31. World Federation of Public Health Associations. <http://www.wfpha.org/about-wfpha>; September 30, 2015.
32. Accenture. The impact of the economic downturn on the nonprofit sector. 2009.
33. American Public Health Association. Annual Report 2014. <www.apha.org/~/media/files/pdf/about/2014_annual_report.ashx>; September 30, 2015.
34. American Physical Society. Lucibella M. Federal Travel Restrictions Impact Scientific Meetings. June 2013;8(2). <http://www.aps.org/publications/capitolhillquarterly/201306/travelrestrict.cfm>; September 30, 2015.
35. US Centers for Disease Control and Prevention. CDC Virtual Platform Initiative. <http://www.cdc.gov/virtual/>; September 30, 2015.

CHAPTER

18

Linking Clinical Medicine Data with Public Health Surveillance for Mutual Benefit

Noelle M Cocoros, Michael Klompas, Gillian Haney, Alfred DeMaria, Jr., Richard Platt

The primary factor in the securing of morbidity reports is the physician who comes into contact with cases of sickness … The practicing physician therefore is of fundamental importance in any scheme of public health administration.
JW Trask (Assistant Surgeon-General, USPHS, 1912)[1]

KEY WORDS

Clinicians
Pay for performance
Electronic laboratory reporting (ELR)
Electronic health records (EHR)
ILINET

INTRODUCTION: THE CURRENT ENVIRONMENT FOR COLLABORATIONS BETWEEN CLINICAL MEDICINE AND PUBLIC HEALTH

Clinical medicine has become much more technologically complex and multidisciplinary, but the fundamental reality remains the same. Diseases are diagnosed by **clinicians**, who are persons such as a doctor or a nurse who works directly with patients rather than in a laboratory or as a researcher.[2] Therefore, clinical practice and public health surveillance are intrinsically linked. Without the cooperation and collaboration of clinical practitioners and clinical facilities, public health surveillance as we know it would be impossible.

The goals and responsibilities of public health and clinical medicine are disparate, and not inherently congruent. Public health surveillance is done to acquire data and interpret it in pursuit of maintaining and promoting public health; the primary responsibility is to the population's health and welfare. The goal of clinical medicine is to serve the best interests of the individual patient; the primary responsibility is to the patient. These differing foci and responsibilities must be recognized and acknowledged—and ultimately addressed—if public health surveillance and interventions are to be timely, effective, and impactful.

In this chapter we lay out a framework for developing strong, fruitful collaborations between public health and clinical medicine via bidirectional, mutually beneficial relationships aimed at improving surveillance and clinical care. We provide suggestions and examples for enhancing partnerships between clinical medicine and public health to take advantage of current opportunities. By addressing the competing interests of clinicians, developing solid communication between the two groups, and utilizing technological advances, public health surveillance can be more efficient and effective. While public health surveillance is performed on a broad spectrum of conditions and health indicators, we focus primarily on public health surveillance in the context of infectious disease surveillance. The details and specifics of this chapter are written from the perspective of clinicians and public health practitioners in the USA, but the overarching points are relevant to other countries.

Current Activities that Could Contribute to a Better Future of Public Health Surveillance

In the USA, the Centers for Disease Control and Prevention (CDC) designate the Council of State and Territorial Epidemiologists (CSTE) to determine the nationally notifiable diseases or conditions, and define what constitutes a "case." In order to conduct investigations and determine case classifications, key data are required by state and local health departments, such as laboratory results, clinical symptoms, treatment, and outcomes. Clinicians and health care facilities collect these data. Effective and efficient communications between health departments and clinicians expedite the information exchange. Clinical laboratories are responsible for reporting key information regarding specimens, testing, and test results to health departments. An ongoing trend toward **electronic laboratory reporting (ELR)** is enhancing timeliness and completeness of this reporting. ELR is the automated transmission of laboratory-related data from commercial, public health, hospital, and other laboratories to state and local public health departments through an electronic health records (EHR) system or Laboratory Information Management System (LIMS).[3] Similar electronic means of communicating clinical data is now increasingly possible.

Beyond clinician-based disease reporting, the critical interdependency between clinicians and public health practitioners is most obvious when patients present with rare syndromes that may be attributable to unusual, highly contagious, or emerging pathogens such as novel coronaviruses, avian influenza virus, and Ebola virus. In these cases, clinicians rely on public health agencies for guidance on how to test for these pathogens and how to reduce risk for health care workers, patients' close contacts, other hospitalized patients, and society at large. Public health agencies may provide diagnostic testing for select organisms and sometimes also provide access to difficult-to-obtain medications to treat these conditions such as artemisinin compounds for malaria and other selected antiparasitic medications. Clinicians also turn to public health agencies to investigate rare syndromes and unusual diagnoses. Clinical reports of encephalitis and fungal meningitis, for example, led to the discovery of West Nile virus in New York City and widely distributed, contaminated pharmaceutical products, respectively.[4,5]

More broadly, clinicians rely on public health agencies to provide context for more common clinical challenges, such as diabetes, obesity, cancer, and influenza. Surveillance data provided by public health agencies help clinicians characterize the prevalence, incidence, risk factors, and common outcomes for patients with these types of conditions. For example, during the 2009 H1N1 influenza pandemic, cases of severe illness were observed among pregnant women and reported to state and local jurisdictions, and CDC was ultimately notified.[6] This led to investigation and confirmation of the association, and guidance was provided for clinicians treating suspect and confirmed cases.[7] Such rapid publication of assessment of situations of public health concern has become the norm in instances of emergent infectious diseases and other emergencies. Epidemiological context enriches clinicians' understanding of individual cases and helps inform counseling, prognosis, and management, and the feasibility and utility of incorporating local surveillance data into patient-specific clinical decision-making has been demonstrated.[8,9] Many health departments also provide educational materials and programs for weight loss, smoking cessation, and free vaccines to help clinicians manage and inform patients.

While the above examples make clear why clinician reporting is important to public health and ultimately useful to the clinician and her or his patient, clinician reporting is often incomplete and not always timely. Reasons for this include lack of awareness of reporting requirements and method, a mistaken sense that someone else is doing it, inconvenience and lack of time, concern about patient privacy and confidentiality, and undervaluation of the utility of public health surveillance.[10-13] Lack of incentive may factor into incomplete case reporting by clinicians, as well as, the burden of manual case reporting as cumbersome and time-consuming. These factors can be addressed through education regarding surveillance requirements, implementing policies and procedures that assure privacy and confidentiality, and by taking proactive measures to make reporting easier.

A primary goal of public health outreach and education is to make clinicians aware of the value of surveillance and how they and their patients benefit from public health activities based on surveillance data. Adapting evolving technology such as web-based data entry systems and creating forms embedded in **EHR** systems can help facilitate reporting. EHR is a longitudinal electronics health record of patient health information generated by one or more encounters in any care delivery setting. Included in this information are patient demographics, progress notes, problems, medications, vital signs, past medical history, immunizations, laboratory data, and radiology reports.[14]

Clinicians should also be aware of the potential risk arising from not reporting. Failure to report is a contravention of both state and local legal mandates and could be construed as furtherance of an ongoing threat to public health, with preventable morbidity and mortality.

In an era of accountable care and "pay for performance" in clinical medicine in the USA, data generated from public health surveillance have the potential for providing quality indicators and benchmarks for population health across an entire spectrum of health care delivery systems and payers.[15] In health care, **pay for performance** gives financial incentives to clinicians for better health outcomes, such as lowering blood pressure or counseling that results in cessation of smoking.[2] This is already happening in many states in the realm of health care-associated infections, but there is also potential for community-wide, population-based surveillance of reportable and nonreportable, communicable and noncommunicable conditions, to be used to assess quality of care. This is now being explored for conditions such as diabetes mellitus, human immunodeficiency virus infection (HIV), and hepatitis C virus (HCV) infection, in the assessment of control of hyperglycemia, computation of HIV "community viral load," and in measures of adherence to evidence-based clinical guidelines for diagnostic testing and treatment.[16-18]

Achieving Goals of Surveillance

Timely, accurate, and complete case information is critical for achieving the goals of surveillance. Until relatively recently, public health was dependent solely on clinicians for such data. While the advent of electronic laboratory reporting and electronic health record (EHR)-based automated reporting has diminished this dependency, clinicians still play a vital role in surveillance and remain the initial source of all case information (e.g., electronic laboratory reports are initiated by a clinician ordering the test). It is therefore necessary to identify and respond to the distinct obstacles to clinician participation.

The adoption of evidence-based medicine, commitment to quality measures to assess processes and outcomes, and huge advances in information technology (with "meaningful use" requirements for clinicians in the USA), have provided opportunities—and some challenges—for improvement in public health surveillance completeness, timeliness, accuracy, relevance, and impact.[19] Health care providers and public health agencies have different priorities, and changes in health care delivery in use of time and resources have only exacerbated the differences in priorities. In the USA, the requirements of public health reporting are not reimbursable by insurers; an "unfunded mandate." Much effort is now directed to maximizing efficiency and minimizing cost, often to the detriment of public health needs. In any situation where the needs of the patient and practice are balanced against the needs of public health, the patients and practice will take precedence. To the extent public health surveillance requirements can be made easier, and even be automated, the more likely surveillance goals will be achieved. It is critical to develop systems that can improve data exchange and communication between clinicians and public health practitioners, without adding extra work to already overburdened practitioners. While clinicians do acknowledge the importance of public health, they prioritize immediate patient care over communicating with health departments or facilitating population-level investigations. Shifting the onus of reporting from clinicians to allied health professionals has been one way that has been used to overcome this barrier. But an even better way, that avoids this shift of burden, is using electronic systems to serve both clinicians and public health agencies by decreasing reliance on clinicians or allied health professionals, while simultaneously improving the timeliness and completeness of reporting. This improves the amount and quality of surveillance information available to public health agencies, and it does so while reducing the clinical workload.

ELR for selected infections and conditions is a common, current example. The institution of ELR dramatically enhances both the timeliness and completeness of notifiable disease surveillance.[20] However, in many cases, public health officials need supplementary data on selected cases that cannot be gathered from electronic laboratory reports alone. Electronic laboratory reports provide little or no contextual data on clinical presentations, epidemiologic risk factors, treatments, or outcomes. Public health agencies must still reach out to clinicians directly through telephone calls, faxes, or mailings to gather these data. Limiting the number of reporting requirements, and regularly reviewing them to be sure that they are high-yield, yet as parsimonious as possible, can help prevent clinician reporting fatigue, resentment, and failure to participate and improve surveillance data.

Other changes in health care delivery can also have consequences to surveillance systems. It was recognized in the 1980s and 1990s that most cases of acute gastroenteritis were managed in the same way irrespective of the etiology; stool examination and culture did not affect management unless signs and symptoms persisted, and therefore were not cost-effective on initial presentation of the patient. This resulted in decreased utilization of stool examination and culture in the initial workup of gastroenteritis. However, at the same time, health departments were becoming more and more dependent on laboratory reports for ascertainment of cases of gastroenteritis and case cluster identification. Since most patients with gastroenteritis have self-limited disease, laboratory testing is not ordered and an etiologic agent is typically not identified; hence, most cases do not come to the attention of public health. In some instances, worried patients contacted health departments to ask what they were doing to follow-up on the "food poisoning" their health care provider told them they had. Other evidence-based practice recommendations and clinical pathways may have similar impact on public health surveillance. Application of such cost-effectiveness measures to clinical care will continue to require adjustment of surveillance practices to new realities.

Similar distortions can result from the introduction of new test technology. Introduction of laboratory testing methods that do not result in an organism being isolated may cause surveillance consequences since no clinical isolate is sent to the public health laboratory for further investigation. An example is gonorrhea detection using nucleic acid amplification tests. These tests reliably establish a case but do not assess for antimicrobial susceptibilities. This hinders health departments' capacities to detect and manage the emergence of new antibiotic resistant strains. Changes in the ways that test results are reported can also have impacts if the results are not recognized as indicative of disease because the case definition does not include them or if the ELR system is not updated to flag and report these results. It is important for surveillance programs to keep abreast of developments in diagnostic testing, as well as changes in health delivery policy and procedures. One possible approach to assure adequate surveillance in the face of these challenges is to engage selected clinicians and practices as sentinel sites that will systematically send samples for culture in all patients with suspected disease. This requires additional resources, but may be more feasible for providing critical data.

On occasion, clinicians or patients may perceive that reporting cases to the surveillance system may compromise patients' welfare. For example, a patient with a communicable disease living in a small community may have concerns about disclosure and embarrassment when his or her condition is reported to the local public health jurisdiction, and ask his or her provider to not be reported. Or, it may be that the health care provider is concerned about violating the Privacy Rule of the Health Insurance Portability and Accountability Act (HIPAA). It is, therefore, obligatory that health departments have rigorously sustained systems to assure privacy and confidentiality, and that they promote an understanding of these policies and procedures among clinicians in their jurisdiction. Clinicians need to be assured that they are serving their patients' best interests when they meet their obligation to public health surveillance, and that the HIPAA Privacy Rule specifically allows for legally authorized reporting to public health (45 CFR 164.512(b); US Department of Health and Human Services).

Sometimes clinicians fail to report diseases in cases where they perceive little or no benefit for either the clinician or the patient (e.g., Lyme disease). One solution to this problem is to find ways to routinely "give" something back to clinicians in exchange for reporting. Examples can include timely data on disease rates in their community, guidance on how best to manage their patient, or an update on what public health agencies are doing to combat the patient's disease at the community level. Identifying ways to communicate with clinicians in order to "give" something back for their time and energy can be daunting in terms of identifying a reward that would be of interest to clinicians.

Information technology (IT) solutions are often the answer to reporting challenges, though IT-based solutions also have their own challenges, particularly with respect to financial and human resources. Furthermore, informatics- and IT-heavy goals mean small clinical practices may be late adopters and will need their own specific solutions.

In light of this, health departments as well as national agencies like the CDC must work with vendors to incorporate public health surveillance needs into EHRs and leverage the resources available through health information exchanges (HIEs). In addition, long-term, informatics-heavy goals and systems level changes can be hard for government agencies to achieve, given resource limitations. While these challenges currently engage the developed world, the developing world is moving toward incorporation of technology in clinical practice.

In order to leverage current evolutions in clinical and public health technologies—and changes in attitude around the utility of electronic data—we must first ensure a solid foundation of collaboration is in place. As we describe in the next two sections, building long-term sustainable systems that provide valid surveillance data requires certain conditions to be in place (Box 18-1).

Current Best Practices

In this section, we describe examples of current best practices on three levels of engagement for infectious disease surveillance: routine activities and responsibilities, enhanced and/or sentinel surveillance projects, and special projects.

Routine Relationships, Responsibilities, and Practices

There are a variety of routine surveillance activities that build the foundation for more advanced collaborative work. Routine communications from health departments to clinicians include clinical advisories and alerts, which provide guidance on new, emerging, or re-emerging infections. Such advisories, sent to hospitals, infection control practitioners, large clinical sites, medical societies, and others provide up-to-date information about situations of concern. As an example of the impact of a clinical alert, a recent report demonstrated that electronic messages sent to clinicians during a *Cyclospora* outbreak helped to identify new cases associated with the outbreak, and helped improve treatment and outcomes for some patients.[21] Information from public health agencies to clinicians should be designed to aid in case identification, prevent further transmission, and improve outcomes for cases.

For select reportable conditions such as suspect measles or meningococcal meningitis, many health departments in the USA require an "immediate" disease report via phone by the case's clinician. For this to occur appropriately, public health must ensure clinicians know when, why, and who they need to call, and the appropriate individual

BOX 18-1 Challenges and Solutions to Achieving Public Health Surveillance Goals

Challenges:

- Competing responsibilities and priorities for clinicians
- Lack of direct benefit to clinician and her or his patient
- Lack of understanding of the requirements and/or importance of case reporting
- Case reporting by clinicians can be time-consuming, inconvenient, and cumbersome
- Information technology-based reporting activities will not be feasible in all clinical settings
- Building technologically advanced capacity requires resources and intense engagement of both parties

Solutions:

- Educate clinicians on reporting requirements and public health importance of reporting
- Build strong collaborative relationships through routine activities to lay the groundwork for more resource and time-intensive activities
- Take advantage of times of crisis to build relationships and communicate public health goals (e.g., during an outbreak or case of an unusual disease)
- Develop automated reporting capabilities that leverage existing infrastructures (e.g., electronic laboratory reporting and utilization of electronic health records)
- Critically examine reporting requirements on a regular basis and make appropriate changes to eliminate unnecessary reporting burden
- Make the case that adequate surveillance provides the kind of population-based information that can be used for comparison metrics to assess populations in care under accountable care organizations or other global payment methods and thereby improve diagnostics and care

must be responsive when contacted. Easy-to-follow summary sheets can be posted on agency websites. When immediate contact is required, system credibility requires reasonable measures for success of two-way communication.

Public health agencies issue clinical advisories when new high-priority conditions need to be reported, but jurisdictions' core reporting requirements must also be conveyed. When changes to reporting requirements are made, those changes must be communicated. This is where existing relationships play a critical role. The health department that maintains an ongoing collaboration with clinical medicine knows the stakeholders and how to reach them. It is in times of acute need for information exchange that these mature communication channels developed over the course of years of routine day-to-day communications really prove their value. Health departments can also sponsor or participate in educational programs to bring information to clinicians. The goal is to provide useful information based on health department experience—the surveillance data provided by the clinicians and from national and international sources—to assist the clinicians in their ability to care for their patients and recognize emerging clinical situations. These communications make the clinicians aware of the public health agency as well as allowing them to identify programs and individuals who they can turn to for assistance. Clinicians can also serve as codevelopers and advocates for public health policies and practices, such as immunization registries and reporting requirements. (See Box 18-2 for how advisory committees can be utilized to improve public health reporting.)

Public health programs and/or departments that build relationships with key clinical staff at large facilities can reap enormous benefits. There are multiple examples of these kinds of relationships that have been successful. Most health departments have close working relationships with infection preventionists and health care epidemiologists working in their jurisdictions. Senior public health staff can provide guidance and support for hospital policies, essentially ratifying hospital policies in some situations. Likewise, in many places, school nurses interact with their local and state health departments on multiple issues, such as communicable diseases, head injury, and substance use. Health departments also communicate with outpatient clinical staff to assure vaccine supply and accountability through federal and state programs. Large group practices may have designated infectious disease/infection control officers who can be important contacts for surveillance and other public health issues, as the example in Box 18-3 indicates. There is a nexus of interest between health departments and accountable care organizations (ACOs); both are responsible for the health of populations and these populations overlap. Having close communication between

BOX 18-2 Improving Public Health Reporting Through Advisory Committees

When modifying public health reporting regulations, convene an advisory committee comprising stakeholders from the broad clinical community including professional societies and hospital associations. Benefits include:

- Obtaining expert opinion from those directly impacted by regulations
- Improving clarity of language
- Using consensus to obtain support for adoption and implementation of new measures
- Eliciting support for dissemination through represented organizations

BOX 18-3 Turning Relationships into Action During the 2009 H1N1 Influenza Pandemic

During the early weeks of the 2009 H1N1 influenza pandemic, the Massachusetts Department of Public Health communicated with a designated, long-term, infectious disease single point of contact in a large group practice that covered approximately 10% of the population. This resulted in:

- Identification of individuals at this large clinical organization who would be responsible for specimen collection, testing, and result reporting
- State public health laboratory conducting testing for the novel pathogen
- Development of a novel reporting mechanism for hospitalized cases of H1N1 infection cared for in the practice
- Early recognition of groups at risk for severe illness (e.g., pregnant women)
- Rapid dissemination of new and updated clinical guidance and situational awareness to a large group of practitioners
- Availability of stockpile antivirals and state implemented vaccine distribution when available

developing ACOs and health departments offers an opportunity to align population health responsibilities in an ongoing way.

Relationships with key clinical organizations such as medical societies, nursing associations, public health nursing organizations, and school nurse groups can enhance communication for surveillance activities. Communications with wider clinical audiences can be achieved through organization membership and buy-in from senior members of these organizations can assist with building support across the group.

Case investigations conducted by health department staff are routine activities that involve both public health staff and clinicians. Whenever possible, such case investigations should be mutually beneficial. For example, investigating a case of pertussis as outlined in Box 18-4. However, not all reportable conditions are investigated, meaning the communication is in one direction only, from the clinician to public health. This is the situation for many high-volume reportable diseases, such as Lyme disease in parts of the USA and chronic HCV infection. In some jurisdictions, clinicians are expected to report key clinical information but they do not receive anything in return (e.g., guidance from epidemiologists). Thus, these conditions are often not reported by clinicians, information is not returned in a timely manner, or the case reports are incomplete. One approach to address this is by providing surveillance or epidemiology reports to clinicians and related organizations, ensuring these partners know that the information they provide is utilized and meaningful. If complete reporting and high-quality data are required by public health, the burden is on public health to convince clinicians that reporting is important and to take care to limit the amount of information collected.[22] It may be necessary to incentivize reporting in some way. Or perhaps, consider altering the surveillance system to sentinel site reporting with select clinicians and/or enhance reliance on information that can be reported electronically. In Massachusetts, public health regulations established a mandate for all clinical laboratories to participate in the health department's ELR initiative. Once implemented, this mandate allowed the health department to stop requiring clinicians to report those diseases that could be adequately ascertained through laboratory testing.

Sentinel and Enhanced Surveillance Activities

Sentinel surveillance is a supplement and/or alternative to population-based surveillance methods and can serve as an early warning system. Sentinel surveillance utilizes relevant data from a subset of institutions, sites, or settings that are either randomly or purposefully selected; typically, sentinel sites are sought that are representative of the larger population. Enhanced surveillance activities are utilized on an as-needed basis for specific situations, providing information not captured via routine surveillance activities. Many expanded, enhanced, or sentinel surveillance activities require more intensive collaboration between clinicians and public health. In Box 18-5, we highlight examples of efforts whose success was rooted in strong, ongoing relationships between the two groups. For instance, in New York City, collaborative work between city health department staff and a group of clinics resulted in the re-engagement of individuals with HIV who had been lost to medical care.[23]

BOX 18-4 Case Investigation as an Opportunity for Mutual Benefit

Investigating a case of pertussis (whooping cough) can be an occasion for the health department and clinician to collaborate to the benefit of the health department, the practitioner, and the patient.

The clinician can receive:

- Treatment guidance
- Assistance with further testing
- Help with answering patient questions
- Contact prophylaxis advice (who to treat and how to treat)

The health department receives:

- Case details not available elsewhere
- Timely information about contacts of the case
- Information that assists with case classification for national notification

The **US Outpatient Influenza-Like-Illness (ILI) Surveillance Network (ILINet)** is a CDC surveillance system based solely on voluntary reporting by clinical providers.[2] Implemented by state health departments, clinical sites are recruited and encouraged to participate in the national system, which entails weekly reporting of ILI activity by each reporting site. The ILINet data are a core component of the country's respiratory illness surveillance and were considered among the most useful during the H1N1 pandemic. These data are used for more advanced surveillance analyses and serve as a standard against which other ILI surveillance systems are measured.[24,25] In return for their weekly reports of ILI visits, participating clinical sites are typically provided with free testing of a subset of respiratory specimens per influenza season and regular updates on the progression of the season by public health departments. Such two-way communication builds a close relationship with participating clinical providers.

The District of Columbia Department of Health designed an intervention similar to that in New York City and its successful implementation was also dependent on the relationships and partnerships between the health department and the clinics.[26] In HIV surveillance and care, these novel methods are setting examples for the rest of the country. Other conditions might also be candidates for such collaborative approaches.

In Massachusetts, health department staff worked with clinicians at two different facilities to conduct a small validation project of the state's HCV infection surveillance system.[28] The clinicians generated a list of nearly 200 clinically diagnosed acute cases of HCV infection over the study period and the state epidemiologists queried the surveillance data to see whether the individuals were reported to the state and appropriately classified. They found that less than 1% of the cases were appropriately classified and reported to the CDC, indicating substantial systematic underreporting of acute HCV nationally. This project's results will likely influence policy on a national level, with both the clinical staff and health department staff engaging stakeholders. Such analyses, usually developed out of long-term relationships, can be valuable for evaluating and improving public health surveillance systems across a number of conditions of public health significance.

Special Projects to Build Long-Term Systems-Level Improvements

In this chapter so far, references have been made to harnessing current technological advances to serve public health surveillance. Emerging technologies can ease some of the reporting burden on clinicians, while simultaneously advancing further the quality and quantity of data available to public health. The increasing sophistication and dissemination of electronic health record systems, for example, make them highly attractive tools to improve communication between clinicians and public health agencies. EHRs offer several advantages over ELR systems (Box 18-6) and may offer the opportunity to facilitate bidirectional communication between public health and clinicians. The ability to use EHR data for public health surveillance, as described below, requires buy-in—in various forms—from the clinicians/clinics who own the EHR data and the public health agency who wants to utilize the data.

The rich array of clinical data routinely captured by EHRs can provide public health agencies with information about a far broader array of conditions than ELR systems. EHRs include patient demographics, vital signs, diagnoses, prescriptions, and laboratory tests from both current and prior encounters. Algorithms that integrate these different data streams can help identify conditions that are undetectable using laboratory data alone (e.g., culture-negative tuberculosis or asthma), they can provide more granular clinical diagnoses (e.g., acute versus undifferentiated HCV infection), and help public health agencies triage their responses (e.g., flagging pregnant patients with sexually transmitted infections for high-priority follow-up).

BOX 18-5 Enhanced Surveillance Using Strong Clinical Partnerships

Several surveillance-based interventions for HIV/AIDS have been implemented in New York City by embedding health department staff at numerous clinical sites.[27] In its first 2 years of implementation, the program was successful in:

- Contacting exposed sexual and needle-sharing partners and bringing them to testing and prevention education
- Aiding clinicians in understanding reporting requirements and improving reporting
- Leading to the implementation of a program to identify and contact HIV-positive individuals who appeared to be out of clinical care based on surveillance data.[26]
- The core element to the success of the program was the relationship between the health department staff and the facilities.

BOX 18-6 Using Electronic Laboratory Reporting (ELR) and Electronic Health Records (EHR) to Advance Public Health Surveillance

Electronic laboratory reporting benefits:
- Rapid ascertainment of key information
- Definitive laboratory data for many case definitions (e.g., for some reportable conditions, only a positive laboratory test is necessary for case confirmation)

Electronic laboratory reporting limitations:
- Demographic information, especially race and ethnicity, is often incomplete
- Detailed information about ordering clinician may be incomplete, delaying case investigation
- Laboratory test results may be hard to interpret out of context of additional clinical data

Electronic health record data benefits:
- Complete and detailed demographics more likely compared to ELR
- Data on diagnoses, prescriptions, vital signs, pregnancy status, concurrent test results, and prior test results can add context to current test results
- Clinician contact information should be complete
- Clinical detail likely available, though completeness varies by element of interest (e.g., symptoms, vital signs, diagnoses, treatment, and pregnancy status usually available)

Electronic health record data limitations:
- Specific risk history information often incomplete or not documented (e.g., vaccination status may be incomplete if case was vaccinated outside of the practice; risk history may not be systematically collected)
- Narrative clinical notes may be hard to access

For example, EHR data can help to reliably distinguish between type 1 and type 2 diabetes, between acute and chronic hepatitis B virus infection, and between true- and false-positive hepatitis A virus laboratory results.[29-31] EHR-based surveillance systems also have the potential to allow health departments to provide point-of-care data to clinicians, such as preventative health recommendations or information about emerging pathogens in the patients' community. Point-of-care messages can be customized to patients' particulars. For example, a public health agency with access to information about a patient's age, sex, medical history, vital signs, and recent laboratory test results could make recommendations regarding missing vaccines, treatment strategies for hypercholesterolemia, referral information for alcohol dependency counseling, and/or community resources to enhance exercise and physical activity.

Electronic Medical Record Support for Public Health (ESPnet) is a model system that proves the feasibility of electronic-based surveillance systems built on clinical and public health collaboration (Fig. 18-1).[32] ESPnet is an open-source surveillance platform that facilitates automated case detection and reporting using EHR data. ESPnet currently tracks and reports four different kinds of events: notifiable diseases, influenza-like illness, chronic diseases, and vaccine adverse effects. The system can be configured on either a stand-alone server or as a cloud-based data repository. Data from every encounter managed by the host practice is exported to ESPnet at least once every 24 h. These include patients' demographics, vital signs, diagnoses, laboratory test orders and results, prescriptions, allergies, and social history. Once on ESPnet, they are organized into tables and then continually scanned with custom algorithms to detect events of public health interest. The disease detection algorithms are designed to leverage the full breadth of data in an EHR feed in order to render more sensitive and specific diagnoses than might be possible using diagnosis codes or laboratory tests alone. Conditions are transmitted to the state health department as either individual case reports with fully identifiable data or as aggregate population-level summary data for chronic diseases and ILI. There are currently three active ESPnet installations in Massachusetts and one in Ohio. Since inception, they have collectively transmitted more than 20,000 case reports to the Massachusetts and Ohio state health departments. ESPnet is the product of long-standing collaborations between an academic/clinical group and the Massachusetts Department of Public Health. The entities worked together to secure funding, create the first incarnation of the system, develop the system in new directions, expand its reach to other clinical sites, and to develop strategies to assure sustainability.

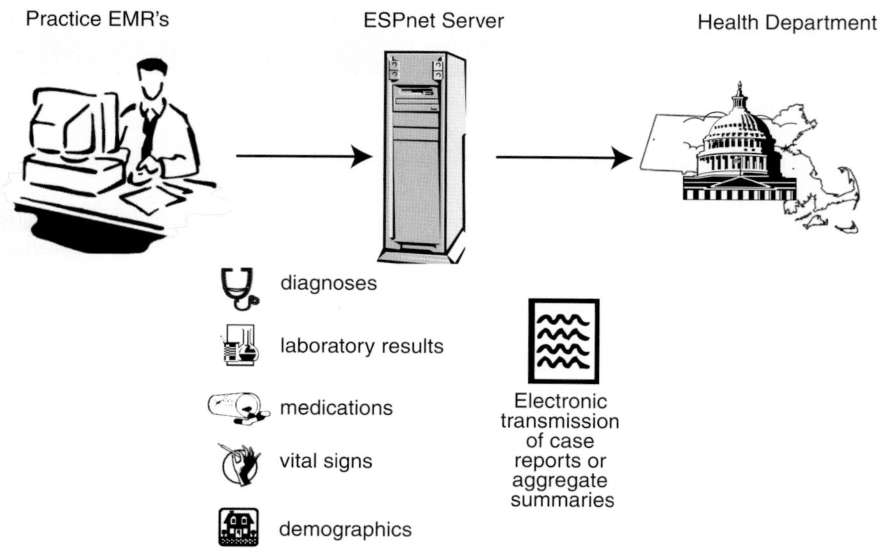

FIG. 18-1 Electronic medical record Support for Public Health (ESPnet) as an example of an electronic-based system for public health reporting.

ESPnet was originally designed to facilitate one-way flow of data from clinical practices to health departments, but over the past few years, Massachusetts Department of Public Health and ESPnet's core developers have taken a significant leap forward by joining separate ESPnet instances in a distributed network that enables health departments to initiate custom queries against participating practices' EHR data via ESPnet. This advance promises to further improve the breadth, speed, and efficiency of data exchange between clinicians and health departments without further burdening clinicians or practice reporting personnel. This will extend the information reach of health departments beyond predefined reportable diseases and notifiable conditions. Historically, health departments have had to make special requests to practice officials to generate custom data for new surveillance targets. These requests were made gingerly and sparingly, and typically only to large practice groups with reporting departments, so as not to overburden clinical practices. ESPnet revolutionizes this model by making it possible for health departments to initiate queries against practices' EHR data with little extra work required of participating practices other than formally giving permission for the query to proceed.

Conclusions

While a comprehensive, responsive, and timely surveillance system could be difficult to implement due to a range of reasons (Box 18-1), we have described a variety of ways to address and build such a system by paying attention to the critical role of clinicians in public health surveillance. From developing relationships through basic activities such as clinical advisories and case investigations to using those relationships to engage clinicians in more advanced surveillance activities, there are a number of activities that can create a mutually beneficial collaboration that contributes to achieving the goals of surveillance. In an era of limited resources, these collaborations and relationships can be attractive to funding agencies in support of novel projects to improve surveillance.

Although we concluded the discussion of best practices by describing a sophisticated, technology-rich surveillance system developed between an academic clinical group and health department, we also outlined many non-IT-heavy approaches to improve surveillance such as minimizing reporting requirements to the minimum data necessary for public health action, fostering strong relationships between public health agencies and clinicians, initiating sentinel surveillance networks, and providing clinicians with useful information in exchange for reporting. Large-volume diseases may ultimately require technology-based solutions in the long term, but much core public health surveillance is rooted in basic communication, analysis, and creative responses to disease-specific problems.

This chapter described how health departments can work to build relationships with clinicians for a variety of reasons, including long-term systems to improve public health overall. Technology dissemination in the developing world is happening and will happen, often skipping steps that occurred in the developed world. However, in light of the 2014 Ebola outbreak in western Africa, it is important to keep in mind the most prominent role of public health: to respond to and prevent the spread of disease. Strong relationships between government health agencies and clinicians are relied upon most conspicuously in emergent and urgent situations in all countries and regions of the world.

KEY SUMMARY POINTS

- Public health departments rely on a number of entities for complete and effective surveillance; clinicians and clinical facilities are the key partners in surveillance activities.
- When these collaborations are fully realized, they support effective case reporting, case investigations, disease prevention and control activities, and ultimately, the development of policies and programs that support population-based health.
- Most collaboration between public health and clinical medicine are mutually beneficial, though the mutual benefits are not always fully appreciated or adequately emphasized. It can be a challenge to elicit full participation from clinicians in surveillance activities; even those that are required, when they or their patients do not in some way benefit or recognized the benefit from participation.
- Buy-in from clinicians into the public health system is essential since clinicians are using time, and therefore resources, to participate in public health surveillance. One example of how public health departments can create such buy-in is providing clinicians with regular reports and materials that can enhance their patient interaction.
- There are many examples of routine and enhanced activities between public health and clinical medicine that contribute to a strong surveillance system. Such a system will be primed for advanced development.
- System level changes to surveillance that affect both public health and clinical medicine can best be achieved when the core relationship between the entities is strong.

DISCUSSION QUESTIONS

1. Identify challenges to clinician reporting of notifiable diseases.
2. Discuss strategies that can be used by health departments to engage clinicians who are not routinely reporting to surveillance.
3. Identify a research study or surveillance activity you would like to conduct that would be dependent on a strong collaboration between public health and a clinician or clinical group.
4. Identify challenges inherent in implementing electronic surveillance methods in a health department.
5. Discuss ways surveillance programs can be mutually beneficial to clinicians and health departments.

REFERENCES

1. Trask JW. The relation of morbidity reports to public health administration. Am J Public Health (N Y) 1913;3(5):421–30.
2. Definition provided by the chapter author.
3. National Notifiable Disease Surveillance System (NNDSS). U.S. Centers for Disease Control and Prevention, <http://wwwn.cdc.gov/nndss/>. [updated August 19, 2015; cited September 25, 2015].
4. Weiss D, Carr D, Kellachan J, Tan C, Phillips M, Bresnitz E, et al. Clinical findings of West Nile virus infection in hospitalized patients, New York and New Jersey, 2000. Emerg Infect Dis 2001;7(4):654–8.
5. Pettit AC, Kropski JA, Castilho JL, Schmitz JE, Rauch CA, Mobley BC, et al. The index case for the fungal meningitis outbreak in the United States. N Engl J Med 2012;367(22):2119–25.
6. Jamieson DJ, Honein MA, Rasmussen SA, Williams JL, Swerdlow DL, Biggerstaff MS, et al. H1N1 2009 influenza virus infection during pregnancy in the USA. Lancet 2009;374(9688):451–8.
7. (CDC) CfDCaP. Novel influenza A (H1N1) virus infections in three pregnant women - United States, April-May 2009. MMWR Morb Mortal Wkly Rep 2009;58(18):497–500.
8. Fine AM, Reis BY, Nigrovic LE, Goldmann DA, Laporte TN, Olson KL, et al. Use of population health data to refine diagnostic decision-making for pertussis. J Am Med Inform Assoc 2010;17(1):85–90.

9. Fine AM, Nizet V, Mandl KD. Participatory medicine: A home score for streptococcal pharyngitis enabled by real-time biosurveillance: a cohort study. Ann Intern Med 2013;159(9):577–83.
10. Schramm MM, Vogt RL, Mamolen M. The surveillance of communicable disease in Vermont: who reports? Public Health Rep 1991;106(1):95–7.
11. Standaert SM, Lefkowitz LB, Horan JM, Hutcheson RH, Schaffner W. The reporting of communicable diseases: a controlled study of Neisseria meningitidis and Haemophilus influenzae infections. Clin Infect Dis 1995;20(1):30–6.
12. Doyle TJ, Glynn MK, Groseclose SL. Completeness of notifiable infectious disease reporting in the United States: an analytical literature review. Am J Epidemiol 2002;155(9):866–74.
13. Friedman SM, Sommersall LA, Gardam M, Arenovich T. Suboptimal reporting of notifiable diseases in Canadian emergency departments: a survey of emergency physician knowledge, practices, and perceived barriers. Can Commun Dis Rep 2006;32(17):187–98.
14. Electronic Health Records: HIMSS, <http://www.himss.org/library/ehr/>. [cited 2015].
15. Shapiro JS, Mostashari F, Hripcsak G, Soulakis N, Kuperman G. Using health information exchange to improve public health. Am J Public Health 2011;101(4):616–23.
16. Chamany S, Silver LD, Bassett MT, Driver CR, Berger DK, Neuhaus CE, et al. Tracking diabetes: New York City's A1C Registry. Milbank Q 2009;87(3):547–70.
17. Das M, Chu PL, Santos GM, Scheer S, Vittinghoff E, McFarland W, et al. Decreases in community viral load are accompanied by reductions in new HIV infections in San Francisco. PLoS One 2010;5(6):e11068.
18. (CDC) CfDCaP. Vital signs: evaluation of hepatitis C virus infection testing and reporting - eight U.S. sites, 2005-2011. MMWR Morb Mortal Wkly Rep 2013;62(18):357–61.
19. Lenert L, Sundwall DN. Public health surveillance and meaningful use regulations: a crisis of opportunity. Am J Public Health 2012;102(3):e1–7.
20. Overhage JM, Grannis S, McDonald CJ. A comparison of the completeness and timeliness of automated electronic laboratory reporting and spontaneous reporting of notifiable conditions. Am J Public Health 2008;98(2):344–50.
21. (CDC) CfDCaP. Notes from the field: use of electronic messaging and the news media to increase case finding during a Cyclospora outbreak - Iowa, July 2013. MMWR Morb Mortal Wkly Rep 2013;62(30):613–4.
22. Heisey-Grove DM, Church DR, Haney GA, Demaria Jr A. Enhancing surveillance for hepatitis C through public health informatics. Public Health Rep 2011;126(1):13–8.
23. Udeagu CC, Webster TR, Bocour A, Michel P, Shepard CW. Lost or just not following up: public health effort to re-engage HIV-infected persons lost to follow-up into HIV medical care. AIDS 2013;27(14):2271–9.
24. Biggerstaff M, Reed C, Epperson S, Jhung MA, Gambhir M, Bresee JS, et al. Estimates of the number of human infections with influenza A(H3N2) variant virus, United States, August 2011-April 2012. Clin Infect Dis 2013;57(Suppl. 1):S12–5.
25. Schirmer P, Lucero C, Oda G, Lopez J, Holodniy M. Effective detection of the 2009 H1N1 influenza pandemic in U.S. Veterans Affairs medical centers using a national electronic biosurveillance system. PLoS One 2010;5(3):e9533.
26. Sweeney P, Gardner LI, Buchacz K, Garland PM, Mugavero MJ, Bosshart JT, et al. Shifting the paradigm: using HIV surveillance data as a foundation for improving HIV care and preventing HIV infection. Milbank Q 2013;91(3):558–603.
27. Udeagu CC, Bocour A, Gale I, Begier EM. Provider and client acceptance of a health department enhanced approach to Improve HIV partner notification in New York City. Sex Transm Dis 2010;37(4):266–271.
28. Onofrey S, Aneja J, Haney GA, Nagami EH, DeMaria A, Lauer GM, et al. Underascertainment of acute hepatitis C virus infections in the U.S. surveillance system: A case series and chart review. Ann Intern Med 2015;163:254–261. doi:10.7326/M14-2939.
29. Klompas M, Eggleston E, McVetta J, Lazarus R, Li L, Platt R. Automated detection and classification of type 1 versus type 2 diabetes using electronic health record data. Diabetes Care 2013;36(4):914–21.
30. Klompas M, Haney G, Church D, Lazarus R, Hou X, Platt R. Automated identification of acute hepatitis B using electronic medical record data to facilitate public health surveillance. PLoS One 2008;3(7):e2626.
31. Allen-Dicker J, Klompas M. Comparison of electronic laboratory reports, administrative claims, and electronic health record data for acute viral hepatitis surveillance. J Public Health Manag Pract 2012;18(3):209–14.
32. Klompas M, McVetta J, Lazarus R, Eggleston E, Haney G, Kruskal BA, et al. Integrating clinical practice and public health surveillance using electronic medical record systems. Am J Public Health 2012;102(Suppl. 3):S325–32.

CHAPTER

19

Engaging Communities to Transform Public Health Surveillance

Paul A Biedrzycki, Anna S Kushnir

Gettin' good players is easy. Gettin' 'em to play together is the hard part.

Casey Stengel

KEY WORDS

Community engagement
Nontraditional partners

INTRODUCTION

Many disciplines, sectors, and practices inform public health surveillance systems through collaborative partnerships. Public health is beginning to integrate data from veterinary, clinical medicine, and military medical systems to understand trends in disease occurrence and progression. These types of linkages are critical to creating a more robust public health surveillance model that can validate and enhance confidence in subsequent public health decision-making. However, the sustainability and resilience of public health surveillance systems will depend on engaging broader and more diverse communities that reduce system vulnerability, accommodate innovation, and readily adapt to external changes in population-driven behavioral and technological evolution. There are several benefits to engaging diverse disciplines, including improvements in early warning and detection, situational awareness, and statistical description of population-based disease morbidity and mortality—particularly important for detecting novel, emerging, and re-emerging disease threats.

This chapter describes how engaging both traditional and nontraditional communities can create the next generation of public health surveillance systems, practitioners, and leadership. There is, unfortunately, little research or study focusing on sociobehavioral aspects or influences on public health surveillance; this chapter is, instead, based on local experience gathered over two decades of work.

Earlier public health surveillance relied on limited and often passive relationships with traditional communities including diagnostic laboratory networks and clinical practitioners for receiving information of possible public health importance. In contrast, the past 10 years of biosurveillance focused on technological improvements to collecting, analyzing, and transmitting data primarily to improve timeliness and quality. This approach requires public health practitioners to think in innovative ways about mining, extracting, and retrieving data and information available from nonclinical sources and nontraditional communities, such as the corporate sector and law enforcement.

Current Status of the Public Health System

Current public health surveillance relies on clinical and epidemiology limited by health care provider and laboratory inputs. This traditional approach does not include a wealth of information available from a much larger community. **Community engagement** is the process of working collaboratively with and through groups of people affiliated by geographic proximity, special interest, or similar situations to address issues affecting the well-being of those people.[1] Community engagement currently is done either as a reaction to unanticipated events, such as disease outbreaks, or to meet stakeholder engagement requirements, such as required for grants or other funding. This approach to community engagement is inevitably short-lived and unproductive.[2] Such superficial interactions with the community can leave community members wary of future participation, leaving health information and data inaccessible to public health; yet, there are data within these communities that can help public health surveillance function more effectively. The catalyst for transforming public health surveillance lies in the practitioner who adopts a vision of wide texture, layering data from clinical, sociobehavioral, environmental, economic, and cultural sources that are prevalent in, and representative of, the community. State and local public health agencies are well positioned to successfully engage their communities, leverage their unique networks, and create trust that can lead to improved public health surveillance and related systems.[3]

Partners and Communities for Public Health Outreach

In the context of examples and related discussion presented in this chapter, communities can be viewed conceptually as networks of individuals, groups, and organizations represented in and by various government agencies, nonprofit organizations, private sector entities, and citizen groups (Fig. 19-1). Connecting to these networks

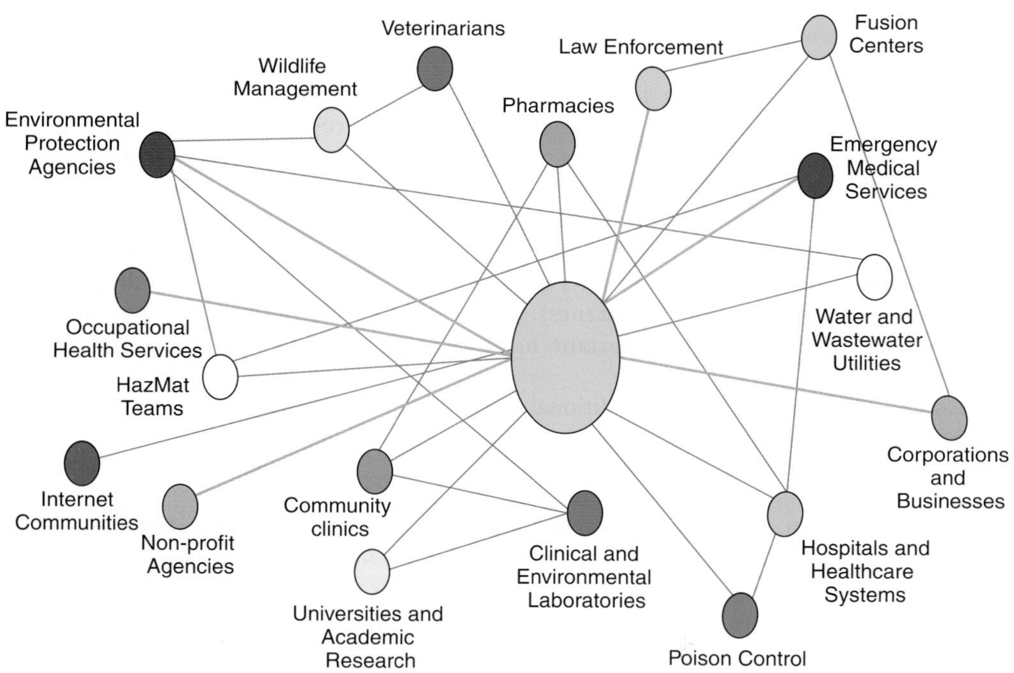

FIG. 19-1 Network of communities involved in public health surveillance.

can allow public health surveillance to move outside traditional and empirical models to assess community health and achieve relevant situational awareness faster, better, and more cost-effectively, which can potentially transform public health surveillance. Community networks hold considerable information relevant to disease and injury surveillance. Specifically, such networks can provide data related to potential threats, exposures, or other significant events.[4] Public health surveillance can use such data to minimize preventable population morbidity and mortality—but only through active, timely, and effective community collaborations. This chapter focuses on the experiences of public health officials in Milwaukee, Wisconsin. Milwaukee is in many ways representative of many cities across the USA in terms of the diversity of the population and types of traditional and nontraditional communities that potentially can be engaged in expanding the scope and depth of public health surveillance. From local first responder agencies (e.g., police and fire departments) to quasi-governmental entities (e.g., drinking water and sewage treatment plants) to community-based agencies (e.g., neighborhood health clinics and faith-based organizations), urban centers like Milwaukee can find fertile ground in mining data from a variety of available and diverse communities of interest that are potentially useful to public health surveillance data.

Nontraditional partners are partners outside a given sector or field.[5] Nontraditional partners for public health surveillance can include academic or research institutions involved in community-based public and environmental health studies; corporations that monitor employee wellness and occupational health; law enforcement agencies that have developed intelligence fusion center capabilities; or nongovernmental organizations (NGOs) such as Humane Societies that monitor and respond to wildlife and/or domestic animal complaints (Box 19-1 and Table 19-1).

For example, the City of Milwaukee Health Department (MHD) convenes stakeholders from a variety of social service, public safety, educational, and health care agencies as part of its Extreme Heat Health Task Force. Stakeholders work together to contribute to review and update plans to reduce seasonal heat-related morbidity and mortality in the community. The group focuses on understanding how information from stakeholders who have regular contact with the elderly (e.g., food, medical, and behavioral health services) can be gathered and rapidly shared with all partners during an Extreme Heat Advisory or Warning in order to implement appropriate prevention and response measures. Such interventions include media messaging, extending public swimming pool hours, and opening public cool spots (Box 19-2).

BOX 19-1 Fusion Center Models as an Example of Public Health Collaboration with Law Enforcement[6]

Fusion centers were developed by the US Department of Homeland Security (DHS) to layer intelligence from an array of data sources to strengthen situational awareness and prevention of terrorism or other criminal events. Data sources include:

- Traditional law enforcement agencies at the federal, state, and local level
- Nontraditional community sources, such as:
  - Fire departments
  - Public works department
  - Hospitals
  - Private sector retailers

DHS developed and promoted guidance to assist medical and public health organizations to both conceptually and practically understand and become involved in fusion centers being stood-up within state and local jurisdictions throughout the USA.[1]

Challenges to public health agencies in participating in fusion center operating models include:

1. Lack of familiarity and training in contemporary intelligence community methodology
2. Lack of security clearances necessary to participate in law enforcement classified threat briefings and discussions
3. Privacy and confidentiality issues surrounding public health exchange of data and information with non-health-care personnel

TABLE 19-1 Examples of Nontraditional Communities that can Inform and Benefit Public Health Surveillance Activities Around Communicable Disease Trends, Population Preparedness, and Environmental Health

EXAMPLE COMMUNITIES	POTENTIAL DATA STREAMS
Fusion centers, first responders, police	• Community threat assessments • Risk-vulnerability analyses • Terrorist/criminal investigations involving Weapons of Mass Destruction • State and national threat-security intelligence
Veterinarians, wildlife services	• Wildlife illnesses/die-offs • Domestic animal morbidity • Unusual or rare animal illness events • Species migration or introduction trends • Pet shop inventory and sales trends • Animal quarantine orders/notices • Unusual veterinary practice disease encounters (agricultural stock and domestic pets)
Local departments of commerce, economic development commissions	• Social and geographic information (population income, race, educational status by zip code, census tract) • Brownfields environmental assessment and remediation data (groundwater, soil contaminants) • Housing stock (age and condition) • Public green-space locations
Water providers, water treatment facilities	• Wastewater and drink water treatment plant data (quality, operational integrity, online monitoring of microbial, chemical, and physical properties of influent and effluent) • Customer complaint logs • Sewer infrastructure (cross-connections, sanitary and combined sewer overflows) • Energy consumption, power plant operational integrity (nuclear and coal-burning environmental discharge/release)
Green business programs, US Green Building Council	• Environmental watchdog reports/scorecards (air, water, land use) • Environmental sampling and monitoring results trends (locally, regionally, nationally) • Unusual occurrences (contamination events, spills, etc.) • Urban agriculture trends (urban chicken and beekeeping activities, community garden activities) • Local community complaints, concerns, and agenda
	• Occupational health and employee wellness trends • Employee absenteeism • Customer complaints • Environmental management practices • Select customer service delivery (flu shots, community health screening programs) • Trends in sales (over-the-counter medications, medical devices) • In-store medical clinics (acute care)

BOX 19-2 Benefits of the Milwaukee Extreme Heat Task Force

The Milwaukee Extreme Heat Task Force represents multiagency trust that is validated each year through member participation, and Heat Plan update and review. That trust is realized through progressive reductions in heat related morbidity and mortality within the community.

This Task Force coordinates roles and responsibilities in preparedness and response without any formal documentation or additional funds. Its effectiveness is dependent on member trust, equity, integrity, commitment, and respect. The establishment of the Task Force required several face-to-face meetings with member agency representatives to identify potential goals and prospective outcomes that could be achieved through participation and engagement. The Milwaukee Health Department, through consensus vote by all participating members became the ad hoc coordinating agency responsible for maintaining membership lists, notification protocols, task force minutes, and written plan maintenance. Challenges to this model included sustaining engagement through member agency representative turnover; assuring equitable distribution of responsibilities across all agencies; disparate resource availability across member agencies; political restrictions with regard to select policy and protocol development; and disparities in interjurisdictional authority.

BENEFITS OF COMMUNITY ENGAGEMENT IN ADVANCING PUBLIC HEALTH SURVEILLANCE

Active and sustained interaction can result in short- and long-term benefits for public health agencies and the communities they serve. These benefits include:

- Improved early warning and detection of significant potential disease outbreaks, clusters, and/or widespread injury;
- Enhanced public health situational awareness;
- Enriched granularity of community-wide common operating picture for first responders;
- Refined public health agency strategic plans and ability to accomplish outcomes;
- Increased diversity in partnerships fueling innovation in prevention and intervention approaches;
- Maturing emergency preparedness and response modeling;
- Informing public health surveillance research and practice; and
- Strengthened community resiliency.

These benefits can be force multipliers within a new paradigm of public health surveillance that better preserve and protect the population's health. Similarly, such engagements improve citizen awareness of health issues within a community and bring citizens in as partners in problem-solving and prevention strategies. Raising awareness of these issues can lead to better solutions in the control and mitigation of communicable disease and adverse environmental exposures.[7]

There are several advantages to integrating and/or overlaying multiple data streams into state and local biosurveillance activities. Such fusion, or combining, of data has become a standard practice in federal, state, and local law enforcement intelligence operations and has been put into practice at the US Department of Homeland Security's National Biosurveillance Integration Center (Box 19-3). A key benefit of this approach can be measured through achieving more comprehensive situational awareness through creation of multidimensional data overlays (e.g., West

BOX 19-3 Examples of Community Partnerships and Collaborations Aiding Public Health Efforts

1. The high incidence of sexually transmitted infections (STIs), such as gonorrhea and chlamydia, in cities is often centered on impoverished minority populations. Curbing the spread of STIs requires a coordinated and concerted effort among:
   - Public and private health care providers
   - Schools and universities
   - Detention facilities
   - Job placement offices
   - Community outreach organizations
   - Churches and advocacy groups

   Target activities can include:
   - Counseling and treatment alternatives
   - Field-delivered antibiotic therapy
   - Targeted peer outreach campaigns
2. Childhood lead poisoning programs in many older and formerly industrialized "rust belt cities" across the USA are centered on non-owner-occupied low-income rental properties with a high degree of deteriorating lead-based paint. Efforts to reduce the prevalence of blood lead levels in young children require the partnership and collaboration of the following:
   - Building owner associations
   - Realty management firms
   - Community clinics
   - Private health care providers
   - Developers
   - Housing rehabilitation contractors
   - Environmental advocates

   Their significant contributions to the public health effort include increasing the capacity for screening and testing of children and housing units for dangerous levels of lead.

Nile virus incidence, mosquito breeding sites, and senior living centers) to informing and sustaining successful partnerships with nontraditional public health agencies (e.g., joint public health/law enforcement bioterrorism threat assessments). In addition, fusion models can link seemingly disparate data sets in a community through temporal and/or spatial orientation to create a new dimension and perspective that can strategically guide subsequent prevention and intervention activities (e.g., urban heat vulnerability index linking tree foliage coverage, housing age/density, and extreme heat morbidity within a community).

Along with the benefits of community engagement through collaboration come inevitable risks. Risks in this context are often more perception than reality and can include lack of confidentiality and data exchange security; technological incompatibilities; Freedom of Information Act noncompliance; overriding political agendas; public misperception; incompatible partner mission and goals; and indemnification and related liabilities. If these risks are acknowledged up front, discussed, and resolved, trust and transparency will be bolstered and the collaborations will not be affected.

IMPORTANT CONSIDERATIONS FOR ENGAGING COMMUNITIES

Collaboration refers to partnerships, cooperative agreements, and mutual aid. Collaboration is strongest in a "win-win" arrangement in which all parties benefit. Building relationships and partnerships with various communities can be initiated and fortified by routine communication, face-to-face meetings, feedback, and equitably assigning roles and responsibilities, as well as identifying realistic resource needs. There are several aspects to establishing and maintaining successful community relationships.

First, fostering trust and process transparency are essential, which requires patience and the ability to listen and hear each other. Trust can be improved through transparency in processes and participant motivation that is further enhanced by omnidirectional feedback during the entire collaboration.[8]

Next, the role of motivating participating organizations or individuals must be recognized. Well-run organizations and highly competent staff are typically immersed in and focused on daily and weekly goals, objectives, and activities. Identifying common goals and meaningful incentives to collaboration that do not conflict with an organization's mission can be used to motivate collaboration. Routinely sharing information and feedback loops are often used in collaborations to motivate and create incentive. Seeing tangible results and outcomes of the collaboration increases the incentive for community members to engage with public health practitioners. If, on the other hand, the incentives decline, community members may feel their input is ceremonial or perfunctory, thus decreasing productive collaboration.[9]

Third, individual and organizational cultures and practices need to be respected. Understanding and respecting the diversity inherent in each community, including cultural, experiential, educational, and other factors contributes to how people interpret and form the foundational building blocks of successful community engagement.[9] These aspects of organizational behavior represent the technological, social, administrative, and economic drivers of a given business, sector, or operation. Awareness and respect for these drivers and differences will limit the potential for pitfalls of miscommunication and misunderstanding.

Finally, partners should identify the mutual benefits wrought from collaborating. Each party should have a stake in the partnership and be allowed to innovate. This type of flexibility not only further stimulates motivation to collaborate through the potential development of new and improved processes but also creates a level of engagement self-sustainment. Partnership growth and evolution is fueled by both prospect and eventual validation of creative solutions that meet mutually desired outcomes.

HOW TO ENGAGE NONTRADITIONAL PARTNERS

Nontraditional partners such as water treatment facilities and community organizations (e.g., social service groups) rarely know what public health surveillance is and does. These partners may not be familiar with the public health system or be calibrated in practice or mission to interact with public health, but they may have information or access to information that is useful for public health surveillance. Local public health practitioners must engage in a lot of outreach to educate and build awareness about what information can be of value and why that information is important. When making requests for information and data, public health agencies should be aware of an organization's hierarchy, structure, policies, and culture. Public health agencies often underestimate the labor, time, commitment, and overall effort required to collect, filter, and transmit seemingly readily available information or data. In addition, the scope and potential legal challenges of collaboration should be understood by all parties. Data sharing agreements (DSUs) are often used between public health agencies and external organizations to formalize such a relationship by explicitly stating the terms and conditions under which information will be exchanged, including privacy and confidentiality provisions. DSUs should not be used as a substitute for building trust and transparency with potential partners but rather to provide clarity in expectations and meet any necessary legal requirements imposed by either party.

Email

Monthly emails describing current public health concerns, prompts for input, upcoming events, and contact information for public health representatives keeps partners aware of issues in public health and enables them to easily contact public health representatives, facilitating the reporting of relevant events.

Seminars

Topics for regular seminars can include the current public health climate, public health programs, and issues in public health. As much as possible, making the seminar topic relevant to the targeted community will improve attendance and community engagement. Seminars can be advertised on social media, through monthly emails, on public health agency websites, and through local publications such as newspapers and trade magazines.

Workshops

Periodic workshops serve to educate the community and, at the same time, allow for the development of personal relationships and trust. Workshop topics may include how to report diseases or how to identify diseases or conditions that may lead to outbreaks (such as a drop in water quality or an increase in a vector population). One example of a productive workshop is presented below.

Joint Criminal and Epidemiological Workshops

In 2003, the US Centers for Disease Control and Prevention (CDC), along with the US Department of Justice and Federal Bureau of Investigation (FBI), developed a curriculum and training model directed toward promoting joint local public health and law enforcement collaboration around assessment and investigation of incidents involving suspected bioterrorism.[10] The resulting workshop, "Joint Criminal and Epidemiological Investigations," has been conducted both nationally and internationally with a wide range of audiences and disciplines, including first responder agencies, hospitals, and emergency management officials. The workshop encompasses a number of interactive exercises designed to actively engage participants in problem solving, especially involving interdisciplinary communication barriers and identification of opportunities for improved exchange of intelligence that is mutually beneficial to everyone involved. Law enforcement's and public health's organizational culture and practices involving surveillance activities, whether from a criminal or communicable disease context, are examined for reporting timeliness, content and accuracy, and assessing threat credibility. Strategic decisions on joint investigations and joint client interviews are then conducted, depending on mutual agreement and urgency. A key principle emphasized throughout the 2-day curriculum is the importance of routine and early information sharing through early relationship building and establishing trust between parties. This synergizes engagement to successfully achieve a common mission and goal.

Social Media

Maintaining a lively and up-to-date Facebook page and Twitter account maintains community engagement and can deliver early warning of a threat to specific communities.[11] Unlike email, which is best used sparingly to avoid overburdening the community, social media facilitates easy and continual communication and engagement.

Big Data Analytics Approach to Surveillance and Engagement

Two significant developments have had profound impacts on public health surveillance over the past decade: the continued conceptual design, implementation, and refinement of electronic health records (EHR) by managed the health care sector and the federal focus and integration of public health emergency preparedness in the USA following the events of September 11, 2001. Each has not only shaped how public health surveillance is practiced but has also provided some evolutionary framework for public health informatics and related data analysis. Benefits of these types of collaborations usually centered on improving early warning and detection of disease events within the community, but they also have residual dividends in more closely calibrating clinical findings against local public health epidemiology.

Most EHR and public health emergency preparedness models require a collaborative approach to surveillance that incorporates both traditional and nontraditional stakeholders. The merits of collaboration in this regard become readily transparent as "passive surveillance systems" such as reporting by laboratories and medical providers is complemented by "active" data mining and synchronous reporting to public health agencies (e.g., BioSense, ESSENCE, and other syndromic data feeds). In turn, these emerging systems provide a level and rapidity of data transference for public health epidemiologic use in analysis, trending, and proactive response.

For example, using syndromic surveillance data feeds from private health care by governmental public health agencies requires close collaboration with hospitals, laboratories, acute care facilities, and other managed care organizations.[12,13] This was typically started through DSUs, which were essential in defining types and categories of data, file coding, privacy and security standards (e.g., the Health Insurance Portability and Accountability Act of 1996), and analysis algorithms. Fundamental to the collaboration were feedback loops to medical professionals that underscored their contribution to understanding trends in community population illness, which further informed individual clinical practice (e.g., through diagnostics and treatment). In return, public health received additional information that could be used for potential early detection of clusters or widespread illness in the community before laboratory confirmation.

CASE STUDIES HIGHLIGHTING COMMUNITY ENGAGEMENT AS THE CORNERSTONE OF PUBLIC HEALTH SURVEILLANCE

The 2003 Monkeypox Outbreak

In 2003, an outbreak of monkeypox affected 71 patients across multiple states in the Midwestern USA. An in-depth investigation by CDC traced the source of the infection to pet prairie dogs housed and sold by an animal distributor in Illinois; the prairie dogs were likely infected with monkeypox when they were co-housed with giant Gambian rats imported from Ghana.[14] Following this monkeypox outbreak, the City of Milwaukee Health Department formed the Veterinary Surveillance Network (VetNet), comprising private sector domestic and agricultural veterinarians, domestic animal control organizations, humane societies, state wildlife agencies, retail pet stores, and animal research laboratories, among other groups (Fig. 19-2).[15]

The initial purpose of the project was to enhance communications with local public health agencies in preparation and response to emergencies involving zoonotic disease. It was later expanded to include assessment and coordination of interdisciplinary training workshops and exercises. The system was also designed to be used for "drop-in"

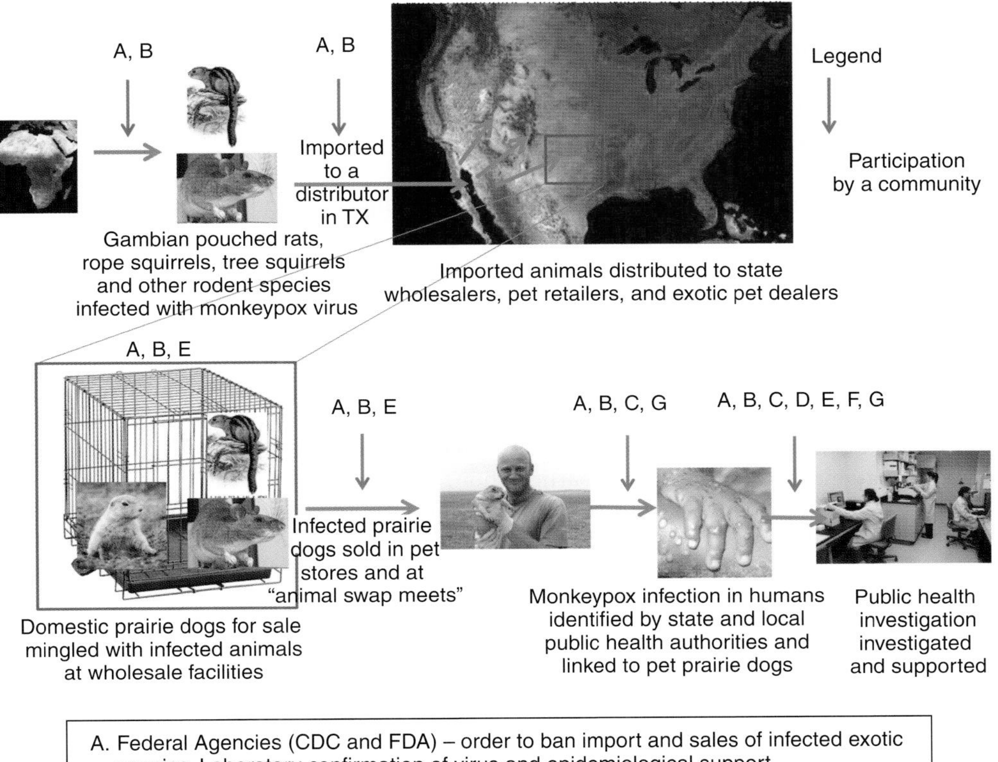

A. Federal Agencies (CDC and FDA) – order to ban import and sales of infected exotic species. Laboratory confirmation of virus and epidemiological support.
B. State and Local Public Health Agencies – laboratory identification, epidemiological investigation, isolation and quarantine of exposed and infected human and animal cases, alert messaging to animal health professionals and healthcare providers
C. Private Sector Veterinarians- identification of animal and human cases at shelters, humane societies and practice settings, exposure control measures.
D. Humane Societies, Domestic Animal Control, Wildlife Management Agencies – assistance in surveillance for infected animals and reporting of employee exposures.
E. Pet Stores, Exotic pet dealers, General public – identification of potential infection in variety of animal species including existing pets
F. Schools of Veterinary Medicine – assist in laboratory testing, animal seroprevalence surveys, occupational heath
G. Private Healthcare Providers (hospitals, acute care settings, etc.) – surveillance for human infection, public messaging.

FIG. 19-2 Points of public health intervention and engagement with communities during the Midwestern US spread of monkeypox in 2003.

surveillance or animal-related disease or injury that may be of public health importance or convey early detection and warning related to a zoonotic outbreak.

In the course of the monkeypox outbreak and review of VetNet operations in the months that followed, a number of gaps and areas for improvement were identified that highlight the challenges of community outreach and coordination between communities with different organizational structures, priorities, and goals. The system continues to be used sporadically as a means to provide health alert updates on information of direct interest to this community but has not been successful for drop-in or active surveillance of animal disease. Some of the lessons learned in the course of launching VetNet, as well as training and exercises with the human and animal public health communities, include the following:

- Differences in organizational cultures should be addressed to improve collaboration. Animal health professionals in the region were not interconnected in ways that could easily be leveraged by local public health agencies to create an effective animal disease surveillance network. Many of these stakeholders were unfamiliar with the organizational culture and practices of other animal health professionals, which complicated information sharing.
- Familiarity with communicable disease surveillance and emergency response models is important for all partners. Many of the animal health professionals targeted for the VetNet initiative were not familiar with communicable disease surveillance systems and reporting requirements commonly used by human public health professionals. The models used for outbreak and cluster investigations and response differ between human and animal health professionals.
- Data management capabilities and capacity are necessary for disease reporting. Most animal health professionals did not have the reporting system infrastructure necessary to collect, collate, and transmit data in aggregate to state and local public health agencies. Many animal health professional organizations and practices did not have the human or material resources needed to design, develop, or implement such systems either.
- Resource limitations can restrict partner participation. Though many animal health professionals were interested in and open to collaborating with public health authorities for disease surveillance, they raised concerns about staff time, cost, and effort that could potentially compromise their current business practices and operations.
- The legal framework and authority for conducting animal health surveillance should be clarified. Some animal health professionals inquired about the legal requirements and authority for conducting animal disease surveillance at the local public health level and how the data would be used in the context of decision-making. This included concerns over future government regulation of animal health organization practices (e.g., licensing, permits, or registrations) that would economically impact current business practices.

The VetNet example demonstrates the benefits and challenges of engaging animal health communities in human health surveillance. The lessons learned from the launch of VetNet can be used to bolster future efforts aimed at integrating human and animal health.

The 2009 H1N1 Influenza Pandemic

During the 2009 H1N1 influenza pandemic, public health surveillance was used by state and local public health agencies to rapidly characterize the first wave of infections by number of cases, susceptibility profile, and severity of disease in local communities.[16,17] This information was used to inform vaccination strategies in preparation for a second or possibly third wave of infection. In the interim, social distancing, including temporary closure of schools, was instituted in many jurisdictions with significant social and economic implications.[18]

While H1N1 severity was eventually found to be similar to seasonal influenza epidemics, early community containment compliance by citizens, nonprofit organizations, businesses, and local policy makers was generally believed by public health authorities to be essential to limiting the spread of disease.[19,20] In many instances, community participation in the public health mitigation strategies was the direct result of successful pre-event community engagement, outreach, and awareness as part of pandemic preparedness programs run by state and local public health agencies. Without the relationship between public health and the community, effective prevention strategies could not have been realized.

For example, to reach student populations in schools and universities during the H1N1 outbreak, the Florida Department of Health formed a working group with elementary, middle, and high schools; universities; community colleges; the education department; and the board of governors. The working group, with representation from a wide collection of education stakeholders, included the education community in the public health response to H1N1.[21]

Local public health agencies are usually both familiar with and well connected to an array of other governmental, academic, nonprofit, and community-based organizations whose partnerships are essential to meeting the core public health functions of assessment, assurance, and policy development. Local public health agencies, as trusted agents in ensuring community health, can serve as an entry point to dialogue and new opportunities for collaboration with traditional (e.g., medical and academic sectors) as well as nontraditional partners (e.g., law enforcement and corporate sectors).

The 2013 *Legionella* Infection Outbreak and Response in Milwaukee, Wisconsin

Between June and August 2013, the MHD received reports of approximately 50 confirmed cases of *Legionella* infection.[22] Many onsets of illness were reported during the 4 weeks of July. Typically, between 20 and 30 cases of *Legionella* infection are reported annually in Milwaukee County, with some seasonal trends noted in September and October. State-wide reports of illness also increased during summer 2013, with the majority of cases in metropolitan Milwaukee (Fig. 19-3).

The 2013 legionellosis outbreak in Milwaukee resulted in a multifold increase in confirmed disease, which fostered collaboration with heating, ventilation, and air conditioning (HVAC) consultants, contractors, and building owners to identify contaminated cooling towers. MHD worked with National Weather Service data to examine precipitation and temperature variations and their possible association with disease incidence. Early epidemiologic evidence indicated a cluster within a specific area of the city, including primarily homebound individuals. The MHD and the Wisconsin Division of Public Health began enhanced surveillance activities including alert messages to health care providers about diagnosis, specimen collection, laboratory analysis, and reporting to public health authorities.

The MHD provided information to the community about the outbreak through several channels. The media was used to build public awareness, maintain transparency, and identify additional cases. Media messages consisted of regular updates to print and televised media, websites, and Twitter, press conferences to provide investigative results to the general public (e.g., number of cases, basic demographic information, key risk factors, suspect exposure reservoirs, and the overall public risk of illness). Televised media interviews were conducted to further underscore the

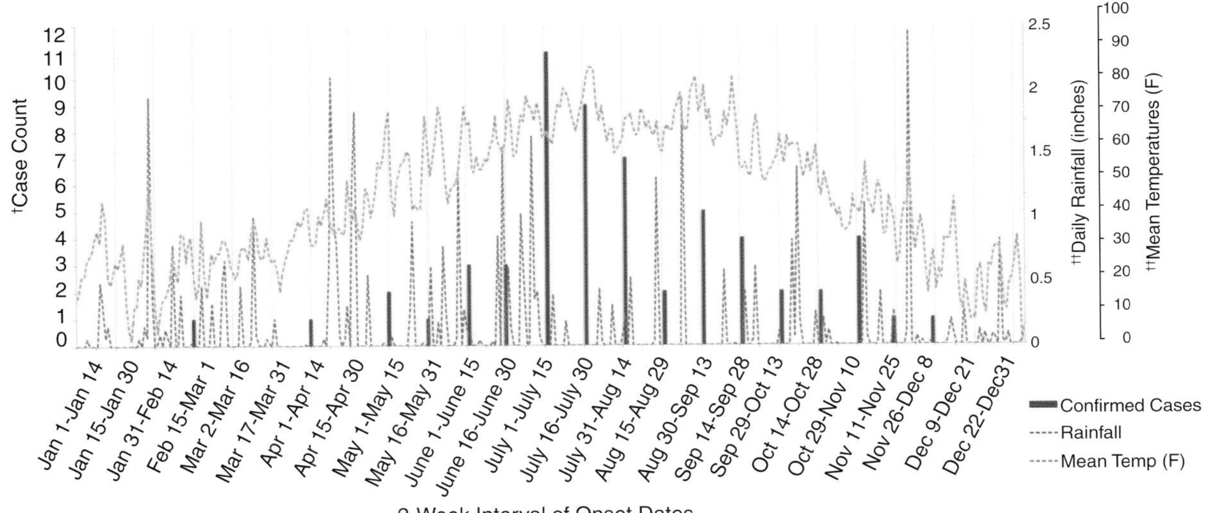

Prepared by the City of Milwaukee Health Department
Disease Control and Environmental Health Division

†Case data provided by the Wisconsin Electronic Disease Surveillance System (WEDSS)
††Mean temperature and rainfall data collected from the National Weather Service

FIG. 19-3 The 2013 epidemiologic curve of reported legionellosis cases. Two-week intervals with daily rainfall and mean temperatures by onset date.

BOX 19-4 Enhanced Biosurveillance

In the course of an outbreak, biosurveillance can be enhanced by the following:
- Analysis of all electronic laboratory reporting for cases of relevant illness.
- Periodic review of syndromic surveillance signals (such as emergency department visits for relevant syndromes).
- Messaging to a broad group of community stakeholders.
  - Messaging content can include case definition, testing and diagnostic algorithms, and public health reporting protocols.
- Contacting the medical examiner and several large hospitals in the metropolitan area to ensure retrospective and prospective reporting of any suspect cases in patients or decedents.

department response and findings, and the local newspaper ran articles about the investigation during the outbreak. MHD also provided information to the public about reporting and testing atypical pneumonia or severe respiratory illness cases in the community.

The MHD initiated an environmental investigation immediately after reviewing the initial confirmed cluster of cases and ruling out potential common indoor sources. Outdoor reservoirs were investigated for possible contamination, including building cooling towers, large decorative water fountains, and community water parks with large water aerosolizing devices in kiddie splash and play areas. The MHD then met with representatives of cooling tower chemical and maintenance contractors to review startup protocols earlier in the season and identify unique factors that could influence *Legionella* amplification and dissemination in the region (Box 19-4).

Environmental sampling (both swab and water specimens) of preidentified and potential environmental reservoirs in the community, based on guidance from the industry sector, did not lead to a definitive source. Meanwhile, laboratory testing of clinical specimens revealed at least four disparate strains of the *Legionella* bacterium associated with confirmed infections, suggesting multiple sources of exposure. As an intervention measure, the MHD engaged several businesses and private sector organizations, including metropolitan building owner associations, realty management groups, and building HVAC contractors, to distribute building water system maintenance protocols, including how to disinfect cooling towers to control *Legionella* growth. The MHD saw a decrease in rate of confirmed infection case reports within 2 weeks of distributing the protocols to established private sector partners.

MHD leveraged its private sector relationships and included these partners in outbreak planning and response. It relied on previously established credibility with media outlets to disseminate disease risk messages. Finally, previous efforts to promote transparency and trust with the public facilitated community sharing of outbreak-related information that included risk, severity of disease, sources of exposure, and mitigation measures. All of these collaborations allowed for targeted environmental assessment and sampling, as well as the initiation of preventive measures in the community.

Effective community engagement extends beyond improving disease surveillance. In this example, reliance on principles of trust (with private health care and business), transparency (with the media and public), partnership incentives (with consultants and contractors invested in maintaining clients), and an agreed upon strategy and outcome (between the local health department and the private sector) were essential for effective outbreak investigation and control.

COMMUNITY ENGAGEMENT IN CURRENT AND FUTURE PUBLIC HEALTH SCENARIOS

Global Climate Change and Public Health

Community engagement has the potential to reach beyond tracking and awareness of the effects of local events on public health. Consistent and in-depth communication with local communities may bring to light the effect of global changes on the local environment and community public health. One global issue that has an effect on local public health is global climate change. Systems that have sufficient sensitivity and specificity necessary to detect, measure, and predict changes and emerging threats to the ecosystem and, inevitably, human health will become increasingly important as the global climate continues to evolve and change. To keep pace with the public health issues that may appear as a result of global climate change, it will be even more important to engage communities across multiple agencies and organizations.

CDC's Climate-Ready States and Cities Initiative assists state and local public health agencies in preparing for and anticipating the public health effects associated with climate change.[23] The initiative advocates the use of the Building Resilience Against Climate Effects framework that delineates potential weather-based scenarios and impacts on public health as a means of catalyzing strategic foresight planning.[24] A key component of this framework is integrating meteorological data and climate projections into public health epidemiologic analysis and planning. Building Resilience Against Climate Effects promotes the development of public health surveillance efforts to predict disease incidence and distribution, focusing on the most vulnerable populations, such as children, the elderly, persons living in poverty, and those in certain geographic areas. Engaging partners such as the National Weather Service, University Atmospheric Science programs, state social service agencies, and regional urban planning commissions is important, as these partners are all potential sources of data and information to support public health surveillance and strategic decision-making for prevention (Box 19-5).

To meet the challenges presented by global climate change, public health surveillance needs new and different partnerships to go beyond relying on data derived solely from clinical diagnoses and/or laboratory analysis. Engaging and collaborating with new communities and building relationships with new partners is an increasingly important part of disease surveillance systems designed to characterize and predict human health consequences. Public health must collaborate with environmental (air, water, and geological) partners, researchers in entomology, meteorology, wildlife, and forestry, and socioeconomic (housing, land use, and civil engineering) entities. Challenges remain in achieving this ideal: there is increased competition for funding between government, research institutions, and NGOs; political leaders must be energized; public apathy must be overcome; and the community must recognize the mutual benefits of collaboration.

Airport and Airline Communicable Disease Surveillance

The emergence of several novel pathogens in the past decade with alarmingly high case fatality rates, such as severe acute respiratory syndrome (SARS), H5N1 and H7N9 influenza subtypes, and Middle East Respiratory Coronavirus (MERS-CoV), represent not only a new era of potential global public health threats but also advancement in public health surveillance (see case studies).[26] Both the World Health Organization (WHO) and CDC have developed response teams and laboratory assets to rapidly respond to early clusters and outbreaks of novel diseases that emerge almost anywhere in the world.[27,28] Importantly, global economic, political, and social forces create significant challenges for the public health system. One of the biggest challenges to public health response is the mobility of individuals through airline travel and the ability to quickly and unknowingly transport a communicable disease anywhere in the world within 24 hours.

BOX 19-5 Future Climate Change And Public Health[25]

Extreme heat events are projected to be of greater frequency with continued climate change, necessitating additional and specific public health programs focused on surveillance of heat-related morbidity and mortality to inform subsequent preventive and intervention measures.[12] Public health surveillance systems will need to mesh with environmental, social, and health disciplines in monitoring:

- Greenhouse gas emissions
- Population demographics and vulnerability
- Clinical presentation of heat illness
- Reporting of heat associated deaths

Engaging agencies involved in the following activities will be essential in crafting a successful community-wide extreme heat surveillance program:

- Air permit/monitoring
- Programs for the elderly
- Mental/behavioral services
- Homebound outreach
- Acute health care

While the CDC has developed international travel guidance since the 2003 global SARS outbreak, similar recommendations do not exist for domestic flights, regardless of their connection with overseas airline routes.[29] This gap in public health control creates vulnerability for state and local public health agencies should they receive passengers on domestic flights who are symptomatic or are incubating novel pathogens. It also creates a substantial and complex scenario for effective epidemiologic response to mitigate disease transmission both within the airports and beyond. Engaging communities affected by potential domestic flight public health threats is essential to instituting procedures and protocols that fortify public health surveillance under these scenarios. Creating a surveillance system that is both meaningful for public health use and reasonable from airlines' and consumers' perspectives is challenging. As a result, many stakeholders must be involved in crafting an approach that protects the public's health while not unduly jeopardizing the continuity of airport operations.

There are a number of transportation and law enforcement agencies that play an important role in the early detection and identification of a communicable disease and related illness on an aircraft whether in flight, at a gate, or terminal, including the passenger screening, preboarding, and deplaning processes. Each stakeholder includes public safety in its mission and agency goals. As such, constructing a public health surveillance model that recognizes and incorporates these communities is essential to coordinate data retrieval for public health use in assessing a disease threat and initiating epidemiologic follow-up. These agencies are distinct in their organization mission, employee education, skills, experience level, and interest. Therefore, it is important to engage these communities early in discussing and building scenario-based protocols that integrate public health surveillance into planning and each agency can contribute to and strengthen disease surveillance by coordinating with public health authorities on reporting (pilots and air traffic control), observation and notification (Transportation Security Administration [TSA] screeners and airline agents), intelligence sharing (airport security, law enforcement fusion centers, customs and border protection, and emergency management), and medical evaluation and confirmation of illness (emergency medical services, hospitals, and the Occupational Safety and Health Administration).

Currently, CDC's Division of Global Migration and Quarantine (DGMQ) leads disease surveillance on airplanes and in airports that serve as ports of entry to the USA.[30] DGMQ representatives respond to reports of ill passengers on airplanes, provide travelers with essential health information, and oversee the screening of arriving passengers at 18 ports of entry that have a CDC Quarantine Station. The DGMQ also liaises with multiple federal, state, and local partners, as well as with international airline organizations, airport planners, and first responders to contain communicable disease in the airport setting. Though much is being done currently, public health surveillance at airports and on airliners can be enhanced by advocating for diverse participation and engagement of various communities by local public health and emergency management agencies. Advocacy and outreach activities can include the following:

1. Training air traffic controllers in response to in-flight public health emergencies declared by the airline pilot/captain, including collecting brief and relevant information on crew and passenger age, gender, symptoms, onset, and underlying medical conditions.
2. Training commercial airline carrier crew, including pilots and flight attendants, to recognize passenger or crew symptoms of potential communicable disease and facilitating appropriate medical care and support as available.
3. Training ticket and gate airline agents to recognize passenger and crew symptoms that may require local public health notification and how to execute preboarding and deplaning processes in such circumstances.
4. Training TSA screeners, customs and borders officials, airport security, and air marshals to recognize crew and passenger symptoms that may pose a threat to other passengers, crew, or airport employees. (Some international airports already have capabilities to screen passenger temperatures for fever prior to boarding, as was the case during the SARS and H5N1 influenza outbreaks overseas.)
5. Building awareness and familiarity among airport and airline employees and federal agencies about basic epidemiologic protocols followed by state and local public health agencies in the surveillance and control of communicable disease, including types of data collected, legal authority, and medical confidentiality.

6. Developing and refining information- and intelligence-sharing protocols between airport authorities and public health agencies to expedite early epidemiologic investigation, such as airliner passenger manifest, control tower communication logs, and in-flight crew assessments.

Engaging communities involved in airport operations, administration, and security in communicable disease surveillance, like SARS or MERS-CoV, can occur through various collaborations already in place. The Federal Aviation Administration's requirements for airports include developing emergency operations plans (EOPs) for various catastrophic scenarios. Public health officials should work with airport administrators to develop a specific addendum or appendices to airport EOPs that specifically address disease threats. In addition, annual exercises typically conducted with local first responders and other stakeholders can be modified or amended to include novel pathogen introduction via an arriving domestic air flight. These exercises can stimulate discussion about what measures and systems can be adopted, including surveillance and intelligence sharing opportunities, to assist public health response. Finally, memoranda of understanding (MOUs) can be formed with public health and airport authorities to facilitate planning and response to disease threats with provisions for improving surveillance and overall index of suspected illness under certain circumstances, alerts, or notifications.

COMMUNITY ENGAGEMENT AS A FUNCTION IN THE PUBLIC HEALTH WORKFORCE

Increasingly, community engagement is becoming a core competency embedded in the mission of state and local public health agencies with responsibilities shared by all levels of staff, including administration. Shrinking budgets and realignment of public health programs and priorities have necessitated the development of new models of community engagement by public health authorities. These models demand more rapid and frequent involvement of diverse communities in both meeting the mission of public health and sustaining innovative practices. Some degree and expectation of community engagement is being added explicitly to almost every job description in public health agencies or implicitly in job duties and responsibilities. Similarly, new skill sets are being defined that leverage social media skills, analysis of near real-time news feed data, collaboration with nontraditional partners (e.g., corporate entities), and creation of public transparency (e.g., web-based access to department databases on communicable disease trends, food inspection reports).

CONCLUSIONS

Timely and accurate disease and injury surveillance has long been the cornerstone of sound public health practice. Prompt detection and analysis of emerging events and trends that threaten population health are essential to develop effective public health prevention or intervention strategies. Achieving a robust and comprehensive public health surveillance system requires collection, analysis, and integration of data streams across a wide array of sources within a defined jurisdiction. Engaging diverse communities, as described in this chapter, will enhance public health situational awareness by leveraging traditional and nontraditional partners to more quickly and accurately describe communicable disease threats, incidence, and distribution.

Transforming public health surveillance necessitates integrating not only new information technologies and analytics but also new stakeholders to broaden and expand imagination. A variety of communities beyond the readily identified medical community can yield new information that can be useful for public health surveillance. This type of data fusion can result in a return on investment that eclipses more traditional models. The success of these types of endeavors, however, will rely on building relationships through engaging diverse communities and building trust, transparency, respect, and mutual benefits.

Successful collaborations begin with a shared vision by all parties involved to achieve a whole that is greater than the sum of its parts. This demands leaders who are innovative and imaginative beyond dependence on technological solutions. Meaningful collaboration speaks to a deeper understanding of community dynamics, including interacting and communicating with the public. Public health surveillance cannot rely on the status quo if it is to adequately confront the communicable and emerging disease challenges on the horizon.

Effective public health surveillance relies on the rapid and accurate detection of illness, injury, or other events that threaten or influence the morbidity and mortality of a defined population. As a core competency and practice within public health agencies and organizations it is being both challenged and transformed by unprecedented and remarkable advancements in the fields of medicine, biotechnology, and informatics. In addition, it is being simultaneously influenced and shaped by shifting cultural and economic forces such as social media and the advent of EHRs and the related consolidation of health data sharing systems. This places public health surveillance on the cusp of new frontier in terms of the potential for interdisciplinary collaboration as well as geographic reach and scope. Global events such as SARS, avian influenza, pandemic H1N1, MERS-CoV, and Ebola have all relied on sound public health surveillance and prompt information exchange across international cross disciplinary networks to provide situational awareness and inform early strategic response. This has become the hallmark of the new era of global health security.

At the forefront of success in this new frontier is collaboration and specifically engaging diverse communities in achieving a more robust and flexible public health surveillance model of practice. The magnitude and diversity of available information and data that can be leveraged by exploring and leveraging nontraditional partnerships provides opportunities that should not be ignored or discounted.

Several examples provided in this chapter highlight the array of possibilities in improving surveillance, establishing productive relationships and rethinking traditional practices. This can enrich and inform emerging sciences such as predictive modeling and forecasting of disease or other events that have the potential to result in adverse population health outcomes. More importantly, engaging communities in collaboration to transform public health surveillance provides visibility in mission, sparks innovation through diversity of perspective, and builds trust in relationships that can further advance future strategies that are protective of community health.

KEY SUMMARY POINTS

- Engaging communities is essential to improving public health surveillance in the context of leveraging a greater diversity of information that may be predictive or indicative of population health.
- Communities are unique in their economic, social, and political fabric. Assessing and understanding these variables is essential to building trust and providing opportunities for successful engagement of communities.
- There are many benefits to engaging communities for the improvement of public health surveillance. These include improved early warning and detection, situational awareness, and the building of stronger relationships with key community partners such as academia, private health care, law enforcement, and corporate entities.
- Successful engagement of communities relies on creating mutual trust between all parties. Recognizing the role of incentive and motivation as well as unique organizational cultural attributes is essential to achieving win-win partnership and meaningful collaboration.

DISCUSSION QUESTIONS

1. Discuss the connection between community engagement and collaboration. How can community engagement improve public health practice and outcomes including public health surveillance?
2. What are the unique characteristics of the community in which you live or work? How might these characteristics affect public health surveillance or interventions?
3. Describe how some existing community networks share information formally and informally.
4. List several factors that influence successful collaboration through community engagement. What are some ways to build trust when engaging communities?
5. Discuss the benefits of engaging the community to improve public health surveillance.
6. How have public health emergency preparedness activities influenced community engagement? How can community engagement be improved in this regard?

REFERENCES

1. Community Engagement. Definitions and organizing concepts from the literature: U.S. centers for disease control and prevention, <http://www.cdc.gov/phppo/pce/part1.html/>; February 13, 2015.
2. Balcazar H, Rosenthal EL, Brownstein JN, Rush CH, Matos S, Hernandez L. Community health workers can be a public health force for change in the United States: three actions for a new paradigm. Am J Public Health 2011;101(12):2199–203.
3. Consortium CTSA. Community engagement key function committee task force on the principles of community engagement. Principles of community engagement. NIH Publication; 2011.
4. Cohen A, Lopez A, Malloy N, Morello-Frosch R. Our environment, our health: a community-based participatory environmental health survey in Richmond, California. Health Educ Behav 2012;39(2):198–209.
5. Definition provided by the chapter author.
6. US Department of Justice Global justice information sharing initiative. Health security: Public health and medical integration for fusion centers. 2011.
7. Adalja AA, Sell TK, Bouri N, Franco C. Lessons learned during dengue outbreaks in the United States, 2001-2011. Emerg Infect Dis 2012;18(4): 608–14.
8. Vangen S, Huxham C. Nurturing collaborative relations building trust in interorganizational collaboration. J Appl Behav Sci 2003;39(1):5–31.
9. Ansell C, Gash A. Collaborative governance in theory and practice. J Public Admin Res Theory 2008;18(4):543–71.
10. Hayashi K, Papagiotas S. The federal bureau of investigation/centers for disease control and prevention joint criminal and epidemiological investigations course: enhancing relationships to improve biothreat readiness. Prehosp Disaster Med 2010;25(Suppl. 1):S23.
11. Newkirk RW, Bender JB, Hedberg CW. The potential capability of social media as a component of food safety and food terrorism surveillance systems. Foodborne Pathog Dis 2012;9(2):120–4.
12. Center for Disease Control and Prevention. BioSense: public health surveillance through collaboration, <http://www.cdc.gov/biosense/files/13_242388_K2_DHNDI_Biosense_topic_remediated508.pdf/>; February 13, 2015.
13. Lombardo JS, Burkom H, Pavlin J. ESSENCE II and the framework for evaluating syndromic surveillance systems. MMWR Morb Mortal Wkly Rep 2004;53:159–65.
14. Centers for Disease Control and Prevention. Update: multistate outbreak of monkeypox—Illinois, Indiana, Kansas, Missouri, Ohio, and Wisconsin, 2003. MMWR 2003;52(27):642–6.
15. National Association of Country and City Health Officials (NACCHO). Program Details - VetNet: integration of veterinary and animal health professionals, <http://www.naccho.org/topics/modelpractices/database/practice.cfm?PracticeID=137/>; February 13, 2015.
16. Centers for Disease Control Prevention. Update: novel influenza A (H1N1) virus infections-worldwide, May 6, 2009. MMWR Morb Mortal Wkly Rep 2009;58(17):453–8.
17. Jhung MA, Swerdlow D, Olsen SJ, Jernigan D, Biggerstaff M, Kamimoto L, et al. Epidemiology of 2009 pandemic influenza A (H1N1) in the United States. Clin Infect Dis 2011;52(Suppl. 1):S13–26.
18. Lessler J, Reich NG, Cummings DA, Nair HP, Jordan HT, Thompson N. Outbreak of 2009 pandemic influenza A (H1N1) at a New York City school. N Engl J Med 2009;361(27):2628–36.
19. US Department of Health and Human Services. HHS Pandemic Influenza Plan. 2005.
20. van den Wijngaard CC, van Asten L, Koopmans MPG, van Pelt W, Nagelkerke NJD, Wielders CCH, et al. Comparing pandemic to seasonal influenza mortality: moderate impact overall but high mortality in young children. PLoS One 2012;7(2):e31197.
21. The Center for Infectious Disease Research and Policy. Meeting the needs of at-risk populations during the 2009 H1N1 pandemic response a look at key strategies, successes and challenges. University of Minnesota; Minneapolis, MN, 2011.
22. Biedrzycki PA, Stanley M, Radmer F, Lauf S. Notes from the field: increase in reported legionellosis-Milwaukee, Wisconsin, June-September 2013. MMWR Morb Mortal Wkly Rep 2014;63(3):63.
23. Centers for Disease Control and Prevention. CDC's climate-ready states & cities initiative, <http://www.cdc.gov/climateandhealth/climate_ready.html/>; February 11, 2015.
24. Centers for Disease Control and Prevention. CDC's building resilience against climate effects (brace) framework, <http://www.cdc.gov/climateandhealth/brace.html/>; February 11, 2015.
25. Centers for Disease Control and Prevention. Climate change and extreme heat events. National center for environmental health. Atlanta, GA, 2013.
26. Balkhair A, Al Maamari K, Alawi FB. The struggle against MERS-CoV (The Novel Coronavirus). Oman Med J 2013;28(4):226–7.
27. Centers for Disease Control and Prevention. CDC global disease detection and emergency response, <http://www.cdc.gov/globalhealth/gdder/>; February 12, 2015.
28. World Health Organization. Global outbreak alert & response network, <http://www.who.int/csr/outbreaknetwork/en/>; February 11, 2015.
29. Centers for Disease Control and Prevention. CDC health information for international travel 2014: The yellow book. Oxford University Press; New York, NY, 2014.
30. United States department of transportation office of the secretary national aviation resource manual for quarantinable diseases. 2006.

4 SECTION

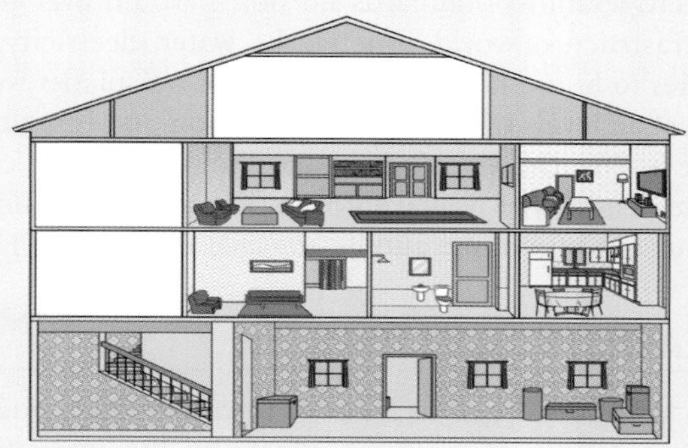

Informatics Enables Transformation

J Mark Conde

Section Outline

Informatics enables public health and PHS and is poised to be even more integral as standard practices are implemented globally and new ideas about working with information are developed. Interoperability is a mantra and there is a good understanding of what the term means. However, achieving interoperability will take diligence in implementation of lower level concepts such as data quality while connections are created fusing heterogeneous data together to achieve higher level knowledge.

The reality of being able to receive data in massive quantities and from many different domains is here; it is an opportunity for PHS capabilities to grow. A wider understanding of "connections" will allow us to see patterns, derive knowledge, and interact with data in a way not possible in the past. This syncs the experts in the public health domain with each other and with new nonhealth domains. The data aggregation for simple observations that is currently common must now grow to a deeper interaction with the information at the next level, combining the strength of humans and technology. The next level of challenges for informatics involves truly using standards globally, finding creative ways to bring heterogeneous data together rapidly, and creating infrastructures that sustain the connections we seek. This will finally create an "ecosystem" of PHS that serves public health, clinical health, and many other human endeavors for a healthy population.

Informatics concepts explored in these chapters drive some new and old thinking with the construction of our PHS house. Without interoperability standards no home would ever be square and fit together. Much less remain connected to our infrastructure world of networks, water, electricity, and sanitary systems. When we look forward to building mega cities to house the overpopulation of our planet we will see an ecosystem of homes can exist to work in unison to meet all levels of the human condition and function in the environment we have created and live in on the earth. We are on the verge of creating homes that are completely controlled by computing devices. This includes our interaction with visual information and interaction with our home environments. Imagine how much data will pour out of a home and be engaged to run the PHS home of the future. It will be daunting!

LEARNING OBJECTIVES

- Define the three types of interoperability and its importance to PHS.
- Identify the current efforts by the international community and WHO on interoperability and system standards.
- Describe the benefits of the standardization of EMR/EHR.
- Define and describe the classifications of Big Data (the V's of Big Data).
- Define data storms and identify some of the new data sources that are now a part of the data storms.
- Describe the importance of data quality as data pools and data streams grow exponentially.
- Define the general enterprise technology principles.
- Describe the benefits of ecosystems in local-level PHS.
- Describe current approaches and advances in data manipulation and data visualization.
- Describe how machine learning approaches are relevant to public health surveillance.

CHAPTER

20

Art and Science of Interoperability to Create Connections

Ramesh Krishnamurthy, J Mark Conde

To develop a complete mind, study the science of art, study the art of science. Learn how to see. Realize that everything connects to everything else.

Leonardo Da Vinci

KEY WORDS

Interoperability
Technical interoperability
Semantic interoperability
Process interoperability
Integration
Electronic health records
Standards
eHealth
Data exchange
Health information systems (HIS)
Electronic medical records

THE BASIC CONCEPTS OF INTEROPERABILITY

Interoperability[1] is defined through three attributes in the context of health and public health. Interoperability is not as simple as just following a set of data standards. Ensuring systems can connect and correlate involves three areas of interoperability: technical, semantic, and process. Tim Benson challenges that interoperability is hard to achieve, considering that all three of these areas are interdependent and must deliver business benefit.[2] In order to meet total interoperability between systems, technical, semantic, and process must be understood and executed consistently with balance between them, otherwise the informatics ecosystem will not function as one. This functioning ecosystem is the business benefit that translates to intended public health outcomes. The most common misconception is that interoperability is simply setting up the technical connections using a common pipe. There are many layers to consider when trying to achieve the goal of being able to exchange, query and interpret, and protect data across many points of existence. We would not worry about interoperability at all if the data and information were simply in one place and all handled the same way.

Technical interoperability ensures that we have computing, network, and software platforms all using the same technology architectures and protocols so that systems can move data around reliably.[3] This layer is usually seen as the hardware and software that follows standards such that machine-to-machine communications can take place. We can fail to achieve the goals of interoperability if we do not consistently share programmatic approaches that can trade data along the same transport mechanisms and network protocols. One example is the declaration that SOAP communication protocols be deployed so that all messages carrying data can have the same conversation to deliver their payloads of semantic HL7 messages. SOAP stands for Simple Object Access Protocol, which is a language for sending information messages between informatics systems that ensures we all talk to each other in the same way. That is an example of software technical message interoperability that would need to ride on the same physical networks or be able to see each other on a network. We can easily have issues when different types of technical networks are established that do not use the same software for carrying messages. In this situation all the parties involved need to reach agreement on what technical deployment they will use to solve this layer of interoperable connections.

Semantic interoperability moves up the hierarchy of moving data around by requiring that the communicating systems can interpret the payloads of data sent between them in the same way.[3] There are variants to how semantic standards are applied. The structure of the message that rides on the network should be consistent; for example, everyone should use an HL7 message format with a specific version to send specific messages in an XML data structure. There are problems even with this example; different versions of HL7 message structures can cause problems, since Version 2.x will not sync with interpreters of Version 3.x. Specific atomic data elements, or fields, follow semantic interoperability rules by using the same coding systems. This is another level inside the semantic interoperability problem that must follow standards or we cannot interpret sections or fields of the message sent consistently. One example is applying the identity of specific lab assays by using the LOINC coding system. Without using something like LOINC we would not really be able to say that a test in one laboratory was done exactly the same way as in a second laboratory even if they both claim to be testing for the same analyte. These subsections or fields have to follow similar format structures, such as the MM/DD/YYYY date format, or we are open to misinterpretation on either side. A larger scale problem is how the structure of the relationships of data records is represented. Often this is a semantic problem, where both sides need database structures that hold multiple related records that can be interpreted the same way between pools of data in separate database systems.

Process interoperability can be the most difficult, because it follows business concepts within each organization that drive how data are interpreted, shared, and executed in an environment.[4] Another term used for this level is Legal Interoperability because laws and policies govern this aspect as well as process.[3] For example, two public health departments might share perfectly transmitted, consistently coded results from a lab test for hexavalent chromium in drinking water. If they examined the data using different thresholds of contamination, one group would open an investigation, whereas the other would not consider this level a threat. This discrepancy may lead to a major misunderstanding among the public, media, and others about a potential drinking water problem. Process interoperability is more difficult to understand but must follow significant discussion with all parties using the data exchanged. A situation at the Minnesota Department of Health[5] illustrates the failure of process interoperability. In this example, process was never discussed and children were put at risk. "The injured school children arrive at an Emergency Department (ED). The provider uses several different [electronic health records] EHRs and assumes that all the systems provide alerts for allergy. This particular ED system does not have alerts implemented and thus the provider is not aware of this different process. A drug is prescribed with potential allergic reaction to an injured child."

As we have demonstrated through this introduction to basic interoperability concepts, creating connections on many levels is critical for successful exchanges and use of surveillance data.

EXPANDING THE INTEROPERABILITY SCOPE

Reliable and timely health information is an essential foundation for health systems strengthening and public health action, both nationally and internationally.[6] Population- and institution-based data are two major sources of data for national health information systems. Population-based sources include censuses, civil registration, public health surveillance, and population surveys. Institutional-based data include individual, service, and resource records.

Functional health information systems depend on harmonized and interoperable data elements between and within systems through the adoption of health data and information technology (IT) standards. This is the semantic layer of interoperability. In order to achieve interoperability, seamless health **data exchange** must occur between devices, from device to EHRs, and between diagnostics platforms and electronic medical records (EMRs). **Data exchange** is the process of sending and receiving data in such a manner that the information content or meaning assigned to the data is not altered during the transmission.[7] Both the terms EMR and EHR can be interchangeable but often they represent different systems. EMR can contain personally reported patient data and the EHRs are mostly designed to drive information flow in the clinical operations. Both are patient-centric systems.

There is a critical need for strengthening eHealth[8] systems and services, including **health information systems**, at national and subnational levels. **Health information systems (HIS)** is a system that provides the underpinnings for decision-making and has four key functions: (1) data generation, (2) compilation, (3) analysis and synthesis, and (4) communication and use. The health information system collects data from health and other relevant sectors, analyzes the data and ensures their overall quality, relevance and timeliness, and converts the data into information for health-related decision-making.[6]

There is also a need for a systematic approach in implementing a health data standards-based "public health information architecture" that could serve as a rubric to achieve timely data exchange through interoperable information systems for disease surveillance, outbreak threat reduction, and compliance with International Health Regulations (2005)—IHR (2005).[9]

There is a sense of urgency for establishing interoperable health information systems using health data standards and health information technology (HIT) standards. This is largely due to fragmented eHealth systems that lack interoperability, and thereby pose a threat to health care delivery (Fig. 20-1). Sectors within countries also depend on accurate and timely health information for decision-making, but such systems are largely absent due to lack of interoperability between and within systems.

In a recent article by eight global health agencies, Chan et al.[10] argue for developing a common data architecture for exchanging health data. They emphasize the need for developing norms and standards for all aspects of a common data architecture and promoting interoperability standards for the health sector at both the individual and aggregate record levels.

Two classes of standards[11] need to be considered for data interoperability between and within health information systems and between information systems and medical devices and diagnostics platforms: (1) health data standards, which include subclasses such as terminologies and data standards, information content standards, information exchange standards, entity and person identifier standards, and privacy and security standards and (2) information technology standards, which include telecommunication, machine-to-machine communications (e.g., from medical device to device), and other technical standards related to information and communication technologies (ICTs). Greater emphasis needs to be placed on interoperability through standardization in areas such as individual medical records and EHRs, population surveillance, public health emergencies, medical devices, laboratory diagnostics, geographic information systems, and telemedicine. This expanse of informatics systems exemplifies how complex

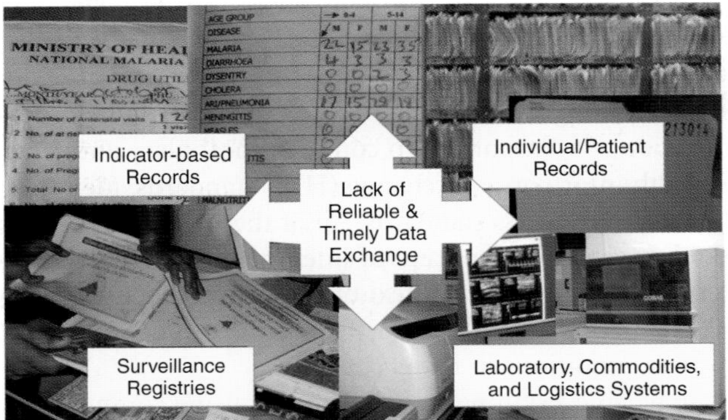

FIG. 20-1 Illustration of fragmentation of public health data collection systems and lack of reliable and timely exchange of data leading to lack of interoperability between various systems. Source: Created by Ramesh Krishnamurthy, picture sourced from internal presentation, 2009.

the problem can be to reach interoperability. Just creating EHR systems that follow interoperable standards does not create the critical surveillance ecosystem that has value to both the patient and the population.

In 2012, the World Health Organization (WHO) convened the first forum on Health Data Standardization and Interoperability.[12] The forum's primary objective was to facilitate dialogue among health data standards development organizations (SDOs), standards maintenance organizations (SMOs), academic institutions, subject matter experts, and member states toward the ongoing efforts to develop a comprehensive roadmap for full implementation of health data standards for interoperability within countries. The forum concluded that, to achieve both semantic and syntactic interoperability, various categories of standards must be implemented to strengthen the overall eHealth systems and services at national and subnational levels. In addition, a competency-based workforce is essential for successful implementation of standards at national and subnational levels. WHO convened the second Forum on eHealth Standardization and Interoperability in Geneva in 2014[12] to facilitate continued dialogue among stakeholders toward the development of a policy framework for full implementation of health data standards for interoperability of eHealth systems within countries.

Countries need to have a national eHealth strategy to implement standards. To achieve semantic and syntactic interoperability at all levels of health information systems, various categories of standards must be implemented as part of strengthening the overall eHealth systems and services at national and subnational levels. An eHealth policy for standardization and interoperability in a national context should include two objectives. First, it should ensure the safety of interoperable medical devices and ensure security, defining privacy and security policies addressing technology use in health care delivery. An eHealth policy should also set health data and HIT standards to ensure interoperability at data, device, and system levels. These standards should contain a fixed core set of standards that also allow for a degree of innovation outside that core and development based on the capacity and maturity of eHealth systems and services. The standards should also regulate an appropriate degree of adoption in the country context.

THE IMPORTANCE OF HEALTH DATA STANDARDIZATION FOR INTEROPERABILITY OF HEALTH INFORMATION SYSTEMS

The 2012 WHO Forum on Health Data Standardization and Interoperability report explains that "interoperability is widely recognized as essential to achieving the full potential of seamless data exchange using information and communication technologies (ICTs) and medical devices in support of health systems."[12] Transmitting personal or population data across ICT-driven health information systems requires adherence to health data standards and related technology standards for timely and accurate exchange of data for health care decisions. A wide range of activities require data interoperability within and between systems based on a given set of standards—from counting the health workforce to providing patient care through digital image review to managing patient information through **EMRs** to conducting public health surveillance. **EMRs** are digital versions of paper charts that contain all of a patient's medical history from one practice. An EMR is mostly used by providers for diagnosis and treatment.[13] Without data standardization, meaningful interoperability cannot be achieved.

As part of data standardization, it is important to consider vocabulary and terminology standards, health information content standards, health information exchange (HIE) standards, identifier standards, privacy and security standards, as well as functional and business standards. All of these categories must be addressed for full interoperability of eHealth systems and services. This concept of interoperable eHealth data actually applies even if we never use technology or computers. Even though the context of this chapter focuses on the application of interoperability applying technology, the base concepts are critical for the health realm even where there are no computers. This is often the case with low resource conditions in many countries.

How could this be the case when everything we talk about is using computers?

Consider the fact that at the most basic point of care service we record in a notebook a patient encounter. We may record any lab results or syndromic data gathered during that encounter that when viewed across encounters or across a population would be valuable for surveillance. This is not saying that a practitioner has to know all the

LOINC codes for every lab test and record that exact code in the hand annotated notebooks. Consider that if the notebooks referenced the tests for a specific infectious agent or indicated temperature in the same way, all the notebooks could be read or interpreted the same way in the clinic and across the points of care elsewhere.

So why would we want this "manual" interoperability? Just consider that people go to different points of care all the time and this physical recording of data could be shared verbally or by paper exchange essentially creating an eHealth record system.

There is even a place for discussing process interoperability in this example. Would finding records for a patient in a clinic or between clinics be easier if they were at least stacked alphabetically? Imagine going between clinics to gather data on an infectious outbreak that you are trying to find an origination point for and finding that all the notebooks were sorted by jurisdiction where the patient lives. Life would be much easier for the epidemiologist to gather data even from this nontechnology nondigital data system. The point is that eHealth strategies that support both point of care services and population surveillance must be formulated under all resource conditions to really move forward with modern surveillance concepts.

It is important to recognize that strengthening health information systems depends on national ownership, multisectoral engagement, appropriate use of ICT, and adequate workforce capacity. National policies for eHealth and HIT standardization must be mandated in order for interoperability to be fully implemented at all levels of the health care delivery chain. A global financial support mechanism must be created to assist member states, especially low- and middle-income countries (LMICs) to adopt standards at all levels of eHealth systems and services. A competency-based workforce is also essential to successfully implement standards at national and subnational levels. National governments must engage academic institutions and health-related nongovernmental organizations to offer specialized training programs about standardization for existing health care and public health professionals (Table 20-1).

United Nations (UN) Commission on Information and Accountability Women's and Children's Health.[14]

The commission stated in its Recommendation 3 that "by 2015, all countries [should] have integrated the use of Information and Communication Technologies in their national health information systems and health infrastructure." The document further emphasized that "the use of eHealth and mHealth should be strategic, integrated and support national health goals. In order to capitalize on the potential of ICTs, it will be critical to agree on standards and to ensure interoperability of systems. Health Information Systems must comply with these standards at all levels, including systems used to capture patient data at the point of care." The document emphasized that "Common terminologies and minimum data sets should be agreed on so that information can be collected consistently, easily and not misrepresented. In addition, national policies on health-data sharing should ensure that data protection, privacy, and consent are managed consistently."

INTEROPERABILITY: CASE IN POINT ABOUT ELECTRONIC MEDICAL RECORDS

Among individual records, patient medical records are integral to well-functioning public health systems and serve as essential data sources. Patient medical records are crucial for reporting notifiable conditions to national and international authorities and complying with the IHR (2005). While most patient medical records are still paper-based in most health facilities worldwide, there is a gradual global trend toward EMR systems. EMRs and other computer-based health information system components are becoming essential tools at health facilities to address routine patient-centric health care needs and provide other eHealth services.

The adoption of EMRs at health facilities can greatly enhance the storage, retrieval, transfer, and analysis of patient information for health care and public health surveillance purposes.[15] This greatly benefits longitudinal patient data collection, for example, in identifying evolving health needs throughout the life cycle or caring for large numbers of patients who may need complex or long-term care. Implementing reliable computer-based health information system and EMRs depends upon adequate human and financial resources and the appropriate use of ICT.[15]

TABLE 20-1 Sample List of Standards Development and Maintenance Organizations
European Committee for Normalization Technical Committee for Medical Informatics (CEN/TC 251)
Digital Imaging and Communications in Medicine (DICOM), managed by American College of Radiology (ACR) and National Electrical Manufacturers Association
Health Level Seven (HL-7)
International Labour Organization (ILO)
International Organization for Standardization (ISO)
International Telecommunications Union (ITU)
International Health Terminology Standards Development Organization (SNOMED—Systemized Nomenclature of Medicine)
Regenstrief Institute (LOINC—Logical Observation Identifier Names and Codes)
World Health Organization and WHO Collaborating Centers (International Classification of Diseases)

Although numerous EMR and EHR systems exist, the lack of seamless data exchange (interoperability) between computer-based health information systems remains a major problem and impediment to health systems strengthening efforts.[15] Without interoperability, much of the electronic health-related data stored in electronic systems are left unused or underused by public health agencies.[15]

When health information systems do not have the seamless data exchange that interoperability enables, health care services can suffer. For ICT to be best utilized in health systems, interoperability must be improved at all levels of the health system.

Exchange of personal, administrative, and clinical data between EMR systems cannot occur without utilizing appropriate standards for interoperability.[15] Therefore, eHealth standards are needed as part of electronic systems for EMR interoperability. This enables health facility data to be transferred to and used at all levels.

The Benefits of EMR Standardization

The benefits of EMR standardization cannot be overstated. Aggregate data from standardized EMRs can be used for disease surveillance, containment, and response, and data from facilities can be reported easily and seamlessly to the appropriate national and international authorities. In addition, IHR (2005) compliance by transmitting reportable data becomes easier at the national level. Through standardized health information systems, and especially through standardized EMRs, health workers can access more complete patient information at the point of care, pharmacies can receive prescriptions, laboratories can transmit test results, and imaging and diagnostic centers can send high-quality digital images—all electronically. Standardization also facilitates data analyses to be completed with greater speed and accuracy and to be transmitted seamlessly within and between various facilities. Through interoperability of health data systems, public health authorities can receive electronic reports on vital events and emergencies in a timely manner, and individuals can access their personal medical information more easily. Through standardized EMRs, national surveillance and response capacities can also be strengthened.

In a person-centric national electronic health information system, it is important to standardize all data elements for full interoperability. When data elements are standardized within EHRs, EMRs, laboratory information management systems, logistics management systems, and other similar systems, countries can harness the enormous potential of quality data through systematic analysis and use the results to address various public health needs. Realizing this vision requires long-term planning and stakeholder engagement. This vision realizes many of the concepts discussed in the feedback channels in Chapter 18 of this book.

EFFORTS TO STRENGTHEN INTEROPERABILITY AT WHO

As the UN agency for health, WHO has recognized the importance of health data standardization and its relevance to 'eHealth' systems and services. WHO has a normative and standard setting function as part of health system strengthening. Through systematic work with SDOs, global health partners, and international organizations, WHO provides leadership in coordinating the adoption of eHealth standards at national and subnational levels. WHO also offers technical assistance to countries in developing architecture, policy frameworks, and implementation guidance to ensure standards-based interoperable eHealth systems.

Efforts are underway to develop repositories of resources on eHealth standards, including an existing eHealth standards compendium, norms, and registries developed by different SDOs; develop a roster of eHealth standardization experts and institutions; use cases of eHealth enterprise architectures and communities of practice for standards adoption.

Through the global network of WHO Collaborating Centers for Health Informatics, standards-based specifications are being developed for EMRs to enable authorized health care providers to securely access content and provide advice and support to member states on developing statistical data, metadata exchange, and clinical data exchange standards.

THE IMPORTANCE OF IMPLEMENTING EHEALTH POLICY FOR STANDARDIZATION AND INTEROPERABILITY IN A NATIONAL CONTEXT[16]

- Should be embedded in a national health plan and an eGovernment plan, if one exists. Its view must be long term, provide continuity, and commit to long-term investment. Development and implementation of national eHealth policies for standardization and interoperability should be a national effort and must include stakeholders from the health sector, nonhealth sectors of national governments, and nonstate actors.
- Should be patient-centered, emphasizing service quality, equity, patient outcomes, patient safety, and population outcomes.
- Should be based on mutual trust and understanding and genuine collaboration between all stakeholders from lawmakers to patients, facilitated from the start by a participatory approach to policy making, and encompassing public and private partnerships where necessary.
- Should support an evidence base for the socioeconomic benefits of eHealth, and encompass user utility and outreach programs to ensure that all stakeholders, including patients, are aware of the uses, benefits, and risks of eHealth and are engaged in related discourse and decision-making, and its implementation.
- Should adopt appropriate electronic HIE technology, including at national and subnational levels, in vertical programs, and in public and private health care facilities.
- Should set health data and HIT standards to ensure interoperability at data, device, and system levels, in a framework containing a fixed core set of maintained standards allowing for a degree of innovation outside that core set and allowing for development based on the capacity and maturity of eHealth systems and services; and regulate an appropriate degree of adoption in the country context.
- Should use existing international standards where possible and adapt specific standards to suit national contexts, taking necessary care to ensure interoperability and backward compatibility, as applicable.
- Should provide unique identifiers for patients, health care workers, and health care facilities, with verification and authentication procedures.
- Should ensure the safety of interoperable medical devices, and ensure security, defining privacy and security policies addressing technology use in health care delivery.
- Should build capacity from country and ministry level down to that of frontline health workers. This includes financial and academic capacity as well as technical and human resource capacity.
- Should ensure good governance, balancing top-down and bottom-up approaches, encompassing: equity and accessibility; legality; user rights in line with human rights; privacy; responsibility; and accountability to citizens and to the state.

- Compatibility of technologies, efficiency, open dialogue, and a shared vision on use of data are necessary for implementation.
- In monitoring compliance, clear goals, and key indicators for monitoring and evaluation are needed, with mechanisms for social participation.
- Should support competency-based education and capacity building in health informatics, with standardized curricula and measurable learning objectives at national and subnational levels. Training should be for the health workforce, including social workers, and should cover eHealth policy development and planning, communications, and leadership as well as technical content. Training, including in-service training, can provide a valuable opportunity for partnership with academia, technical colleges, and other relevant bodies.
- Should encourage relevant ministries of national governments to include eHealth core competencies in job descriptions for relevant posts.[16]

CONCLUSIONS AND DIRECTION

Achieving interoperability is not a simple process, but it is a critical goal for every system created for clinical and public health interests. The implementation of full interoperability between and within health information systems is also a global requirement, as indicated by the significant commitment by WHO to promote the use of standards and policies that ensure success. Interoperability is seen as the key to making connections at all levels of health care delivery, using data for advancing quality health. This chapter created the vision that connecting systems is critical and has to follow standards. In the next chapter, interoperability becomes the highway on which heterogeneous data can travel together to answer our surveillance questions.

KEY SUMMARY POINTS

- When a system or framework is comprehensively interoperable, effective exchange of data leads to advanced analysis and use of surveillance data for decision-making.
- Reliable and timely health information is an essential foundation for health systems strengthening and public health action, both nationally and internationally.
- There is an urgency to achieve true interoperability between PHS systems. Clinical system and public health systems are being created at a rapid pace and are often unable to exchange useful data between themselves and with partners.
- Interoperability can create connections at the lowest level (i.e., between veterinary health and human health at the local level) of data exchange as well as create connections at the highest level (i.e., scientific communities) of human understanding around a global event.
- Standards Development Organizations and Standards Maintenance Organizations are critical in the creation of interoperable systems. Engagement with these organizations is critical on a global scale.
- The interoperability of electronic medical record or electronic health record systems is critical for achieving any modern surveillance strategy.

DISCUSSION QUESTIONS

1. What is the difference between technical and semantic interoperability when exchanging disease case reporting data?
2. List some of the benefits of interoperable EMRs to facilitate public health surveillance missions.
3. Are there "essential health data standards" for interoperability that are necessary for effective health systems performance and if so why are they essential? What problems do these "specific standards" would solve in health systems performance?
4. Based on your experience, what issues you are facing in implementing health data standards? What successes have you experienced?
5. How can we improve access, dissemination, and adoption of health data standards?

6. Name examples of best practices in policy and governance mechanisms for health data standards adoption and use that you have read about or experienced.
7. What kinds of policy and governance mechanisms promote appropriate data sharing while also ensuring health-data protection, privacy, security, and confidentiality?
8. List some of the "core competencies" for people who deal with the area of health data standards implementation and maintenance at national and subnational levels.
9. How do we increase in-country capacity of health workforce who can manage issues related to health data standardization and interoperability?
10. What are the most important elements and components of a policy framework?

REFERENCES

1. IEEE Standard Computer Dictionary. A compilation of IEEE standard computer glossaries. IEEE Xplore; 1991.
2. Benson T. Principles of health interoperability HL7 and SNOMED. 2nd ed. London: Springer-Verlag; 2012.
3. Initiative eG. On semantic and technical interoperability. 2012.
4. Amos P. Interoperability within health & social care systems. Information standards board for health and social care. 2008.
5. Health MDo. Health information exchange – interoperability. 2008.
6. Network HM. Framework and standards for country health information systems. 2nd ed. Geneva: WHO; 2008.
7. OECD Glossary of Statistical Terms. Data Exchange, <http://stats.oecd.org/glossary/detail.asp?ID=1355/>; 2015.
8. Assembly WH. WHA58.28 resolution on eHealth. 2005.
9. Assembly WH. WHA66.24 Resolution on eHealth standardization and interoperability. 2013.
10. Chan M, Kazatchkine M, Lob-Levyt J, Obaid T, Schweizer J, Sidibe M, et al. Meeting the demand for results and accountability: a call for action on health data from eight global health agencies. PLoS Med 2010;7(1):e1000223.
11. Public Health Data Standards Consortium, <http://www.phdsc.org/>; 2014.
12. Organization WHO. WHO forum on health data standardization and interoperability. Geneva; 2012.
13. Benefits of EHRs. What is an Electronic Medical Records (EMR), <http://www.healthit.gov/providers-professionals/electronic-medical-records-emr/>; 2015.
14. Health WHOColaAfWsaCs. Keeping promises, measuring results. Geneva: World Health Organization; 2011.
15. WHO. Consolidated strategic information guidelines for HIV in the health sector. Geneva; 2015.
16. Organization WHO. Joint inter-ministerial policy dialogue on eHealth standardization and second WHO forum on eHealth standardization and interoperability. Geneva; 2014.

CHAPTER

21

Data Storms Are Growing, Everywhere, and Have to Work Together

J Mark Conde, Arun Kumar Srinivasan

Maybe stories are just data with a soul.

Brene Brown

KEY WORDS

Data exchange
Causation
Interoperability
Data fusion
Big data
Data streams
Data storms
Next-generation sequencing
Data warehouse
Data pools

DATA STORMS ARE THE NEW SURVEILLANCE WEATHER PATTERN

Public health passive surveillance systems focus on examining an aggregate collection of one set of events or data usually designed to answer relatively simple questions about case counts, rate, and basic correlations for one disease or condition. Now public health is asking more complex questions that require bringing together heterogeneous data to generate correlations across domains and to discover causation. **Causation** is the relationship between cause and effect.[1] These more complex questions create a new pattern, where we realize that just as wind patterns, air pressure, global temperature changes, pollution, and land masses impact our weather in a systems manner, so too must surveillance be designed as a system that combines many heterogeneous domains of data. The complex questions being asked now can be tied to global migration, emerging infectious conditions, environmental quality issues, and society behavior changes that have triggered PH surveillance to go over and beyond the traditional data sets.

Today's public health is facing the challenge of simultaneously comprehending data from dozens of dimensions. Meaningful and holistic interpretation of data requires generation of higher level explanations based on knowledge and expertise from multiple principles.[2, 3] Context is essential to illustrate a big picture view of the dynamic and complex problem.[4] The new forms of questions we are asking require a system's view across many domains such as climate, human symptoms, disease outbreaks in humans, animal disease, environments, changing molecular structures, and others. Data from each of these domains can be brought together to generate views of correlation, discovery of patterns, and derivation of causes for human disease. Bringing these data sets together is best thought of as "data storms," all interacting with predictable outcomes. **Data storms** describe what is happening now as a part of big data when data are coming in high velocity from many different directions at once into a surveillance system or analysis.[5] This process is similar to watching a weather radar map that shows us where the storm is going to hit and with what velocity. There is a great deal of information buried under this simple imagery we can easily understand. The idea of interoperability creating connections discussed in Chapter 20 is a key concept to understand and execute this data fusion in order to answer our questions. Otherwise we will never really be able to take advantage of the enormous volume of data now available to public health to discover these interrelationships. **Data fusion** is a process dealing with the association, correlation, and combination of data and information from single and multiple sources to achieve refined position and identity estimates, and complete and timely assessments of situations and threats as well as their significance.[6]

Imagine a surveillance question we might tackle today that would require a data storm be assembled to find the answer. Suddenly in Midwestern Ohio, certain types of cancer have started to appear in the population and the rate is increasing. We can start setting up surveillance to track the specific cancer rates in the population and where it is being found but can we really answer why it is suddenly starting to appear and how to slow it down? When you examine the area of exposomes you may have a clue that we need to look at what was buried in the environments in that part of the country and what may have changed to release the agent causing the issue (see case studies*).

For this example, assume we start to realize it is an unknown heavy metal causing the cancer. Perhaps the trail was picked up by an epidemiologist who started to see this metal in the blood of the patients tracked in the surveillance system. What data do we think we need to explore the hypothesis that something has occurred to start releasing this heavy metal that is causing the cancer to appear in the population? The data storm now needs to assimilate data from toxicology data from various sources like water and food. When starting to think about what may have changed, and assuming this heavy metal was buried in the mud from the industrial days of that region, we will then want to bring in data from events that could have caused the mud to release the metals into the water causing active exposure such as climatic data that could show storms in the area. Thus, being able to monitor data from the local Department of Natural Resources (DNR) would become critical. In this example, there are many heterogeneous data sources that we want to start bringing together to answer this one question, but it makes sense to do the same thing for future surveillance challenges.

A great deal of data manipulation and translation will be needed to just investigate the theories for this one event. Moving forward with modern surveillance systems, we should be discussing that all data sources across domains be designed to bring data together to answer any questions we may have. That means they must achieve some level of interoperability (see Chapter 20).

In this chapter we will examine some of the developing data storms and how they can be brought together to answer progressive public health questions. Data storms have characteristics that require a method to match them to the questions being asked and to address the problem of bringing them together. Data are coming fast and furious at us as well as structured in many variations. Public health practitioners often have to determine the value of data as they formulate the questions about the public health and health needs that impact which data are chosen, how much is used, and how the data are assembled. Data storms are now brewing for public health that will change how we use data in the new world of surveillance. Finally, clinical health is automating data into electronic health record (EHR) systems that will inundate public health with population data at volumes not previously available for public health surveillance.[7] Molecular data are also now available that is changing our understanding of disease. The molecular data being derived are huge, unwieldy, and require many correlated data sets to understand the relationships to disease, infection, and genetic tendencies.

SETTING THE STAGE

The key to selecting and manipulating the data for the purposes of modern surveillance is to understand what data are needed through the dissection of public health questions. To set the stage we will examine some public health scenarios.

Zoonotic Disease

Many diseases are blurring the line between animal and human disease, and many factors can influence when this occurs. Chapter 14 further explores these concepts through the One Heath project. This situation causes public health practitioners to ask questions such as: When does this occur? What animals are carriers and how does exposure occur?

*Available at http://booksite.elsevier.com/9780702063374/

Why are we seeing these new diseases now, and what environmental factors influence transmission? What human behavior might allow for a molecular change in the animals' infectious organism to increase human virulence?

Thinking through these questions demonstrates the nature of this new surveillance environment. We are not just looking at reported confirmed cases collected at the local public health department. In this new surveillance world, we need to bring data together that track animal infections or identify the animals' ability to carry a disease under changing environmental factors that can lead to human exposure. Economic factors that have changed farming practices may now expose disease-carrying animals to humans through a common vector such as water. Access to this data might be assembled to solve how the human exposure is occurring. The One Health (see Chapter 14) initiative is doing exactly this type of surveillance.[8] This data storm is not a traditional public health surveillance approach. We usually wait until the human population indicates something is wrong and then back track to derive causation. Instead, we should bring heterogeneous data streams together to anticipate threats and use systems thinking to find these patterns and disease causations before they strike.

Exposomes

Exposomes correlate long-term exposures to many variations of environmental conditions over our lifetimes, which change our molecular engine and possibly cause chronic disease or susceptibility to other conditions (see case studies*).[9] This concept may prompt us to ask questions based on this long-term surveillance. For example, based on higher cancer rates among populations living in certain areas, if Tom lived in Cleveland, Ohio, in the 1970s when steel mills poured industrial slag into our waterways, does Tom have a higher likelihood of contracting cancer? Why? Can that impact his children, who have never lived there? The science of epigenetics suggests we do harbor long-term effects that can be passed down to our children, and therefore it now makes sense to look at data to find related patterns. Again, this necessitates a higher level of data brought together in a long-term surveillance program in order to start answering these questions. For this example, we would need environmental toxicology data, industrial activity information, cancer registry data, and inherited molecular propensities correlated to predict possible causation of cancer that is not obvious. The Emory University Hercules Center is building the surveillance system of the future to explore exposomes.

DATA QUALITY

In the examples above, deriving data sources involved at a high level is easy to see, but these data do not tell us if a data source is capable of being used to answer the questions we are asking. We need to look closer at the characteristics of the data in the storm. Can each data source described above be interoperable so that we can ask cross-domain questions? Is the volume of one data source huge but without common linkage, such as temporal or spatial linkages? We decide if the data usability is found through a concept of deriving dimensions in data classically used in data warehousing systems to solve this. Data quality concepts are critical to support the possible interoperability needed to answer these questions. Data quality characteristics, such as those in Table 21-1, must be followed for high-quality

TABLE 21-1 **Characteristics of Data Quality**

CHARACTERISTICS	DESCRIPTION
Data fields or attributes	Are consistently named and typed
Standard coding systems are used for the fields	Such as LOINC for laboratory test identification
Granularity of data can be correlated	The measures of data are derivable or similar such as time
Relationships of data are held in stand schemas	Data are placed in a structure that tells the story how data relate across themselves
The data are complete	No missing data

*Available at http://booksite.elsevier.com/9780702063374/

data that meet interoperable states between **data pools. Data pools** describe when we have aggregated or closely integrated sets of data usually located in the same computing center or servers. The term is most useful when discussing federated integration of data across many data pools to create one data view from many sources.[5] Data quality is best understood by realizing that we cannot have missing data or data that are represented in varied ways.[5] Unless we use coding standards such as every laboratory assay identified by a LOINC code we can never know a laboratory result was derived exactly the same way. The table shows other data quality aspects that have to be considered.

OLD MICROSTORMS HAVE US SPINNING IN OUR OWN SPACE

We have created silos with public health data and surveillance services. This environment is consistently found for the various surveillance systems we have created to support our endeavors. These pools of centralized data are usually created for a specific purpose and often only answer specific questions or microstorms. Looking forward, we realize that the data in these data microstorms have a great deal of value when correlated with other microstorms. This is particularly true when we try to answer questions that require data from multiple domains. For our data discussion purposes, a domain is a concentration in a field of science, such as toxicology, or a more granular area of public health, such as reportable infectious disease cases.

Current surveillance data systems are silos that work reasonably well for their specific purposes. The National Electronic Disease Surveillance System (NEDSS) is an example that persists aggregate data at the US Centers for Disease Control and Prevention (CDC) and in almost every state that stores reportable disease cases (see Chapter 3). However, the NEDSS system tends to be a silo of data for just infectious reportable patient event disease and does not link to other data pools. We discuss this microstorm first because it is an evolutionary step in the right direction to create a basis for a modern surveillance system. We need to be able to bring all the data together as one active and interacting "organism" of data that can answer more complex questions. In our quest to make data interoperable, we had to start building each single system with consistency. NEDSS and the NEDSS Base System (NBS) standards ensured that these systems were coded consistently, used the same data fields, and held data relationships the same way across all deployments of this type of system. However, these are deployed all over as single microstorms and do not talk to each other yet. The modern surveillance informatics "organism" has to be able to talk to all of these NEDSS systems through a network and a query engine that can ask a question and return the aggregate view of the results back to the epidemiologist.

There are a number of other national systems at the CDC that are examples of this silo structure. NETSS is the aggregate disease data system that was developed in the 1990s and is still running. The overall aggregate disease data collection system is NNDSS. The CDC National Notifiable Diseases Surveillance System (NNDSS) is a nationwide collaboration that enables all levels of public health (local, state, territorial, federal, and international) to share health information to monitor, control, and prevent the occurrence and spread of state-reportable and nationally notifiable infectious and some noninfectious diseases and conditions. NNDSS has two data streams: NETSS and NEDSS HL7 Data. The NETSS system includes 22 core data elements for reportable disease conditions. NETSS differs from NEDSS in several ways. NETSS was case based; NEDSS is person based. However, NETSS used proprietary ontology coding whereas NEDSS is based on standards, so it can capture data already in electronic health care data streams. The NEDSS initiative uses standards to advance the development of efficient, integrated, and interoperable surveillance systems at the state and local levels. This initiative facilitates the electronic transfer of information from clinical information systems in health care, reduces the provider's burden of providing data, and enhances the timeliness and quality of information provided. These further examples show where some evolution of surveillance systems has occurred but not really moving beyond specific use data analysis.

We have discussed needing available data for multiple domain questions that touch heterogeneous databases, but we cannot even ask homogeneous questions across similar databases yet. Large aggregated data pools of all data will not work for our modern surveillance needs (see Chapter 22).

Explaining the Problem of Multiple Surveillance Systems with Pandemic Influenza

The pandemic influenza scenario* illustrates the obvious questions that need to be answered quickly when we discover an outbreak. Public health practitioners ought to be able to use multiple sources of data (like many separate NEDSS systems others such as general disease surveillance, laboratory data, quarantine management, and clinical systems) all talking to each other to tell them that confirmed cases of H1N1 are appearing, how fast they are showing up in a region, and the pattern of spread. Using this network, epidemiologists should be able to ask additional questions about the molecular variances of this virus in each region and track both virulence and antiviral use. This hypothetical system should pull data from many separate data microstorms into an analytical and visualization engine anywhere that it is needed. However, our current surveillance informatics systems now would take weeks to pull, aggregate, and manipulate the data, even though it is all built from the same data quality standard. Interoperability should be driven by data quality compliance but there are more dimensions to interoperability.

The systems have to be able to "talk" to each other through architecture standards. Often that is missing in the design of a surveillance system. When the current silos of data have been created we did move forward with using interoperability code, specific use like data structure, and message standards but the architecture of fusing the data together was not always considered. That is the architecture standards for data linking across nonspecific domains (such as vital data infectious disease data brought together) and query message architectures that allow the data to move around.

OLD AND NEW SOURCES FROM ALL DIRECTIONS

As indicated above, we have been pooling a lot of data in many different areas. Part of the epidemiology challenge to answering modern questions is knowing what data pools exist. Box 21-1 is derived from a CDC National Center for Environmental Health web site listing.[10]

After looking at this massive list of data microstorms one can start asking modern surveillance questions. Discovering that many of these sources could be very useful for finding answers and seeing patterns if they were

BOX 21-1 List of Available Data Sources for Public Health Surveillance

Health data

1. CDC Behavioral Risk Factor Surveillance System (BRFSS): http://www.cdc.gov/brfss/

Childhood lead poisoning data and surveillance resources

1. National Ambulatory Medical Care Survey (NAMCS): http://www.cdc.gov/nchs/ahcd/about_ahcd.htm
2. National Environmental Public Health Tracking Network
3. National Hospital Discharge Survey (NHDS): http://www.cdc.gov/nchs/nhds/about_nhds.htm
4. National Health and Nutrition Examination Survey (NHANES): http://www.cdc.gov/nchs/nhanes/about_nhanes.htm
5. Bureau of Labor Statistics Survey of Occupational Injuries and Illnesses, US Department of Labor: http://stats.bls.gov/iif/oshsum1.htm

Biomonitoring data

1. CDC
   - National Report on Biochemical Indicators of Diet and Nutrition
   - National Health and Nutrition Examination Survey (NHANES): http://www.cdc.gov/nchs/nhanes.htm
   - National Report on Human Exposure to Environmental Chemicals

Environmental data

1. EPA air data
   - Acid Rain Emissions Tracking System
   - Air Quality System (AQS): http://www.epa.gov/air/data/aqsdb.html

*Available at http://booksite.elsevier.com/9780702063374/

BOX 21-1 List of Available Data Sources for Public Health Surveillance—cont'd

- National Emission Inventory (NEI) Data: http://www.epa.gov/ttn/chief/net/neiwhatis.html
- Envirofacts Data Warehouse: http://www.epa.gov/enviro/html/ef_overview.html

2. EPA toxics data
   - Toxics Release Inventory (TRI): http://www.epa.gov/tri/
3. EPA ambient water data
   - Beaches Environmental Assessment and Coastal Health (BEACH): http://www.epa.gov/waterscience/beaches/about.html
   - Watershed Assessment, Tracking & Environmental Results (WATERS): http://www.epa.gov/waters/about/overview.html
   - STORET (short for STOrage and RETrieval): http://www.epa.gov/storet/about.html
4. EPA drinking water data
   - Safe Drinking Water Information System/Federal Version (SDWIS/FED): http://www.epa.gov/safewater/databases/sdwis/basicinformation.html
   - Safe Drinking Water Information System/State Version (SDWIS/STATE): http://www.epa.gov/safewater/sdwis_st/aboutstate.html
5. FEMA Flood Hazard Mapping (Digital Flood Insurance Rate Map [DFIRM] Database)
6. FDA Total Diet Study (TDS): http://www.cfsan.fda.gov/~comm/tds-toc.html
7. NOAA National Oceanographic Data Center (NODC): http://www.nodc.noaa.gov/
8. National Climactic Data Center (NCDC): http://www.ncdc.noaa.gov/oa/ncdc.html
9. National Geophysical Data Center (NGDC): http://www.ngdc.noaa.gov/index.html
10. USGS National Water-Quality Assessment Program (NAWQA): http://water.usgs.gov/nawqa/
11. National Stream Quality Accounting Network (NASQAN): http://water.usgs.gov/nasqan/
12. National Atmospheric Deposition Program/National Trends Network (NADP/NTN): http://bqs.usgs.gov/acidrain/
13. National Water Information System: http://waterdata.usgs.gov/nwis
14. National Geospatial Data Clearinghouse: http://nsdi.usgs.gov/

Census data: http://www.census.gov/

Query engines

1. Agency for Healthcare Research and Quality (AHRQ)
   - Healthcare Cost and Utilization Project (HCUP): http://www.hcup-us.ahrq.gov/
   - Medical Expenditure Panel Survey (MEPS): http://www.meps.ahrq.gov/mepsweb/
2. CDC
   - Behavioral Risk Factor Surveillance System (BRFSS): http://apps.nccd.cdc.gov/brfss/index.asp
   - Cancer Control PLANET: http://cancercontrolplanet.cancer.gov/
   - CDC WONDER: http://wonder.cdc.gov/
   - Data FERRET (Federal Electronic Research and Review Extraction Tool): http://www.cdc.gov/nchs/datawh/ferret/ferret.htm
   - TheDataWeb: http://www.thedataweb.org/
   - Work Related Injury Statistics Query System (Work-RISQS): http://www2a.cdc.gov/risqs/default.asp
   - Web-Based Injury Statistics Query and Reporting System (WISQARS): http://www.cdc.gov/injury/wisqars/index.html
3. EPA
   - AirData: http://www.epa.gov/air/data/info.html
   - Air Information Retrieval System AQS: http://www.epa.gov/aqspubl1/select.html
   - AIRNow: http://airnow.gov/
   - Envirofacts Data Warehouse: http://www.epa.gov/enviro/html/ef_overview.html
   - EnviroMapper: http://www.epa.gov/emefdata/em4ef.home
   - Resource Conservation and Recovery Act Information (RCRAInfo) http://www.epa.gov/enviro/html/rcris/
   - Search your community: http://www.epa.gov/epahome/commsearch.htm
   - Sunwise: http://www.epa.gov/sunwise/
   - Surf Your Watershed: http://cfpub.epa.gov/surf/locate/index.cfm
   - TRI Explorer: http://www.epa.gov/triexplorer/introduction.htm
   - Windows to My Environment (WME): http://www.epa.gov/enviro/wme/
4. National Institutes of Health, National Cancer Institute
   - Surveillance Epidemiology and End Results (SEER): http://www.seer.cancer.gov/

brought together is the key. Drilling down into each of these data sets one would find wide variation in data quality. In many cases, the data simply could not be integrated at all due to varying context, granularity, and representativeness—this is where we need to evolve. The list is provided to show that there are data sources that can be used to answer our multidomain questions. However, the challenge of drilling into each of these data sets to confirm the data quality still needs to be addressed as it creates an interoperable state.

Thinking about where data sources might be needed as we dissect our more complex surveillance questions, we examine the following list of domain areas for sourcing our guidance to find data. This list can be used to define a set of domains you may need to answer questions and be a guide for where to look.

- Vital records (death and birth records)
- Molecular data from humans, animals, and lower level phyla
- Political data: Political influences can change health behavior and events
- Financial data, including health insurance payment data, pharmaceutical company spending, and funding for major health programs
- Manufacturing/logistics data critical to finding vectors in etiologies
- War data where social disruption may be taking place or has existed
- Veterinary data, especially with regard to the intersection of animal and human disease
- Natural resources data, including wild animal and environmental data
- Clinical patient data from treatment, confirmed disease, and behavior
- Laboratory order and results data for raw qualitative and quantitative experimental data
- Environmental data, including toxicology, materials, air, water, earth, and industrial data
- Census data about where people live and with whom they live
- GIS data indicating layered views of spatial information
- All Payer-Claims data provide insight into systematically collected health care claims data, which can in turn provide insight to prevalence of diseases in the population, type and use of drugs, effect of health reforms, etc.

THE STORMS ARE BIGGER, MORE COMPLEX, AND EVERYWHERE

Data microstorms are everywhere, and it is clear they have to evolve in order to be used for more complex surveillance questions. New data storms are forming to which public health has never had access, and they are changing our ability to start answering more complex multidomain questions. The two most significant data storms brewing come from clinical automation and molecular analytics. These storms are not only producing massive volumes of data but also offering new ways of thinking about our surveillance approaches. Molecular data alone now give us a tremendous view of the population changing not just at the symptom and phylogeny level but also at the molecular level.

EHR and clinical systems are finally being brought online, and these systems hold massive amounts of valuable data for population health surveillance. Point-of-care data from emergency rooms, hospitals, and local clinics, when used in aggregate, will tell us a great deal about what is happening in our populations. One system, BioSense, is designed to pool syndromic data from all of these clinical sources to examine precursor patterns for outbreaks.[11] The use of the BioSense detection algorithms has been proven valuable through a number of software systems, but the central BioSense engine has been troubled, mostly because of the speed at which data can be processed, aggregated, or analyzed. As the EHR systems are brought online and emergency room data are quickly moved into BioSense-like engines, we can finally use data from syndromic surveillance to answer many of our public health questions and actually see emerging patterns in a population.

EHRs can provide many data we will use for public health surveillance questions. Even using results from laboratory tests that are ordered can be used for public health benefits. For example, using clinical laboratory test results about cholesterol levels can help public health agencies understand their populations' risk for chronic disease. Imagine having de-identified access to every HIV test conducted in real time via EHR data; we would know many aspects about the HIV population very quickly that would make more efficient interventions possible, such as shifting treatment supplies to new locations or populations.

However, EHR data, just like those from the data microstorms above, are in danger of becoming unobtainable to the public health surveillance and analytics communities, locked in their silos. These EHRs must use consistent data quality standards for the first step in their evolution. Second, they should be part of a data exchange and query system that allows public health to ask population- and public health-related surveillance questions. Once again, we know that trying to pool all the data into one big analytics engine will simply not work. Instead, we need to ensure this isolation does not happen (see Chapter 22).

The other monster data storm coming is from molecular data. Public health continues to prove that molecular analysis of organisms is very valuable in determining what specific virus is the causative agent in an outbreak and what its source is.[12] It has only been recently that the cost and speed of full DNA sequencing has fallen, so we can test more organisms and, soon, humans. The data storm coming from these analytics is huge and is referred to as next-generation sequencing. **Next generation sequencing (NGS)**, massively parallel, or deep sequencing are related terms that describe a DNA sequencing technology, which has revolutionized genomic research. Using NGS an entire human genome can be sequenced within a single day.[13] One run of full sequencing for a bacterium can hold 50 GB of data! Furthermore, if you mix this molecular analysis with protein and expression data analysis, a major storm will continue to grow.

There is one more storm we should pay attention to—the unstructured data from social media and general communication sources. It is becoming apparent that mining these massive amounts of data from sources such as Facebook can actually tell us many things about our behavior and can provide signals about the health of the population. These data are massive, complex, and may not ever follow a data standard. We therefore need new tricks to use these data in public health surveillance.

THE VS OF PUBLIC HEALTH SURVEILLANCE DATA

Both EHR and molecular data are classified as "**Big Data**," meaning they have different characteristics than our classic surveillance data pools in the past. The connotation of Big Data only suggests that we are dealing with large volumes,[5] but this type of data is much more than that and that is why we have the four Vs to describe this data. The four Vs of Big Data[14] are volume, velocity, variety, and veracity and are very useful in understanding how Big Data fit into modern public health surveillance. There are many descriptions of the four Vs; one of the original definitions comes from IBM (Fig. 21-1). Examining where modern public health surveillance is evolving using Big Data, the Vs have to be described in terms of the characteristics of the domain data we will be using and the questions we want to answer.

Volume

Volume is already discussed above and will quickly reach levels of multiple petabytes in each data source or system (e.g., EHRs, laboratories, and disease reporting systems). We have to accept that a computing infrastructure has to be designed to hold these data volumes and allow access by surveillance query engines to answer our complex questions. For example, in order to perform a molecular analysis, we now have to download a Genome-Wide Association Study (GWAS) data set to our local computers. Just the base data sets can take up terabytes of local computer disk storage and significant computing power to do the analysis. We need to rethink moving so much data around redundantly and move computing to data pools, as data are becoming too big for us to move and store locally. From a surveillance perspective, we want to hold a great deal more than just a sequence; we have to store what the sequences mean, phylogenies, and eventually how they influence causation. Now that is complex data!

Velocity

Velocity is often referred to as streaming data. In surveillance it also represents data that are coming from all directions and quickly. Without centralized data pooling, expecting that a public health department can handle all of the

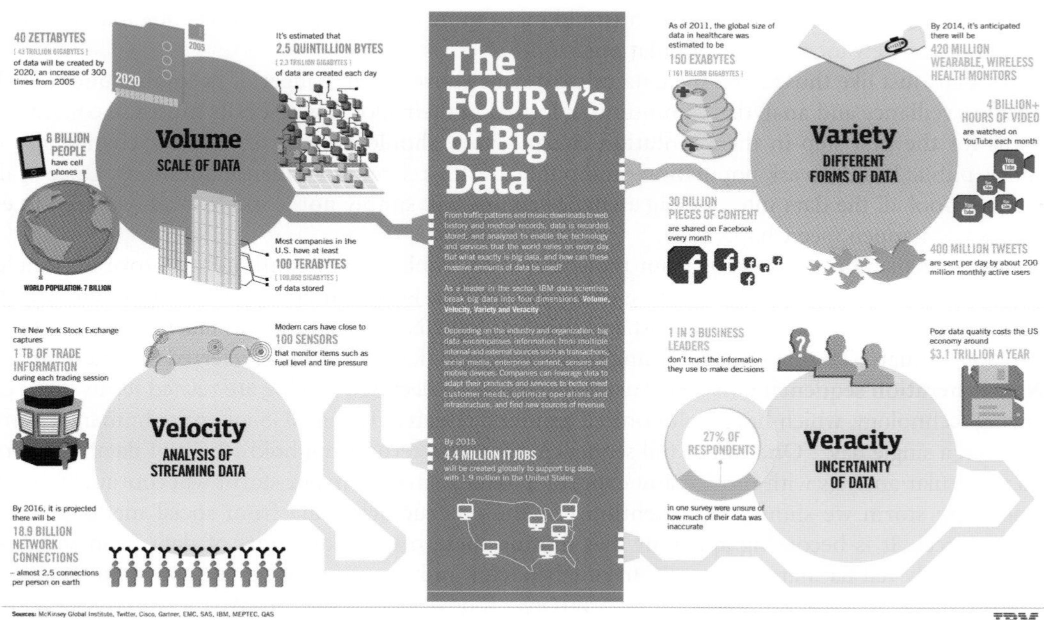

FIG. 21-1 The four Vs of big data. Source: http://www.ibmbigdatahub.com/infographic/four-vs-big-data.

data streams coming from just EHRs, for example, we are in trouble. **Data streams** tend to describe data that are in motion.[5] Surveillance data are now valuable to examine in real time while these are moving between systems. Think for a moment about how much data are collected from patients in just one emergency room everyday, and then imagine data from all of the emergency rooms in just one state. We are very far away from having a computing infrastructure at a public health department to handle that much volume, much less analyze it. This example establishes more support for the distributed storage of fast-moving data that we can access with fast-moving multidomain questions across all of the data pools. There is another concept we will explore below that touches on velocity as related to streaming data that could be critical for surveillance systems.

Variety

We are used to the idea of data variety in public health surveillance. Many of our questions require bringing together heterogeneous data. However, the level of data complexity is increasing as we evolve into a new surveillance realm. As discussed above, we are starting to ask population and public health surveillance questions that can only be answered by combining different forms of data from different domains. These different forms of data are becoming more available, such as social media data or magnetic resonance imaging (MRI) archive data. MRI image data represent a growing arena of epidemiologic studies that use image data, such as predicting the risk of breast cancer from breast MRIs. Indeed, variety is one of the interoperability curses we have to face. There are standards for each type of data but not always cross-domain interoperable.

Veracity

Veracity refers to the uncertainty and the quality of data. It is not a new concept to a public health professional that data have veracity. This will never really disappear with our data. Public health professionals cannot expect that every domain will create perfect and high-quality data all the time that work perfectly for surveillance use. Public health has developed proven methods to apply statistics and mathematical certainties about the veracity of the data with which we work. The modern catch now is, again, the volume problem of data. A statistical analysis tool, like SAS, is quite efficient, but it will be overwhelmed when we really start trying to solve veracity problems across huge volumes of data. We need to be thinking differently about how to solve the problem of so much variable quality data.

A NEW WAY OF THINKING

The new surveillance system of systems will require combining the strength of data management systems like database technologies (e.g., SQL) with more advanced statistics analysis integrated close to data engines and data pooling systems. The concept that we are combining many systems together to operate as one organism is generally called systems of systems. This suggested architecture change is a departure from our current thinking that data are stored in a big pile, and pulled out into a mathematical engine, and then stored again. This process simply will not work with the issues of volume and veracity we are facing. The data management side of the engine would handle active translation, transformation, and basic statistical verification of the data. Then a level of data quality could be reached that meets the rigors of the more advanced mathematical manipulation that requires cleaner and consistent data. Another possibility is to create a centralized engine that can perform higher order mathematical analysis for smaller amounts of data in the distributed query system that will process data that have been bulk processed by local data management systems that will resolve veracity issues.

DATA FUSIONS ARE DATA STORMS WORKING TOGETHER

This discussion of Big Data is exciting—but wait a moment. We need to figure out how to bring these data together to answer our modern surveillance questions. It does not matter if we do so in a giant mega database or a type of hybrid distributed engine—the same problems exist. The data have to somehow be "fused" together to find correlations and eventually causations across domains.

We also have to expect that the data we need are not found in just one data pool and that fusing will be required. A simple example of this is pulling immunization events from all EHRs into an immunization registry. Immunization registries are often critical in surveillance to determine the level of protection against vaccine-preventable diseases that a population may have. While the concept of having a massive flow of point-of-care immunization data to a central processing engine is wonderful, there are data missing. For example, clinical record keeping does not require familial linkages that are important for public health to identify epidemiologic links, but those analyzing data from immunization registries require such information for public health purposes. Those linkages therefore need to come from another data source that needs to be fused or integrated into immunization registry data.

Data Warehouse Techniques

There are significant rigors to data fusions in the very effective data warehousing methods developed over the years. These take a great deal of time and tend to use massive, passive data pools. Another aspect of data fusion is to understand how to break apart a question into pools of subquestions. These subquestions often align with data pools within a domain, and we would use techniques (e.g., parallel computer processing) and tools (e.g., Hadoop and MapReduce) to ask subquestions and then fuse the smaller refined data together to answer the question.

Some of the simpler concepts of data warehouse (DW) techniques can help us create a fast way to determine how data should be fused to answer a question. A **data warehouse** is an integrated information-storage area that consists of a data repository bringing together multiple databases from various data sources, and a report-generating facility.[15]

First, we will examine how we can quickly discover data domains in a surveillance question, or "dimensions." "It may help to think of dimensions as things or objects. A thing such as a product can exist without ever being involved in a business event."[16] The dimension, according to this definition, is the noun in our question. In many of the questions posed above the dimension we want to discover is the patient or the location. Its also implies that a dimension can be a verb in the question as well, such as an event or action that we are tracking in our surveillance question that is acting on the noun. The third type of dimension is often a measure that forms a scope inside the question.

Let us look at a complex surveillance question we may have about an outbreak as an example of this type of thinking. We have some sort of outbreak occurring in two countries where people are showing up to emergency rooms with a specific set of symptoms. We start asking where these people are coming from, who or what they have been near recently, and what they have been doing and how long ago. The dimensions in this situation, therefore, are the symptomatic patients, their locations and health care facilities, time of illness onset and other time measures, and their behaviors. Usually we try to capture all of this in the epidemiologic process, but can we find the people we do not know to talk to? By integrating and fusing data sources, systems, and other information, we can find those additional dimensions, or people.

We create case definitions to describe how to look for these dimensions in an outbreak that others can use, but we want to know where to look, across data pools, and to find others who might be at risk. We can map the dimensions of our questions to the data pools available. EHR data may give us the symptoms of people in whom we are interested. Local census data may tell us who else may be nearby. Social media data could give us clues about behavior. We may find a possible source to food or animals as the carrier for our outbreak.

Data Pools

Generally, it is not hard to know where to find data pools. But it is hard to know how to fuse the data together unless we start looking at the field and attribute level where these dimensions are represented in the data. Most or all of the data pools will have some sort of time dimension in order to find correlation with the event being investigated. We know that some data are held in domains such as census bureaus, clinical points of care, and logistics systems for food processing. The trick now is to find the dimensions we need within those domains to bring the data together.

We can quickly come up with sample data fields that equal the derived dimensions, and then reach out into the distributed query engine network to find data correlated to our questions. Since massive volumes of data could exist in all the various domains, we want to take advantage of distributed data pool ideas above keeping in mind data quality.

We use this simple example to think about data that need to come together to answer our questions and to use traditional methods for collecting and fusing data into an aggregate database. We have to ask ourselves about what the future surveillance engine should be doing instead of just collecting and storing massive amounts of data.

THE TRANSFORMED SURVEILLANCE SYSTEM

The transformed surveillance system may be very different from the passive aggregator of data we think belong together. Instead, it may be a system that maps common dimensions to the possible data sources and is designed to create varied analyses against all the data to answer our questions. The new surveillance system would also understand how to break down the questions and ask subquestions in a parallel approach and in the right order to meet the challenges in the complex queries found in our questions.

Other ideas need to evolve into the various domains of data we might use. One is that not all of the same data quality will exist to ensure successful fusions. Therefore, we have to be ready to translate data on the fly while queries are being processed. This idea suggests that the data pools need to show us what their data look like, and the surveillance engine should know how to do these translations—commonly called "metadata" or, data about data. This is a very different way of thinking about informatics and how a surveillance system might actually meet the challenges of our complex questions.

Does the modern surveillance system hold any data? It would store data used to show the history of queries run in the past. It would also hold temporary data just for the period of analysis processed for visualization or further derivation of questions. In some cases, data fusion may have to be done locally after raw data subsets are pulled. Either way, the surveillance system is now really an engine for analysis and visualization, not a massive pooling place for data with static views.

DATA WITHOUT STRUCTURE

As discussed above, we are increasingly finding value in working with social media and image data. These data tend to be unstructured and, although useful, can be daunting to use. To define unstructured data, let us look at what is meant by structured data. Structured data have specified identities, and each specific identity holds a value. For example, "Name = Smith" is a structured field and piece of structured data. Unstructured data would be the open-ended text in a chief complaint field that a clinician types into an EHR system when a patient visits the doctor.

Although image or sound data appear to have structure, their interpretation is not well defined, and we need to create an interpretation in order to derive value from it. Public health has been applying qualitative analytics to unstructured data for a while, such as open-ended survey text responses. Interpretations of chief complaint data have been coded through an ontology, such as Medical Subject Headings (MeSH),[17] to create a consistent interpretation of the text. This type of ontology would ensure that all permutations of "heart attack" are discovered, despite the many ways of describing this condition (e.g., myocardial infarction, necrosis of the myocardium, cardiac event, etc.). Basically, we use methods to interpret the unstructured data by overlaying it with some sort of structure. Another method for processing textual data is to use natural language processing (NLP) methods.[18]

We are finding many more ways to use what the data can tell us to answer surveillance questions. When looking to the surveillance system of the future, we have to start incorporating more unstructured data.

IS THE FLOW OF A CONSTANT DATA USEFUL?

Thus far, our discussion has focused on finding and manipulating data somewhere at rest. We may be moving some data around to find our answers, but basically it is data parked in a data repository and not streaming while we examine them. To further evolve the concept of a new surveillance platform, we should continue to revert to our basic goal we have to process data as quickly as possible to aid in our search to find answers to public health problems or discovery of significant public health events.

Data are moving all the time from their generated source to passive storage domains. Deciding to process data while they move can have significant advantages, particularly when dealing with Big Data. We talk about data quality issues to meet a consistent interpretation; if we place real-time data engines in front of our surveillance systems receiving data and then translate those data on the fly to a data quality we can process, everything speeds up.

Using data stream analytics we could decide whether to store everything that comes at the surveillance system or apply a policy to select just what we need for the purpose of the system or the specific question being asked. We will soon see that storing all of the molecular data that we are generating will be massive and hold quite a bit of redundant information. If we run an entire sequence and then filter the related sequences for an organism, just storing the variances we need, we can save having to build immense computing infrastructures.

Not all surveillance analysis has to be done with a passive pool of data. If we start building streaming analytics engines driven by models derived from our surveillance system to watch for patterns, then very fast detection can occur. For example, we may be watching a stream of data that is moving around all of the laboratories in the country back to their EHR units. We may start to see a pattern of a lot of *Escherichia coli* infections. Do we wait for the laboratory to report it to the public health department or do we automatically start running data to the public health department for further analysis and investigation across jurisdictions?

Adding surveillance analytics to streaming data can be very powerful and used in many ways we have not even begun to explore. It is another new way of thinking about how informatics has to change with new directions in population and public health informatics.

THE FINAL WIND

There are many directions we can explore when discussing the changing data landscape for future of public health surveillance. It may be obvious that there needs to be a new way of thinking about how we handle so much data now (or soon) available to public health. As the complexity of our questions increases so does the complexity of the data, technology, and level of human interaction. One area for future discussion is what the technology would look like to create the architectures needed to support future surveillance systems—an entire book could be written on how these technologies could be designed and deployed.

KEY SUMMARY POINTS

- The old way of thinking about aggregating piles of data and only letting one set of people look at the data does not, nor did it ever, achieve the maximum global public good.
- PHS data sources involve much more than just data from passive surveillance of the diagnosed sick. Our data sources now include data about the environment around the population, predictive surveillance, and searching for the unknown.
- Data sources are classified with the following behaviors, also called the Vs of Big Data: volume, variety, velocity, and veracity.
- Data streams will continue to be plentiful; therefore, we need to understand how to find the data, organize the data, and use the data to create information for decision-makers.
- Our data needs must be conveyed to those creating technologies in order for the technologies to best support decision-making.
- Data are no longer small, clean and, able to be analyzed from a structure. Dealing with unstructured data will enable us to take advantage of an entirely new source of information; however, data quality becomes increasingly important.

DISCUSSION QUESTIONS

1. How would you find the appropriate data sources to provide data for a multidomain, multidimension public health question?
2. Is fusing data the same as creating a data warehouse? Why or why not?
3. Describe a situation, from the scenarios in Appendix 3 or from your own experience, which could benefit from streaming data analytics.
4. Explain the 4 Vs around advanced public health data when building a surveillance system to track a long-term chronic disease.
5. How might unstructured data be used in public health surveillance?
6. What technology is needed to support these new types of surveillance systems?

REFERENCES

1. Oxford Dictionaries. Causation, <http://www.oxforddictionaries.com/>.
2. Mirhaji P, Richesson R, Srinivasan A, editors. Public health surveillance; a semantic approach. In: Multisensor, multisource information fusion: architectures, algorithms, and applications. SPIE; 2004.
3. Mirhaji P, Richesson R, Smith J, Zhang J, Srinivasan A, editors. Knowledge based public health situation awareness. In: Sensors, and command, control, communications, and intelligence (C3I) technologies for homeland security and homeland defense III. SPIE; 2004.
4. Mirhaji P, Zhang J, Smith J, Majid M, Casscells S, Lillibridge SR. Informatics critical to public health surveillance. In: Sensors, and command, control, communications, and intelligence (C3I) technologies for homeland defense and law enforcement II. SPIE; 2003. p. 151–63.
5. Definition provided by the chapter author.
6. White FE. Data fusion lexicon. San Diego: CA; 1991.
7. Kukafka R, Ancker JS, Chan C, Chelico J, Khan S, Mortoti S, et al. Redesigning electronic health record systems to support public health. J Biomed Inform 2007;40(4):398–409.

8. Dixon MA, Dar OA, Heymann DL. Emerging infectious diseases: opportunities at the human-animal-environment interface. Veterinary Record 2014;174(22):546–51.
9. Rappaport SM. Implications of the exposome for exposure science. J Expo Sci Environ Epidemiol 2011;21(1):5–9.
10. US Centers for Disease Control and Prevention. National Center for Environmental Health Atlanta, GA, <http://www.cdc.gov/nceh/data.html/>. [cited 2014].
11. Buehler JW, Whitney EA, Smith D, Prietula MJ, Stanton SH, Isakov AP. Situational uses of syndromic surveillance. Biosecur Bioterror 2009;7(2):165–77.
12. Foxman B, Riley L. Molecular epidemiology: focus on infection. Am J Epidemiol 2001;153(12):1135–41.
13. Behjati S, Tarpey PS. What is next generation sequencing? Arch Dis Child Educ Pract Ed 2013;98(6):236–8.
14. Marr B. Big data: the 5 Vs everyone must know, <http://www.linkedin.com/today/post/article/20140306073407-64875646-big-data-the-5-vs-everyone-must-know/>; 2014. [cited 2014].
15. Network HM. Framework and standards for country health information systems. 2nd ed. Geneva: WHO; 2008.
16. Mundy J, Thornthwaite W, Kimball R. The Microsoft data warehouse toolkit: with SQL Server 2008 R2 and the Microsoft business intelligence toolset. 2nd ed. Indianapolis, IN: Wiley Publishing, Inc.; 2011. p. 696.
17. Bodenreider O, Nelson SJ, Hole WT, Chang HF. Beyond synonymy: exploiting the UMLS semantics in mapping vocabularies. Proc AMIA Symp 1998: 815–9.
18. Townsend H. Natural language processing and clinical outcomes: the promise and progress of NLP for improved care. J AHIMA 2013;84(3): 44–5.

CHAPTER

22

Surveillance Informatics Builds an Ecosystem for Transformation

Arthur J Davidson

It is not how much empty space there is, but rather how it is used. It is not how much information there is, but rather how effectively it is arranged.

Edward R Tufte

KEY WORDS

Ecosystem
Standards
Modularity
Collaboration
Meaningful use
Interoperability
HAI
National Healthcare Safety Network
Sociotechnical ecosystem
eMeasures

INTRODUCTION

This chapter explores public health surveillance issues from an informatics perspective. The ultimate goal is to suggest ways that public health surveillance may transform public health practice and for informatics to transform the conduct of surveillance. Comparative studies of informatics systems are virtually nonexistent; thus, through pilots, demonstrations, and practical experiences, the informatics field defines and suggests new surveillance approaches. Often such informatics systems remain disparate when it comes to being interoperable. Significant resource gaps between countries and regions may challenge effective dissemination and implementation of innovative informatics solutions, further creating an ineffective surveillance **ecosystem** that is not interoperable. An **ecosystem** is a system, or a group of interconnected elements, formed by the interaction of a community of organisms with their environment.[1] Differential technology approaches will be necessary based on regional opportunities. Regardless of resource wealth or challenges, local assets should be aligned to create progressively more complex yet functional "ecosystems."[2] Cost-effective, highly adaptive solutions are desirable and should increase capacity to efficiently share surveillance information, creating public health value.

In a recent literature review, most published reports from US local health departments (LHD) described use of standard terminologies to communicate data, interventions, and outcomes; this compilation identified primarily best practice descriptions with few experimental studies.[3] Few journals publish negative LHD informatics studies; thus, descriptions here will be empirical or anecdotal. Cost-effectiveness[4] or return on investment analyses[5, 6] for implemented information systems are sorely lacking, as are comparative studies. This chapter will focus on and primarily describe practical approaches to surveillance informatics applications and their sustainability.

General enterprise technology principles (i.e., standards, modularity, parsimony, and trustful collaborative relationships) will be reviewed as they should inform and guide public health surveillance system transformation. **Modularity** is where a system is created from subcomponents that can be reused in different configurations or independently replaced to change the characteristics of technology systems without complete systems redesign.[7] Using a common **healthcare-associated infection** (*Clostridium difficile*), as a case study, this chapter will explore some emerging alternatives to current processes and systems. **Healthcare-associated infection (HAI)** is a localized or systemic condition resulting from an adverse reaction to the presence of an infectious agent(s) or its toxin(s). There must be no evidence that the infection was present or incubating at the time of admission to the acute care setting.[8]

To date, limited technology investments mean most existing architectures fall far short of idealized surveillance systems. Emerging informatics advances (e.g., health information exchange, standards adherence, and growth of cloud services) create both opportunities and challenges in the fragmented and resource-limited US public health system. Combining multijurisdiction resources may ultimately create more sustainable surveillance systems, where information and tools are appropriately and efficiently shared across a complex ecosystem, enabling progress toward common goals.

A CASE STUDY OF HEALTH CARE-ASSOCIATED INFECTIONS IN THE USA

Ever-expanding communicable disease challenges include organisms highly resistant to current antibiotics. Key monitoring focuses on occurrence and outcomes of communicable events within high-use antibiotic environments. HAI surveillance monitors health care practice and effective disease control. For decades, the Centers for Disease Control and Prevention (CDC) has organized public health surveillance (PHS) and clinical surveillance efforts through the National Healthcare Safety Network (NHSN)[9] with case reporting from more than 12,000 medical facilities (i.e., acute care hospitals, long-term acute care hospitals, psychiatric hospitals, rehabilitation hospitals, outpatient dialysis centers, ambulatory surgery centers, and nursing homes). Hospitals and dialysis facilities represent the majority of reporting facilities. The example of NHSN and this type of surveillance reporting is used as a use case for this chapter to show a successful **integration**[7] and feedback loop of clinical operations and public health surveillance effectiveness. This is one of the few systems that have created an effective informatics "ecosystem" between the two domains serving the personal and population goals for health quality. A goal we have been suggesting is the new direction and transformation of surveillance and informatics. The effectiveness stems from applying public health surveillance analytics and provides targeted feedback interventions and training across the clinical domain to measure and change the infections. This also allows for a population level of measurement and reporting on the effectiveness of intervention methods that can reinforce or change the clinical process.

NHSN HAI reporting focuses on five areas: (1) central line-associated bloodstream infections, (2) ventilator-associated events, (3) surgical site infections, (4) catheter-associated urinary tract infections, and (5) *C. difficile* infections. For this discussion, we will focus on *C. difficile* infections as an organism of growing health care importance in the health care and hospital setting. While most HAI have been declining as a consequence of effective NHSN monitoring, *C. difficile* remains at historically high levels with nearly threefold increase in infection-related hospital stays over the last decade and 94% of those associated with some prior medical care.[10] Typically, *C. difficile* causes serious diarrhea and has been linked to as many as 14,000 American deaths annually. Risk factors include age, previous use of antibiotics, and receipt of medical care. Antibiotic usage results in suppression of favorable intestinal flora, which protect against infection. During the postantibiotic recovery period, patients may acquire *C. difficile* from environmental contamination and also from exposure to health care providers. About one quarter of *C. difficile* infections present in hospital patients, while the rest first show symptoms in patients in nursing home facilities or those recently cared for in medical facilities (e.g., doctors' offices and clinics). Annual health care cost estimates for *C. difficile* infection exceed US$1 billion.

Reduction of *C. difficile* spread relies on health care providers and facilities taking proper environmental precautions; from a surveillance perspective, knowing health care facility infection rates aids in monitoring intervention effectiveness. Efforts to adopt and implement certified electronic health record (EHR) technology, as a result of the **meaningful use**[11] incentive program,[12] offer a unique opportunity to leverage unprecedented federal investments to improve *C. difficile* surveillance. This EHR deployment expansion increases the opportunity for more, faster, and more accurate data to flow into a system like the NHSN.

CURRENT PUBLIC HEALTH SURVEILLANCE INFORMATICS OPPORTUNITIES

Meaningful use (MU) includes a focus on public and population health measures. In 2014, as US federal agencies (Office of the National Coordinator for Health Information Technology and Centers for Medicare and Medicaid Services) consider MU criteria, NHSN reporting has been suggested as a way to comply with a registry objective. MU is a phased set of compliancy criteria for the deployment of technology standards and functional capabilities for specific interfaces to public health from EHR systems. Currently the focus is on electronic laboratory reporting, syndromic surveillance, and registry reporting. Considering one of the major health informatics goals is to increase health quality and care the extension of MU for the enhancement of existing reporting to more automated processes and reporting of HAI (e.g., *C. difficile*) to NHSN can inform public health officials and make that information available to advise clinical and community providers to meet the goals.

These ongoing federal health care information technology investments expand technology adoption by health care providers and in turn permit greater public health access to health information. Across the nation, thousands of health care facilities need to accurately and efficiently communicate with multiple public health jurisdictions (e.g., local, state, and federal). This information exchange web is considered **a sociotechnical ecosystem**; like the internet, it is composed of decentralized systems[2] where people and organizations develop technologies and implement policies to support the cultural and economic goals of those producing and using the system. Participants set operational policies to govern the system and then design the system to meet those needs. Interdependencies among players, systems, and activities are significant and there is need to relinquish control, acknowledge the needs of others, and create more value. This change in information system design and thinking from silo services to ecosystem services is the only way surveillance goals can be accomplished. For instance, public health officials depend on effective and comprehensive reporting from providers and providers seek minimal reporting burden (e.g., data collection, chart review, and completed case reports). Decreased burden should result in more timely, complete, and accurate surveillance reports (see Chapter 18).

Infection control practitioners consider identifying and reporting these hospital cases a significant burden. These practitioners spend time aggregating data from multiple data sources (e.g., laboratory and medical record); however, aggregation could automatically occur based on clinical triggers (e.g., positive *C. difficile* test). Once identified, an EHR could populate the standard *C. difficile* case report form with additional information stored in the EHR (e.g., history of recent antibiotic use) or retrieve additional clinical or operational data (e.g., patient exposure to specific staff). Achieving this automation requires interoperability. Data need to be standardized and shared through common message structure and content. Both data sender (e.g., hospital) and receiver (e.g., NHSN) use computers to share and pragmatically use information. Both parties need agreement and explicit rules on how detailed content, structure, and transport will be standardized for interoperability to be achieved. Mapping HAI surveillance needs to these specific informatics concepts and methods is essential for computers to efficiently interact and use exchanged data. Practitioners of surveillance and informatics each may have a unique perspective and be seeking to answer slightly different questions with divergent goals, as described in Table 22-1.

TABLE 22-1 **Distinct Public Health Perspectives on Communicable Disease Reporting Messages**

MESSAGE	PERSPECTIVES: SURVEILLANCE	PERSPECTIVES: INFORMATICS
Content	Is the infection newly hospital acquired or was it present on admission and thus community acquired? For how long was the patient hospitalized before the infection was noted? What antibiotics has the patient received and in what temporal sequence?	What standard terminologies and data formats are used to describe the infection, its onset date, where it was first diagnosed, associated symptoms, and what/when antibiotic exposures have occurred?
Format	Is the case report form completed?	What are established data and message standard formats? How should the message be formatted to assure that the receiver can parse and retrieve the electronically transmitted information?
Transport	What is the mechanism for exchange of the case report form (e.g., letter, fax, or email)?	What is the automated mechanism for exchange of the message (e.g., email, direct message, web service)? What are the security requirements for transmission?

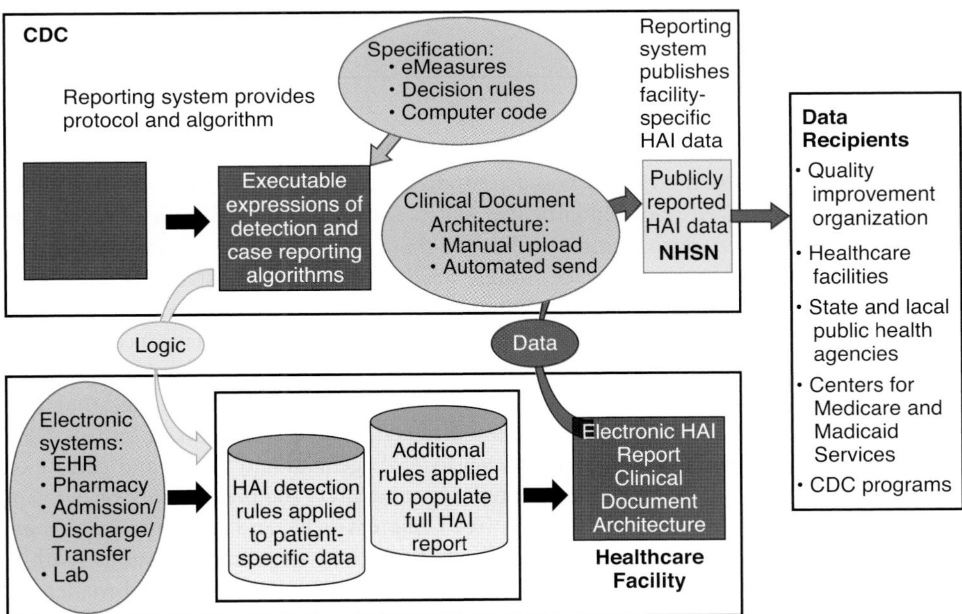

FIG. 22-1 HAI reporting schema to the NHSN. (Slide modified and used with permission, CDC.) Source: Pollack D. CDC's National Healthcare Safety Network (NHSN). 2012 HAI Data Summit, Kansas City, MO, May 30–31, 2012. http://www.health.gov/hai/pdfs/final_plenary_one_master_slide_deck_final.pdf

Health care facilities using certified EHR technology for MU need to establish basic health information exchange. For MU, if a hospital reported to NHSN as a registry activity, successful health information exchange would require the EHR vendor to understand reporting requirements, to build appropriate triggers, and then to compile a machine interpretable surveillance message with high-quality data. The surveillance message is the automated data feed channel out of the EHR into surveillance systems that generally does not exist today.

TABLE 22-2 Examples of Networks, Focus, and Architecture used for Public Health Surveillance

DESCRIPTION	FOCUS	ARCHITECTURE
Primary Care Information Project[12] (NYC Department of Health and Mental Hygiene) 2500 providers 2.5 million residents	Chronic disease, reportable, syndromic	Distributed
Mini-Sentinel[10] (Federal Drug Administration, Harvard Pilgrim, and Health Maintenance Organization Research Network) 17 large health care systems, 126 million covered lives	Diagnoses, drugs, procedures	Distributed
MDPHnet[13-15] (Massachusetts Department of Public Health, Massachusetts Leagues of Community Health Centers, and Atrius Health)	Influenza-like illness, diabetes mellitus surveillance	Distributed
BioSense 2[11] (Centers for Disease Control and Prevention, and the Association of State and Territorial Health Officers) Cloud-based system across 35 jurisdictions	Syndromic surveillance	Centralized
National Healthcare Safety Network[6] (Centers for Disease Control and Prevention) 12,000 health care providers across the USA	Health care associated infections	Centralized

Fig. 22-1 describes data flow and methods for HAI reporting to NHSN. Noteworthy is that all health care providers report to one CDC data repository. NHSN serves a centralized function rather than replicating this function in each state or jurisdiction. Authorized and authenticated states and local public health entities, federal payment programs, and health care providers retrieve information for their jurisdiction, reimbursed facilities, and practice sites, respectively. Using this cloud-based approach, public health enterprise infrastructure investments are minimized. More importantly, one site means one set of standards; reporting burden and implementation costs are decreased for EHR vendors and health care providers. When each jurisdiction implements its own instance, standards subtly vary from one jurisdiction to another. These subtle variations result in increased integration, deployment, connectivity, and maintenance costs; the EHR vendors or their customers will then incur additional financial burden. The Federal Health Architecture[13] principle of interoperability standards are reinforced by this NHSN model to assure seamless and secure exchange of health data between federal agencies and public and private organizations.

Public health surveillance in the USA and internationally is generally a fragmented mix of overlapping government organizations building program-specific solutions (see Chapters 2, 15, and 16). Infrequently, an architecture or infrastructure might span multiple countries or programs but program-specific applications (within one agency) are more common; the result is ineffective integration. Both local and national examples of broader, more collective and trusting approaches are described in Table 22-2. Agencies have built or invested in tools to solve a programmatic need (e.g., CDC-NHSN[9]; FDA Mini-Sentinel[14, 15]; and CDC-BioSense 2.0[16]), which have been effectively deployed to multiple stakeholders. However, the rule is highly fragmented systems (often imposed by categorical funding), which means that jurisdiction- or program-specific informatics solutions are replicated in thousands of jurisdictions across the USA. This repetitive public health surveillance/informatics approach operates at extremely high cost (both human resources and technology). Overall, there has been relatively little emphasis on sustainability and transferability of knowledge and infrastructure.

Enthusiasm to build “in-house” program-specific solutions should be reassessed from the public health enterprise or learning systems[17] view—what makes sense? One systems view is fostered by the Federal Enterprise Architecture,[18] in which guiding principles include (1) future-readiness, (2) strategic investment support, (3) shared services,

(4) interoperability standards, (5) transparent information access, (6) emphasis on security and privacy, and (7) decoupled (i.e., modular) technology adoption for maximum flexibility to cope with change. Decoupled technology or architecture allows components to remain completely autonomous and unaware of each other. By integrating decoupled modules, each with its own specific strength, opportunistic architecture may blend "best of breed" tools rather than rebuilding a list of functionalities into one unwieldy product.

Consider a few pointed questions when systems are designed, procured, or deployed to avoid some of these traps. Do in-house public health program solutions typically address or consider these important principles? Are these even considered during requirements gathering for the in-house solution? For instance, what are the security and privacy requirements for the program or agency? How do surveillance systems meet public expectations for transparency, adhere to internationally adopted Fair Information Privacy Principles,[19] and are accountable to and compliant with varying state and federal (e.g., the Health Insurance Portability and Accountability Act) regulations. Similarly, agencies should avoid being locked into vendor-specific or proprietary solutions where more standard surveillance business process definition[20] would drive to economically sustainable informatics solutions.

Sustainable surveillance systems, despite being highly utilized, would never be used up and should last for a long time. The idea that a surveillance system should contain useful data from the day it is created to forever is often not a consideration. Myopic design, missing integration architecture, and overly specific context of data often leaves an investment in a surveillance system very limited in scope and life. For a public health informatics infrastructure environment, those are exceedingly challenging requirements. Software and hardware technology have been constantly evolving for the past several decades. Finding an adaptive architecture that addresses rapid change and embraces short life cycles is essential to effective surveillance infrastructure investments. Most public health agencies have limited capacity to revise their architecture or infrastructure on a frequent basis. Working across jurisdictions on a flexible, common platform allows funding to be aggregated and resources shared. Establishing a common platform requires a set of integrated functional (e.g., what the platform does—exchanges information) and nonfunctional (e.g., what the platform is—secure and interoperable), requirements. A flexible infrastructure should easily adapt to changing technologies and conform to a spectrum of jurisdiction-specific policies. Shared systems have already demonstrated increased return on investment for many public health jurisdictions.

MU rapidly accelerated broad public health interest in accessing a stream of syndromic surveillance data from a majority of eligible US hospitals.[21] BioSense 2.0[16, 22] now offers a secure, cloud-based, common platform to solve a common multijurisdiction public health need. Given widespread hospital participation, virtually every jurisdiction needed ready access to a high performance, secure environment that respects jurisdictional boundaries and political variations leading to the emergence of BioSense 2.0.[16] While authority and responsibility to conduct disease surveillance is established jurisdiction-by-jurisdiction, rapid adoption of shared, cloud-based systems means less cost to that jurisdiction. While uncommon, this parsimonious, shared, multijurisdictional method, which adheres to standards, will accelerate and build public health informatics capacity. The approach is worthy of study and potential replication.

In the conceptual model (Fig. 22-1) for reporting of *C. difficile* infection to NHSN, there are some valuable lessons and parallels to be observed. The CDC (upper box) serves several key functions. The CDC helps (1) establish common reporting needs, (2) define the protocol, (3) design executable expressions for *C. difficile* infection detection, and (4) designate triggers or algorithms. These drive the development of computer tools or "**eMeasures**" that support executable expressions. The rules are open-source and may be imported by health care facilities to be used internally to detect HAI. **eMeasures** are standardized performance measures in an electronic format. eMeasures help ensure that measures are consistently defined, implemented, and compatible across clinical IT systems to promote higher quality and more appropriate care delivery.[23] Facility data from multiple sources are exposed to rules for case identification. For example, (1) knowing a patient's culture was positive for *C. difficile* (laboratory), (2) determining whether a patient had been on antibiotics (pharmacy), (3) calculating time in the hospital (registration system), and (4) verifying no prior *C. difficile* diagnosis (EHR) all contribute information for an algorithm to evaluate infection, onset, and precipitating factors.

Each clinically relevant system needs to use a common vocabulary or standard set of terminologies for the algorithm to execute properly. Once an incident case is identified, the health care facility packages the information that may come by message from these various sources into a common structure (i.e., clinical document architecture[24]) that organizes the information in a format the receiving computer at NHSN can anticipate, understand, and manipulate as a completed case report. Data transmitted to the CDC in Fig. 22-1 may be in a manual or automated fashion, depending on the capabilities of the sending system.

NHSN uses this basic process for all of its five major areas of interest. Many aspects of this model are extensible; other surveillance systems that seek to establish interoperability between senders and public health surveillance systems might consider this as a successful model. A key feature of this nationally developed system is that it requires little effort by state or LHD to maintain, yet they are the recipients of reports from the central repository.

CONCLUSIONS

Public health needs to design, implement, and maintain practical informatics systems that by ease of use and dissemination increase the likelihood of sustainability given resource limitations at local, state, and federal agencies. Achieving interoperability and data availability is necessary but insufficient for true transformation. The real potential for a transformed surveillance system will be through useful, highly effective, and sustainable informatics infrastructures.

The public health community has made progress in learning to apply business process analysis but limited joint or cross-jurisdiction analyses for multijurisdictions planning, data modeling, and standards adherence. Determining pertinent requirements[25] and how proposed and implemented solutions fit critical parameters is key to managing an informatics investment portfolio.

Several surveillance systems exist as successful examples for governance and technical models. As accreditation of public health agencies accelerates in the USA, emphasis should be placed on improving informatics skills and a work force capable of leveraging new opportunities and avoiding informatics failed investments due to limited use of standards and ineffective information exchange. By working collaboratively with other jurisdictions, agencies should focus on key public health enterprise informatics principles, which value (1) standards, (2) modularity, (3) parsimony, and (4) trustful collaborative relationships. Public health agencies should define standard surveillance business processes and how to best address them through thoughtful and economically sustainable informatics solutions.

As twenty-first century epidemiologists, technology advances, and new architectures create opportunities for significant transformation in how we use data to drive daily public health practice. Epidemiologists will need ready access through a host of devices. Getting devices (e.g., laptops, smartphones, tablets, and voice interaction) to work well together means using the web to provide data and information. Health departments should expand their skilled workforce and through their broad networks engage the open source community, build common platforms, and leverage enterprise resources. Focused on joint application development of adaptable, flexible, and extensible tools, public health surveillance should be ready to truly leverage emerging technology opportunities from a burgeoning world of interoperable health information stakeholders.

KEY SUMMARY POINTS

- Architectural decisions should be based on clear understanding of all the functional and nonfunctional requirements.
- A variety of infrastructure solutions are available; decisions about which solution to pick should be based on simultaneously considered the resources and requirements within the target program, agency and broader public health enterprise.
- Shared architectural solutions require relinquishment of control and a more challenging governance solution; while more difficult to build those cultural and business alliances, they are often more rewarding as they promote greater standards adherence and reduced development and sustainability costs.

DISCUSSION QUESTIONS

1. How long must data persist in any environment? Must massive database systems hold data for many years to achieve the surveillance goal?
2. How do solutions compare (e.g., centralized data storage systems versus distributed data that reside at the source)? Neither extreme will likely serve all use cases; the real answer probably lies somewhere in the middle with hybrid systems.
3. Give some examples of centralized data storage and why are they particularly good for some situations. By enhancing data types (e.g., PulseNet includes genomic identity data for *E. coli* and *Salmonella* sp. along with phenotypic data), epidemiologists can quickly identify food-borne sources during an outbreak. Limited resources suggest that most public health programs would benefit from extensive sharing of technology and data. More importantly, technology projects have an enormously high risk of failure if proper project management (e.g., risk control and mitigation) are not implemented early in development.
4. What are typical ongoing maintenance and enhancement costs and how should a program plan for these over time? Can programs easily identify resources to support those costs with challenging and highly fluctuating budgets? How do sustainability cost compare with initial development and implementation? How should baseline resources be used to project recurring costs to support the technology?
5. Imagine you are a public health leader of either a jurisdiction's communicable disease or chronic disease surveillance unit. Engage in a discussion with your counterpart of how you define sustainability of your surveillance information system. How does your definition impact on the work of your unit? What would be worthwhile infrastructure investments for your unit and how does sustainability influence these decisions and solutions? What changes (i.e., technology, politics, and funding) are necessary to achieve an enterprise perspective?

REFERENCES

1. Ecosystem. Dictionary.com. The American Heritage® New Dictionary of Cultural Literacy, Third Edition. Houghton Mifflin Company, 2005. <http://dictionary.reference.com/browse/ecosystem>; October 02, 2015.
2. Software Engineering Institute. Ultra-large-scale systems: the software challenge of the future. Pittsburgh, PA: Carnegie Mellon; 2006.
3. Olsen J, Baisch MJ. An integrative review of information systems and terminologies used in local health departments. J Am Med Inform Assoc 2013;21:e20–7. Published Online First: October 26, 2013.
4. Kempe A, Saville A, Dickinson LM, Eisert S, Reynolds J, Herrero D, et al. Population-based versus practice-based recall for childhood immunizations: a randomized controlled comparative effectiveness trial. Am J Public Health 2013;103:1116–23.
5. Walker J, Pan E, Johnston D, Adler-Milstein J, Bates DW, Middleton B. The value of health care information exchange and interoperability. Health Aff 2005;(Suppl.):W5–18.
6. Mays G. Public health return on investment: making the case" Kentucky Department of Public Health, Forum on the Future of Kentucky's Public Health System. Frankfort, KY; <http://works.bepress.com/glen_mays/65/>; 2012. [accessed March 30, 2014].
7. Definition provided by the chapter author.
8. Horan TC, Andrus M, Dudeck MA. CDC/NHSN surveillance definition of health care-associated infection and criteria for specific types of infections in the acute care setting. Am J Infect Control 2008;36(5):309–32.
9. Centers for Disease Control and Prevention. National Center for Emerging and Zoonotic Infectious Diseases, Division of Healthcare Quality Promotion. National Healthcare Safety Network, <http://www.cdc.gov/nhsn/about.html/>. [Last updated January 27, 2015].
10. Centers for Disease Control and Prevention. Making healthcare safer: Stopping C. difficile infections. Vital signs, <http://www.cdc.gov/vitalsigns/>; 2012.
11. Meaningful Use, <http://www.cdc.gov/ehrmeaningfuluse/introduction.html/>; 2015.
12. US Congress. American Recovery and Reinvestment Act, Health Information Technology for Economic and Clinical Health Act or the "HITECH Act", <http://www.healthit.gov/sites/default/files/hitech_act_excerpt_from_arra_with_index.pdf/>; 2009.
13. Office of the national coordinator for health information technology. Standards and interoperability framework, Federal Health Architecture, <http://healthit.gov/policy-researchers-implementers/federal-health-architecture-fha/>. [Last updated July 31, 2015].
14. Curtis LH, Weiner MG, Boudreau DM, Cooper WO, Daniel GW, Nair VP, et al. Design considerations, architecture, and use of the Mini-Sentinel distributed data system. Pharmacoepidemiol Drug Saf 2012;21(Suppl. 1):23–31, <http://www.ncbi.nlm.nih.gov/pubmed/?term=Raebel%20MA%5BAuthor%5D&cauthor=true&cauthor_uid=22262590/>.
15. Platt R, Carnahan RM, Brown JS, Chrischilles E, Curtis LH, Hennessy S, et al. The U.S. Food and Drug Administration's Mini-Sentinel program: status and direction. Pharmacoepidemiol Drug Saf 2012;21(Suppl. 1):1–8, <http://www.ncbi.nlm.nih.gov/pubmed/?term=Nelson%20JC%5BAuthor%5D&cauthor=true&cauthor_uid=22262586/>.
16. Centers for Disease Control and Prevention. BioSense Program: The Community, <http://www.cdc.gov/biosense/community.html/>. [accessed January 15, 2014].
17. Senge PM. The fifth discipline. New York: Doubleday; 1990.
18. Office of Management and Budget. The common approach to federal enterprise architecture, <http://www.whitehouse.gov/sites/default/files/omb/assets/egov_docs/common_approach_to_federal_ea.pdf/>; 2012. [accessed January 5, 2014].
19. Organization for Economic Cooperation and Development. OECD guidelines on the protection of privacy and transborder flows of personal data, <http://www.oecd.org/document/18/0,2340,en_2649_34255_1815186_1_1_1_1,00.html/>; 1980.
20. Public Health Informatics Institute. Taking care of business: a collaboration to define local health department business processes. Decatur, GA: Public Health Informatics Institute; 2006.

21. Centers for Medicare and Medicaid Services. Medicare & Medicaid EHR Incentive Programs, Report to HIT Policy Committee, <http://www.healthit.gov/FACAS/sites/faca/files/HITPC_Feb2014_HITPC.pdf/>; 2014. [accessed March 1, 2014].
22. Centers for Disease Control and Prevention. BioSense 2.0 Community forum, <https://sites.google.com/site/biosenseredesign/?pli=1/>. [accessed May 24, 2014].
23. Electronic Quality Measures (eMeasures), <http://www.qualityforum.org/Projects/e-g/eMeasures/Electronic_Quality_Measures.aspx/>; 2015.
24. Centers for Disease Control and Prevention. National Healthcare Safety Network. Clinical Document Architecture. [accessed March 30, 2014].
25. Lombardo JS, Ross D. Disease surveillance, a public health priority. In: Lombardo JS, Buckeridge DL, editors. Disease surveillance: a public health informatics approach. Hoboken, NJ: Wiley; 2007.

CHAPTER

23

The Human Interaction Required for Visualizing and Manipulating Information

Matthew D Dollacker

For good ideas and true innovation, you need human interaction, conflict, argument, debate.

Margaret Heffernan

KEY WORDS

Visualization
Analytics
Data quality
Reporting
Big data
GIS
Spatial analysis
Information processing
Open question and answer system
Dengue trends
HITECH Act

PUBLIC HEALTH IS A DATA-DRIVEN DISCIPLINE NEEDING DISCOVERY AND VISUALIZATION OF THE HIDDEN KNOWLEDGE

The public's conception of the field of public health is of myriad scientists in lab coats scurrying around laboratories performing tests to identify a mysterious infectious disease. Although that certainly occurs, it is only one part of what it takes to protect the population's health. Arguably, the precise identification of a given infectious disease is at a lower immediate importance than understanding its current transmission rate, mortality rate, prevalence, and other factors relative to a given population. The low importance of identifying any given disease becomes even lower for chronic disease, injury, and other public health concerns, where many decades can pass without significant medical breakthroughs relative to these afflictions.

The big questions in public health have always been data driven, beginning with John Snow's analysis of data on cholera deaths in nineteenth-century London. The manipulation and visualization of data that was otherwise uninteresting from a medical perspective provided crucial new insights that saved many lives. Though Snow's laboratory examination of samples yielded no conclusions, by taking data that were already being collected and *visualizing* them in new ways, Snow made his key realization that the cases clustered around a particular well (Fig. 23-1).[1]

Our ability to gather, analyze, manipulate, and visualize information is every bit as important as understanding the mechanics of disease transmission and epidemiology. As even laboratory science becomes data driven with genomic analysis (see Chapter 26), it will be even more important to develop new and better ways to organize and visualize data.

The rest of this chapter will detail some of the ways that these approaches are evolving to enable the next generation of capabilities in data manipulation and visualization. These capabilities follow broader revolutions in the tools, technologies, and approaches for working with and understanding data that are occurring across many industries.

They go far beyond just a new type of chart; rather they involve dramatic new capabilities to look deeply into data and process them via computer analysis that mirrors (and maybe even exceeds) human abilities to derive conclusions and knowledge from raw information.

CURRENT STATE AND HISTORY OF TOOLS SUPPORTING PUBLIC HEALTH

To understand where the field is going, it is important to understand where we are and have been. Before Snow and the modern field of public health, the understanding of health-related impacts on a population was minimal. In the 1850s, there was a commonly held belief that disease was caused by "bad airs." The basic biologic and medical breakthroughs had not yet occurred to enable understanding of the mechanics of pathogens and disease transmission; this was the period of rumor, myth, and oral history—and it was not that long ago.

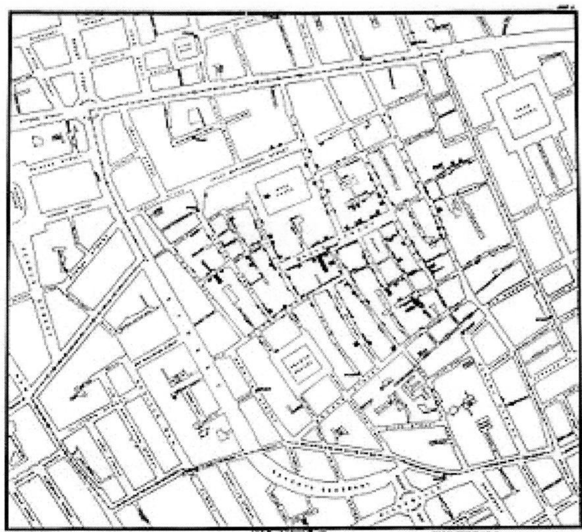

FIG. 23-1 John Snow's map showing cholera cases clustering around the Broad Street well in nineteenth-century London. Updated source: Snow. Wikipedia. Public domain.

Perspectives on Data

When we think about **data visualization**, we often immediately jump to thinking about computer systems and **databases. Database**s are technology architecture components that specialize in the persistence and manipulation of data in specific technology structures allowing many types of inquiry systems to manipulate the information stored.[2] Though they are important tools, many important paradigm shifts in the way people interacted with data came before the modern era of computers. As discussed above, a simple written log of morbidity reports and a map were enough to draw fundamental conclusions about the nature and causes of disease, changing the way disease transmission and control occurred forever. What seemed like "bad air" randomly passing through the streets of London was suddenly and obviously clustered around one particular water source when viewed from a different perspective. **Data visualization** is the graphical display of abstract information for two purposes: sensemaking (also called data analysis) and communication. Important stories live in our data and data visualization is a powerful means to discover and understand these stories, and then to present them to others.[3]

The power of new perspectives on data should not be lost with human understanding, but often is. Massive data **analytics** have to involve the interaction of human intuition and comprehension or we quickly lose the value of the analytics results. **Analytics** is the systematic computational analysis of data or statistics.[4] Though computer analysis has brought down the cost and effort associated with tabular collection and analysis of data, there have been relatively few changes to the fundamental way we interact with data until quite recently. Even today, the humble tools of spreadsheets, charts, and maps form the foundation of how we typically interact with public health data.

Fig. 23-2 offers a powerful example of how data visualization can provide new perspectives on data. This view shows the impact of troop movements, geography, engagements, and Russia's cold temperatures (bottom) on the size of Napoleon's army as it invaded and retreated from Russia (in black). It is a reminder that visualizing data in new ways is not always a technology problem. We often forget this in public health.

Computer Analysis, Spreadsheets, and Databases

Computer analysis shifted the scale and mechanics around our interaction with data and significantly sped up the processing of the calculations that previously were processed by hand. Spreadsheets now allow for the almost

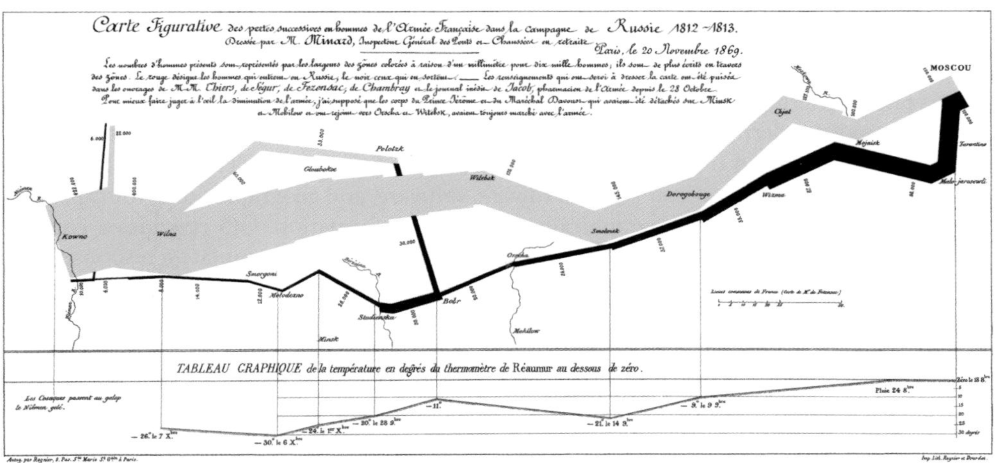

FIG. 23-2 Charles Joseph Minard's chart of Napoleon's march into Russia. Source: Tableaux Graphiques et Cartes Figratives de M. Mindard, 1845–1869.

immediate sorting, filtering, summarization, and calculation of hundreds of thousands of rows of tabular data, with dozens of varieties of charts and graphs. Pareto analysis, statistical computation, and Monte Carlo simulations can be performed at the speed of thought with essentially zero cost of computation.

Databases have enabled us to capture even larger data sets stretching into the many millions (and even billions) of rows, with relational structures that allow for the collection of complex and highly structured data entities. The classical database concept of a foreign key relationship provides the ability to capture varying ordinalities between different data entities, resulting in much richer mechanisms for portraying varying perspectives on a given set of data. By normalizing data and then using database joins to combine entities, a user is no longer limited to analyzing data using only the columns and rows in which they were captured (Fig. 23-3). With a normalized model, it is trivial to identify all of the persons or laboratory reports associated with a given investigation. Alternatively, with the same data and data structure, we can analyze laboratory reports relative to individual cases, providing a view into which tests are confirming the incidence of disease. Database concepts that support where we need to go can be learned through more exposure and practice of information technology (IT) methods. These skill capacities are often not taught in public health settings and are critical to understand how to take advantage of these new data perspectives. The advent of the new role called the informatician is working to bridge these missing competencies with people who understand public health, science, and IT.

Databases are powerful tools that work best with highly structured data. The sorting, filtering, combining, and calculation logic in common database platforms assumes that information is stored in strictly typed fields (e.g., integer, floating point, string, and date), which puts some constraints on the methods and types of information analyzed with these tools. Considerable effort has gone into creating systems, processes, and information sources that impose and maintain these structures on data. As anyone who has spent any time analyzing data knows, a database sees "Positive," "Pos," "Y," and "10828004" (a SNOMED-CT value for positive) as completely distinct values, though they may be storing the same positive result of a given test. This has been a particular challenge in efforts to incorporate clinical information (which historically has been largely unstructured) into the practice of public health. Though we may have better emerging tools to deal with less structured data in the future, it will be an ongoing struggle to impose order on our data.

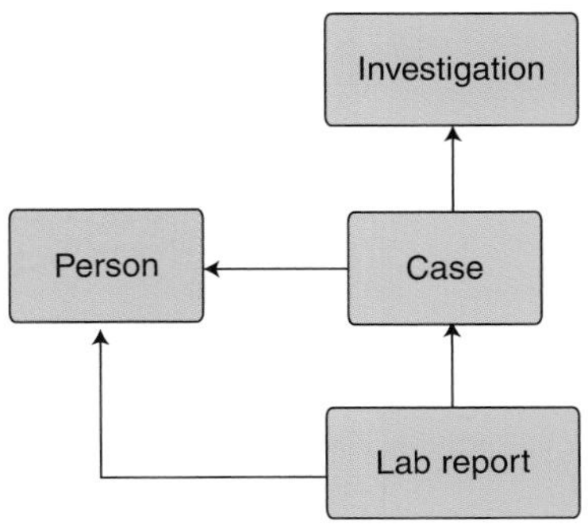

FIG. 23-3 Typical surveillance modeling entities in a Third Normal Form database model.

Geographic Information Systems and Spatial Analysis

Geographic visualization is a powerful analysis technique for uncovering spatial patterns within data. It is of particular importance to public health, since much of our work involves the movement and interaction of populations (of both people and vectors). Modern **geographic information systems** (**GIS**) include the ability to quickly and efficiently plot and geocode data and overlay various data sets onto a geographic view to understand relationships between data sets. **GIS** is a collection of computer hardware, software, and geographic data for capturing, managing, analyzing, and displaying all forms of geographically referenced information. GIS provides a common analytical framework in which public health authorities can understand problems and formulate a response, improving incident management and health planning.[5] **Spatial analysis** is the process of examining the locations, attributes, and relationships of features in spatial data through overlay and other analytical techniques in order to address a question or gain useful knowledge. Spatial analysis extracts or creates new information from spatial data.[6]

The Dartmouth Atlas of Health Care (Fig. 23-4) is a great illustration of the power of geographic analysis. This study utilized Medicare billing claims data to better understand and visualize the regional variations in health care across the USA. By looking at these Medicare data across regions, new patterns emerged that brought fresh understanding to this already highly analyzed data set. The Dartmouth Atlas provided new revelations on the delivery of health care in the USA, such as that seen in Fig. 23-4, which illustrates the remarkable variation in the use of surgery to treat back pain. Further investigation showed a relationship between the number of surgery treatments in a region and the prevailing methods taught in each region's medical schools.

Reporting and Visualization

The Morbidity and Mortality Weekly Report published by the US Centers for Disease Control and Prevention (CDC) is one of the primary reference reports in public health. It is a great example of both the power and limitations of

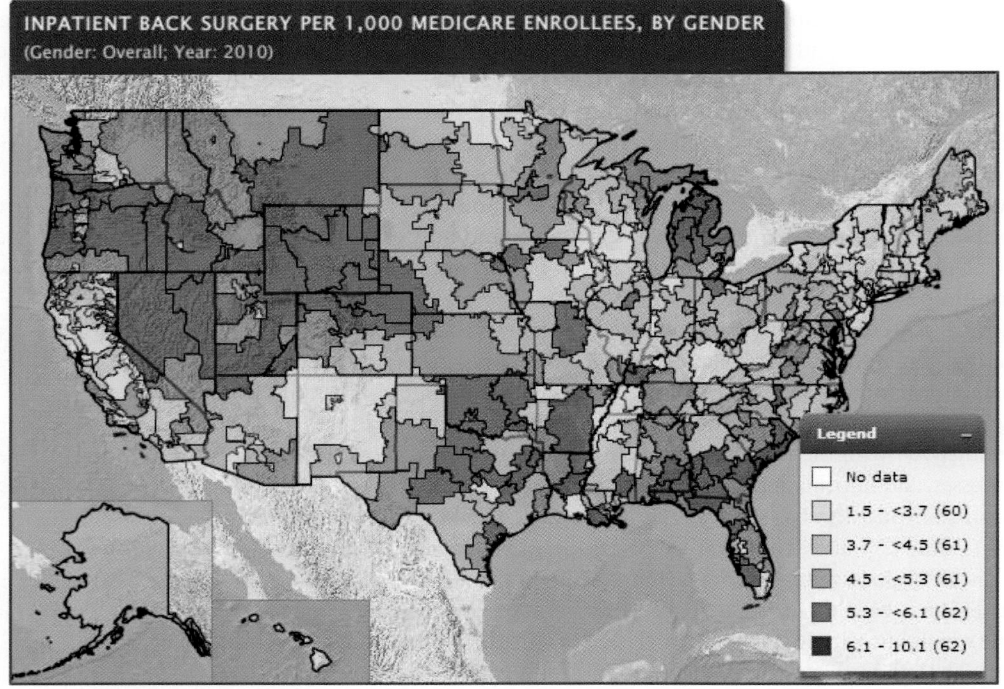

FIG. 23-4 Inpatient Back Surgery Data from The Dartmouth Atlas of Health Care.

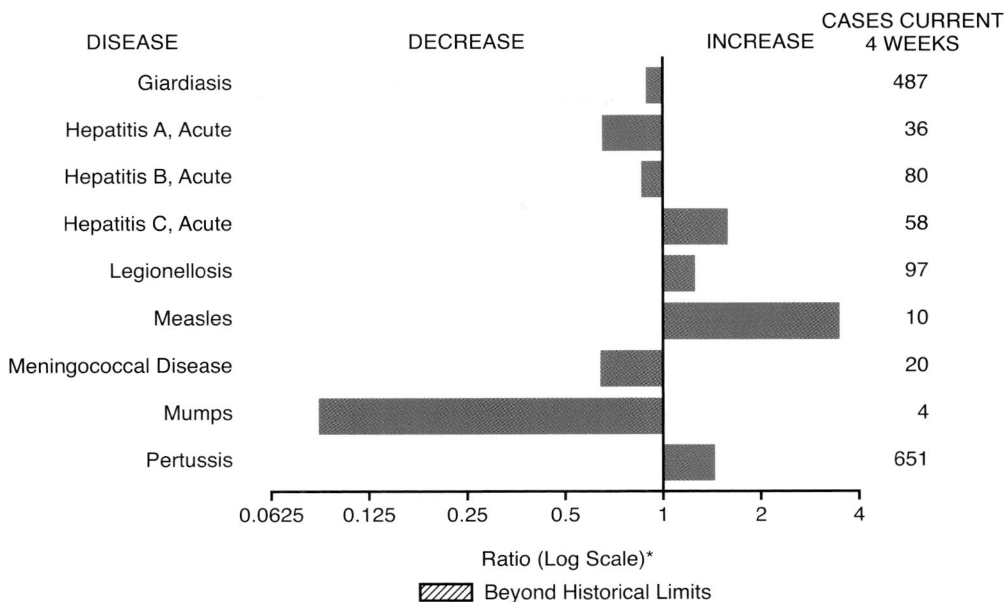

*Ratio of current 4-week total to mean of 15 4-week totals (from previous, comparable, and subsequent 4-week periods for the past 5 years). The point where the hatched area begins is based on the mean and two standard deviations of these 4-week totals.

FIG. 23-5 Selected notifiable disease reports, the USA, comparison of provisional 4-week totals February 22, 2014, with historical data.

our current approaches to public health data visualization. While Fig. 23-5 provides an intuitive view of the relative changes in the prevalence of key infectious diseases compared to previous years, much of the information remains comparatively locked away in large tables like those in Fig. 23-6 that are difficult to analyze or to import and process via automated tools.

FUTURE VISION

The broader field of **information processing** is undergoing a revolution, with dramatic new capabilities emerging, of which we are only just starting to take advantage. These emerging capabilities have been driven primarily by the availability of large amounts of computer processing capacity as well as new tools to manage that capacity and make it available for convenient use. These new tools and technologies have only just begun to be applied to the public health space and include a variety of new approaches to access and manipulate data. These include more accessible machine learning and artificial intelligence, predictive modeling, new "Big Data" tools to deal with extremely large data sets, unstructured data processing and language analysis, voice interfaces, pattern analysis, **open question and answer**, and more. The new tools available combine with new neuroscience insights into the ways the human brain processes information to help us structure information for optimum human understanding and cognition, enabling the next generation of public health breakthroughs. **Information processing** is the science concerned with gathering, manipulating, storing, retrieving, and classifying recorded information.[7] **Open question and answer system** describes technology systems that allows the human to interact with information and derive knowledge and understanding in a normal way. The human asks questions and technology systems should enable that to be as easy as possible to advance the human understanding.[2]

	Babesiosis					*Chlamydia trachomatis* infection					Coccidioidomycosis				
	Current	Previous 52 weeks		Cum	Cum	Current	Previous 52 weeks		Cum	Cum	Current	Previous 52 weeks		Cum	Cum
Reporting area	week	Med	Max	2014	2013	week	Med	Max	2014	2013	week	Med	Max	2014	2013
United States	3	15	140	10	13	11,741	27,683	29,773	161,849	223,470	21	197	307	896	1,803
New England	—	4	79	5	8	520	900	1,155	4,907	7,353	—	0	0	—	1
Connecticut	—	1	36	1	3	—	235	379	1,046	1,960	N	0	0	N	N
Maine	—	0	6	1	—	41	69	110	532	462	N	0	0	N	N
Massachusetts	—	2	48	3	4	392	427	680	2,571	3,382	—	0	0	—	—
New Hampshire	—	0	1	—	1	—	57	71	47	533	—	0	0	—	1
Rhode Island	—	0	26	—	—	80	81	118	486	657	—	0	0	—	—
Vermont	—	0	1	—	—	7	33	96	225	359	N	0	0	N	N
Mid. Atlantic	3	7	56	5	4	2,110	3,378	3,732	23,507	26,048	—	0	0	—	—
New Jersey	—	0	24	1	2	145	558	680	3,716	4,313	N	0	0	N	N
New York (Upstate)	2	3	41	2	2	655	734	1,699	4,471	4,672	N	0	0	N	N
New York City	1	0	12	2	—	471	1,080	1,261	7,692	9,088	N	0	0	N	N
Pennsylvania	N	0	0	N	N	839	1,001	1,324	7,628	7,975	N	0	0	N	N
E.N. Central	—	0	11	—	—	1,244	4,834	5,594	21,858	42,821	—	0	3	9	3
Illinois	—	0	0	—	—	19	2,039	2,508	3,386	19,475	N	0	0	N	N
Indiana	—	0	1	—	—	179	560	793	3,388	4,181	N	0	0	N	N
Michigan	—	0	0	—	—	333	838	1,092	5,094	6,934	—	0	3	6	1
Ohio	N	0	0	N	N	436	1,021	1,152	6,650	8,509	—	0	2	3	—
Wisconsin	—	0	11	—	—	277	427	517	3,340	3,722	—	0	0	—	2

FIG. 23-6 Provisional cases of selected notifiable diseases, the USA, weeks ending February 22, 2014, and February 23, 2013 (8th week) (Export data).

The fundamental shift enabled by these new technologies is that we will increasingly be able to outsource more of the information processing tasks that humans have performed to computers (or clusters of computers). While we are still some ways off from the singularity technology popularized by Ray Kurzweil and others, we are already undergoing some fundamental shifts in the way we deal with information on a day-to-day basis.[8] As shown in Fig. 23-7, by preprocessing information for easy consumption and access, Google saves the steps of having to navigate to a weather website, search for one's location, and then navigate to the next day's forecast. More importantly, Google is performing a complex analysis of the words we used and has understood that we likely want to know the weather forecast, not retrieve articles with the words we have typed in the search bar. New services such as Google Now go a step further in using predictive models to proactively bring forward information that the algorithm predicts would be relevant to you, based on a variety of factors, including what types of data you access and when, your location, and email traffic (to determine whether you are expecting a package, are about to take a trip, etc.). This type of information preprocessing is becoming more prevalent and will be important to future access to public health information, both for the public and for researchers. So imagine Google using this technology to discover searching behaviors on the web over time to start showing increased interest in a particular disease. This has been done to indicate support discovery of an increasing flu outbreak.

These tools have much more power than just simplifying your web searches. For example, IBM's Watson is capable of beating the best human players at the game of Jeopardy by processing a large corpus of reference documents, books, and scholarly articles and analyzing the cryptic clues provided to give the best response.[9] Applying this power to other open question and answer problems, such as medical diagnoses, or analysis of scholarly research and studies is an area of active investigation. By processing huge amounts of data and better understanding the human language and concepts (both those used in asking about the data and within the data itself), these tools will eventually become powerful partners in research. We are not far off from being able to ask these types of computer systems questions like "Has the NS1 influenza protein ever been found in bats?"

Open question and answer systems (which are as they sound: systems designed to answer unstructured human language questions) are powered by machine learning and large-scale distributed data analysis tools, both of which will be important on their own in the processing of data for public health purposes. In the case of machine learning, there are a number of generalized tools now available to predict or extrapolate values based on historical data using a variety of predictive modeling approaches. These tools have evolved from bespoke implementations, such as Amazon's recommendation engine, to generalized tools that can be applied to a variety of problems and data sets, including spam filtering, traffic analysis, and weather prediction.

It is not hard to imagine a future where sophisticated models track a variety of data to develop local forecast models for the incidence of communicable disease. If we can develop forecast models for the weather, pollen, and pollution, why not also for influenza or other communicable diseases? There are a variety of data available now

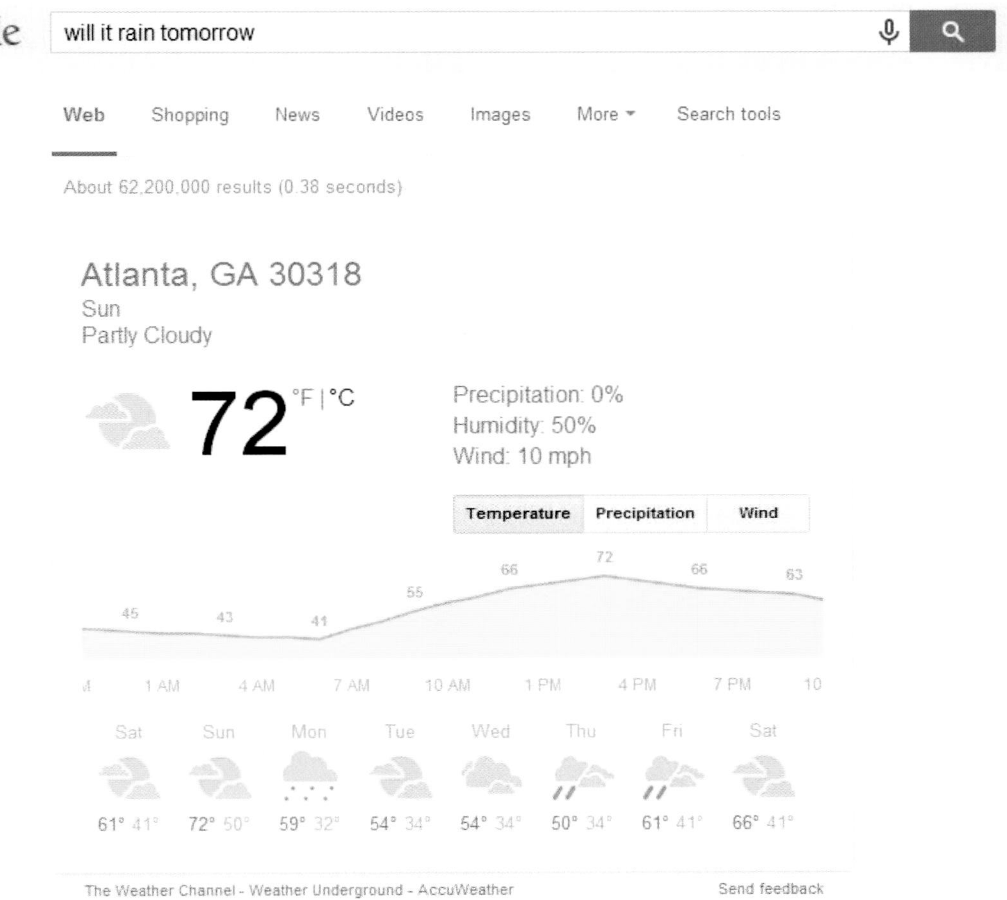

FIG. 23-7 Google search for "will it rain tomorrow."

(e.g., weather, school and work schedules, vaccination rates, laboratory tests, health care provider chief complaints, and search terms) that would be useful in training such models to deliver localized forecasts. With new approaches for large-scale data storage and analysis (including "Big Data" technologies such as Hadoop), the prior constraints on available computational and storage capacity are no longer barriers.

Supplementing these powerful new analysis technologies is the growing trend of data "mashups" where data are combined on a variety of platforms for social discovery and collaboration. The US federal government's Open Data Initiative[10] has been a key contributor to this trend, which has been driven by increased open access to a number of significant data sets. With these tools, it is becoming easier to combine even large data sets for new context and meaning. Supplementing this is a new wave of Silicon Valley startups and other technology firms enabling social discovery and sharing of data science problems, visualizations, approaches, and data sets. Kaggle's data science competitions[11] and Tableau's public data exploration platform[12] are interesting emerging examples.

The future of our public health data manipulation and visualization approaches will continue to follow that of broader industries pioneering these technologies and tools. The economic incentives for investment in public health data analysis will likely not match these other industries in the near future (which is unfortunate, given the significant societal global public good through public health informatics). The obvious downside is that public health tends to utilize older approaches than those common in a number of industries. The benefit, however, is that we can pick and choose the best technologies and approaches for use in public health problems after many of the initial technical hurdles have been overcome and clear patterns are in place for their use and application. The key question is how we can at least reduce that gap and bring the benefits of these tools to public health problems sooner.

Adoption in the Public Health Field

Despite the economic barriers for adoption, there are places where the technologies, tools, and approaches outlined in this future vision are being used today in public health. Google's Flu Trends and **Dengue Trends** tools are great examples where machine learning algorithms were applied to correlate the incidence of a variety of search terms to traditional influenza and dengue surveillance models (which typically take some time to be compiled). The benefit is that these search term-driven models are updated continuously and can be segmented down to detailed city and regional levels with statistical significance, given appropriate search volume. There are limitations to this approach, but by looking to alternate data sets and combining them in interesting ways using predictive modeling, public health has valuable new tools available. **Dengue trends** is a Google application that uses near real-time search query data to create an index of dengue incidence that is a linear proxy for traditional surveillance. Studies have shown that Google Dengue Trend correlates highly with dengue incidence in multiple countries on a large spatial scale.[13]

Another example is MIT researchers John Guttag's and Collin Stultz's study of electrocardiogram (EKG) data.[14] They utilized otherwise discarded EKG data from heart attack patients to look for new signals that might predict the likelihood of a patient having a repeat heart attack. They utilized machine learning to perform pattern matching on a large data set of EKG data and were able to identify three new markers that correlated with a 2–3 times higher risk of dying from a second heart attack within 1 year. These markers were impossible to identify via human observation and inspection of these EKG data. New EKG software is being developed to look for these subtle markers and signal physicians of this risk and the need for additional observation and treatment. As suggested above, this new perspective using older data for new discoveries is a critical new way of thinking about our surveillance systems and what questions they can answer or patterns we can discover.

Emerging Data Sets

As we can see from the examples above and from the discussion in Chapter 21, many new and unconventional data sets are emerging that have significant value to public health. This is in large part due to the dramatic changes occurring across society in the quantity of data collected and available on almost every aspect of our lives. Some estimates show data growth tripling from 2003 to 2008 to 14.7 EB (10^{18} bytes, or 1 billion GB) of new information,[15] and this trend will continue.

These new data sets differ from conventional sources in two significant ways: they are often much larger and they typically have only limited data structure and typing. They also generally represent a move from summary and manually collected data to detailed source data, be it from machine interfaces, sensors, or other sources (Fig. 23-8). In dealing with these new data sets, there are new approaches that become more important to deal with when data are more loosely structured in larger and larger volumes.

In the case of Google's Flu trends, Google has taken a very chaotic and loosely structured data source—search terms—and applied a combination of natural language processing and predictive modeling techniques to derive meaning and a useful signal. For example, distinguishing between searches for "flu research studies" and "urgent care in Atlanta" is important for deriving meaning from this data set. While the first would trigger a simple text search for "flu," the individual performing the search is likely not ill. However, in the second case it is much more likely that the person or someone in his or her household is currently ill. Distinguishing between the two searches is key to deriving value from this data set and can only come about by training predictive modeling algorithms using large sets of source data correlated with the known signal for which we are looking.

With increasingly large data sets becoming prevalent, we need new techniques to efficiently store, query, analyze, and process this information. As data sets grow far larger than the largest available storage systems, different approaches have been required to enable efficient processing. These techniques have been broadly labeled "Big Data," which is primarily defined by the ability to efficiently harness the power of clusters of computers to process data. The MapReduce pattern and similar functional programming techniques have formed the technology foundation of a new generation of data storage and analysis tools that offer nearly linear processing and storage capacity growth with the addition of computing capacity.[16] This fundamental breakthrough is still at its early stages of being applied to technology problems, but it will be the foundation of new data storage systems and will eventually replace most applications of conventional database technology.

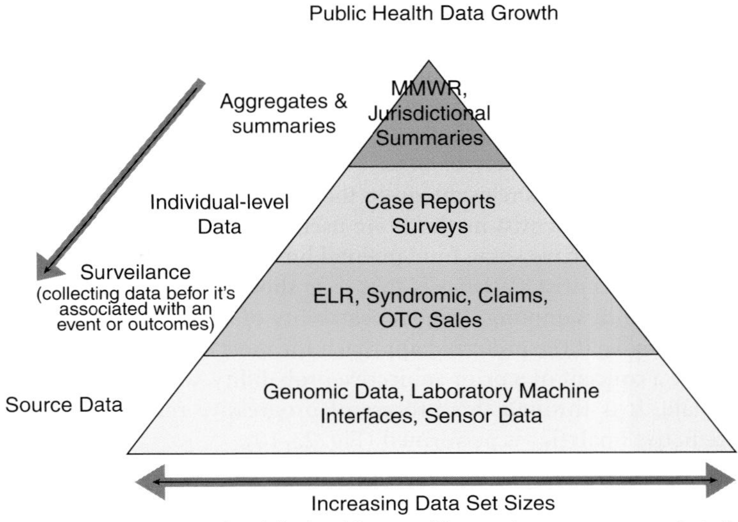

FIG. 23-8 Diagram of public health surveillance data sources and their relative sizes.

These diagrams illustrate the need for new approaches to data storage and processing as well as the fundamental difference between "Big Data" approaches and conventional database technology (Fig. 23-9).

Transition to Bayesian from Frequentist (Classical) Statistical Models

Although this chapter does not focus on statistical methods, it is important to understand their role in how we perceive, visualize, and understand data and the tools and technology that we will use in the future. Our particular

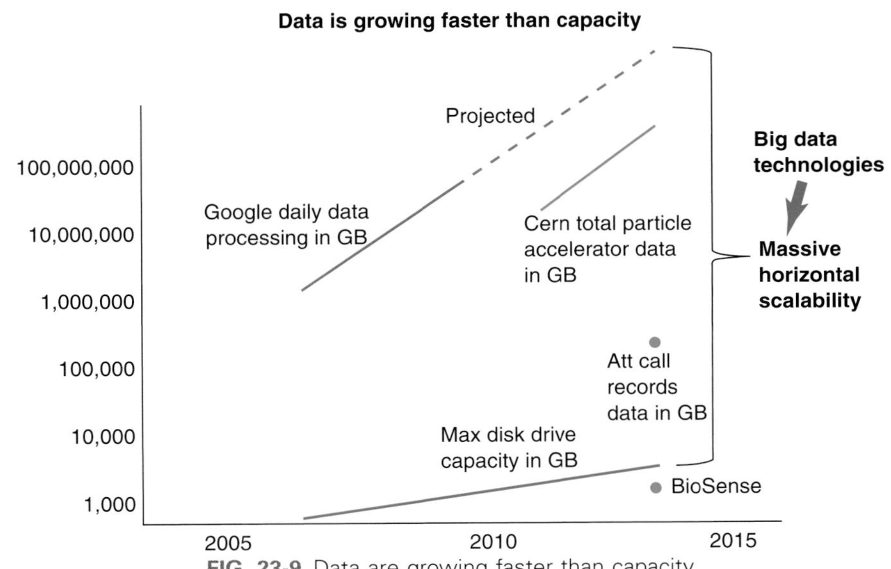

FIG. 23-9 Data are growing faster than capacity.

focus here is on the relationship of the two primary schools of statistical methodology and how Bayesian statistics is a key enabler of many of the machine learning and predictive modeling technologies we have already discussed. This is important since the move to Bayesian methods represents a shift from the dominant approach to public health statistics, based on frequentist (i.e., classical or Fisher school) statistical methods.

This debate has been made popular by Nate Silver and others and featured prominently in changes to political forecasting and a variety of other fields. The debate itself is outside the scope of this book, but the move toward Bayesian statistics is relevant, given the role it plays in most machine learning approaches.

Though frequentist methods are useful for a number of important problems and are comparatively simple to calculate, they have some fundamental limitations in their ability to represent the messy real world. The core idea behind frequentist statistics is that tests should be repeatable and that uncertainty in a model arises solely from limitations in sampling.[17] The repeatability of frequentist statistical analysis and its lack of the use of a subjective "prior" make it the preferred approach for most experimental science to date. In contrast, Bayesian models incorporate a concept of a prior subjective probability, which is progressively refined through the incremental addition of data. It is through this process of progressive refinement that much of the work of machine learning and predictive analytics is performed (Fig. 23-10).

You may be familiar with this process of Bayesian incremental refinement when using email spam filtering tools. Spam filters use the probability that a given email is spam based on a user's prior indication of whether an email from a given address, text, or subject has been marked as spam. As more and more emails are categorized as either spam or not spam, the probabilities are further refined. They do not encode a single view of what spam email is, and they evolve as techniques change to try to evade them. These filters have gotten so good that it is increasingly rare that they make incorrect predictions, necessitating new training.

Machine Learning Approaches and Their Relevance to Public Health

At its most basic, machine learning is the discipline of building computer systems that automatically improve with experience.[18] For our purposes, experience is a direct corollary with data, which is why machine learning and large quantities of data go hand in hand. With more data comes more "experience" and better performance, be it predictive or analytic.

Machine learning can be decomposed into two primary subfields: supervised learning and unsupervised learning.[19] (Note: there are others, but their applications are more esoteric.) Supervised learning is what we are familiar with in spam filtering and other similar tools that utilize a set of training data to make a prediction based on some piece of new data. At a high level, this prediction can include classification (e.g., is this spam or not) or regression (e.g., give me a numeric

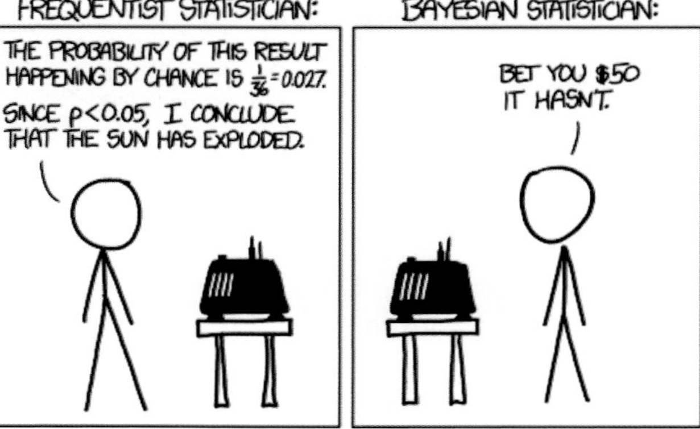

FIG. 23-10 xkcd comic comparing frequentist versus Bayesian schools. Source: xkcd.com.

value). Unsupervised learning is the general approach of running an algorithm against a data set to determine patterns or structure. Commonly unsupervised learning includes some type of clustering analysis (such as *k*-means), where data are grouped or clustered into a number of buckets based on patterns present in the data. In practice, supervised learning algorithms tend to have more practical applications than unsupervised. In public health, we could envision training a supervised Bayesian model with the frequencies of positive laboratory reports for a variety of conditions against any number of possible predictors, such as the temperature and vector populations.

There are now a variety of tools available to apply these algorithms, including the R statistical software package, data mining add-ins for Excel, and even the Google Prediction API, which can be accessed via Google Drive. More advanced-use cases may require programming tools such as Apache Mahout, though additional algorithms are being added to standard business intelligence suites as well. By starting to experiment with these approaches and incorporate machine learning tools into our systems, we will be able to find new and creative ways to apply this type of analysis toward key problems in public health.

Future Human–Computer Interfaces

Although some of the most impactful changes to the way we work with data will happen "under the covers" with the various machine learning and predictive modeling approaches discussed above, there are also important changes to the way we will physically visualize this information and present it to optimize our understanding and the data's value (Fig. 23-11). As we deal with more and more data, and analytics becomes more important to public health decision-making, we will need to develop better ways to sort through these various sources of information to bring forward the right information at the right time. We have already talked about Google Now as an example of a new breed of systems that looks at patterns in data use (including time of day, location, email contents, and calendar appointments) and tries to optimize our access to these sources at the right time. Applied to public health, this may include understanding whether a user is doing research or doing a field outbreak investigation and bringing forward information based on this context.

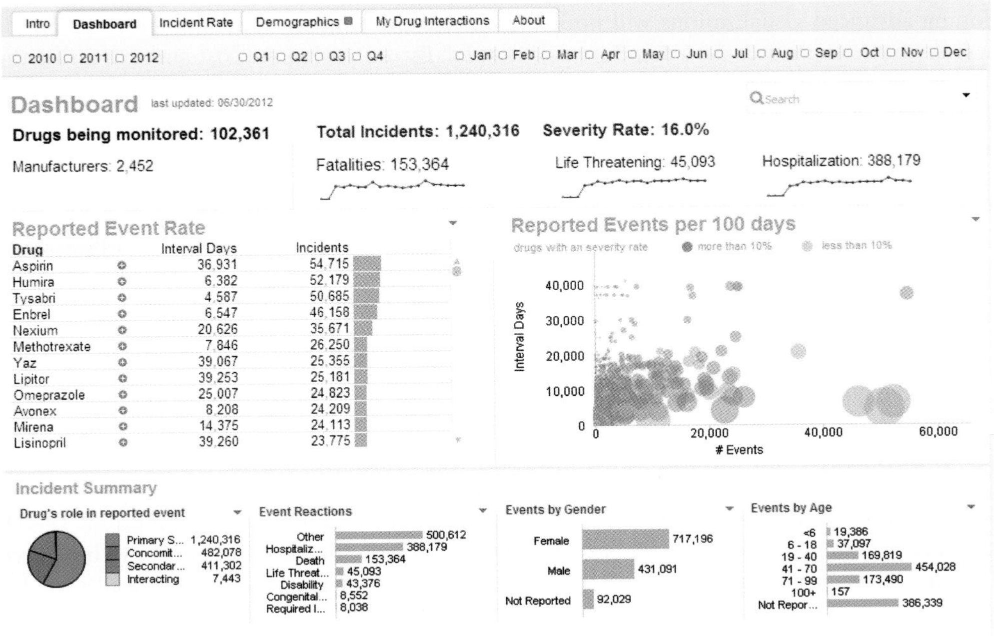

FIG. 23-11 An example of a modern self-service business intelligence tool. Surce: Qlik.

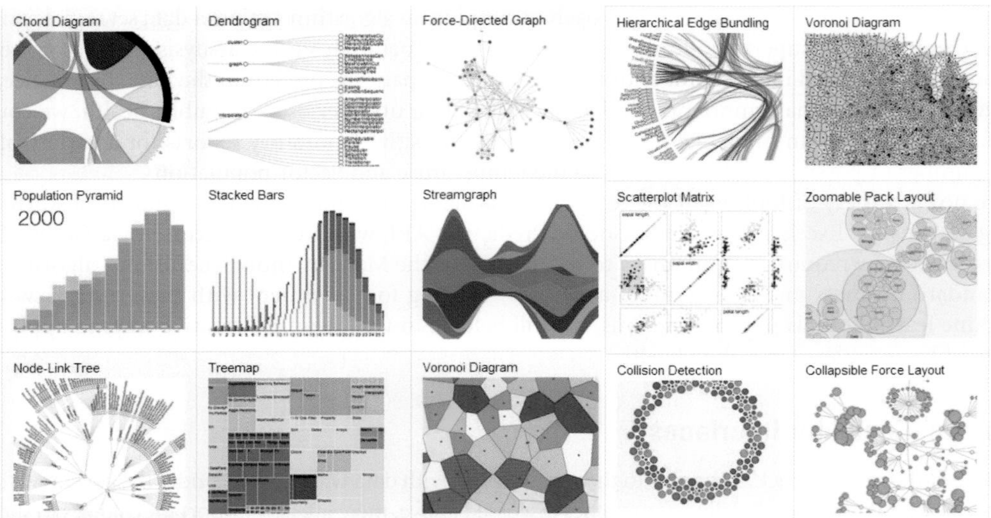

FIG. 23-12 Example visualizations from the D3 JavaScript visualization library. Source: d3js.org.

This vision presumes the continued evolution toward ubiquitous computing where our smartphones or Google Glass-type devices deliver information to us all of the time. Recently, there have been many opportunities in public health to customize systems, workflows, and processes to mobile-oriented and ubiquitous computing. Given the field-oriented nature of so much public health work, it is surprising that more has not been done in this area.

Supplementing these approaches will be continued incremental advances in charting, graphing, and display technologies and their ease of use, bringing down the costs of and barriers to visualizing data in new and relevant ways. Developing advanced visualizations will no longer require investment in coding and software development but rather will be increasingly user driven and user developed. By decreasing the cost and increasing the speed and depth of our analysis, we will be able to make better public health decisions with the data we collect.

New libraries and tools will make advanced charting and visualization increasingly accessible to end users (Fig. 23-12). It is no wonder that we think in terms of the built-in charts in common data analysis tools such as Excel—the additional effort to utilize any other visualization tools is typically too high for the net benefit. Increasingly, as common visualization libraries mature and are incorporated into core data analysis tools, we will have more opportunities to use visualizations like those below with a few clicks of a mouse, rather than requiring the development of custom software code.

GOALS TO ACHIEVE

It is easy to lay out a vision, but the real work is in how we get there. This section will lay out a roadmap, describing some of the specific objectives we can aim for in public health and the enablers needed to meet those objectives.

Short Term (1–5 years)

Public health is faced with an avalanche of new types of data ripe for analysis and consumption. The HITECH Act and accompanying Meaningful Use measures have paved the way for public health agencies to have access to much more data than they have in the past (see Chapter 2). The short-term challenge for public health will be to manage the incoming tidal wave of integrations and data and to store and make sense of all of this information.

Databases that used to comfortably fit on a single server will require rethinking to be adapted to run-on clusters. This will necessitate new data architectures, be they extensions of the relational database management system

(RDBMS) pattern or new implementations using fully distributed NoSQL (Not Only SQL) architectures. This change in data architecture will be needed not only for the quantity of data stored but also to support efficient querying and analysis of this data. For example, many provider syndromic surveillance feeds typically send multiple HL7 Admission Discharge Transfer (ADT) messages for a given patient encounter. Normalizing these requires querying existing data to determine matching patient records (potentially using advanced patient-matching predictive models) as the new records are inserted or updated; this can happen for millions of transactions a day on data stores of many tens of millions of records.

Meaningful Use is only one prominent example of the dramatic increases in data volumes we will see in coming years. Once we have systems in place to efficiently store and query these data sets, the next major objective is to do something useful with this information. Increasingly, these data sets are more "raw," meaning that additional post-processing will be necessary to derive insights to inform action. It will become increasingly difficult to simply export all records to Excel for quick and dirty analysis, and the potential exists to even increase the difficulty of analysis and visualization for some time until new tool sets are available. This is where self-service data analytics and data mining platforms start to become necessary to do meaningful research and studies using these large, sparse, and somewhat dirtier data sets.

Toward the end of this period, we will have more effective tools to deal with these larger data flows and be able to analyze them and manipulate them in even more powerful ways than is possible today. Combining these data sets via data sharing platforms and other data "mashups" will drive even more value from these siloed data sources. Eventually we should aim toward breaking down the barriers between data sources for more complete and timely visualizations of the broader risks to public health to inform our interventions to avoid them.

Long Term (5+ years)

Furthermore, we should look to develop integrated visualizations *and predictions* of public health risks in much the same way we forecast the weather currently. While this may seem like an audacious goal, it is likely achievable with today's technology. Meteorology is a great example of how immense quantities of data and new distributed analysis techniques and predictive models have come together to dramatically improve our ability to understand the environment around us. These models evolved quickly as new sources of data from satellites were made available and now incorporate a variety of data sources from thousands of ground monitoring stations, local radars, ocean temperature sensors, and others.

With larger quantities of more timely data, public health will be able to adopt, train, and customize models to better understand the patterns and risk factors for impacts to our health. This will not only take the form of predicting tomorrow's risk of influenza for a given location but will also enable deeper insights into forecasting and measuring the public health impacts of any number of policy decisions. We can then answer questions such as "what should the allocation be for free influenza vaccine distribution between two locations?" or "what is the impact of spending more on a marketing campaign to encourage vaccination versus providing free or low cost vaccines?" In industry, similar probing questions are asked and answered—why don't we do the same in public health?

By focusing more of public health funding on IT and by directing more of our IT dollars on processing, visualizing, and modeling data (versus just trying to get it in the door), we will be able to make dramatic leaps in the effectiveness of our public health interventions. Increasingly, we will be able to utilize the processing power of large computer clusters effectively to do more of the hard work of data analysis, not just the simple storage, transmission, and calculation done today.

Key Barriers to Overcome

While this vision may be compelling, with other industries having done much of the heavy lifting against the truly difficult computer and data science problems in this area, there are several material barriers to achieving these objectives in public health. The most significant is the chronic underinvestment in information systems in public health.

Other industries where data and information systems have been more completely integrated allocate significantly more of their budgets to IT. For example, the finance industry allocates approximately 6% of gross revenues to IT.[20] Few complete statistics exist for public health, but for the broader health care industry, that figure is closer to 3–4%.[20] Looking at CDC's budgets, this figure is even worse. This underallocation of funding to IT is all the more surprising given public health's roots in data and creative data visualization.

Other significant challenges include the difficulties in simply receiving, exchanging, and transmitting data between agencies and organizations for public health use. Longstanding ambiguities in core information standards underpinning much of health care and public health integration are to blame for these high costs and slow progress. Clarifying these standards to enable true pluggable interoperability will be key to allowing public health to gather relevant data in sufficient quantities to begin to apply some of the techniques described in this chapter.

Finally, our core academic training is still somewhat stuck in the methods of classical statistics. By beginning to adopt Bayesian methods and already available predictive modeling tools in our academic settings, we can ensure there is a workforce able to implement this vision. These tools are disruptive in their nature and represent a sea change of new capability, but we need to be ready to change all of our roles in the practice of public health to achieve their promise.

KEY SUMMARY POINTS

- Data visualization is not just about technology. Creativity and inquisitiveness is needed to see new perspectives in raw information that we often already have at hand.
- Creative data analysis has defined the field of public health since its inception.
- The innovation, sophistication, and importance of our data analysis tools and focus have not always reflected this.
- Public health will follow the broader trend across industries of having to deal with dramatic increases in the quantity of data in the near future. In the public health field, this is driven by changes in lab science toward genomic-based versus assay-based analysis, as well as broader increases in the quantity of available digital information from clinical health care and other sources.
- Data will increasingly transition from summary level and human entered to automated feeds and sensor data.
- The technology to deal with these increasing data volumes ("Big Data") is defined by its ability to efficiently harness the power of clusters of computers against a given data storage, analysis, or manipulation task.
- Emerging predictive modeling and machine learning techniques will allow computers to take more of the burden in pattern recognition, forecasting, and analysis that humans have performed to date.
- The transition from classical to Bayesian statistical methods is foundational to many machine learning and predictive modeling approaches. Bayesian methods are well suited to progressive refinement using new data.
- Interorganizational data exchange and insufficient budgets are the primary barriers to realizing more value from public health data using data manipulation and visualization technologies already in use in other industries.

DISCUSSION QUESTIONS

1. List some interesting data visualizations you have seen outside of public health. How might they be applicable to a public health problem?
2. List some of the key limitations of relational database management system (RDBMS) technology in analyzing and manipulating data.
3. What might we want to show in a weather map (or forecast) for public health threats? What data would we use? What techniques would you use to manipulate the data set for display? How would you translate this into a forecast?
4. How can we encourage creativity and innovation when working with data?
5. What are nontraditional data sources that impact public health? What kinds of problems could you address with these data? How would you go about collecting, formatting, and analyzing them to test your hypotheses?
6. What research studies could be revisited using Bayesian statistical approaches and incremental data to better approximate and forecast real-world behavior?
7. Many researchers turn to web search tools like Google as a key tool to access and discover information. How would you improve Google to better serve your research objectives?

REFERENCES

1. Markel H. Happy birthday, Dr. Snow. JAMA 2013;309(10):995–6.
2. Definition provided by the chapter author.
3. Few S. Data visualization for human perception. In: Soegaard MaD, Rikke Friis, editor. The encyclopedia of human-computer interaction. 2nd ed. Aarhus, Denmark: The Interaction Design Foundation; 2014.
4. Analytics. Oxford Dictionaries. Oxford University Press. <http://www.oxforddictionaries.com/us/definition/american_english/analytics>; October 02, 2015.
5. Glossary of public health informatics organizations, activities, and terms. National Association of County and City Health Officials, <http://www.naccho.org/topics/infrastructure/informatics/glossary.cfm/>. [cited 2015].
6. GIS Dictionary. Spatial Analysis, <http://www.esri.com/>. <http://support.esri.com/en/knowledgebase/GISDictionary/term/spatial analysis/>. [cited 2015].
7. The Free Dictionary. Farlex. Information Processing, <http://www.thefreedictionary.com/>.
8. Eden AH, Moor JH, Soraker JH, Steinhart E, editors. Singularity hypotheses: a scientific and philosophical assessment. Springer; 2012. p. 300.
9. Brown E, Epstein EJ, Murdock W, Fin T-H. Tools and methods for building Watson. IBM; 2013. [Contract No.: RC25356 (WAT1302-021)].
10. Open Government, <http://www.data.gov/open-gov/%5D/>. [cited 2014].
11. Kaggle. About, <http://www.kaggle.com/about/>. [cited 2014].
12. Tableau Public, <http://www.tableausoftware.com/public/>. [cited 2014].
13. Gluskin RT, Johansson MA, Santillana M, Brownstein JS. Evaluation of Internet-based dengue query data: Google Dengue Trends. PLoS Negl Trop Dis 2014;8(2):e2713.
14. Syed Z, Stultz CM, Scirica BM, Guttag JV. Computationally generated cardiac biomarkers for risk stratification after acute coronary syndrome. Sci Transl Med 2011;3(102):102ra95.
15. Bounie D, Gille L. International production and dissemination of information: results, methodological issues, and statistical perspectives. Int J Comm 2012;6:21.
16. Dean J, Ghemawat S. MapReduce: Simplified data processing on large clusters. Google, Inc.; 2004.
17. Fisher RA. Statistical methods for research workers. Edinburgh: Oliver and Boyd; 1925.
18. Mitchell T. The discipline of machine learning. Carnegie Mellon University; 2006. [Contract No.: CMU-ML-06-108].
19. Grudic G. Machine learning [PowerPoint slides]. <http://www.cs.colorado.edu/~grudic/teaching/CSCI4202/>; 2002. [cited 2014].
20. Guevara J, Stegman E, Hall L. 2014 IT Enterprise Summary Report. Gartner Consulting; 2014.

REFERENCES

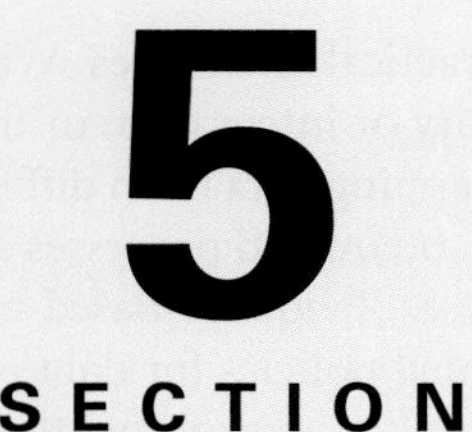

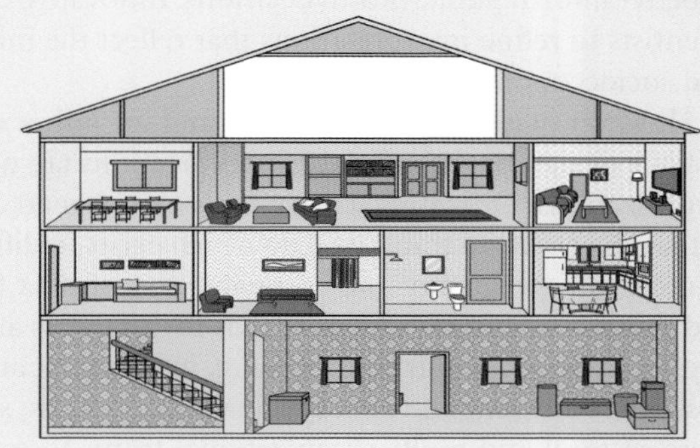

New Data, Analytics, and Intelligence (Knowledge) Enlightens Transformation

Meeyoung Park

Section Outline

Public health surveillance requires timely and factual data for public health organizations to (a) effectively monitor the health of the populace, (b) prioritize, implement, and evaluate public health programs, and (c) mount appropriate interventions during outbreaks or other public health emergencies. As methods and models of public health surveillance evolve, so too do approaches for validating and processing surveillance data. Interoperable electronic technologies enable real-time, bi-directional data exchange based on standards for data content, structure, and messaging. These data and messaging standards facilitate data quality and computational analyses for merged data sets. Some systems may employ data mining and public health modeling algorithms to systematically collect, manage, and manipulate data so as to identify risk factors and predict the burden of disease. Some epidemiologists have invented the means of analyzing novel streams of data, such as pathogen genetic sequences, social media, or climate patterns, to enrich public health information. With increasing frequency, multidisciplinary teams are needed to apply new analytic tools, such as 3D graphics, multivariate modeling, geovisual animation, and artificial intelligence. Moreover, public health surveillance systems increasingly trend towards integration of environmental and veterinary health data to heighten our understanding of risk exposure and disease burden and to better inform public health decisions. Innovative combinations of technology and multidisciplinary research allow scientists to refine interpretations that reflect the inherent complexity of our interwoven environmental, biological, and socioeconomic systems.

However, with new technologies and an influx of data come analytic and practical challenges. When merging systems or data, standardized IT specifications are needed to enable interoperability or integration of the databases. Organizations integrating data systems may expend considerable effort towards mapping data from different sources, as they may need to translate data which exists in different formats. In addition, standardized processes are necessary to maintain the quality and comparability of data for accurate and robust analyses. Evidence-based best practices and promising cutting edge methods for analytics are established upon foundational policies for data privacy, security, governance, acquisition, sharing, integration, and standardization. Enabling policy environments are necessary to support efficient and effective analytic practices; strong collaboration and communication is therefore needed for cross-sectoral and multi-organizational teams to establish common goals and align policies for public health data analytics.

LEARNING OBJECTIVES

- Discuss the balance of key attributes in a surveillance system.
- Identify potential sources of error in surveillance data systems.
- Describe best practices for validation and verification of surveillance system data.
- Explain how transmission models can be used to inform disease prevention and control programs.
- Describe and compare different classes of transmission models.
- Describe an optimal process for policy makers, surveillance personnel, and academic modelers to collaboratively inform policy decisions.
- Describe how pathogen sequence data can enhance traditional epidemiologic analysis.
- Explain the three levels of systems analysis that use genetic data.
- Identify a health-related scenario (other than HIV) in which genetic surveillance could be applied and describe specific analyses, possible genomic patterns that define populations by geography and risk behavior, and subsequent inferences.
- Discuss the benefits of using genetic surveillance to guide disease prevention and control programs and policies.
- Discuss how descriptive, predictive, and prescriptive analytics provide actionable information to public health professionals.
- Identify and discuss the importance of each of the building blocks of public health analytics.
- Describe potential economic and logistical barriers to effectively analyzing and using electronic surveillance data.
- List the primary considerations of predictions in a predictive surveillance system.
- Identify a health-related scenario and discuss what types of data and analyses would be useful to develop a predictive surveillance system for that scenario.

CHAPTER

24

Necessary Challenge of Verifying and Validating Public Health Data

Richard S Hopkins

If it's worth doing, it's worth doing right.

Anonymous

KEY WORDS

Data
Data representativeness
Positive predictive value
Data quality
Flexibility
Utility
Data integrity
HL7
National Institute of Standards and Technology (NIST)
Acceptability
Data stability
Data sensitivity
Data timeliness
Simplicity
Cost

BACKGROUND AND CURRENT ENVIRONMENT

Any surveillance system depends critically on the quality and integrity of the data on which it is based. Important public health decisions are, or should be, based on surveillance data, and poor data may lead to inappropriate decisions. Practical reportable disease surveillance systems have always had some degree of quality control and error-checking, as has seemed appropriate to their managers. Such quality control consumes resources, and may slow down the availability of data to its users; the appropriate degree of investment in assuring quality and integrity is an important decision for surveillance information system managers.

At the Montana Department of Health in the late 1970s, case reports arrived primarily as paper cards in the mail. Each case report was reviewed by an epidemiologist to assure that the reported diagnosis was plausible and that sufficient information was included on the case report; occasionally additional information was sought from the submitting local health department or physician. Each accepted case report was entered into a logbook with a separate line list for each disease, with name, county, age, sex, and date of onset, while the original case reports were physically filed for possible later reference. Missing data were easily identified by scanning the line list visually. Any deduplication was done by simple inspection of the line list and by stapling duplicate case report cards together. The weekly and annual summaries of reported cases of disease were tallied by hand from the logbook. For a state of fewer than a million people, before computers became ubiquitous in the USA, this was a perfectly reasonable system.

The current situation is that most jurisdictions in the USA, and many elsewhere in the world, have computerized systems for storing, managing, and analyzing case reports, and often for supporting case and contact follow-up as well. These systems are used for acute reportable diseases (infectious and toxic) as well as for cancer and, in many states, for birth defects. A large fraction of case in the USA now arrive at state health departments as electronic laboratory reports, and an increasing proportion will in future be arriving as electronic case reports from physicians or from electronic health records. Both the volume of reports and the amount of information received with each report have increased greatly, for most reportable diseases and most jurisdictions. In the near future, we will likely see development of new automated systems for case detection, with an as yet unclear role for human review of candidate cases. The current and future situations present great opportunities for more timely and in-depth analysis of surveillance data, followed by appropriate action, and also present challenges for assuring data quality. The focus of this chapter is on such data validation and verification.

SURVEILLANCE SYSTEM PARAMETERS

The United States Centers for Disease Control and Prevention (CDC) identified the following important attributes of public health surveillance systems that should be addressed in evaluations of such systems[1]:

- **Simplicity** is the amount and variety of data, users, organizations receiving case reports, and integrated systems; level of effort to collect, manage, analyze, and disseminate the data; staff training requirements; as well as time needed for system maintenance that contribute to the ease of operation of a public health surveillance system.
- **Flexibility** is the ability of public health surveillance system to adapt to changes in operation or information requirements quickly, with minimal investment of additional resources.
- **Data quality** refers to the "completeness and validity of the data recorded."
- **Acceptability** is the "willingness of persons and organizations to participate in the surveillance system" that may be ascertained by measuring the participation rate of subjects and agencies, completeness of interview and forms, reporting rates, and timeliness of reports.
- **Sensitivity** is the proportion of cases or events that are targets of surveillance that are detected.
- **Positive predictive value** is the proportion of cases or events detected that are actually the target of the detection system.
- **Representativeness** of a system is high if it accurately describes the occurrence of a health-related event over time and its distribution in the population by place and person.
- **Timeliness** is the measure of speed between timed intervals between various steps in the surveillance process, such as the interval between the onset of a health-related event and the initial report to the public health agency responsible for follow-up.
- **Stability** of a surveillance system is its ability to operate and provide data without system failure. Measure of stability includes the amount of time and resources needed for system maintenance and operation, including any system outages and lags.
- **Cost** of a surveillance system may refer to direct costs of operation, including the staff, equipment, training, software, etc. involved in operating the surveillance system, and indirect costs related to case-related follow-up, such as treatment or outbreak investigations.
- **Utility** of a surveillance system is based on its ability to detect and characterize health-related events and subsequently inform the development of prevention and control programs, policies, and research.

All of these attributes relate to some degree to data quality, but in this chapter we will pay special attention to representativeness, stability, sensitivity and positive predictive value, as well as data quality in the sense that the CDC guidelines define it.

Surveillance data will never be perfect, and always will need to be interpreted with local, regional, and national contexts in mind. In any surveillance system, there is an inevitable trade-off between data timeliness and data quality: if one is willing to wait longer, one can almost always get higher quality data. This is because there is more time for data quality checks and editing, because diagnostic tests and procedures take time to be processed and be posted to health records, and because the nature of an illness often becomes more clear after the patient has been sick longer. Modern electronic health records and new laboratory and other diagnostic techniques may reduce the absolute amount of time it takes for reliable information to be available for inclusion in a surveillance system record, but the general relationship still holds: a surveillance system that puts a premium on timeliness will tend to pay a price in terms of sensitivity, positive predictive value, or record-level completeness and accuracy.

There is a well-known tension between sensitivity and positive predictive value for screening tests that also applies to surveillance systems. For any given detection system, increasing one of these parameters will tend to decrease the other. For example, if a surveillance case definition is modified to require more definitive diagnostic information before a case is counted, in order to avoid unnecessary responses to noncases, some of those excluded from the new case definition are likely to be true cases, and sensitivity will go down. Conversely, if the surveillance case definition is modified to allow inclusion of less definitive cases, in an effort to assure that no true cases are missed, some noncases will be counted as cases and positive predictive value will go down.

Timeliness is related to both sensitivity and positive predictive value. Very rapid collection of case reports or other surveillance data is very likely to lead to collection of case reports, which, on further review, turn out not to be valid cases, and thus reduce positive predictive value in the surveillance system. Allowing more time to pass between health events and case reporting may allow additional or more accurate information to be added to each record, and thus reduce the number of false-positive case reports. Allowing more time to pass may also allow additional cases to be detected (because additional information is available), and thus increase sensitivity. Thus, increased timeliness of a surveillance system tends to be in tension with both sensitivity and positive predictive value, which are already in tension with each other.

A surveillance case definition might depend on data that are often missing in real-world medical records, such as exposure to arthropod vectors, travel history, or occupational exposures. This situation could be ameliorated by changing the case definition (though perhaps with some loss of sensitivity or positive predictive value), by modifying the data system so that the critical data elements are less likely to be missing, or by gathering supplemental information from the patient. For example, if being classified as having a probable case of a disease depends on having had recent exposure to a particular arthropod vector, as well as various clinical findings, and that information is often missing, then probable cases will be missed. On the other hand, dropping the requirement for such exposure may result in larger numbers of lower probability cases being detected or reported. Similar considerations apply for other data quality issues such as duplicate records, merged records, miscoding, unannounced changes in coding systems, and dropped records.

When missing or incorrect information, in combination with surveillance case definitions or other algorithms to classify events as events of interest, leads to failure to recognize cases or events that a surveillance system is designed to detect, the sensitivity of that surveillance system goes down, but more importantly the public health agency misses opportunities to intervene to prevent further disease. When missing or incorrect information, in combination with surveillance case definitions or algorithms, tends to falsely identify people as having cases of a disease of interest, or to falsely identify outbreaks, then the positive predictive value of that surveillance system goes down, and public health agency time and effort are spent on responses that will not have any beneficial effect. A public health agency must balance these two types of errors. The correct balance will differ according to the condition, disease or risk factor under surveillance. For example, in conducting surveillance for meningococcal disease, missing true cases is very undesirable because the disease is so serious and has epidemic potential, so the system should maximize sensitivity and timeliness. A somewhat lower positive predictive value is acceptable. Conversely, in a surveillance system for acute hepatitis B, where the focus is more on outbreak detection and patterns of disease rather than on individual case response, there is a danger of the public health system being overwhelmed by low-probability reports if hepatitis B surface antigen positivity alone is reportable. Such reports rarely indicate acute infection.

SOURCES OF ERROR IN SURVEILLANCE DATA SYSTEMS

Analysts must be familiar with the characteristics and limitations of the data they are working with, including possible sources of error in the data. These errors may be of many types: data may be unrepresentative, slow to arrive, or miscoded, contain systematic errors leading to biased estimates of incidence in the population or in subgroups, contain incorrect diagnoses or be incorrectly assigned to syndromes, be incomplete at the record level, miss cases or events that are intended for inclusion, or contain duplicates. Many key information systems in government and business depend critically on accurate and timely data. There are general approaches to assuring data quality, and numerous software products have been developed to support monitoring of data quality and detection of changes in quality.[2] These more general approaches and products are beyond the scope of this chapter, which is focused on the special case of data quality in public health surveillance systems, and would likely need considerable modification for use in such settings.

Data quality and integrity in public health surveillance data can be looked at from many points of view, some very general and some very specific. Here are some examples of questions an epidemiologic analyst might ask related to data quality:

- Are the data (if they are collected as intended and if they are as timely as planned) suitable for addressing the public health questions that motivate the operation of the surveillance system?
- Are the records sufficiently representative of the events for which surveillance is desired?
- Are there changes over time in how the records are obtained or processed, that would change the representativeness and thus make inferences about events or trends in the data unreliable?
- Is the data flow regular?
- Is the data flow timely?
- Are the data collected in a systematic and reproducible way?
- Are the individual records in the data flow complete—that is, do the records consistently have information in all fields of importance?
- Are the data in the records accurate?
  - In particular, when clinician diagnoses are included, are these diagnoses correct or complete?
- Is there a process for quality control of the records?
- Is there an automated system to detect and flag possible issues with data quality (timeliness, completeness, accuracy)?
- Is there a system in place to detect, flag and/or resolve likely duplicate records (whether of laboratory results, case reports, or people)?

Suppose that, for example, you desire to establish surveillance for illness due to infection with a novel coronavirus in the population for which you have public health responsibilities. You have four main options (not mutually exclusive) for setting up such surveillance. Formal systems can be based on (1) case reporting by physicians (or others), (2) reporting of laboratory results, (3) tabulations of visits to health care facilities for care of an illness that clinically resembles the target illness, or (4) recording of deaths. You also will receive informal, unstructured reports of illness, from many different sources, that need to be triaged and investigated.

First, if the illness is clinically distinctive, or has a distinctive exposure history, clinicians may be able to make a reliable clinical diagnosis based on symptoms, signs, and exposure history, follow a surveillance case definition developed by the public health authority, and make timely case reports that have a high positive predictive value. Second, if there is a specific laboratory test for the infection, then laboratories can be asked or required to report positive laboratory results. Laboratories can also report requests for testing for this agent, as an early and somewhat less specific indicator of likely infection with the agent. Third, if the illness is reasonably clinically distinctive, counts of visits to primary care sites (such as medical clinics or emergency departments) for a syndrome resembling the disease can be collected on a frequent basis (syndromic surveillance). Finally, if your jurisdiction has uniform and timely death registration, it may be possible to detect fatal cases from review of death certificates. In the worst case, surveillance may have to be based on changes in total numbers of deaths—this is how the summer 2003 heat wave mortality event was initially detected in France, as a striking increase in the weekly number of funerals of older people.

UNDERSTANDING YOUR POPULATION, HEALTH CARE SYSTEM, AND HEALTH-RELATED BEHAVIORS

Interpreting surveillance data of any of these types also requires (among other things) an understanding of how health care is organized and used by residents of your jurisdiction. For example, if there are large segments of the population (e.g., the poor or an ethnic minority) who almost never receive care through the formal health care system, or receive it only when very ill, and if members of these populations are at risk for the disease of interest, then a surveillance system based entirely on the formal health care system will give an inaccurate picture of the incidence, distribution, or risk factors for the disease, no matter how well run it is, and analysts will need to take account of the unrepresentativeness of the data. Deaths may in some circumstances (unfortunately) be the best indicator of a possible epidemic affecting medically underserved groups.

In the course of an episode of illness, people may go through several stages before they present to a setting where a definitive or laboratory diagnosis is made: they may seek the advice of friends, family members, traditional healers or elders, seek information from various other sources including the internet, obtain over-the-counter medications from a pharmacy, stay home from work or school, make a physician visit in which no laboratory testing is obtained, or eventually visit an emergency department or be admitted to a hospital. At each stage, various selection factors influence whether the behavior occurs at all, or whether the combination of the clinical syndrome of interest and the environmental exposure (e.g., travel to a region where there is an epidemic) is recognized as a possible case of the new infection, whether the event or case is reported to public health before laboratory testing is done, whether any or appropriate laboratory testing is obtained, whether the laboratory identifies the agent correctly, and whether the laboratory result is reported to public health authorities.

Through numerous field and analytic investigations, experienced public health epidemiologists gain an understanding of the process by which people in their jurisdiction decide to seek health care, and then obtain it, and thus can work with and interpret data that are to some degree unrepresentative. They also are aware of local events that may result in increases or decreases in reported cases or health care visits for specific syndromes, but are not of great public health significance or are already accounted for. To detect anomalies due to data quality changes, they must be alert for possible changes in the health care system or in health care-seeking behavior that may lead to spurious increases or decreases in reported cases of a disease. For example, if many people in the population come to believe that doctors and hospitals can do little for people who are ill with a new infection, they may become much less likely to seek care, and the number of cases in an epidemic may appear to be abating, while the average severity of observed cases appears to increase. For example, in late 2014, when the Ebola surveillance data showed that the number of people being admitted to hospitals for Ebola Virus Disease in Monrovia, the capital of Liberia, and the number dying of the disease had reached a plateau, considerable effort was needed to rule out the possibility that people with the disease were simply not being brought to the hospitals.[3] Conversely, in the first few weeks (April 2009) of the 2009 H1N1 influenza A pandemic in the USA, there were large increases in emergency department visits for influenza-like illness by worried people with mild illnesses that were not due to the novel virus.[4]

PROCESSING SURVEILLANCE DATA AT A PUBLIC HEALTH AGENCY

Once a clinical or laboratory diagnosis of the new disease is made, a case report can be generated. Until fairly recently, in the USA such case reports were very brief (consisting of perhaps a name and address for the ill person, a physician or laboratory name, the name of the disease, and the date of onset) and were submitted to public health agencies as postcards, paper forms, or (more recently) faxes of forms or lists. Newer technologies have allowed increases in the amount of data per record that public health agencies can absorb. If the case report record is generated from an electronic health record, emergency department information system, laboratory information management system, or electronic death registration system, the number of fields it can contain is limited only by the information in the electronic record that is the source of the case report. In addition, information that is only incidental to patient care but of great public health importance may get automatically transferred to the public health case report. Such information could be in error without affecting patient care significantly but prompt erroneous public health conclusions. While electronic systems often have built-in error and range checks that reduce the average number of errors per record, when more different pieces of information are collected for each record the risk that there will be error in some field of each record goes up.

A public health agency that receives paper or electronic reports (of physician diagnoses, laboratory results, visits for particular syndromes, or deaths) must have a plan for how to assimilate these records and how to monitor changes that could affect their representativeness or other aspects of their quality. If such monitoring is not done, erroneous public health inferences may be drawn and public health action may be too little, too much, or wrongly directed. Although most current surveillance information systems carry out this function to some degree, the advent of new types of information and of automated transmission of this information makes it critical to do explicit planning for this function as systems are improved or replaced.

In the late 1990s, the Florida Department of Health initiated annual surveillance of tobacco attitudes and use among middle- and high-school students. Surveys were carried out in classrooms using familiar bubble-sheet technology. One year, in a critical item used to stratify the data, there were 13 possible response options, but the data structure into which the data were to be imported allocated only a one-character field. The result was that response options 10, 11, 12, and 13 were all interpreted as "1". The net effect was to underestimate the true prevalence of tobacco use in the population. The error was identified only after a preliminary report, prepared under great time pressure, had been disseminated. A corrected report was issued. This incident was an object lesson in the importance of careful scrutiny of the methods for moving raw surveillance data (in this case, the bubble sheets) into an analytic environment.

Errors may creep into the data in several different ways as follows:

- Transcription errors at the sending facility, from their records to the case report form (whether carried out manually or automatically).
- Transcription errors at the receiving agency, as information is transferred from a paper or faxed case report into the surveillance information system, or from an electronic message into a database.
- Transcription errors introduced by software that automatically reads handwriting or bubble sheets, or transcribes recorded audio information.
- Mixing of data from more than one patient into a single record, either at the sending facility or the receiving public health agency.
- Unrecognized duplicate records on the same case, either from the same facility or from different ones.
- Multiple laboratory results from the same specimen from the same testing event, or from different tests on the same specimen, or results from different specimens on the same person not accounted for by the algorithm that parses electronic laboratory results.
- Missed and lost records, either in paper or electronic systems.
- Misunderstanding on the sending end of what is wanted in various fields, leading to data that are in the wrong field or incorrectly coded or formatted.
- Local coding systems in various facilities, unknown to the receiving agency. (For example, in the first year of operation of CDC's BioSense syndromic surveillance application, records from some Veteran's Administration facilities for people with congestive heart failure were being coded locally as "CHF," and being handled by the receiving application as though they were for cases of Congo–Crimean Hemorrhagic Fever, a potential bioterrorism agent.)
- Changes in coding systems at sending facilities without notifying the receiving public health agency. For example, a laboratory may change the local codes it uses for certain laboratory tests or results.
- Operational changes at a facility that result in no data being sent even when there are records that meet sending criteria.

To verify and validate data received by a surveillance system, managers of surveillance systems should have systems in place to verify data from each entity that is contributing data to the system when it first starts contributing and on a periodic basis, and to monitor data quality in real time once data flow is established.

Processes for both initial and periodic assessment of data streams should address the following:

- Are the records correctly formatted?
- Where coding or a structured vocabulary are required at the sending facility, are all codes that are received valid codes?
- Is information stored in the correct fields (e.g., physician address and patient address in their correct locations in the record, and never substituted for each other)?

- Are records being submitted as timely as protocol requires, on a regular schedule?
- Are any records that meet inclusion requirements not being submitted? (This requires review of records at the facility that did NOT generate case reports or records.)
- Are any duplicate records for the same case being submitted?
- In what ways are records received from this facility representative or unrepresentative of cases of the disease or syndrome under surveillance? (This requires review of information about the community as a whole, from sources other than the source under review.)
- Do the distribution of age, gender, race, residence location, and other variables make sense from what is known about the epidemiology of the disease in this community and the patient population served by this facility?

In the USA, CDC and the National Institute of Standards and Technology (NIST) have established web-accessible tools for testing both syndromic surveillance and electronic laboratory report messages against Health Level 7 (HL7) version 2.5.1, to assist both sending hospitals and receiving health departments in determining whether messages containing reports are consistent with standards established as a requirement for meaningful use of electronic health records.[5,6] **NIST** is a US federal agency involved in the development and application of technologies, measurements, and standards.[7] **HL7** is an organization that develops electronic health data exchange and integration standards and frameworks to facilitate interoperability between surveillance systems.[8] Syndromic surveillance or laboratory report records that are compliant with this tool are almost always correctly formatted and coded, but other issues (as enumerated above) may remain to be resolved before a sending facility can be deemed to be ready for production for this type of report.

The European CDC has developed a set of recommendations for the type and frequency of data quality reviews in surveillance systems, including triggers for when these reviews should be carried out.[9]

Ongoing real-time review of records from each facility should address the following:

- Are there gaps in submission of records? For example, has a facility had no records submitted for one or several reporting cycles? (Under some conditions, it may be desirable to require sending facilities to send a "nothing-to-report" message if they have no eligible reports in a particular reporting cycle.)
- Is there a sudden reduction in the number of case reports received?
- Is there a sudden increase in the number of case reports received, either in one cycle or in a sustained manner? Such an increase always needs to be evaluated as to whether it is due to a real change in the incidence of disease, which would require public health action, or whether it is due to an artifactual change in how data are being managed.
- Is there a sudden change in the proportion of records with particular values in any field that would suggest a change in data coding or management practices at the sending end?

In the early 1990s, a review of mother's cigarette smoking information on Florida birth certificates revealed that (1) the prevalence of cigarette smoking during pregnancy reported on the birth certificate was consistently lower in the Miami area than in the rest of the state and (2) in some Miami-area hospitals, the reported prevalence was zero for years at a time. Review of multiple data sources suggested that the low prevalence of cigarette smoking during pregnancy in the Miami area was real, as similar patterns were seen for the general youth and adult population in other data sources: the **Youth Risk Behavior Surveillance System (YRBSS)**—a surveillance system that monitors six types of risk behavior in adolescents linked to the leading causes of mortality and morbidity in youth and adults; the **Behavioral Risk Factor Surveillance System (BRFSS)**—a telephone survey conducted to collect state-specific data on health-related risk behaviors, chronic conditions, and use of preventive health care services; and the **Pregnancy Risk Assessment Monitoring System (PRAMS)**—a surveillance system to monitor maternal attitudes and experiences from before to shortly after pregnancy.[10-12] But there were a few hospitals at which the cigarette smoking item on the birth certificate worksheet was always left blank. After keypunching, these records were interpreted in the birth certificate dataset as a "no" response. Corrective action was taken with these hospitals.

SYSTEMS FOR DATA QUALITY CHECKING—CURRENT BEST PRACTICES

The Florida Department of Health's web-based Merlin system for managing reportable disease case reports has multiple types and levels of data quality checks built into it (personal communication, Leah Eisenstein, Florida

Department of Health, November 2013). For as many fields as possible, there are logical checks. For example, an onset date cannot be later than the laboratory result report date. Zip codes are compared to street addresses and discordances must be resolved. For some diseases, each reported case is automatically classified as to whether it is confirmed, probable or suspect, or not a case, using the Council of State and Territorial Epidemiologists (CSTE)/CDC surveillance case definition, applied algorithmically to the laboratory, clinical, and epidemiological data supplied by county health department workers.[13,14] For most diseases (though not some of the most common ones), information about every reported case is also reviewed by a central office expert on that disease before it is finally counted as a case.

Automated alerts are built into Merlin, which alert the appropriate central office disease-specific expert whenever certain high-priority laboratory results are received and whenever county health department staff start to enter a case of certain high-priority diseases. Among other things, these notifications help to promptly identify false-positive alerts that are due to misunderstandings of laboratory results by county health department staff or to simple keying or coding errors (e.g., incorrect choice of polio rather than pertussis from a drop-down menu). Merlin tools, which capture information about record-level completeness (e.g., percent of records missing age, race, or zip code), are available to local and central office workers; these indices are built into an overall annual score of county health department performance in the domain of reportable disease epidemiology.

In Seattle-King County, hospital-level heat map displays have been developed for yearly, monthly, or daily review of data completeness and quality in their syndromic surveillance system. These show how each individual ED performs on each of 13 data quality measures. Color change on the heat maps indicates that data quality has shifted over time. The system puts white space on the heat map for periods of time where data were not recorded by the system.[15] Similar displays were developed for the national Distribute influenza surveillance data-sharing project by Distribute collaborators at the University of Washington, especially to assess timeliness, completeness and accuracy in the data submitted by participating jurisdictions in real time.[16,17]

In Florida's ESSENCE syndromic surveillance system, users are given access to numerous pages that show variable-level percent completeness measurements by hospital or county, the percent of time a required value is actually present, the number of input files received from each hospital, and the time each data source was processed. An algorithm and display alert users when these data quality factors have changed significantly.[18]

Surveillance data analysts expect a certain amount of random, nondirectional error in the records they review, and they incorporate this expectation into their analytic approaches. They do need to have a sense for how large this random error is. For example, they need to have a sense on an ongoing basis for how frequently reported cases are reported in the week of or the week before or after their "correct" week. What is critical to recognize is directional error, or bias, leading to incorrect inferences about incidence, the occurrence of outbreaks, or the populations at greatest and least risk of particular conditions, risk factors, diseases, or syndromes.

Some surveillance systems are designed to detect outbreaks directly, by methods other than detection and confirmation of individual cases. Syndromic surveillance systems are a large class of such systems. For these systems, sensitivity and positive predictive value are thought of in terms of outbreaks: what percent of outbreaks that are the target of the system are detected, and what percent of potential outbreaks detected by the system turn out to, in fact, be outbreaks of interest? In this context, verification and validation should be thought of in terms of records representing outbreaks, rather than records representing individual cases. Users may seek to tune outbreak detection algorithms to improve sensitivity, timeliness, or positive predictive value for outbreak detection without too much compromise of the other attributes.[19]

Data items to be captured about outbreaks, which are also subject to error, include the number of cases and their dates of onset, numbers of laboratory confirmations, identification of agent, date of onset of first case, incubation period, mode of transmission, source or vehicle of the outbreak, age group affected, setting, and so on. For example, in a system designed to record information about food-borne outbreaks, information must be reliably recorded about the identity of the contaminated food item, and about the agent (virus, bacteria, parasite, toxin) responsible for the outbreak. Systems that record this kind of information about outbreaks are important tools for quality assurance about outbreak investigations, and thus complete recording of this information—or a clear indication that it is not known—are extremely important for program management.

SUMMARY

Surveillance data must be validated and verified in order to assure that public health decisions are based on as good data as possible. For any given surveillance system design, timeliness, sensitivity, and positive predictive value are in tension with each other. Without any other change in the data collection and analysis methods, steps to improve one of these three parameters will compromise at least one of the others. Improvements in data quality, through necessary validation and verification, can attenuate the effects of such changes. Data quality can be assessed before a data source is put into production, on a periodic basis, and/or on a continuous basis. For surveillance systems designed to support immediate response (as for most systems focused on infectious diseases), continuous data quality assessment should be implemented as well as periodic surveillance system evaluations. Tools and approaches to surveillance data quality that take advantage of the computerization of these data are available and steadily improving.

KEY SUMMARY POINTS

- High-quality data are essential to effective public health surveillance.
- Errors in records received as part of a case-based surveillance information system may result in cases being missed, in noncases being called cases, or in delays in recognition of cases.
- In any given surveillance system, there are inevitable trade-offs among sensitivity (the probability that a targeted event or case will be captured in the system), positive predictive value (the probability that a detected event or case fits the surveillance case definition), and timeliness.
- Major changes in a system (such as improved diagnostic techniques) are necessary to improve one of these three parameters without adversely affecting at least one of the others.
- Surveillance information systems need to have processes in place both to ensure the quality of a new data source and to monitor data quality in a production system.
- Data received in an automated system are not necessarily of higher quality than those in the manual system that it replaced.
- In addition to assessing record-level errors, a thorough approach to data quality means periodically assessing sensitivity, positive predictive value, timeliness, and also representativeness of data.
- Epidemiologists who work with surveillance data must become familiar with the characteristics of the community covered by the system, patterns of health care-seeking behavior in the population, and the health care system from which the surveillance data are generated, so that they can interpret the data correctly.

DISCUSSION QUESTIONS

1. Why are sensitivity and positive predictive value in tension with each other in a surveillance information system?
2. How could inaccurate surveillance data lead to ineffective public health decision-making?
3. How can automation of data capture by surveillance information systems improve the quality of surveillance data?
4. What effects could changes in a surveillance case definition have on data quality (including sensitivity, specificity, timeliness, and representativeness)?
5. How can automation of data capture by surveillance information systems threaten the quality of surveillance data?
6. Name three important potential sources of record-level errors in surveillance data systems, and identify possible steps to reduce those sources of error.
7. Name two potential sources of unrepresentativeness of surveillance data, and identify steps to mitigate or adapt to this type of error.
8. In the surveillance system(s) you are most familiar with, are the processes in place to assure high-quality data adequate?

REFERENCES

1. Centers for Disease Control. Updated guidelines for evaluating public health surveillance systems. MMWR 2001;50(RR13):1–35.
2. Goasdue V, Nugier S, Duqennoy D, Laboisse B. An evaluation framework for data quality tools, <http://mitiq.mit.edu/iciq/pdf/an%20evaluation%20framework%20for%20data%20quality%20tools.pdf>. [Published 2007, accessed January 27, 2014].
3. Sharma A, Heijenberg N, Peter C, Bolongei J, Reeder B, Alpha T, et al. Evidence for a decrease in transmission of Ebola virus—Lofa County, Liberia, June 8–November 1, 2014. MMWR Morb Mortal Wkly Rep 2014;63(46):1067–71.
4. Malone C. Summary of 2009 influenza A H1N1 surveillance. Epi update. Florida: Department of Health Bureau of Epidemiology; 2011. p. 1–13.
5. National Institutes for Standards and Technology 2014 edition meaningful use test tools, <http://healthcare.nist.gov/use_testing/tools.html>. [accessed January 23, 2014].
6. Centers for Disease Control and Prevention. PHIN message quality framework, <http://www.cdc.gov/phin/resources/certification/MQFtool-overview.html/>. [accessed January 23, 2014].
7. National Institutes for Standards and Technology general information, <http://www.nist.gov/public_affairs/general_information.cfm/>. [accessed May 26, 2015].
8. Health Level Seven International. About HL7, <http://www.hl7.org/about/index.cfm?ref=nav/>. [accessed May 26, 2015].
9. European Centre for Disease Prevention and Control. Data quality monitoring and surveillance system evaluation - A handbook of methods and applications. Stockholm: ECDC; 2014.
10. Centers for Disease Control and Prevention. Youth Risk Behavior Surveillance System (YRBSS), <http://www.cdc.gov/healthyyouth/data/yrbs/index.html/>; <http://www.cdc.gov/healthyyouth/data/yrbs/index.html/>. [accessed May 26, 2015].
11. Centers for Disease Control and Prevention. BRFSS, <http://www.cdc.gov/brfss/>. [accessed May 26, 2015].
12. Centers for Disease Control and Prevention. What is PRAMS? <http://www.cdc.gov/prams/>. [accessed May 26, 2015].
13. Eisenstein L, Hamilton JJ. Harnessing the Power of System Automation to Improve Efficiency of Reportable Disease Surveillance through Automated Case Creation. Boston, MA: Paper presented at the annual conference of the Council of State and Territorial Epidemiologists; June 17, 2015.
14. Eisenstein L, Hamilton JJ. Improving Reportable Disease Surveillance Data Quality: 92% Reduction in Selected Data Quality Errors by Implementing Early Checks. Nashville, TN: Paper presented at annual conference of the Council of State and Territorial Epidemiologists; June 24, 2014.
15. Baer A. An information visualization approach to improving data quality. Emerg Health Threats J 2011;4(0)10-10. doi: 10.3402/ehtj.v4i0.11014.
16. Painter I, Eaton J, Olson D, Lober W, Revere D. Visualizing data quality: tools and views. Emerg Health Threats J 2011;4. 10.3402/ehtj.v4i0.11702.
17. Painter I, Eaton J, Olson D, Revered D, Lober WB. How good is your data? Emerg Health Threats J. 2011;4. doi: 10.3402/ehtj.v4i0.11702.
18. Loschen W, Kite-Powell A. Development of automated data quality indicators and visualizations using Florida's ESSENCE System. Online J Public Health Inform 2013;5(1):e17. PMCID: PMC3692820.
19. Centers for Disease Control. Framework for evaluating public health surveillance systems for early detection of outbreaks. MMWR 2004;53(RR05):1–11.

CHAPTER

25

Public Health Modeling and Data Mining

James S Koopman, Prem Singh, Edward L Ionides

When you engage with people, you build your own insight into what's being discussed. Someone else's understanding complements yours, and together you start to weave an informed interpretation. You tinker until you can move on.
Marcia Conner

KEY WORDS

Transmission modeling
Data mining
Assumption
Differential equation models
Agent-based (AB) models
Inference robustness assessment (IRA)
Identifiability analysis
Parameters
Variables

INTRODUCTION

Models of how infection flows through populations are increasingly being used to inform disease control decisions. Technological advances discussed in previous chapters that allow for more and better data are improving how models can relate to reality. Better technology, in terms of software and computers, is also making models more usable and useful. New technologies make it easier to add realism to models and to explore what aspects of a model determine its behavior, which facilitate the formulation of hypotheses and theory about what is determining the behavior of the real world. Better technology also helps test hypotheses and theory by fitting models to surveillance data. Nonlinear dynamics of complex real-world systems generate the patterns seen in surveillance data. Fitting these nonlinear dynamic models to data has been a challenge that is, bit by bit, being met by new algorithms and new hardware.

A major theme of this chapter is the logic of how to use such model fitting to improve disease control decisions. The logic presented demands particular forms of coordination among surveillance personnel, modelers, and policy makers. Accordingly, structured steps are presented in this chapter to improve this coordination. To illustrate the general concepts presented, a real-world example is presented about proceeding to use surveillance data and transmission models to inform polio eradication endgame policies by helping to monitor levels of nonparalytic poliovirus infections that are difficult to observe and count directly.

TRANSMISSION MODELING AND BROADER ANALYTIC CONTEXTS

Two recent analytic advances, data mining and fitting of transmission models to data, help public health surveillance to incorporate more complex data and methods for guiding disease control decisions. The focus in this chapter is on inferring control action effects from surveillance data using causal system models of infection transmission. **Transmission modeling** uses mathematical representations to relate and simulate disease transmission variables for the purpose of analyzing surveillance data and forecasting outcomes of interventions.[1] Data mining is a different approach to complexity that, like classical risk factor analyses, assumes away all system control loops while providing a better way to perceive complex risk factor effects.

Currently both data mining and transmission modeling are applied as special analyses of surveillance data that were not gathered for these purposes. In the future, data mining and transmission modeling have the potential to transform surveillance if they evolve within systems that guide disease control, and feedback is provided by surveillance system users on the effectiveness of their guidance. All surveillance systems need such feedback. Data mining involves machine learning of how sets of factors lead to other sets of factors and the feedback needed is whether the machine is focusing on the right things to learn. Causal system analyses, like those using infection transmission models, build theoretical system models, and feedback is needed on whether those models are adequate to guide public health actions.

Data Mining

Data mining uses computer programs to progressively learn from massive and diverse data about how patterns of single variables or combinations of variables relate to patterns of disease.[1] Diverse strategies and algorithms have been developed for data mining, and new approaches are evolving rapidly. Since our main purpose in mentioning data mining here is to make broad contrasts with transmission modeling, we will not discuss these specific approaches. Data mining either retrieves answers to narrow questions or describes relationships. The relationships of interest might be about how words like "flu" in internet communications or purchases of particular types of medications from pharmacy records indicate disease patterns of infection or disease variables. Or they may be about how patterns of risk factors such as behaviors, genetics, or physiological states relate to patterns of disease. Data mining mostly examines the type of associations that have been the core of mainstream epidemiology since John Snow linked water sources and cholera, but it pursues more complex relationships between predictor variables than is feasible with traditional methods. Data mining is mostly "theoryless"[2] in that it does not currently use mathematically expressed theory about the complex system processes through which disease states at the individual or population level are generated.

The learning programs used by many data mining methods are like those that enabled the IBM computer named Watson to beat the best Jeopardy contestants[3] and represent significant advances in learning theory. These programs can "learn" more effectively if they get feedback as to whether the analyses performed provided an informative inference. In traditional epidemiology, analysts do the learning themselves rather than having a machine do it. In data mining, analysts direct a computer to learn and then guide the computer to learn more effectively by providing feedback on whether it is learning helpful things about risk factors or generating gibberish.

Infection Transmission System Modeling

Mechanistic, causal models of infection transmission systems (called **transmission models** for short hereafter) are used to analyze the dissemination of infections through populations. They differ from risk factor epidemiology models and most data mining models by using systems theory to formulate mechanistic feedbacks between variables and the individuals or populations modeled.[1] Such feedbacks generate nonlinear dynamics that cause the outcomes experienced by some individuals to change the risks experienced by other individuals. Traditional analyses and data mining, in contrast, describe data (not theory) using dynamically linear models of relationships in the data in a manner that preserves the independence between outcomes in different individuals.

One source of a positive system feedback in a transmission model is risk factors for infection transmission, such as drinking from an unsafe water supply. Early in an epidemic, with each new infection there is a new source of contamination for the unsafe water, causing the risk from drinking unsafe water to increase. On the other hand, late in an epidemic or during endemic transmission, immunity acquired from previous infections related to risk factor exposures provides a negative feedback. Those who drank unsafe water have more immunity and lower risks of infection. This might make an exposure like drinking from an unsafe water supply look like a protective factor in a study of endemic infection where individuals' immunity levels are not measured. A transmission model that captures the risk of drinking contaminated water would include variables that specify individuals' immunity status and parameters that govern the risk of infection by immunity status and exposure status. Such a model would require specifying immunity status in the model, even though there might not be such data available. When the model parameters are fitted adequately to exposure and disease experience data, it would make more accurate predictions of ongoing risk than a risk difference because it captures the effects of exposures and immunity.

Traditional surveillance systems describe surveillance data by time, place, and person. These descriptions may identify risk factors directly or stimulate special investigations that identify risk factors. Odds ratios, risk ratios, risk differences, and other epidemiologic measures are used for risk factor identification. For infectious diseases, however, these measures can provide bad predictions of future risk because of the system feedbacks generating nonlinear dynamics such as those arising from risk factors in the previous paragraph. With regard to the positive risk factor example, the traditional measures miss the new infections generated by the person getting the infection from risk factor exposure. The negative risk factor example made a factor that is disseminating infection look like a protective factor. Because transmission models capture these feedbacks, they are more capable of predicting future infection levels if control actions change risk factors.

When a risk difference is used to predict the effect of eliminating an exposure, the assumptions behind that prediction are often poorly specified and understood. One basic assumption is that the infection or disease outcome from exposure in one individual is independent of outcomes in other individuals. Infection transmission and immunity effects violate that assumption.

The assumptions behind transmission model-based predictions are usually better specified than the assumptions behind risk difference-based predictions; however, considerable care, experience, and knowledge are required to specify how assumptions in transmission models differ from real-world situations being modeled. We propose a set of steps to assess the effects of assumptions on inferences made by analyzing data using transmission models. These will be presented later in sections dealing with inference robustness assessment (IRA) and identifiability analyses.

Another important difference between traditional surveillance data analysis and transmission model analysis is what determines the variables used in an analysis. Traditional epidemiology and data mining both determine what variables are used in a model by the availability of data for those variables. In contrast, transmission system model variables are determined by what is theoretically needed to understand an infection control issue—whether or not data for a particular variable are available.

CLASSES OF TRANSMISSION MODELS

Differential Equation Models

Compartmental models based on differential equation (DE), model continuous populations rather than discrete individuals. **Differential equation models** use deterministic approaches that predict expected mean system behavior for very large populations.[1] They break up a population into compartments such as susceptible, infected, or immune, as is the case for the classic SIR (susceptible, infectious, recovered) model and define transmission generating contact patterns between these compartments. DE models assume very large numbers of individuals in compartments so that chance events cannot drive the model behavior. This assumption holds no matter whether the size of the compartment is 1 or 1 billion because the DE form assumes that population or compartmental sizes are continuous, in the sense that between any two values for a compartment there are an infinite number of intervening values.

An example of a compartmental model can be found in Fig. 25-1. Each box in the figure represents a segment of the population. The "S_n" boxes represent susceptible populations, the "I_n" boxes represent populations infected with wild poliovirus (WPV), and the "V_n" boxes represent those infected with live oral polio vaccine (OPV). The arrows represent transitions between population compartments. All new population comes into compartment S_0. There are n levels of immunity and n different natural histories of infection corresponding to OPV or WPV infection that occur in individuals at each level of immunity. Infection with OPV or WPV can occur out of the S compartments

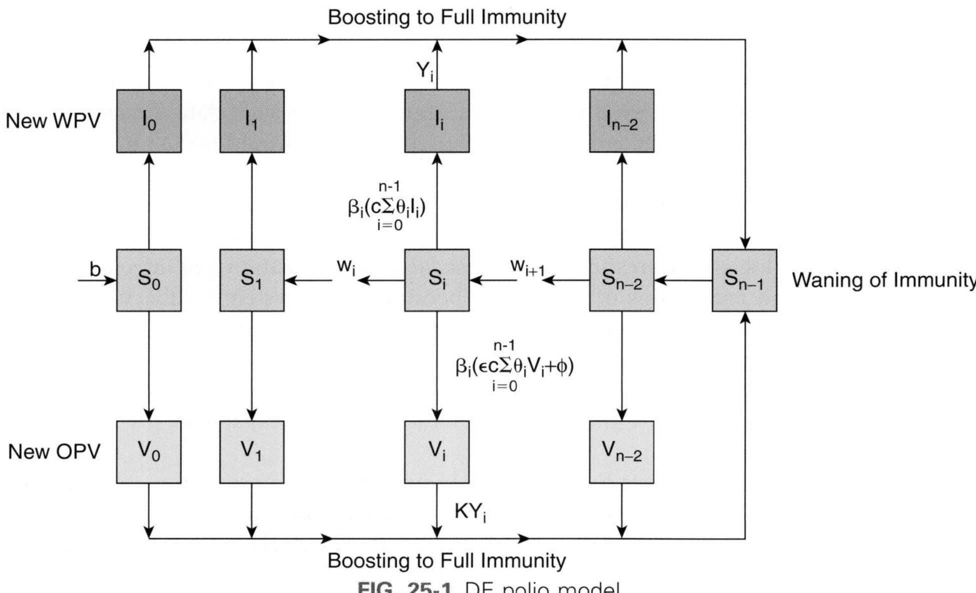

FIG. 25-1 DE polio model.

at the 0 through $n - 2$ levels, but no infection can occur at the $n - 1$ level of immunity. When individuals recover from either an OPV or a WPV infection, they recover into the S_{n-1} compartment. This model was used to generate general insights into the dynamics of poliovirus infection and immunity and how these dynamics are altered by increasing transmissibility, speed with which immunity wanes, the transmissibility of OPV, and the timing and extent of coverage of vaccination campaigns.[4] A radically simplifying assumption of this model is that the immunity levels generated by WPV and OPV infection are identical. A single infection with either OPV or WPV gets one to the maximal state of immunity, and if one gets reinfected after immunity has waned, immunity cannot be boosted beyond that achieved after the first infection.

One does not need to know much about the mathematics of DE to use this modeling approach. Expertise in the social, epidemiologic, and biological processes involved is the most important factor for developing useful models. Computer programs are then utilized to solve the DE tied to the model. Understanding how to translate model assumptions into model structure and equations is a skill almost anyone can acquire, but a capacity to make judgments about the appropriateness or necessity of model assumptions is needed in order to make valid inferences from a model analysis. Gaining such capacity requires experience and a good theoretical foundation of how model structures relate to assumptions. A complete public health surveillance system should include individuals with this capacity.

Agent-Based Models

Agent-based (AB) models use individuals instead of continuous population segments. When an infected and a susceptible individual encounter each other, there is some chance that transmission may take place.[1] Chance plays no role in DE models. AB modeling is one variety of "stochastic" or "chance" modeling. A single run of an AB model provides one possible outcome, but the next outcome might vary greatly from the first. Thus, a model must be run many times to produce a distribution of outcomes in order to make inferences about disease control on the basis of surveillance data. This extra computing work has an important benefit not possible with DE models: one can calculate the chances of different outcomes having different degrees of severity. The real world can be viewed as having experienced such a chance process that might have come from a variety of different distributions; such chance considerations can be an important driver of disease control decisions.

To use the example of polio eradication again, one might want to choose between two different control options that, on average, take the same time and effort to achieve eradication. If one control option has a chance of a very large outbreak that could not be controlled with available resources but the other does not have that chance, the choice of control options may be influenced—such chances could not be evaluated using a purely DE approach.

Similar to that for DE modeling, a growing body of software facilitates AB modeling without requiring specialized mathematical or programming skills. What is required is experience and a broad disciplinary knowledge base that improves judgment capacity when deciding what to include or ignore in a model to make it as simple as possible, but no simpler. Simple models help make clear inferences relevant to disease control, but models that are simpler than necessary lead to erroneous inferences. Later, we will present an inference robustness strategy for finding simple models that lead to good inferences.

Model Complexity and Inferences

Complexity of DE models relates to the total number of compartments in a model as well as the number of interactions between compartments and their variety. Similarly, the complexity of AB models relates to the numbers of individuals, the number of states those individuals might have, and the number and types of things that can happen to individuals, especially the number and type of interactions that might occur between individuals.

Because the social and biological complexities that underlie real-world infection transmission systems are so rich, simpler models in general make more unrealistic assumptions about the real world than more complex models. The simplest models assume that all individuals or all population segments behave identically to all others and have equal contact rates with all others. The classical SIR model makes such assumptions. However, if there is a high-risk group affecting transmission, and mixing between high- and low-risk groups affects the spread of infection, then decisions about resource allocation can be dramatically wrong if the model does not capture these complexities.[5]

One relaxes an unrealistic simplifying assumption by making a model more realistically complex. To relax unrealistic assumptions about large population size in DE models, one can keep most assumptions in the DE model but transition to an AB model. Any such transition also involves adding the analytic task of having to examine distributions of model outcomes affected by chance events rather than just deterministic mean model outcomes. Assumptions regarding networks of interactions between individuals are best handled by AB models, as DE models do not have individuals but rather only continuous segments of population. Consequently, DE models intrinsically assume that if one person makes contact with two individuals, those contacts do not affect the chances that those two people will contact each other. In other words, the chance of two people contacting each other is not influenced by whether they both have a common contact as it is in the real world. To relax this unrealistic assumption, one must use an AB model. In general, however, since it is much faster and easier to explore the effects of relaxing assumptions in DE models than in AB models, one should go as far as one can to relax simplifying assumptions in DE models before transitioning to AB models.

INFECTIOUS DISEASE MODELING: POLIO EXAMPLE

The global strategy for polio eradication is a product of a century of epidemiologic research and 60 years of experience with polio immunization. Since the launch of Polio Eradication Program at the World Health Assembly in 1988, the Global Polio Eradication Initiative (GPEI) has reduced the global incidence of polio by more than 99% and the number of countries with endemic polio from 125 to 3.[6] Of the three types of WPV (type 1, type 2, and type 3), type 2 WPV transmission has been successfully stopped (since 1999), and significant progress has been made toward eradicating type 1 and type 3 WPV.[7]

Until recently, polio transmission modeling has not been very important in guiding control decisions. The polio eradication effort has used an empirical strategy that detects acute flaccid paralysis (AFP) cases and diagnoses polio infections among these. Even though only a small fraction of poliovirus infections result in paralysis, eradication efforts have assumed that AFP surveillance sufficiently detects all places with poliovirus transmission. However, now, in the final stages of eradication, this assumption may no longer be appropriate. It is thus becoming more important to understand what can sustain poliovirus transmission in the absence of paralytic cases and not just what immunization program deficiencies create risks of paralytic poliomyelitis cases. To ensure eradication, it may be necessary to make inferences about whether waning immunity is allowing previously infected individuals to sustain transmission. Before vaccination efforts begin in high transmission areas, waning immunity is continuously boosted by WPV infections that immunity aborts before they become contagious. A major value of OPV transmission is that it allows waning immunity in older individuals to be boosted by OPV infections. But some individuals, due to better sanitation, hygiene, and less crowded living conditions, will not be boosted by OPV transmission. These individuals' immunity will wane so that if they get infected with WPV, their infections will last longer and they will excrete enough virus to be more capable of transmitting.

Immunity affecting transmission wanes much more quickly than immunity against paralysis. Thus, waning immunity could result in reinfected cases transmitting enough to sustain WPV circulation without there ever being paralytic poliomyelitis cases. It is not practical to make observations about WPV transmissions from people who have waned to different immunity states after WPV or OPV infections. However, it is possible to estimate how much waning immunity affects transmission if the right data from the right situations can be fit to models. With such estimates, the models can be used to estimate how much transmission might be occurring in the absence of paralytic polio cases.

Transmission model analyses have recently shown that the polio eradication achieved in high transmission settings like India and Egypt is a tenuous eradication.[4] It is tenuous because waning immunity acquired from WPV infection before OPV vaccination campaigns with eliminated WPV will progressively increase the potential for WPV circulation over time. Since waning immunity mostly affects age groups not getting OPV directly but rather through secondary transmissions, the increase in WPV transmission potential in the absence of paralytic polio could be large.

WPV transmission has been detected in the absence of paralytic polio in Israel.[8] While the waning of inactivated vaccine-induced immunity, rather than WPV or OPV immunity, caused the situation in Israel, the theoretical demonstration of the waning effects of WPV and OPV in high transmission countries[4] makes the Israeli experience more important for two reasons. First, few countries have the type of WPV surveillance used in Israel that could detect asymptomatic infection circulation. The World Health Organization (WHO) is addressing this issue by increasing sewage surveillance. Second, the Israeli situation presents a unique opportunity to estimate waning immunity parameters by fitting models to the available data. Such parameter estimation would increase the validity of modeling estimates to determine where WPV has the best chance to circulate in the absence of paralytic cases. These are the areas where surveillance needs to be set up for nonparalytic poliovirus infections.

At the time this chapter is being written, three endemic countries, Nigeria, Pakistan, and Afghanistan, have never stopped polio circulation. Polio transmission in Nigeria has set off outbreaks widely across Africa but is now coming under control.[9] Some of the outbreaks caused by viruses from Nigeria have taken over a year to control.[9] Pakistan has also set off several significant outbreaks[9] and appears to be the source of cases detected in Israel as well as paralytic cases in Syria.[8] The intensive and ongoing eradication efforts in these countries bring hope for final eradication in the near future, but waning immunity could be making adults from endemic transmission areas more capable of transmitting infections to new areas. For example, a virus in Chad appears to be the source of cases in Cameroon over 2 years after the last paralytic case detected in Chad.[10] Moreover, waning of WPV- and OPV-induced immunity could be making many areas more capable of sustaining WPV transmission when cases arrive from endemic areas. Accordingly, WHO declared an emergency situation in May 2014 urging that all people, adults and children, traveling out of endemic areas provide proof that they have been recently vaccinated.

This emergency situation calls out for a better understanding of waning immunity, of whose waning immunity is likely to be boosted by getting an OPV infection from a vaccinated child, and of the conditions that allow WPV circulation with few or no paralytic cases. Applying transmission models to surveillance data will be essential to generate this needed understanding. Models will be needed to estimate key parameters from the data, after which models can use these parameters to project where silent poliovirus transmission is most likely.

Using Transmission Models to Estimate Unknown Parameters and Unobserved Variables

Models have variables and parameters. A variable changes value over time as a result of system influences. **Parameters** are fixed theoretical relationships in models that govern how the values of variables change over time.[1] The polio example can be used to illustrate how models are used to estimate both unmeasured variables and unknown parameter values.

First, let us consider an example of estimating an unmeasured variable. Current surveillance systems only record paralytic poliomyelitis cases; they do not measure the frequency of nonparalytic infection. The AFP surveillance system has been very successful at detecting these cases because it incorporates good methods for evaluating the completeness of paralytic polio surveillance.[11] The circulation of WPV in the absence of paralytic poliomyelitis in Israel and the theoretical risk of waning creates a need for surveillance systems that also detect nonparalytic WPV infections. Since surveillance to detect nonparalytic polio can be very expensive, such surveillance needs to target the situations in which a high ratio of nonparalytic to paralytic cases can be expected.

An important step toward effective surveillance of nonparalytic polio infections is to describe the joint distribution of paralytic and nonparalytic infections using transmission models that are sufficiently detailed and realistic and that are informed by sufficiently detailed data on diverse aspects of the real world. Since direct surveillance of nonparalytic WPV infection rates is very expensive, surveillance must involve estimating those rates using models informed by other surveillance data. To date, model-based inferences made about nonparalytic WPV rates are still crude,[12–16] but the new methods for fitting models to data to be discussed later in this chapter should improve that.

Next, let us consider a parameter example. Essential parameters in recent polio models establish the patterns over time by which immunity wanes.[4,12–16] No longitudinal data are available about the state of immunity of individuals and how that affects transmission potential that would allow one to infer parameters describing how fast immunity wanes. Nonetheless, waning parameters can be found that are consistent with available observations on different aspects of polio from different parts of the world.[13] The methods used so far, however, have not taken advantage of recent advances in methods for estimating parameters of transmission models discussed in the next section.

Let us put this discussion of variables and parameters back into the context of traditional versus transmission model analyses in epidemiology. The variables used in standard risk factor epidemiology or data mining analyses are determined by what is in the data. The variables in transmission models, in contrast, are determined by causal theories defining what is needed to predict system behavior. When direct data on some variables are not available, transmission models can make inferences about those variables if enough good theory and data on other aspects of the transmission system are available.

The parameters in standard risk factor epidemiology or data mining models describe relationships between variables rather than causal system mechanisms. Thus, they do not allow for projection of future infection transmission levels. When using transmission models to project effects of policy choices, limitations on what is known about parameter values make policy choice projections less precise and less reliable. In order for surveillance systems to better inform policy choices, they should use transmission models to both project the consequences of policy choices and learn more from their data about unknown variable and parameter values.

New Methods for Estimating Parameters from Transmission Models

One fits a model to surveillance data that characterizes patterns of infection over time by finding parameter values that reproduce these patterns in the surveillance data. Statistical analysis of time series data like those collected by surveillance systems traditionally focused on models with linear relationships between observations.[17] Recent algorithmic advances for nonlinear models have made possible the formal statistical analyses that used to be available only for linear models, including confidence intervals for unknown parameters, model selection tests, and the computation of Bayesian posterior distributions. Furthermore, several recent methods have the convenient plug-and-play property that implementing the methodology requires the scientist to specify the dynamic model only via computer code to simulate trajectories.[18,19] Plug-and-play statistical methodologies for imperfectly measured dynamic systems include iterated filtering,[20] particle Markov chain Monte Carlo,[21] synthetic likelihood,[22] approximate Bayesian computation,[23] and nonlinear forecasting.[24] Both maximum likelihood inference and Bayesian inference involve the likelihood of the data given the model. Therefore, it may be counterintuitive that inferences of this kind can be obtained when direct evaluation of the likelihood is unavailable. Nevertheless, theoretical results underpinning iterated filtering (for maximum likelihood inference) and particle Markov chain Monte Carlo (for Bayesian inference) show that this is indeed possible.

All of the plug-and-play methods mentioned above are freely available in the open source R package POMP, which deals with inference for partially observed Markov process models.[25] Examples involving the use of POMP for epidemiological investigations include studies of malaria,[26,27] cholera,[28] pertussis,[29] and pneumonia.[30] Introductions to statistical inference for nonlinear mechanistic models in the context of the pomp package are provided by the pomp package vignettes.

We propose that these methods promise to provide useful estimates of nonparalytic poliovirus infection rates in areas where good data on vaccination program activities and paralytic cases are available. As discussed later with regard to identifiability analyses, data on sanitation conditions and on genetic sequence patterns of isolated polioviruses may also be needed. Surveillance team members other than statisticians will not need to understand the technical aspects of the listed methods, but all team members can and should have an understanding of the general scientific approach.

Because these new methods are being developed in academia and will need modification to meet specific public health practice needs, and because they require a new way of thinking about what one can get from data and how one analyzes data by analyzing systems, collaboration between academics and field epidemiologists is essential in order for analyses of dynamic causal system models to become an important part of surveillance activities. Furthermore, since most academics do not appreciate the needs, flexibilities, and rigidities of a well-functioning surveillance system, the collaboration between service entities and academics must be established in a context where the goals of academics are unified with those of service agencies. After elaborating our polio example to incorporate model fitting for making policy decisions, we will then propose a framework for unifying academic and surveillance system goals for modeling. First, however, we will present a theory-based discussion about the validation of transmission model analyses that lead to policy choices.

MODEL CHOICE, MODEL VALIDATION, AND THE POLICY DECISION PROCESS

In this section, a particular approach to model choice and model validation will be presented. There is no universally valid model for making any possible inference—each policy question requires a model form adapted to the inference addressed. A model is validated with regard to its ability to inform inferences. When pure science is pursued the inference may be what theory is correct, but here we focus on policy choices.

Just finding that a model fits available data does not validate a model for making any policy decision for two reasons. First, different models that lead to different policy decisions could fit the same data. Second, any model that fits the data makes a series of simplifying assumptions about what is important for a decision in the real world—that is the nature of models. In some cases, realistic relaxation of those simplifying assumptions may not change the fit to data dramatically, but it might change the decision chosen. For these reasons, model validation for specific inferences needs to follow the steps in Fig. 25-2, which enumerates all action steps. Step 4 leads to a decision criterion for proceeding to an IRA by proceeding to step 5 or to an identifiability analysis by proceeding to step 6. In many cases it will make sense to pursue both IRAs and identifiability analyses simultaneously.

Inference Robustness Assessment

Inference robust assessment is a type of assessment that is performed by comparing an inference across different model forms.[31] Two questions that should be answered when modeling a transmission system to inform policy include (1) what aspects of a system and what details about processes and feedbacks in that system need to be

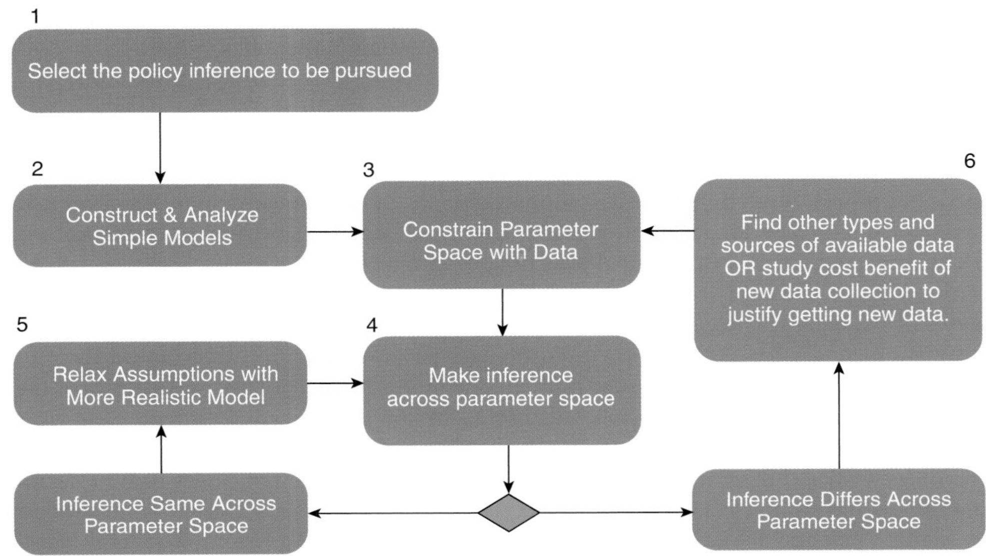

FIG. 25-2 Steps to making valid and robust policy inferences using dynamic system models.

included in a model in order for transmission models to generate good control decisions? and (2) how can a particular model form and a particular set of parameter values in that model be validated with regard to informing policy choices? The answer to these questions should be sought using a set of iterative steps that involve "inference robustness assessment"[31,32] and "identifiability analyses."[33-39] These steps are presented in Fig. 25-2.

The flow chart in Fig. 25-2 has an initial process to reach the decision point after step 4. The decision is to proceed with either further IRA or further identifiability analyses. The figure then has two infinite loops coming through the decision point; the one going through step 5 is the inference robustness loop, and the one going through step 6 is the identifiability loop. These two loops represent the processes by which science continually develops deeper levels of understanding and increasingly verified theories. Policy decisions cannot wait for infinite loops to be completed—decisions must be made wherever one is within these loops. The processes in Fig. 25-2 ensure, however, that the best model currently available for a particular policy decision is being used to make that policy decision.

The IRA process involves finding a simple model that is adequate for informing a control decision but is not too simple in the sense that its unrealistic simplifying assumptions cause the wrong control decision to be made. To ensure that a model is not too simple, one must verify that realistic relaxation of simplifying assumptions is unlikely to change a policy inference. This verification is done in Fig. 25-2 by following step 5 whenever step 4 leads to a single policy choice. Skill in identifying assumptions, finding ways to relax assumptions, and choosing the most important assumptions to pursue are gained mainly by experience and are helped by a good theoretical foundation in both modeling and the relevant scientific, social, or professional disciplines. To identify hidden assumptions, it is helpful to have a diverse and multidisciplinary team involved.

Identifiability Analyses

An **identifiability analysis** focuses on what data are needed to make a control decision using a causal system model.[1] A policy choice is "identifiable" by a set of data if those data are consistent with only parameter values that lead to a single policy choice. Whenever that is the case, an IRA is the next step to help validate the model as appropriate for making the policy choice. When a policy choice is not identifiable using the current set of data, more data are needed. What is the best type of new data to pursue is determined by an identifiability analysis. In Fig. 25-2, identifiability analyses involve looping through steps 6 then 3 then 4.

Types of Data that Can Inform Models

A surveillance system might gather data routinely on some things and might conduct surveys or special studies to gather data on other things. Demographic data are always needed when modeling populations and may be collected by a health agency or others. Sanitation, transportation, economic, or service use data might also increase the identifiability of policy choices. The total data available might cover infection or disease incidence and prevalence, individual risk factors, population structure, patterns of contact between individuals, contacts with environmental reservoirs, control actions, laboratory results affecting the course of infection or transmissibility of individuals, and genetic sequences of pathogens. These diverse sorts of data deserve both standard descriptive analyses and integration into transmission model-based analyses. When the data provide direct information on the parameters of a model, then the transmission model analysis need only run the model to interpret the significance of the surveillance data. The more complete model-based analysis will use all of the data together to help estimate all otherwise unknown parameter values.

An important type of data for analyzing surveillance data across many years includes data on factors that might affect the completeness and accuracy of surveillance data, such as surveillance personnel activities and outbreak investigations. Surveillance personnel have many responsibilities and as different situations arise, they must decrease the time they spend on getting routine surveillance data. This can affect reporting completeness. A model-based inference might not be robust to realistic relaxation of the assumption that surveillance is constant over many years. In other words, adding a term to a model that allows reporting completeness to vary over time could change a control inference made from analyzing the model. If so, in a model with variable reporting rates, the inference sought might not be identifiable. That is to say the inference could depend upon unobserved variability in the reporting rates. However, if reporting rates can be informed by factors affecting reporting completeness, identifiability might be recovered.

Making Control Decisions Involving Policy Choices

The processes in Fig. 25-2 are advisable whenever a model is used to inform policy. These processes represent the general steps of scientific progress that pursue deeper understanding. There is no end point that definitively says no more IRAs or identifiability analyses are needed; science should always seek deeper and wider understanding. Policy choices, however, must be made even when some threats to inference robustness have been identified and when inferences are not identifiable with available data. If policy makers were involved in the initial choice of policy inferences to be pursued, and if the modelers have used the models developed to help the policy makers understand the mechanisms generating infection control outcomes, then the team of surveillance personnel and modelers are in a position to inform policy makers so that they can make decisions in the face of residual uncertainties.

After recently announcing a WHO polio transmission emergency, WHO decided to require vaccination of travelers from polio-endemic regions.[40] This was the first time WHO has indicated that adults could be important in polio transmission. The resulting consternation and resistance in the affected countries might have been mitigated had there been a solid model-based analysis supported by inference robustness and identifiability analyses. The threat to global eradication probably justifies this decision despite not being able to back it up with model analyses incorporating inference robustness and identifiability analyses. A well functioning surveillance system, however, should lessen the chances that choices need to be made in a state of ignorance by identifying at an earlier stage what new data would be most informative for anticipated decisions. For example, an identifiability analysis for potential decisions based on surveillance data might have indicated that better genetic sequence data, population movement data, or sanitation data was needed to make an informed policy decision.

For the policy maker to be comfortable with how model analyses are informing their decisions, step 1 in Fig. 25-2 is the key. Policy makers must be involved in defining the inferences pursued using transmission models, but they cannot dictate those inferences because they are unlikely to fully understand the factors affecting the utility of different choices. The choice must involve an interactive process between the modeler team and the policy makers. One reason for this interaction is that "systems thinking" is required to choose policy options when dealing with infection control. While being adept at envisioning the feedback processes affecting policies is a characteristic of good policy makers, they may not be trained in envisioning the feedback processes involved in infectious disease control. Moreover, they may have little insight into the ability of models and data to inform policy choices. Therefore, a formal meeting to select the precise wording of policy choices to be pursued is advisable.

In such a meeting, policy makers should begin by presenting how they see their policy options, what their objectives are (e.g., minimize infections, deaths, days in hospital, disparities, etc.), what their constraints are (e.g., personnel or other resources), and what would lead them to choose different options. Then, modelers should discuss those options in terms of their possible effects on the behavior of transmission systems. This discussion should modify what the policy makers see as their options and lead to the selection of inferences to pursue. If this crucial first step is not pursued adequately and the goal of the modeling is poorly defined, then the modeling is more likely to wander in the complexity of reality and available data than it is to influence policy. We illustrate the steps of this process and the paths that this process can take with our polio example.

VALIDATING THE TRANSMISSION MODEL-BASED POLIO ERADICATION POLICY CHOICES

Identifying and Selecting Inferences To Be Validated

Beginning with step 1 in Fig. 25-2, the relevant policy makers must be identified. WHO and GPEI officials aggregate and analyze global surveillance data and make policy decisions that could benefit from a transmission model analysis of their surveillance data. One modeling group worked with the US Centers for Disease Control and Prevention and, through them, with WHO and GPEI. One thrust of this group's recent work emphasizes the need for a change from surveillance to detect paralytic polio cases to surveillance to detect poliovirus infections even in the absence of paralysis.[12-16]

For our example, we can consider India, which has been declared polio-free on the basis of no paralytic polio cases being detected for 3 years by a well-functioning AFP surveillance system. The road to eradication in India was difficult. After a seemingly intensive vaccination program knocked paralytic cases to a very low level, there was a big rebound in transmission and extremely intensive revaccination with different OPV formulations once again reduced paralytic cases to a low level. During that time, surveillance was set up in large cities by testing samples from the sewage system for WPV. Some cities without paralytic cases found WPV in their sewage, but the areas where paralytic cases appeared were almost all in regions lacking large sewage systems; in these areas, people defecate in open fields and there are few latrines. Elimination in these areas required very intensive vaccination as well as careful identification of migrant populations that might be missed by vaccination campaigns. Sanitation improvements were not investigated as a policy to improve polio eradication. If such improvements were pursued, the results of the crude system analysis indicate that eradication could be made less fragile.[4]

Fitting models to data from endemic periods when not much is changing often fails to elucidate transmission dynamics in the populations modeled because endemic data cannot identify model parameters. Identifiability is lost because highly diverse models can give the same endemic incidence at parameter values that generate very different patterns during periods of changing vaccination. When the data come from periods when the system was markedly knocked off equilibrium and has since bounced back, just as described for India, the data are much more likely to identify model parameters from available data. Thus, India, with its large population and intensive control and surveillance efforts, could provide estimates for immunity-waning parameters. Models incorporating these parameter estimates could then contribute to choosing between whatever policy options are the focus of analysis. Examples are presented in the following sections.

Inferring Large Nonparalytic Polio Outbreak Potential

While most health officials believe that it is unlikely that polio infections could be persisting in India without paralytic cases, the theoretical case for that belief is weak. Of particular concern is the potential for new occult introductions from Pakistan or Africa; while immunity may be strong in young children, it may have waned in adults since WPV circulation was stopped. Because the places in India where polio persisted the longest have very high transmission potential, it might be easier in those places to surpass the "reinfection threshold."[41] The reinfection threshold determines when WPV transmission can be sustained by individuals who have previously acquired immunity from WPV or OPV infection. On the other hand, more OPV circulates in these areas after vaccination campaigns. Thus, repeated OPV infections transmitted from vaccinated children might keep waning of immunity from causing these areas to pass the reinfection threshold. It could be that the biggest risk of WPV circulation in the absence of paralysis is in areas with good vaccination levels but intermediate potential to transmit OPV. Transmission potential that is too low would not only fail to spread OPV but also fail to spread WPV. What populations are most likely to sustain WPV circulation as a function of vaccination levels is the kind of question where modeling can improve both intuitions and policy decisions. Indeed, relevant modeling insights have recently been published.[4]

To improve intuitions on this issue, simple models could be used where model behavior is easier to explain. Then, one would observe and explain infection patterns as the values of parameters and the initial settings of variables are varied in the model. If a complex model is used where such explanations are difficult to verify, then neither the model system under investigation nor the real world is understood. Once the behavior of a simple model is explained, it is easier to explain the behavior of a model that adds complexity to that simple model. A simple model might have a homogeneous population where all individuals mix evenly with all others and all individuals of all ages have the same risk of dying and the same response to infection. The question we are discussing has to do with first infections versus subsequent infections, because paralysis only arises from first infections. Thus, the model must distinguish first from subsequent infections.

Even in the simplest transmission models, it can be difficult to predict how model behavior will change as parameters and variables change. When a prediction is made and then, upon running the model, the prediction is wrong, one can gain new understanding. This understanding might come from a process of hypothesizing what explains model behavior and testing those hypotheses by setting up special conditions in the model. Or it might be gained by examining model behavior in fine detail to discover what leads to the observed behavior. Modelers should sharpen their intuitions by examining simpler models in this way before pursuing answers about the very complex real world.

In the case of polio, the modeler might run simple models that introduce vaccination programs to eventually eradicate transmission. Then WPV could be introduced once again into the population to examine the ratio of first WPV infections to reinfections. Using the methodology in the last paragraph, insight would be gained into what might cause a high ratio of infections in previously immune individuals in comparison to infections in individuals who have never had an OPV or WPV infection.

Simple models that help develop intuitions may behave quite differently compared to the far more complex real world. The next step in pursuing models that can inform policy is to think of all of the aspects of the real world that would have some chance of changing transmission patterns from those in the simple model. Each of those changes should be explored by using models that add them one at a time and retain them only if they do make a difference. This gets us back to the crucial step 1 in the Fig. 25-2 flow chart.

Settling on Inferences To Be Made through Modeling

Suppose that officials in India or GPEI want to decide whether to set up a surveillance system for poliovirus infection that goes beyond sewage system testing. They might be a little skeptical about the value of this step compared to other investments of time and public health resources. Furthermore, suppose that modelers familiar with poliovirus transmission modeling are available to collaborate with these officials to determine what surveillance methods are worthwhile to pursue. Given this scenario, the first step is to set up meetings to decide on specific inferences about specific control options that will be pursued. This initial meeting should include a broad discussion about how policy makers and modelers view this issue in addition to focusing on the control options and inference statements that will influence the choice of those control actions.

To help clarify the cultural dynamics that are likely to dominate meetings on objectives between policy makers and modelers, we now turn to possible policy maker perspectives and modeler perspectives on what needs to be modeled. We go into considerable detail as to how these will affect the process of choosing inferences to be pursued with modeling because the ability of models to serve public health is so dependent upon this dialogue that leads to the choice of inferences.

Policy Maker Perspectives

There are several options policymakers may choose for polio surveillance. One option is an active guidance system that continuously updates how nonparalytic infection surveillance is focused as new paralytic cases are diagnosed and nonparalytic infections are detected. This option follows the long tradition of the polio eradication initiative of focusing control on wherever problems are detected. Another option is to focus on where rarer but more severe transmission problems might arise. WPV transmission in areas with better sanitation and hygiene might be less likely to experience outbreaks. If immunity has waned significantly in adults in these areas, however, the resulting outbreaks may be larger. Direction of surveillance efforts under this option is dependent upon model-based output that can specify the chances of large outbreaks. Recall that an AB model is required for such inferences. Another option policy makers might choose is not to institute new surveillance of nonparalytic infection until it is observed that apparent eradication based on paralytic polio surveillance led to a false determination of eradication. In this case, modelers might bring up the chances that not adding new nonparalytic case surveillance systems might lead to such widespread infection before an outbreak is detected and control of that outbreak might be exceedingly expensive. The step 1 choice might then be to seek inferences about the risks to ultimately successful polio eradication intrinsic to proceeding with only a paralytic poliomyelitis surveillance system.

Another possible policy maker decision might be that any surveillance beyond sewage testing should focus on populations where the last paralytic cases occurred. In this case, modelers might bring up dynamics issues about OPV transmission and boosting that could alter second infection transmission potential. Policy makers might then be more interested in determining how past frequency of paralytic cases is related to the potential for undetected circulation of WPV after initial elimination of WPV transmission.

A third possibility is that testing diarrhea cases in young children is the surveillance that would be most reasonable, as it would have other benefits to the patient in addition to polio eradication benefits. In this case, modelers might bring up the characteristics of symptomatic patients who are good sentinels for occult polio transmission. That might lead to the pursuit of inferences about whether older individuals with greater chances of waned immunity should be the focus of surveillance.

Whatever policy makers decide, these possibilities need to be discussed when meeting with modelers and addressed in the inferences the modelers pursue in order to ensure that modeling affects policy. The different classes of inferences suggested here would require very different modeling approaches. If the approach chosen does not address policy maker defined issues determined by their concepts, they are more likely to dismiss the model-based inferences as irrelevant.

Modeler Perspectives

We can also look at possible views of nonparalytic infection surveillance from the modeler's perspective. Modelers are likely to be academics who want to discover broad general scientific principles that advance the development of new methods and new theories. They might be interested in whether new theories and description of B-cell dynamics[42] can help predict waning patterns after infection. Thus, they might be particularly focused on estimating waning parameter values through the modeling they pursue. In particular, they might want to test whether the assumptions behind waning patterns in recent polio models are correct.[4,12-16] One assumption in those models is that maximal immunity is achieved after each live virus polio infection, whether a first or a subsequent infection or whether an OPV or a WPV infection. Violation of that assumption might affect whether vaccinations to control outbreaks in the end stage of polio eradication, especially nonparalytic outbreaks, should be directed to age groups other than those targeted by traditional special immunization activities. Pursuing these questions might be a more natural part of pursuing policy maker questions related to the risks from not instituting any new nonparalytic poliovirus surveillance.

The modelers might also have done previous work on how the synchrony of infections across geographic areas offers opportunities to elucidate fundamental parameters of transmission. This approach has been particularly productive for pertussis.[43] For polio, examining synchrony across areas that eliminated poliomyelitis early and those that only did so at the end could greatly increase the power to fit parameter values. To further advance the methodology they have developed, the modelers may be more strongly drawn to addressing questions related to what geographic areas should be targeted for nonparalytic infection detection. If, in contrast, the modelers have been primarily interested in how the natural history of infection affects transmission dynamics, they might be more strongly drawn to the question of what class of patients should be the target of surveillance.

Rather than engaging in a tug of war between policy makers' and modelers' interests, the modelers must accommodate the policy makers' interests. The choice of inference to be pursued must be the choice that will make the most difference to the populations on which the policy makers focus. There will be plenty of reasons for the modelers to pursue their own special interests as they go through inference robustness or identifiability loops in Fig. 25-2.

Pursuing Inference Robustness and Identifiability Loops

Modeling can be pursued to determine whether any nonparalytic polio surveillance beyond sewage testing is indicated. For simplicity of exposition, we dichotomize our outcome to say that current surveillance is either sufficient or it is not. Current surveillance consists of AFP surveillance and WPV detection in sewage systems. Suppose step 1 in Fig. 25-2 settles on the following criterion; note that this criterion requires the use of an AB model. If a model generates only outbreaks that are detected and controlled before a total of 2000 WPV infections occur in 99.5% of runs, then the decision is that current surveillance is sufficient. To answer this question, a model must have a variety of built-in control options that can be instituted given different levels of paralytic and nonparalytic infections in areas that correspond to the populations on which the policy makers focus. Also note that the key policy makers must be involved in setting such a criterion.

For step 2 in Fig. 25-2, building even the simplest possible model in either a DE or an AB framework will entail considerable work, but since this question focuses on the chances of a particularly bad outcome, only an AB model will work. However, to find out what model aspects do or do not need to be included, the initial inference robustness and identifiability loops should be conducted using DE models. For these initial DE explorations, a different criterion will have to be used; the DE model can use the size criterion, but it cannot use the frequency (99.5%) criterion.

Let us say that the first pass at examining this question uses the DE model published by Duintjer Tebbens et al.[13,14] with modifications that allow for introduced outbreaks and outbreak control measures. This model is shown in Fig. 25-3. It adds many dimensions to the compartmental flows seen in Fig. 25-1. It divides the natural history of infection and immunity into categories related to oropharyngeal infection and intestinal infection. It models the reversion of OPV back toward WPV and thus can address the emergence of circulating vaccine derived polioviruses (cVDPV). One reason for doing this is the persistent problem of type 2 cVDPV in Nigeria. These model elaborations are captured in flow diagrams[13] as seen in Fig. 25-3.

These extensive model elaborations add further realism to the model. They enable it to address issues like cVDPV dynamics that could not be addressed with simpler models. However, they have details that might not be needed so we might begin by dropping out model elements we think might not be needed. We can add

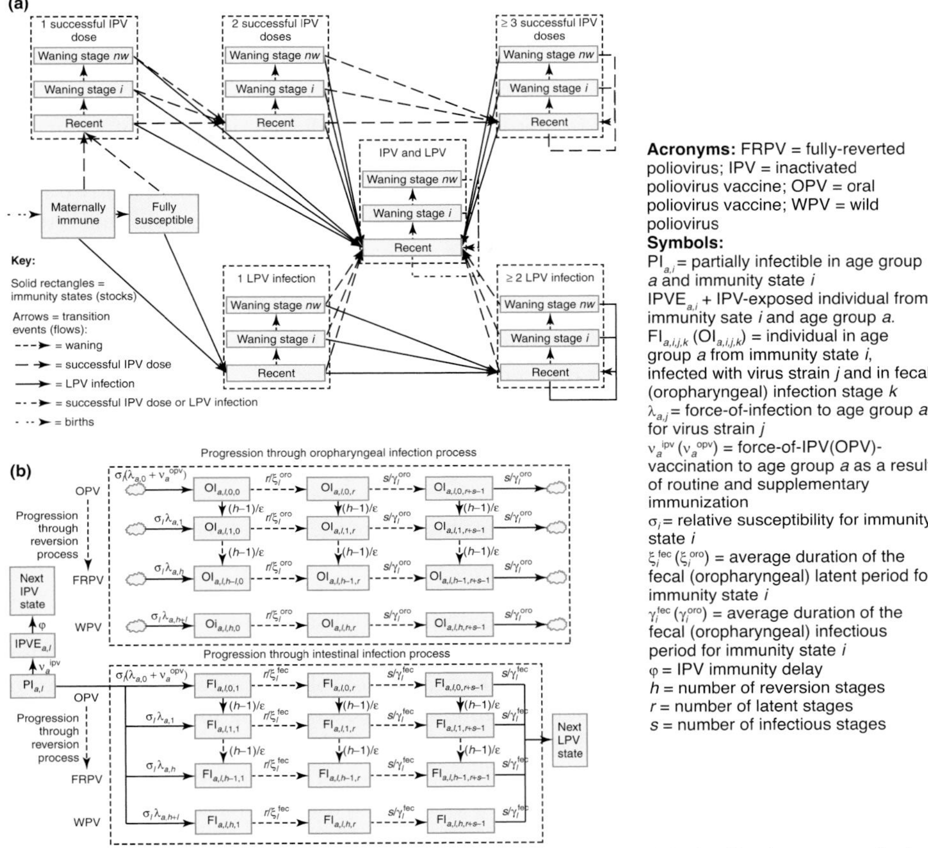

FIG. 25-3 A moderately complex deterministic compartmental model of polio virus transmission.[13] (a) Flows between immunity states as a result of epidemiological events. (b) Infection and reversion processes.

them back during IRA analyses. Even in their complex form, however, they leave the model with many highly unrealistic simplifying assumptions that would deserve evaluation through an IRA if the model were directed toward answering any of the three classes of specific policy inferences discussed earlier. In particular, the assumption that the population is homogeneous with regard to exposure to people or contaminated environments is both highly unrealistic and likely to affect the inferences sought. If a concern arises that special risk populations may be those most capable of circulating nonparalytic WPV, the elaboration of risk or geographic groups would be needed for IRA and for addressing basic policy inferences like where to focus nonparalytic WPV surveillance.

In step 3 of Fig. 25-2 the model space is constrained by the same data used in the original publication,[13] which are very general with overall vaccination and infection rates across broad populations. Suppose that constraining the parameter space so the model outcomes fit with these observed data leads to a model where no large, uncontrollable outbreaks occur anywhere in this parameter space. The decision process coming out of step 3 in this case would lead to “the inference is the same across parameter space”—current surveillance is sufficient to avoid catastrophic eradication failure. For this example we suppose that it is not the case that uncertainty in immune waning parameters leads to different inferences in different parts of feasible parameter space.

One should still question the robustness of this inference from this "simple" model because the model unrealistically assumes no variation in transmission risk between individuals and all individuals mix homogeneously. Geographic and socioeconomic variation in sanitation and hygiene conditions is inconsistent with this assumption. The potential for large outbreaks in this model could be less than in a model where sanitation varies by block or district. Before feeling confident in the inference that the current surveillance system is sufficient, modelers should relax the unrealistic simplifying assumptions that sanitation and mixing are homogeneous.

Relaxing these simplifying assumptions is best pursued using DE models, and there are two reasons why a DE framework for this particular IRA should be used before proceeding to the AB framework. One is the time and effort involved. The other is the potential to gain insights into the mechanisms by which a complex model generates different outcomes. To do so, modelers would add realistic details to the model little by little while exploring how those details generate effects on infection patterns. By exploring explanatory hypotheses of why their model generates different results and by examining in detail the dynamics that generate the observed results, modelers can come to understand what model characteristics explain different model behaviors.

In the inference robustness step 5 from Fig. 25-2, the modelers might add sanitation and contact pattern variation by geography and socioeconomic level. The parameter space for such variation might originally be quite broad. There is a high chance that in some of this parameter space catastrophic epidemics that threaten eradication after reintroduction of WPV are observed, meaning that special nonparalytic WPV surveillance systems are needed. In other words, the inference of low risk made using the simplest model would have been found to not be robust to realistically relaxing the unrealistic homogeneity assumptions. It also means that this latest iteration of step 4 in Fig. 25-2 leads to the need for a new identifiability analysis loop—step 6 in Fig. 25-2.

That lack of robustness on its own might lead to the decision to institute new nonparalytic WPV surveillance. However, it might not lead to such a policy if policy makers believe that the parameter space that leads to catastrophic outcomes is unlikely to exist in reality. In that case the lack of inference robustness could just lead to an identifiability analysis. One possible identifiability analysis would examine the effects of fitting model parameters to new data on geographical sanitation variation by district and to the original Indian data.[13] If it is expensive or politically difficult to get these data, a formal identifiability analysis would show the value of getting them and that the data could make a big difference to the inference in a cost-effective manner. That would lead to data collection and then to data fitting in a new step 3 of our iterative process.

If, in this new step 3, the parameter space is constrained to a region where the current surveillance system results in large outbreaks, then there would be strong reason to implement a new surveillance system for nonparalytic infections. Even if part of the parameter space does not produce large outbreaks, new insights from the modelers into transmission dynamics might convince policy makers that they should pursue new surveillance approaches. Performing an AB model analysis would help in this evaluation.

But, even with the new sanitation data, there would still be uncertainty, and nonparalytic infection detection surveillance could be quite expensive. Additional types of data might be collected to resolve this challenge. One particularly powerful type of data is genetic sequence data available from all WPV isolated in India for several years before elimination was achieved. Newly developed phylodynamic methods[44,45] could constrain parameter space enough to make the inference about the need for nonparalytic infection surveillance identifiable; these methods can use DE models.

Relationships among Surveillance Workers, Policymakers, and Modelers

One reason for describing this analytic path as elaborately as we have is to emphasize how important it is to specify the inference that will influence policy. If all of this work had been done but it turns out that policy makers would have always felt some pressure to set up surveillance for the detection of nonparalytic infection, the control decisions would not be much advanced by all this analysis. In that situation, the most influential and effective analysis would have been to specify in what populations or in what type of patients surveillance should take place. It would probably take an equal amount of modeling work to build the models needed for this inference as for the more general inference, and proceeding directly to this inference could have saved a lot of time and effort.

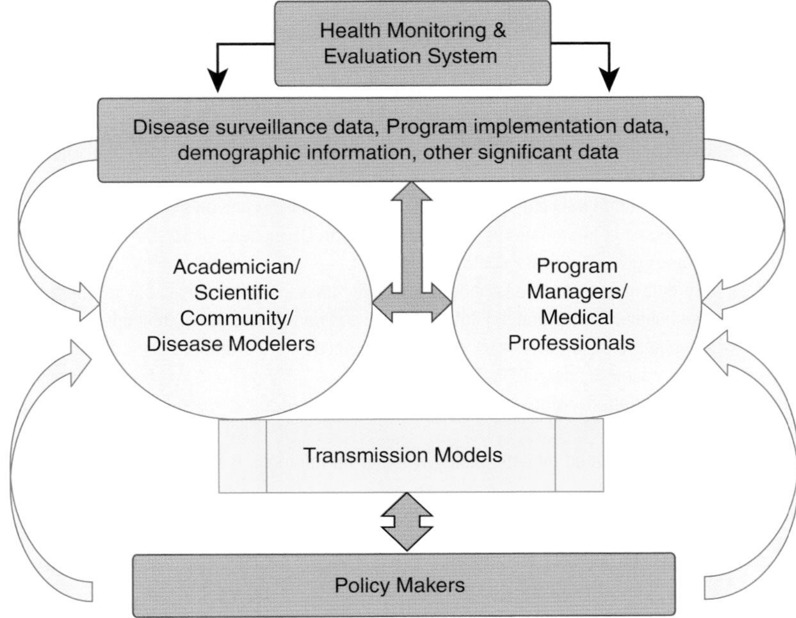

FIG. 25-4 Personnel relationships for integrating transmission modeling into surveillance systems.

Another reason for presenting the example in detail was to provide background about how important the structure of relationships between different classes of individuals is for achieving the goal of making surveillance inform effective prevention efforts. In Fig. 25-4, we revisit concepts regarding such relationships presented elsewhere in this book. The relationships between the groups in the central ellipses are central to integrating transmission models into surveillance systems, but the base of relationships that make such a system serve public health is supported and balanced by the inputs from policy makers. Policy makers can tip the system in one direction or the other. Without their input and collaboration, the system fails to serve public health. Policymakers must heavily influence the dialogue that determines what directions the system tips toward, and both modelers and others involved with public health surveillance must continually seek direction from policy makers.

EPILOGUE

We have presented an idealized vision of how a team of public health professionals and modelers can incorporate causal system modeling into disease control. From a science point of view, this vision is simply a scientific process that pushes theory about the way the real world is closer and closer to the complexity that characterizes the biology, ecology, and sociology that determine the health of populations. From a public health point of view, it is a path for continuous quality improvement in using public health data to guide disease prevention and control activities. From either perspective, the key to success is teamwork and good communication between individuals who might have different visions and goals.

Of course, the real world will not be so idealized. But there is no need to abandon this vision because an academic does not see public health practice as part of his or her research agenda or because a public health administrator sees this process as too difficult and theoretical to achieve within the bureaucratic agency structure. Practical progress may well involve initial pursuit of separate academic and public health practice goals while edging slowly toward a fuller integration of public health science and practice.

KEY SUMMARY POINTS

- Transmission models are built on a base of causal theory about how infection is transmitted and who transmits to whom and specifies needed variables like the number of individuals in different exposure or disease categories and needed parameters like the probability of transmission given contact between individuals or exposure to a source of pathogen.
- Differential equation (DE) models use continuous population segments. They are deterministic and easier to analyze by nonexperts using modern software.
- Agent-based (AB) models are stochastic in that they parameterize the chances of different events occurring. They can relax unrealistic assumptions about large population sizes or about contact patterns that are intrinsic to DE models. Unlike DE models, they can be analyzed to determine the chances of different outcomes given a disease control decision.
- Transmission modeling differs from data mining or traditional epidemiology analyses: mechanistic causal theory defines the variables used; analysis begins by examining model behavior to understand how variables and parameters generate model behavior; a formal process is used to determine what essential knowledge affects a decision; and causal inferences can be validated by inference robustness assessment.
- Transmission models increase policy makers' understanding of what processes generate transmission levels and how policies affect those processes. Models also use surveillance data to estimate parameter values and infer what control actions are favored, and they estimate the values of variables.
- Inferences about control actions can be validated by determining whether an inference is robust to realistic relaxation of simplifying model assumptions.
- The key step in using transmission models to inform public health decisions is to get policy makers, surveillance personnel, and modelers to agree on what inferences should be pursued using the models.

DISCUSSION QUESTIONS

1. Compare and contrast DE and AB models.
2. Describe what would influence the choice of either a DE model or an AB model for making a final determination of the costs and benefits of establishing a nonparalytic poliovirus infection surveillance system that tests specific patients receiving care for illnesses.
3. What makes DE models a good choice for initial analyses to make inferences about infection control decisions? What would lead to using an AB model? When would an AB model not be necessary and when would it be essential?
4. How can transmission models improve our knowledge and understanding of disease transmission?
5. What are the processes through which transmission modeling could change the focus of surveillance for polio eradication from paralytic infections to nonparalytic infections?
6. Why do we want transmission models to be as simple as possible but no simpler? Explain the criteria to determine how simple a model is, what it means to be as simple as possible, and why a simpler model can have a greater effect on public health actions.
7. What is the advantage of having a routine process for analyzing measles surveillance data with a transmission model every time a new summary of results from the surveillance system is prepared? What knowledge could be generated by such an analysis that would not be generated by routine descriptions of surveillance data? How could this knowledge inform policy?
8. What are advantages and difficulties of having policy makers run some analyses? What type of model analyses would be most important for policy makers to perform?
9. How would the analyses performed by surveillance personnel differ from analyses performed by academic modelers?
10. Describe a process to get policy makers, surveillance system personnel, and academic modelers to collaborate to make surveillance data maximally inform policy decisions. Be specific about who should take the lead on what kind of activities and what it would take for those activities to best inform policy choices.

REFERENCES

1. Definition provided by the chapter author.
2. Vaillant L. Probably approximately correct: nature's algorithms for learning and prospering in a complex world. New York: Basic Books; 2013. p. 195.
3. Ferrucci D, Brown E, Chu-Carroll J, Fan J, Gondek D, Kalyanpur AA, et al. Building Watson: an overview of the DeepQA project. AI Mag 2010;31(3): 59–79. [2010, Fall].
4. Mayer BT, Eisenberg JN, Henry CJ, Gomes MG, Ionides EL, Koopman JS. Successes and shortcomings of polio eradication: a transmission modeling analysis. Am J Epidemiol 2013;177(11):1236–45.
5. Koopman JS, Simon CP, Riolo CP. When to control endemic infections by focusing on high-risk groups. Epidemiology 2005;16(5):621–7.
6. GPEI, WHO. Polio Eradication and Endgame Strategic Plan 2013-2018 Global Polio Eradication Initiative World Health Organization, Executive Summary. 2013.
7. WHO. World Health Organization Polio Fact Sheet, <http://www.who.int/mediacentre/factsheets/fs114/en/>; 2013 [accessed 25 September 2015].
8. Shulman LM, Gavrilin E, et al. Molecular epidemiology of silent introduction and sustained transmission of wild poliovirus type 1, Israel, 2013. Euro Surveill 2014;19(7):207–09.
9. CDC. Progress toward poliomyelitis eradication - Nigeria, January 2012-September 2013. MMWR Morb Mortal Wkly Rep 2013;62(49):1009–1013.
10. WHO. Wild poliovirus in Cameroon. <http://www.who.int/csr/don/2013/11/21/en>; 2013 [accessed 25 September 2015].
11. WHO. Performance of acute flaccid paralysis (AFP) surveillance and incidence of poliomyelitis, 2013. Wkly Epidemiol Rec 2013;88(49):528–31.
12. Thompson KM. Modeling poliovirus risks and the legacy of polio eradication. Risk Anal 2013;33(4):505–15.
13. Duintjer Tebbens RJ, Pallansch MA, Kalkowska DA, Wassilak SG, Cochi SL, Thompson KM. Characterizing poliovirus transmission and evolution: insights from modeling experiences with wild and vaccine-related polioviruses. Risk Anal 2013;33(4):703–49.
14. Duintjer Tebbens RJ, Pallansch MA, Kim JH, Burns CC, Kew OM, Oberste MS, et al. Oral poliovirus vaccine evolution and insights relevant to modeling the risks of circulating vaccine-derived polioviruses (cVDPVs). Risk Anal 2013;33(4):680–702.
15. Thompson KM, Pallansch MA, Duintjer Tebbens RJ, Wassilak SG, Kim JH, Cochi SL. Preeradication vaccine policy options for poliovirus infection and disease control. Risk Anal 2013;33(4):516–43.
16. Thompson KM, Pallansch MA, Tebbens RJ, Wassilak SG, Cochi SL. Modeling population immunity to support efforts to end the transmission of live polioviruses. Risk Anal 2013;33(4):647–63.
17. Box GEP, Jenkins GM. Time series analysis: forecasting & control. San Francisco: Holden-Day; 1970.
18. Breto C, He D, Edwards LI, King AA. Time series analysis via mechanistic models. Ann Appl Stat 2009;3:319–48.
19. He D, Ionides EL, King AA. Plug-and-play inference for disease dynamics: measles in large and small populations as a case study. J R Soc Interface 2010;7(43):271–83.
20. Ionides EL, Breto C, King AA. Inference for nonlinear dynamical systems. Proc Natl Acad Sci U S A 2006;103(49):18438–43.
21. Andrieu C, Doucet A, Holenstein R. Particle Markov chain Monte Carlo methods. J R Stat Soc B 2010;72(3):269–342.
22. Wood SN. Statistical inference for noisy nonlinear ecological dynamic systems. Nature 2010;466(7310):1102–4.
23. Toni T, Welch D, Strelkowa N, Ipsen A, Stumpf MP. Approximate Bayesian computation scheme for parameter inference and model selection in dynamical systems. J R Soc Interface 2009;6(31):187–202.
24. Kendall BE, Ellner SP, McCauley E, Wood SN, Briggs CJ, Murdoch WW, et al. Population cycles in the pine looper moth: dynamical tests of mechanistic hypotheses. Ecol Monogr 2005;75(2):259–76.
25. King AA, Ionides EL, Breto C, Ellner SP, Kendall BE. Pomp: statistical inference for partially observed Markov processes, <http://kingaa.github.io/pomp/>; 2009 [accessed 25 September 2015].
26. Laneri K, Bhadra A, Ionides EL, Bouma M, Dhiman RC, Yadav RS, et al. Forcing versus feedback: epidemic malaria and monsoon rains in northwest India. PLoS Comput Biol 2010;6(9):e1000898.
27. Roy M, Bouma MJ, Ionides EL, Dhiman RC, Pascual M. The potential elimination of Plasmodium vivax malaria by relapse treatment: insights from a transmission model and surveillance data from NW India. PLoS Negl Trop Dis 2013;7(1):e1979.
28. King AA, Ionides EL, Pascual M, Bouma MJ. Inapparent infections and cholera dynamics. Nature 2008;454(7206):877–80.
29. Blackwood JC, Cummings DA, Broutin H, Iamsirithaworn S, Rohani P. Deciphering the impacts of vaccination and immunity on pertussis epidemiology in Thailand. Proc Natl Acad Sci U S A 2013;110(23):9595–600.
30. Shrestha S, Foxman B, Weinberger DM, Steiner C, Viboud C, Rohani P. Identifying the interaction between influenza and pneumococcal pneumonia using incidence data. Sci Transl Med 2013;5(191):191ra84.
31. Koopman JS. Infection transmission science and models. Jpn J Infect Dis 2005;58(6):S3–8.
32. Koopman J. Modeling infection transmission. Annu Rev Public Health 2004;25:303–26.
33. Audoly S, Bellu G, D'Angio L, Saccomani MP, Cobelli C. Global identifiability of nonlinear models of biological systems. IEEE Trans Biomed Eng 2001;48(1):55–65.
34. Hengl S, Kreutz C, Timmer J, Maiwald T. Data-based identifiability analysis of non-linear dynamical models. Bioinformatics 2007;23(19):2612–8.
35. Jacquez JA, Greif P. Numerical parameter identifiability and estimability: integrating identifiability, estimability, and optimal sampling design. Math Biosci 1985;77(1):201–27.
36. Jacquez JA, Perry T. Parameter estimation: local identifiability of parameters. Am J Physiol 1990;258(4):E27–36.
37. Komorowski M, Costa MJ, Rand DA, Stumpf MPH. Sensitivity, robustness, and identifiability in stochastic chemical kinetics models. Proc Natl Acad Sci U S A 2011;108(21):8645–50.
38. Meshkat N, Eisenberg M, Distefano JJ. An algorithm for finding globally identifiable parameter combinations of nonlinear ode models using Groebner bases. Math Biosci 2009;222(2):61–72.
39. Raue A, Kreutz C, Maiwald T, Bachmann J, Schilling M, Klingmuller U, et al. Structural and practical identifiability analysis of partially observed dynamical models by exploiting the profile likelihood. Bioinformatics 2009;25(15):1923–9.
40. WHO. WHO statement on the meeting of the International Health Regulations Emergency Committee concerning the international spread of wild poliovirus. <http://www.who.int/mediacentre/news/statements/2014/polio-20140505/en/>; 2014 [accessed 25 September 2015].
41. Gomes MG, White LJ, Medley GF. The reinfection threshold. J Theor Biol 2005;236(1):111–3.
42. Tarlinton D, Good-Jacobson K. Diversity among memory B cells: origin, consequences, and utility. Science 2013;341(6151):1205–11.
43. Rohani P, Zhong X, King AA. Contact Network Structure Explain the Changing Epidemiology of Pertussis. Science 2010;330(6006):982–5.
44. Volz EM, Ionides E, Romero-Severson EO, Brandt MG, Mokotoff E, Koopman JS. HIV-1 transmission during early infection in men who have sex with men: a phylodynamic analysis. PLoS Med 2013;10(12):e1001568; discussion e.
45. Volz EM. Complex population dynamics and the coalescent under neutrality. Genetics 2012;190(1):187–201.

CHAPTER

26

Using Genetic Sequence Data for Public Health Surveillance

James S Koopman, Betsy Foxman

Knowledge leads us from the simple to the complex; wisdom leads us from the complex to the simple.

Anonymous

KEY WORDS

Genotype
Pathogen sequence data
Phylodynamics
Modeling
Genetic surveillance systems
Population sequence patterns
PulsedNet
Multilocus sequence testing
Genetic sequence data
Coalescent theory
Flow model phylogeography
Analytic phylodynamics

INTRODUCTION

Over the past two decades, classifying pathogens based on genetic sequence (genotype) has become standard practice in most public health surveillance systems. To **genotype** is to characterize phenotypes (e.g., physical traits) by determining variations in genetic markers of an organism.[1] Now, technological advances are propelling us into an era of massive genetic data availability at dramatically falling costs. Rather than classification based on differences in frequency of restriction sites across the genome (such as used by PulseNet), it is possible to rapidly and economically sequence parts or the entire genome of viruses, bacteria, and fungi. **Pathogen sequence data** are a record of the whole genomic sequence for pathogens studied for identification of genes whose expression triggers disease in host organisms.[1] For current surveillance systems, these data increase the discrimination of classification at reduced cost, enhancing detection of outbreaks, and local transmission patterns. But when analyzed with new methods to be discussed in this chapter, sequence databases provide new power to understand the complex systems and evolutionary phenomena generating infection transmission. This leads in turn to new power to inform public health decisions at every level.

This new power helps refocus control actions from factors that increase the risks of susceptible individuals for getting infected to factors that increase the spread of infections from infected individuals and to social and structural factors that affect the flow of infection through populations. Routine surveillance data analyses can only make inferences about the characteristics of individuals who increase their chances of getting infected. Analyzing genetic data with the analytic phylodynamic methods discussed later in this chapter can make inferences about the characteristics of individuals involved in transmitting infection[2,3] and about how contact patterns and risk behavior dynamics affect the flow of transmission through a population. Infection control strategies that focus only on infection risks miss major opportunities to stop transmission. Focusing prevention on contagiousness characteristics can be a highly effective control strategy, especially when focused on groups that are major disseminators of infection in a population.[4] Similarly, intervening on structural factors affecting the flow of infection through population, such as sanitation, hygiene, or crowding conditions, has long been recognized to be more effective than intervening on individual factors. While such structural factors can be deduced from either routine surveillance or genetic sequence surveillance, a deeper understanding of their role within overall transmission systems can be obtained when sequences are available. Thus, analyzing genetic surveillance data with transmission models (see Chapter 25) significantly increases the potential to find effective control strategies. **Disease transmission modeling** is conducted using a mathematical causal system model representing infection transmission.[1]

We present a framework in this chapter that allows genetic systems analysts to serve health officials. One foundation for that framework is infection transmission system analysis as discussed in Chapter 25. Transmission system models informed by genetic sequence data have the potential to clarify key complexities in infection patterns, explain why infection patterns vary among populations, and guide control activities. **Genetic sequence data** are a nearly complete genomic record of an organism studied for identification of genes and mechanics for gene expression.[1] Sequence data alone, however, are insufficient. Genetic data need to be linked to surveillance data to establish at least some of the person, time, place, and risk factor exposures of the hosts whose pathogens are sequenced. **Genetic pathogen surveillance** is surveillance of genetic markers in pathogens that can facilitate early detection of outbreaks or clusters through investigation of genetic divergence in chains of transmission, and characterize expression of pathogen behaviors and traits such as antimicrobial resistance.[1]

To illustrate our vision of what the course forward should be, we will describe how genetic sequence data can guide control of two different infections with markedly different epidemiologic and evolutionary patterns. The first is the human immunodeficiency virus (HIV), a leading indicator of the potential of this field.[5] We believe that well-focused control actions, guided by genetic sequence analyses, will first reduce and then eradicate HIV transmission. We will then consider influenza for which the methods we advocate have also made remarkable inroads toward more effective control. While these two ribonucleic acid (RNA) viruses are leading examples of success in the methods we will describe, all pathogen control can benefit from these methods.

HOW GENETIC PATTERNS CARRY INFORMATION ABOUT TRANSMISSION

The genetic sequences of pathogens carry the history of their particular path to the current host. That path cannot be read directly from a single sequence. It must be inferred by comparing large numbers of sequences. A surprising amount of history can be inferred from a small number of sequences because the most recent common ancestor of every pair of sequences can be inferred. Increasing the number of hosts sequenced and the number of pathogens sequenced within each host increases the amount of information that can be extracted. The information arises because every time a pathogen reproduces there is some change in the sequence and most of that change is carried across transmissions.

Fig. 26-1 illustrates the transmission tree for an infection with a constant endemic prevalence. It has many chains of transmission that die out and some that are carried on. The sequences of individuals at one point in time are sequenced resulting in the coalescent tree shown. Transmission events that involve transmission of only a small fraction of the viruses in a host represent bottleneck events that fix some small part of the sequence variation that arose in the source host in a new host. That is a major reason why genetic trees reflect transmission trees. The shape of a coalescent tree depends upon the growth rate of infections in the population as illustrated in Fig. 26-2 for the comparison between the constant growth rate in Fig. 26-1 and an exponential growth rate as seen at the start of a new epidemic.

When characteristics of the hosts from which sequences are obtained are known, the location of different classes of individuals on the genetic trees reflects the mixing patterns between classes of individuals with those characteristics as illustrated in Fig. 26-3. Information about when an individual was infected and how long they remained infectious can add greatly to the amount of transmission system information that can be extracted from sequences. The situation where sequences on a high fraction of cases are available is illustrated in Fig. 26-4 with genetic trees

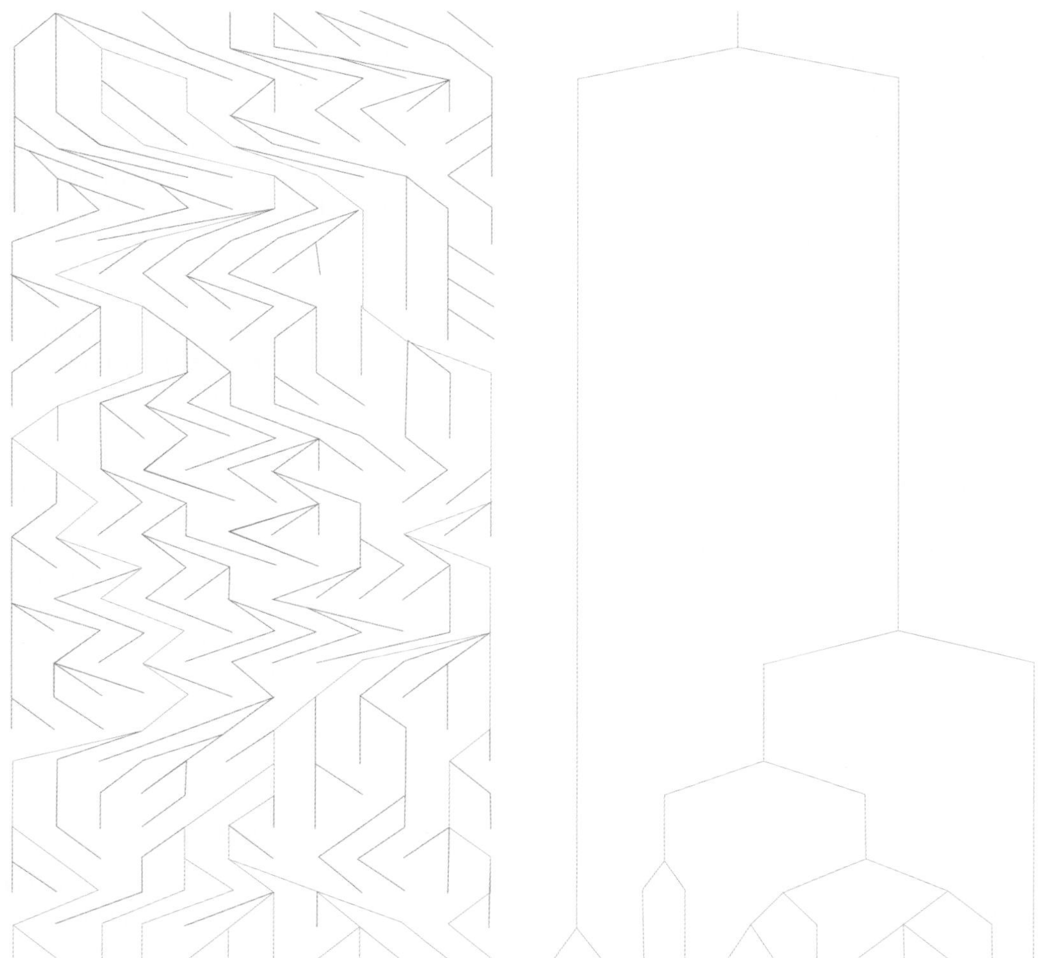

FIG. 26-1 The chance die out of some transmission chains during endemic transmission produces a coalescent tree.

both within and between hosts. In this case, the coalescent tree does not exactly reflect transmission trees so methods not using the coalescent must be used to correctly extract the transmission history.

ANALYTIC FRAMEWORKS FOR INFECTION CONTROL USING PATHOGEN GENETIC SEQUENCES

The analytic frameworks for pathogen genetic sequence data can be grouped into descriptive uses and system analysis uses (Table 26-1). Descriptive uses include classification of pathogens into groups for outbreak detection and for characterizing evolution and transmission patterns. Systems analysis uses include using sequence data to model population dynamics, pathogen flows between populations, and infection transmission systems. The division between descriptive and systems analysis uses is determined by whether the analysis model employed describes a theory-based system for population pathogen behavior. Descriptive analyses are well established, while systems analysis uses are emerging rapidly as the genetic data get more complete, software to handle those data improves, and new theoretical frameworks for using those data to make important inferences are developed.

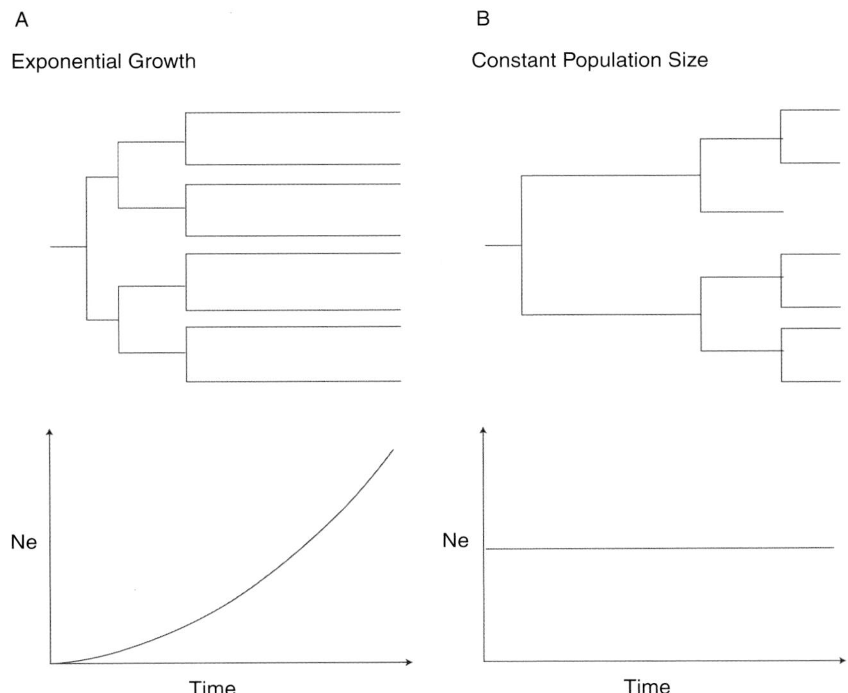

FIG. 26-2 The coalescent tree has different shapes depending on the infection growth history. (*Source:* Volz EM, Koelle K, Bedford T. Viral phylodynamics. PLoS Comput Biol 2013;9(3):e1002947.)

DESCRIPTIVE USES OF GENETIC SEQUENCE DATA

Pathogen Classification Analyses

Pathogen classification analyses use sequence data to group pathogens for epidemiologic analyses. Multilocus sequence testing (MLST) was established with this classification purpose in mind. **MLST** sequences a set of housekeeping genes with slow rates of change to characterize bacterial and parasitic pathogens.[1] The initial logic leading to MLST employed analytical models that assumed all microbial evolution was characterized by a series of clonal expansions.[6] The job of MLST was to identify such clones. We now know that microbial evolution is more of a continuous process with evolution within and between hosts involving processes of diversification and selection. The choice of sequences with slow evolutionary clock rates makes the sequence data look like a set of clones. But the continuous process of change outside of these slow clock genome segments makes the clone definitions seem arbitrary. Analyses of MLST classes that relate them to epidemiologic variables can nonetheless make them valuable.

Phylogenetic analyses of whole genomes are now replacing MLST and other genotyping methods. Given an extensive phylogenetic tree of a population of microbes, one can choose any level of aggregation or refinement of the tree to classify microbes. Fig. 26-5 shows genetic clusters defined by different levels of depth in a genetic tree. The cluster size distribution depends strongly on the depth of the tree chosen to define clusters. For illustration purposes, a small tree is presented. Epidemiologic relationships indicating useful classification criteria might be found at any level.

Classification is used to characterize pathogens with different origins, geographic patterns, natural histories and prognoses, treatment needs, control potential, or transmission routes. Subtype classifications lead to a fuller understanding of transmission patterns and evolution of almost every type of pathogen. Due to the high dimensionality of sequence data, sequence types can be repeatedly refined and then more meaningfully aggregated. This enables existing sequence databases to gain power as new theory is developed that implicates new pathogen characteristics involved in either pathogenesis or transmission. The current rise of pathogen sequence surveillance databases is motivated by the ability to use sequences for classification and is driven by these cost and flexibility considerations.

Characterizing genetic strain patterns without analyzing infection flows can be very informative for public health decision-making, especially in the case of polio, where single introduction events are important. For example, the characterization of genetic patterns over time for polio in Ghana demonstrated how the process of local eradication was related to vaccination efforts and how recrudescence of infection later on was not due to occult circulation of asymptomatic infections but rather introduction from known infection foci outside of the country.[7]

Genetic microbial classification focusing on specific functional capacities can be especially informative, revealing the emergence of resistance to therapy or the emergence of transmissibility or pathogenicity. An interesting pathogenicity case involves the surveillance of live polio vaccines in sewage. A set of genetic changes that transform vaccines back into transmissible pathogens have been identified.[8] Identifying vaccines in sewage with these changes helps identify the emerging threats from circulating vaccine-derived polioviruses (cVDPV). When viruses with these genetic changes are found, it means that cVDPV have transmitted so extensively in a population that they have had time to accumulate mutations making them both more virulent and more transmissible. Polio eradication using the current World Health Organization (WHO) strategies requires that vaccine viruses be transmitted from

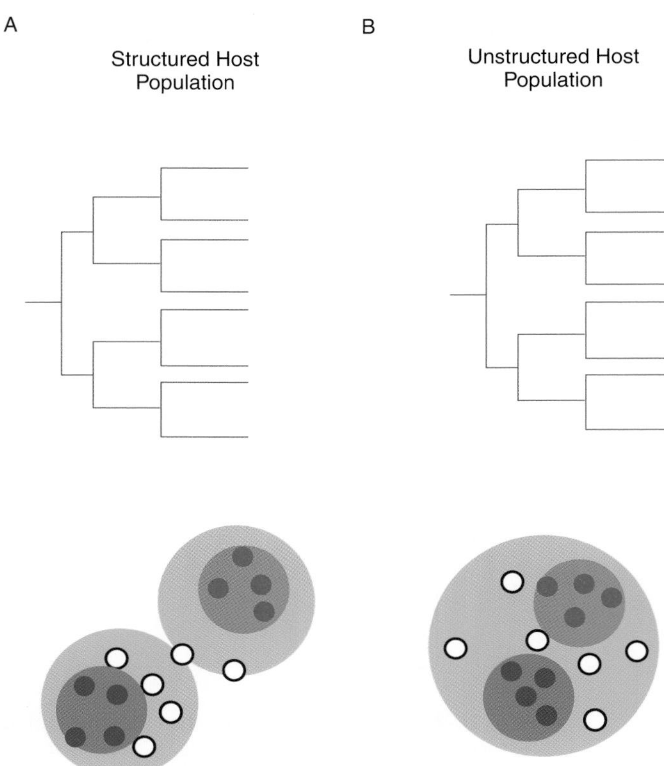

FIG. 26-3 Genetic patterns reflect the mixing patterns generating infection transmissions. (*Source:* Volz EM, Koelle K, Bedford T. Viral phylodynamics. PLoS Comput Biol 2013;9(3):e1002947.)

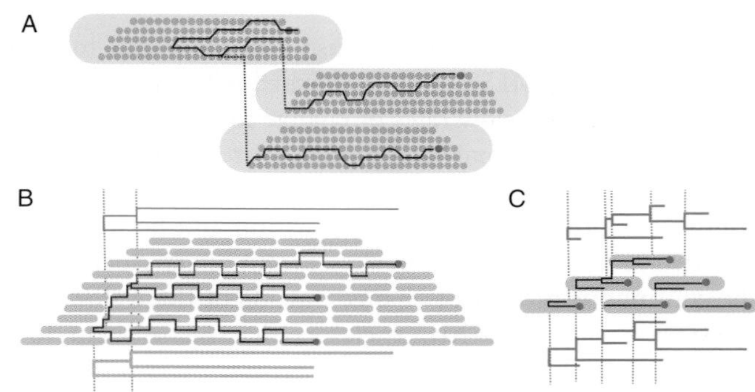

FIG. 26-4 Genetic trees depend upon evolution within and between hosts and on sampling densities. (*Source*: Ypma RJ, van Ballegooijen WM, Wallinga J. Relating phylogenetic trees to transmission trees of infectious disease outbreaks. Genetics 2013;195(3):1055–62)

TABLE 26-1 Analytic Frameworks for Infection Control using Pathogen Genetic Sequences

USE OF SEQUENCE DATA	ANALYTIC OBJECTIVES	IMPLEMENTATION SETTINGS
Descriptive Uses of Genetic Sequence Data		
Classification: group pathogens by genetic sequence patterns	Epidemiologic risk assessments	Well established and growing rapidly in health departments
Descriptive phylodynamics: relate evolution patterns and transmission and disease patterns	Infer how evolutionary patterns explain epidemiologic patterns and vice versa	Still mainly in academic settings or major national agencies
Systems Analysis Uses of Genetic Sequence Data		
Basic coalescent theory: model simple population dynamics using genetic data	Insight into past histories of endemic or epidemic infection	Academic settings or major national agencies
Flow model phylogeography: model pathogen flows between populations	Insight into local or worldwide patterns of disease spread	Academic settings or major national agencies
Analytic phylodynamics: model infection transmission systems	Inferences on biological, social, behavioral, and system determinants of infection flow	Very new and currently only applied in academic settings

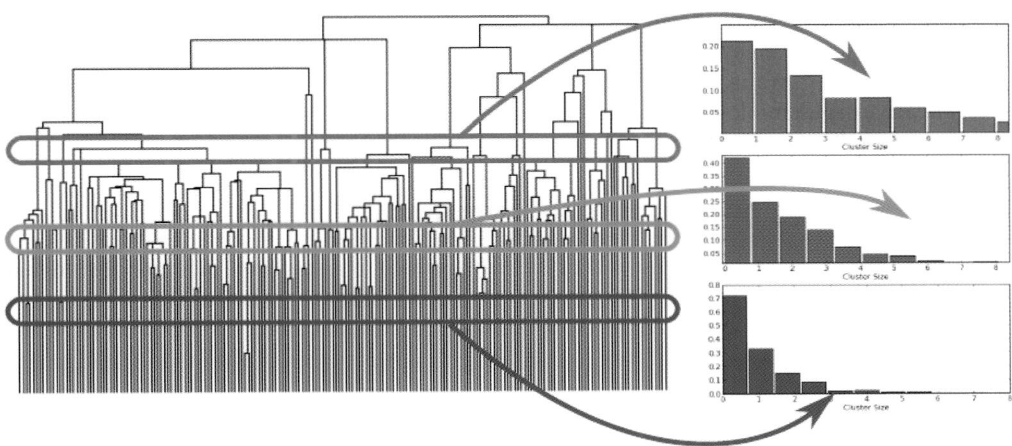

FIG. 26-5 Illustration of making different cluster definitions resulting in different distributions of cluster sizes by defining different depths in a genetic tree. (*Source:* Volz E, Romero-Severson EO, Alam SJ, Stephens DA, Brenner BG, Wainberg MA, Roger M, Koopman JS. Complex epidemiological dynamics generate phylogenetic clustering of HIV in Montreal. Presented at Epidemics 2 - Second International Conference on Infectious Diseases Dynamics 2009, Athens, Greece.).

vaccine recipients to others in the population such that individuals with waning immunity have their immunity boosted by vaccine virus infections. Without such transmission, immunity can wane to the point that wild poliovirus (WPV) transmission can be sustained by individuals who were previously infected or successfully vaccinated (see chapter 25). Vaccine virus transmission, however, presents the threat of emerging virulence in cVDPV so that sewage surveillance for specific genetic changes associated with virulence has become crucial to the eradication effort. Detection of pathogenicity mutations in sewage can lead to focused control actions before cVDPV becomes a more serious problem.[8]

An interesting transmission case where gene sequences show evolution toward increased transmissibility occurs for influenza. Human infections with bird flu strains can be highly pathogenic but they do not spread from human to human. Identifying genetic changes that facilitate human-to-human transmission provides a basis for surveillance to indicate whether a strain is evolving toward greater transmissibility.[9]

Descriptive Phylodynamics

Currently, almost all microbial genetic surveillance is motivated by the classification uses just discussed. The value of sequences is only partially realized, however, by using them for classification; their greater value lies in advancing descriptions and theory about patterns of pathogen spread through populations. Phylodynamics emerged in the twenty-first century as the study of how the interactions among epidemiologic, immunological, and evolutionary processes lead to phylogenies.[10] **Phylodynamics** analyzes how the evolution of pathogens and immune responses to pathogens relate to dynamic patterns of infection within hosts or across populations.[11] Through analysis of phylogenic trees, phylodynamics gives insight into various epidemiologic phenomena such as endemic versus epidemic dynamics, host population structure, and immunological selection processes.[12] Descriptions of tree shapes for pathogens from a defined population thus facilitate hypothesis generation and testing regarding these phenomena.

Descriptive phylodynamic analyses use phylogenetic relationships more fully than classification analyses that describe geographic, age, and risk group relationships related to the spread of infection. Descriptive phylodynamic analyses commonly use a basic unit of measure that reflects genetic distances between individual strains rather than just strain categorization. Specifying the time when a pathogen emerged or became newly epidemic can be an important objective of descriptive phylodynamics. Because descriptive phylodynamic analyses describe more detailed patterns of different pathogen strains over time than classification analyses, they provide a fuller description of how genetic patterns relate to epidemiologic patterns. This greater detail helps investigators develop and test new lines of epidemiologic and phylodynamic theory.

SYSTEMS ANALYSIS USES OF GENETIC SEQUENCE DATA

Systems analyses use formal mathematical models of causal processes to assess and elaborate phylodynamic theory. They integrate evolutionary models used in phylogenetic analyses with models describing the forces spreading infection in populations and fit these to observed genetic patterns. Most studies to date are of viruses, which have sufficient genetic variation with enough overall genome stability to make the task easier than with bacteria. Bacterial genomes are more complicated because they have many insertions and deletions, homologous recombinations, and mobile genetic elements.[13] Moreover, there are more sources of false-positive and false-negative reads with regard to these sources of genetic variation. The expense and work involved for bacteria means that most systems analyses using genetic sequence data to date are for viruses, but that should change over the next decade.[12,14]

Phylodynamic theory explains how the forces affecting pathogen evolution in individuals and in populations affect the spread of infection over time and the patterns of genetic sequences that result from those forces.[1] Pathogen sequences in a human population evolve under the influence of transmission because transmission represents a bottleneck in the pathogen population; only a small number of pathogens are transmitted from the larger population that has grown and accumulated genetic changes within a host. This bottleneck promotes sequence drift because only a small part of the diversity in viable genomes evolving in a host is transmitted to a new host.[15] Because of this drift, sequences in each host can be related to the sequences of other infected hosts to describe high-dimensional clustering patterns that reflect the flow of infection throughout a population. Bottlenecks also occur in infection flow at levels within and above the individual. For example, in foot-and-mouth disease virus, these bottlenecks help genetic sequences reflect infection flow at tissue, individual, farm, and region levels. Thus, systems analyses of infection flow dynamics are possible at all of these levels.[15] Many infections have similar potential for hierarchical systems analyses.

In the bottom part of Table 26-1, we distinguish three types of models representing three levels of theory that use genetic sequences to analyze and estimate the forces spreading infection in populations. These are presented in the order of the realism they add to processes generating infection levels and patterns in a population. These divisions organize concepts useful for our exposition on how systems models can be fit to genetic data.

Basic Coalescent Theory

Basic coalescent theory[16] uses a simple Wright–Fisher model of neutral evolution to construct continuous entity models of the processes by which separate lines of evolution converge in the direction from the present to the past. The assumptions allowing for continuity entail a further assumption that the sample of cases whose sequences are analyzed represents a small fraction of all cases. **Coalescent analyses** make inferences about broad populations from relatively small numbers of samples since each pair in a sample reflects a unique path back to a most recent common ancestor.[1] Coalescent analyses use the information extracted all the way back on these paths to infer population size over time. They are commonly used to describe the past sizes of pathogen populations across human populations.

Coalescent theory inferred sizes of microbial populations are often interpreted in terms of incidence and prevalence of human infection. But because the simple population models used do not correspond to the true processes generating population dynamics, the incidence and prevalence estimates can represent extreme distortions from true incidence and prevalence.[17] One perspective on this distortion is that it arises because a simple model is used that is highly unrealistic and even gross characteristics of the population size patterns generated may not be robust to realistic relaxation of the simple model assumptions. Regardless of this limitation, coalescent analyses allow us to get some vision of past histories of endemic or epidemic infections for which we had no information previously. Hepatitis C in Egypt is a classic and highly useful illustration of coalescent analysis that allowed for the inference of epidemic spread arising undetected in the past from a suddenly higher transmission.[18] In this case, injections related to schistosomiasis control programs were implicated. Other coalescent analyses in different countries with different strains showed different epidemiologic behaviors. Most, however, had epidemics rising in the twentieth century and seem likely to be related to blood transfusions and needle sharing.[19]

Flow Model Phylogeography

Flow model phylogeography is a second level of systems analysis with genetic data that fit models of pathogen flows between populations without modeling the transmission system processes behind these flows.[20-23] Most often, phylogeographic models do not detail population pathogen size, incidence, or prevalence in the populations between which flow is modeled. If they do, they use the simple population models of coalescent theory to do so. They parameterize genetic flows between populations but not human flows that may either carry an infection elsewhere or pick up an infection and bring it back home. The literature on pathogen phylogeography using genetic flow models is large and growing rapidly. Descriptions of influenza flow have been particularly informative and have influenced control actions relating to pandemic control and vaccination. This will be discussed later in this chapter when we use influenza to illustrate the major chapter messages.

Analytic Phylodynamics

Analytic phylodynamics is a third level of systems analyses. It fits models of infection transmission systems to genetic sequence data.[1] Transmission models relax simplifying assumptions in the simple population models usually used for coalescent analyses. They do the same for the infection flow processes of phylogeographic models.

Coalescent theory provides one framework for fitting transmission models to genetic data.[19,24] Multitype birth–death process formulations provide another.[25] Several different groups are working to develop new methods that go beyond these. A virtue of all these new methods for fitting transmission system models to genetic sequence data is that the model parameters and structures allow one to make inferences about the characteristics of infected individuals that make them highly contagious and the characteristics of populations that facilitate the flow infection. Standard surveillance analyses, in contrast, only allow for inferences about what makes individuals more prone to infection.

A significant advance that enables fitting transmission models to genetic data involves a formulation that translates the continuous processes in differential equation (DE) models (see Chapter 25), which are in the past to future direction into the coalescent model direction of present to past that captures coalescent events.[24] This formulation is able to capture the likelihoods of different trees. Thus it facilitates estimation. The framework for a formulation of this type that was used to estimate the fraction of transmissions from different stages of HIV infection[3] is presented in Fig. 26-6. The statistical advances discussed in Chapter 25 for fitting dynamic system models to surveillance data can be adapted to this framework.

Using transmission models facilitates inference robustness assessments in ways that phylogeographic models and standard coalescent models cannot. The amorphousness of the classic coalescent model and the failure to specify transmission events in phylogeographic models makes the path to relaxing simplifying assumptions unclear. In contrast, the wealth of experience with transmission system models provides many more established avenues to determine whether realistic relaxation of simplifying model assumptions will change a key inference.

This model formulation flexibility is illustrated by a phylodynamics study of dengue in Vietnam that used progressively more realistic models and methods.[26] A standard coalescent approach to the genetic sequence data (the Bayesian Skyline plot in the BEAST software) did not come close to reproducing the temporal pattern of dengue hospitalizations over a 7-year period. Using an SIR (susceptible, infectious, recovered) model of transmission had

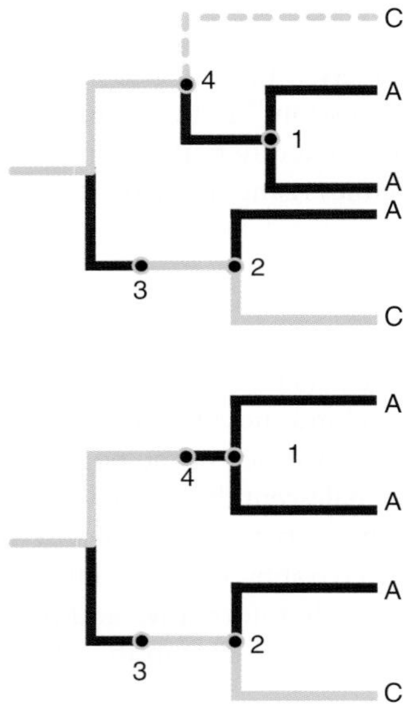

A simple gene genealogy that could be generated by an HIV model. Dark branches with taxa labeled A correspond to stage-1 (early/acute infected hosts). Ligyht branches with taxa labeled C correspond to stage-2 (chronic infections). Event 1 represents the coalescence of two lineages corresponding to early acute infection. Event 2 represents coalescence of an early and a late infection. Even 3 represents the stage transition of an early infection to a late infection. Event 4 represents the transmission by a late infection which is not ancestral to the sample. Top: Includes an unsampled lineage (dashed). Middle: The unsampled lineage has been pruned from the tree. The point where the lineage is pruned corresponds to event 4. The number of lineages as a function of time (NLFT) which correspond to a host with early/acute infection (black) or chronic infection (grey).

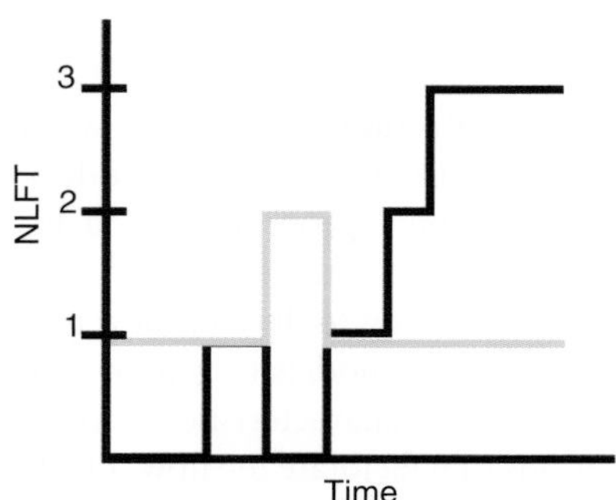

FIG. 26-6 A framework allowing for differential equation models to capture transmission tree likelihoods. (*Source:* Volz EM, Koopman JS, Ward MJ, Brown AL, Frost SD. Simple epidemiological dynamics explain phylogenetic clustering of HIV from patients with recent infection. PLoS Comput Biol 2012;8(6):e1002552.)

minimal effect in improving the pattern. Adding mosquito vectors into the model did, however, make a large improvement, as did adding spatial details or both vectors and spatial details. Note that the only data used in these analyses are the genetic data. The import of this demonstration is that the genetic data are clearly informative to the underlying transmission dynamics, but inferences from such analyses are valid only when model formulations are sufficiently realistic. The inference robustness assessment methods presented in Chapter 25 are needed to validate the inferences by realistically relaxing simplifying assumptions.

The direction for future analyses, however, is not to use genetic data alone, as in this dengue analysis; all data sources that could be informative and strengthen inferences should be used. As commented above, genetic data analyzed with transmission models can make inferences about who is doing the infecting that routine surveillance data cannot—but routine surveillance data may be better able to establish the time course of population infection patterns than genetic data. If the time is short between infection and when the samples sequenced are obtained, and if samples are collected continuously over time, timing will be well established. But for chronic infections where the time when the sequence is obtained can be quite long after transmission, other data that can help establish timing will be helpful. The HIV example discussed later provides an example of how that can proceed.

TYPES OF GENETIC SEQUENCE DATA AND DIFFERENCES IN THEIR ANALYSIS

The two basic types of sequence data are consensus and deep sequence data, some characteristics of these that are relevant to phylodynamic analyses are presented in Table 26-2. Consensus sequences read the dominant nucleotide at each base pair site even though the sample being read may have some strands of sequence that differ from the dominant base pair pattern. If there is a high fraction of nucleotide differences at a base pair site, a consensus read calls that site ambiguous. All of what have been called "next generation" sequences provides deep sequences that indicate how many reads there are for each nucleotide at each base pair site. Almost all new sequence data are now data from deep sequencing. Sometimes these data are summarized, however, as consensus sequences. To date, all analytic phylodynamic studies have been conducted using consensus sequences. But deep sequences, with properties we will describe, should increase the power of analytic phylodynamic studies to fit transmission model parameters.

A basic difference between consensus and deep sequences is that the former only allow for genetic tree inferences between hosts, while the latter can help make within host inferences. In either case, however, the validity and preciseness of genetic tree inferences will be improved by greater accuracy and a greater number of base pairs that are read.

TABLE 26-2 Characteristics of Genetic Sequence Affecting their Contribution to Analyses

CHARACTERISTIC	DESCRIPTION	CONTRIBUTION TO ANALYSES
Consensus from Sanger or deep sequence methods	A single read on the most likely nucleotide at a site with some sites being called ambiguous	Main type of data used to date to make genetic inferences that inform transmission analyses
Characteristics Relevant to Both Consensus and Deep Sequences		
Genome coverage	Number (or fraction) of base pair sites in a genome that are sequenced	Improves precision and validity of genetic tree inferences
Accuracy	Low error on base pair cells	Improves genetic tree inferences
Characteristics Relevant to Only Deep Sequences		
Depth	The number of times a nucleotide is read during sequencing	Increased depth detects rare variants and describes virus diversity within a host
Read length	Number of base pair reads linked across a single deep sequence read	Longer reads improve within host genetic tree inferences

All of the deep sequencing methods make higher error rates per base pair site on a single read than the Sanger chemistry that has been dominant in generating consensus sequences. But when many different sequence strands are read independently in a host (that is to say with greater read depth), bioinformatics methods can improve overall accuracy to a level that is greater than the Sanger chemistry methods.

The methods discussed in the "Analytic phylodynamics" section above have only been applied to consensus sequence data. In the new age of deep sequencing data, however, within host tree inferences will help to determine the direction of transmission when fitting genetic data to individual-based models. Such fitting processes are being pursued by several research groups and there is hope that these will improve inferences about transmission system parameters and conformations from what is possible when fitting only consensus sequence data. To see why this is the case, see Fig. 26-7. The distance between consensus sequences only tells us whether they are close. It does not indicate who the likely source case is. When trees can be constructed from all different haplotypes (sequence patterns) within two hosts, the haplotypes (taxa) within the recipient host will be nested within the diversity of the source host. **Population sequence patterns** are patterns of commonality and divergence in genetic sequences between members of a population.[1] The biggest determinant of whether a particular deep sequencing method will allow for within host genetic tree inferences is the read length. There are marked differences in read length obtained from the currently available deep sequencing technologies.

Another contribution of more and longer deep sequence reads will be in improving inference robustness assessments. To date, phylodynamic analysis has not paid close attention to assessing how different microevolutionary model assumptions affect phylodynamic inferences. Describing within host evolutionary patterns helps to determine what evolutionary process assumptions might need relaxing in order to make valid phylodynamic inferences from population-level genetic sequence patterns.

Technologies Generating Sequence Data with Different Characteristics

Two technologies affect the characteristics of sequence data in Table 26-2: (1) technologies for preparing sequencing libraries and (2) technologies involved in the actual sequencing. A sequencing library is a set of sequences from a sample that have been prepared according to a specific protocol. The protocol may break longer genomes into shorter

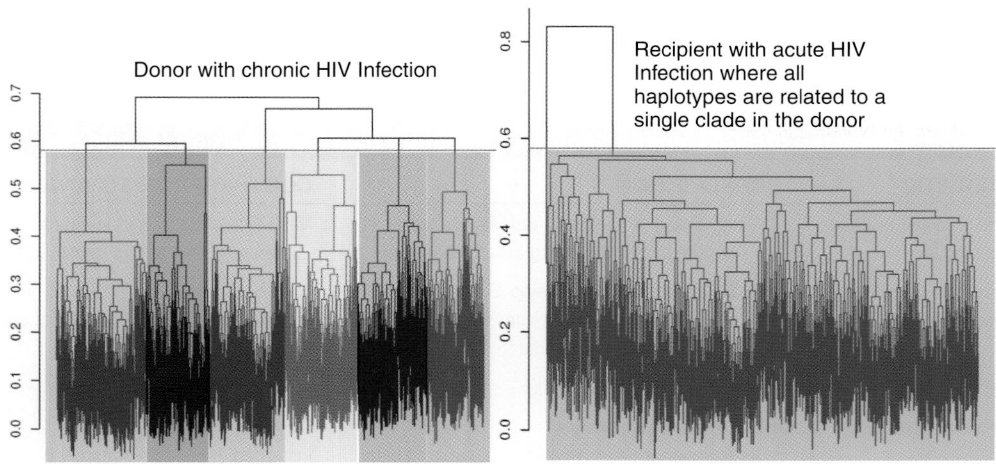

FIG. 26-7 Within host phylogenies across a transmission pair. (*Source:* Figure prepared by Michael P. S. Brown[2], Malinda Schaefer[1], Yan Guo[2], William Kilembe[3], Susan Allen[1], Eric Hunter[1], and Ellen E. Paxinos[2]—Affiliations: [1]Emory University, Atlanta, GA; [2]Pacific Biosciences®, Menlo Park, CA; [3]Zambia Emory HIV Research Project, Lusaka, Zambia.)

ones, generate polymerase chain reaction (PCR) amplicons, and add "bar codes" to the sequences to identify either the subjects they come from or the PCR amplicons that produced a particular sequence. All methods of library preparation for modern deep sequencing generate some bias between the libraries and what was in the host. These can potentially affect phylodynamic inferences. But ways to detect or handle such biases are improving.[27]

One important difference in library preparation is whether one amplifies defined genome regions or starts sequencing reads at random points across the whole genome. Specific region amplification using specific paired primers can help increase the length and number of haplotype determinations that one can compare across different subjects. In other words, it makes the inference of genetic trees within hosts more possible.[28] When sequencing library bar codes identify each separate sequence amplified from the host, this allows for haplotype descriptions across the amplified regions.

Sequencing technology is evolving extremely rapidly and the amount of information generated by this technology for a given cost has grown tenfold over each couple of years. In choosing a technology for generation of data that will inform public health policy using analytic phylodynamics methods, it seems wise to choose methods that will allow for use of data collected now to which transmission models can be fit as long as 10 years from now. By then, methods that generate long unbiased haplotype reads will likely enhance phylodynamic analyses.

HIV SEQUENCES AND HIV CONTROL

Genetic sequence analysis has elucidated the HIV transmission system in a variety of ways. An understanding of this highly complex system should emerge as phylodynamic methods are increasingly applied to HIV sequences and as deep sequences replace consensus sequences. The fact that more sequences are available for HIV than any other pathogen makes it a good case to illustrate the major points in this chapter.

The HIV transmission system is all of the elements and processes that keep HIV circulating in some defined region or population group. HIV transmission systems in different localities are highly diverse. There are differences between heterosexual, injection mediated, and homosexual transmission modes; between ethnic, age, social, and behavioral groups; between regions with different levels of other infections that alter HIV transmission; different medical care structures; and different social structures that affect the interactions between all these factors. Even slight differences in how high-risk behaviors of individuals vary over time can make major differences in infection patterns.[29] This diversity means that control actions that were effective at one time in one place may not be effective at other times or places. Thus, WHO has promoted the mantra "know your epidemic." An alternative to analyzing the complexities of transmission in a population is to find "magic bullets" like broadly protective vaccines that will stop transmission under any conditions. But HIV has been waiting for vaccines that could be just around the corner for 30 years, and a broadly protective vaccine is most likely many years off.

Scientific advances offer powerful new opportunities for HIV control. Antiviral medicines for treatment or prophylaxis stop transmission. Male circumcision can slow transmission among heterosexuals but not homosexuals. Behavioral interventions are sometimes effective. The promise of partially effective vaccines and for a cure offers the hope for additional control tools. These, however, are unlikely to be magic bullets. We will still need to "know our local epidemics" in order to allocate resources in a way that achieves control. To see how HIV genetic data can help with that, we describe how HIV sequence data are being used.

HIV Genetic Data Analyses Affecting Public Health Policies

HIV illustrates the value of genotyping, phylogeographic, and phylodynamic analysis. Phylogenetic analyses also have been quite informative in characterizing HIV infection forces and patterns. Genetic sequencing identified two different groups of HIV, types 1 and 2, which were found to have quite different natural histories of infection and immunity. Phylogenetic analyses show that type 1 (HIV-1) has four subgroups that arose from separate introductions of infection to humans from primates. The M subgroup of HIV-1 accounts for the vast majority of the acquired immune deficiency syndrome (AIDS) epidemic. Subtypes and sub-subtypes of recombinant forms of the M subgroup have strong geographic and risk group distributions that tell a story of how HIV has spread over time at a macro level without having to fit a model to the data. The highest diversity of subtypes is in the regions where the virus was first introduced into the human population.[30] The flow of infection from there and in many local regions has been described based on such analyses. Subtype distributions are useful for distinguishing epidemiologic populations with different modes of transmission. For example, genotypes separate men who have sex with men (MSM) from other risk groups in some situations,[31] but in others, MSM appear to act as bridges to other risk groups.[32]

The major reason for obtaining HIV sequences has been to classify HIV-1 M group strain subtypes by antiviral resistance mutations. Genetic sequences are far cheaper for resistance testing than are assays of biological resistance behaviors. They have the advantage of indicating pre-resistance states because some biological resistance mechanisms occur only after the accumulation of several specific mutations. Because of the life and death value of resistance assays, sequences have become available for most patients under medical care in developed countries and are becoming increasingly available everywhere. The sequences gathered for resistance testing are the sequences that currently constitute most HIV genetic surveillance databases. Thousands of studies have shown informative epidemiologic relationships using sequences in these databases. For example, genetic patterns reveal a unique history of the B subtype in China[33] and highly compartmentalized epidemics in Europe.[34] HIV in South Africa has been largely subtype C, but there is also a focus in Southern Brazil that phylogeography indicates derives from a limited importation at one time with subsequent defined patterns of internal spread.[35]

For epidemiologic studies, however, HIV genome regions not connected to resistance testing have proven to be especially informative about HIV transmission and population patterns.[36-38] Using information theory supported approaches, complex sequence patterns have been related to geographic regions in a manner the promises to be more widely useful to study epidemiologic patterns.[38]

Surveillance for transmission of resistant HIV subtypes is currently the major surveillance program that uses genetic sequences. Initially in the USA, such surveillance used sequences from the residuals of diagnostic specimens paid for by the Centers for Disease Control and Prevention; now only tests ordered by doctors are used. Most detected resistance has arisen as the result of treatment. Detecting transmission of resistant strains is a major reason for resistance surveillance. Finding resistance mutations in individuals who have not received any antiviral medication is presumptive evidence of transmission of resistant strains. Finding resistance mutations throughout genetically linked transmission clusters is more definitive evidence. Transmitted resistance has been relatively infrequent in the era of triple therapy regimens but remains a threat requiring vigilance.

The majority of phylodynamics studies have been conducted using resistance sequence databases. Some patterns of HIV transmission are seen clearly using these databases. In the USA and Europe, phylogenetic clustering alone reveals a story of transmission from early HIV infections in MSM sustaining a broader epidemic.[39-45] Phlyogenetic analysis alone also reveals that most transmission between MSM is in narrow age groups.[3] Clustering presumably indicating early infection transmission has also been noted in African populations.[46]

Analytic Phylodynamic Inference of Early Infection Transmission Fractions

The fraction of transmissions from acute infection is expected to have a big effect on how effective treatment as prevention (TasP) can be in stopping HIV transmission. Until recently this fraction was well estimated in only one study,[47] as directly observing transmissions is extremely difficult and expensive. Now phylodynamic analysis can be used to estimate this fraction. Descriptive phylodynamic studies support the inference that early transmissions represent a high fraction of all transmissions.[40,41,43–45] But the fraction of transmissions from early infection cannot be directly calculated from the frequency of clustering.[3,17] For that, one must use an analytic phylodynamics approach that fits models and then evaluates inferences made from these models using the inference robustness assessment approach presented in Chapter 25. A key first step in that process was performed using a resistance database from MSM in Michigan. Forty-five percent of transmissions were inferred to have occurred in the first year of infection.[2] The analytic approach to making this inference employed multiple different types of HIV surveillance data that are available in most US states together with the sequence data. The way these different data types were integrated into the analysis is illustrated in Fig. 26-8.

This study uses coalescent methods but builds a more realistic HIV population model than the usual coalescent methods would. The model used is a transmission system model. But the complexities of historical, behavioral, biological, spatial, and social factors affecting HIV transmission are not built into the model. Instead a semicatalytic model approach was used. Catalytic models model the force of infection generating incident cases rather than the transmission system processes like contact rates and patterns that generate the force of infection. The forces of infection from early infection and later infection were modeled separately in order to infer the fraction of transmissions from acute infection. The pattern of change over time in the force of infection and the resulting incidence were modeled using splines. The data were informative enough so that there was little variation in the incidence patterns estimated.

Given these semicatalytic model analysis results and the dengue phylodynamics demonstration of the power of the genetic data to inform fairly detailed mechanistic models of dengue transmission,[26] the next steps for analytic phylodynamics analysis of HIV should involve more detailed mechanistic modeling of contact and transmission processes. That will be important because the fraction of transmissions from early infection by itself cannot answer a key public health issue: what that fraction implies about the potential for HIV TasP to stop HIV transmission.

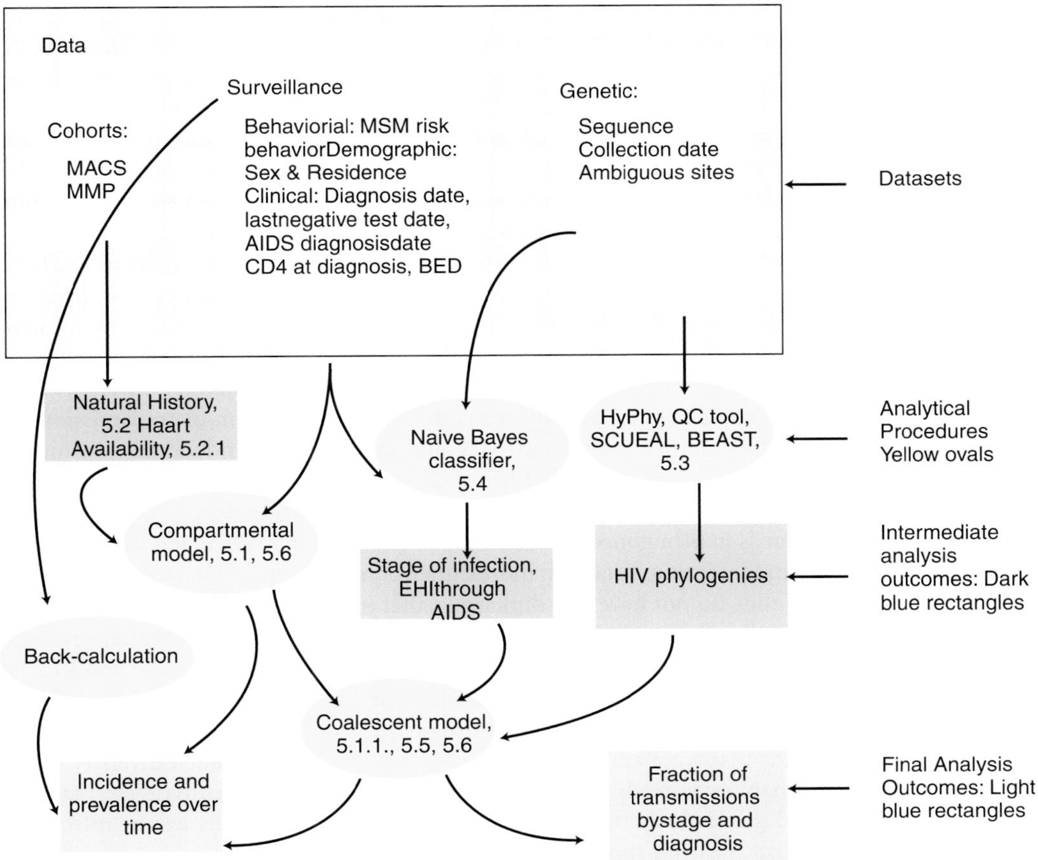

FIG. 26-8 Data and analysis methods used by Volz et al.[2] to infer the incidence of HIV over time and the fraction of transmission during the first year of HIV infection.

To model TasP effects, behavioral dynamics and population contact patterns affecting both the fraction of transmissions from acute infection and the basic reproduction number (R_0) are needed. When the fraction of transmissions during early infection is high, effective diagnosis and treatment rates that make cases noncontagious will have to be higher to prevent the same number of cases. But the number of transmissions that must be prevented to stop transmission can also vary dramatically across different transmission systems. Any given endemic level of infection might be produced by a high or a low R_0. Contact patterns and risk behavior volatility play a big role in the relationship between R_0, endemic prevalence, and the fraction of transmissions from acute infection. To stop transmission, TasP needs to get the R_0 down below 1. An R_0 of 10 means TasP must stop more than 90% of transmissions. But at an R_0 of 1.1, TasP needs to stop less than 10% of transmissions. If a small, tight group of high-risk individuals who do not often change their risk behavior sustains the epidemic by transmitting to lower risk individuals, the R_0 can be very high. If risk fluctuation is the driver of transmission, R_0 can be very low. Analytic phylodynamic studies will help distinguish what the real situation is. Very different control decisions are indicated if a tight, long-lasting high-risk group is driving the epidemic. In that case, pre-exposure prophylaxis (PrEP) could be highly efficacious if focused on this group. On the other hand, if risk fluctuation is driving transmission and new individuals are continuously entering high-risk situations, PrEP will have difficulty reaching a moving target and intensive Test and Treat (T&T) in high-risk settings might be the best TasP approach.

Informative Value of Genetic Data with Different Characteristics

For HIV it appears that deep sequence data with long read lengths should be particularly informative, but it is not yet clear how much value will be added by long reads that allow for construction of within host genetic trees. In this section, we discuss some of the evolutionary dynamics that affect the value of different sorts of genetic data.

Genetic data are particularly informative for HIV analyses because transmission involves only one or a few viruses getting through the eclipse period after infection and causing infection to take off.[48] That, together with the high rate of diversity development within hosts, generates high-genetic diversity. However, the rapid evolution within hosts can make population inferences about transmission using analytic phylodynamics methods more difficult. Genetic sequence data obtained in late infection might differ considerably from the initial infecting strain—and the strains they transmitted. As seen in Fig. 26-9, this is due to the "ladder-like" pattern of HIV within host evolution that is driven by selection processes involving immunity or treatment. That ladder-like pattern is due to strong selection from immunological or antiviral treatment forces that eliminate most of the variations that occurred earlier while allowing viruses with less diversity to proliferate and diversify before the next big selection event creates a new step on the ladder.

The ladder-like history of HIV strains within a host means that if a high fraction of transmissions occur early during infection, the genetic distances between sequenced HIV and the viruses an individual transmitted could be far greater than the average distance between viruses down a chain of early infection transmission. Most likely, however, enough transmitted diversity will remain in deep sequences late in infection to make those deep sequences informative. The informative value is in fitting model parameters much more than deducing whether one individual infected another individual. For model fitting, data with more dimensions are helpful. Consensus sequence data only provide a distance measure, and they do not have any dimension that indicates which of two individuals preceded the other in any chain of transmission between them. Patterns like those from the deep sequences that generated Fig. 26-7 can do that and thus deep sequences will have more power to estimate transmission model parameters.

Deep sequence data could also be used to assess the stage of infection when an individual was diagnosed and had their virus sequenced. Volz et al.[2] found that even with consensus sequences the best indicator of stage of infection was the fraction of base pair reads that were ambiguous. This is a measure of how much diversity there is at base pair sites within a host. Even if haplotype reads were not possible and only individual base pair site diversity was assessed, deep sequencing would give a far better measure of viral diversity and thus age of infection in a host. If haplotype reads are available that measure should be even better.

Another value of haplotype deep sequence reads is in assessing what assumptions for an evolutionary model at the population level are consistent with observed evolutionary outcomes within an individual. Currently almost no

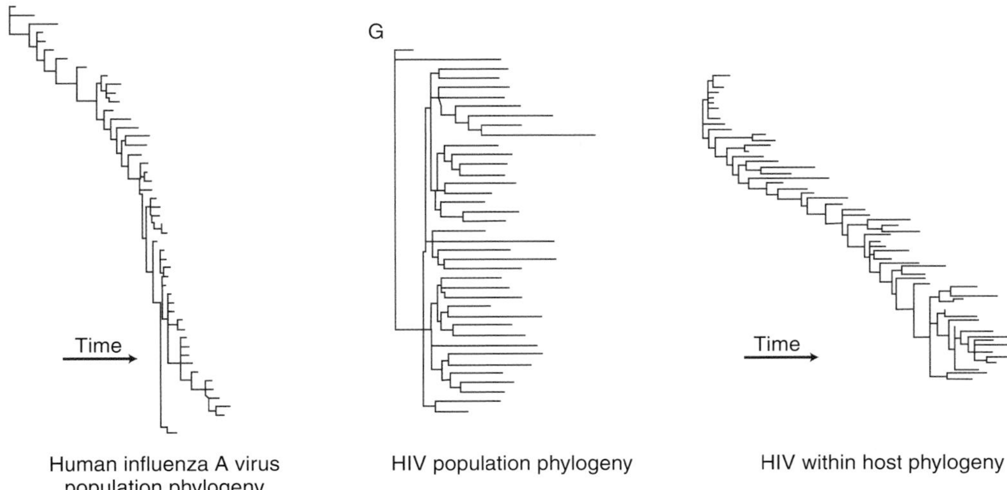

FIG. 26-9 Illustrations of population trees for HIV and influenza H3N2 and a within host tree for HIV. (*Source:* Grenfell BT, Pybus OG, Gog JR, Wood JL, Daly JM, Mumford JA, et al. Unifying the epidemiological and evolutionary dynamics of pathogens. Science 2004;303(5656):327–32.)

attention is paid to the effects of evolutionary model assumptions on the population inferences made from phylogenetic analyses of consensus sequences between hosts. Within host haplotype patterns should help suggest what evolutionary distance measures between hosts would be most informative for population-level analyses.

THE VALUE OF ANALYTIC PHYLODYNAMICS FOR INFLUENZA CONTROL

Genetic surveillance and analytic phylodynamic studies that fit transmission system models to the genetic surveillance are proving just as informative for influenza as they are for HIV, despite the differences between influenza and HIV in its genetic patterns and in the forces affecting those patterns. Whereas acquired immunity plays almost no role in determining HIV population patterns, immunity and evolution to escape that immunity are the dominant factors making influenza a serious and complex health problem. HIV and influenza also differ markedly with regard to the natural history of infection and the degree of genetic bottleneck imposed by infection. Influenza has short infections that are usually fully controlled by acquired immunity in a couple of weeks. The bottleneck imposed by influenza is not as tight as for HIV, so more within-host variants are transmitted by influenza.

Consequently, the contrast of influenza within host versus population genetic patterns is the exact opposite of HIV. As shown in Fig. 26-9, population genetic patterns of HIV are radial with persistent lines of diversity over time, while within-host patterns are ladder-like. Influenza, in contrast, has radial patterns within the host and ladder-like patterns at the population level. The ladder-like pattern at the population level is driven by escape from acquired immunity at the population level, just as the ladder-like pattern of infection within the host for HIV is driven by escape from immune responses.

Phylogeographic studies of influenza are revealing population patterns of spread that help focus on the emerging strains in specific parts of the world that should lead to changes in vaccines' antigenic structures and how control should focus on specific populations in order to decrease infection levels worldwide.[49] A classic study describes the worldwide flow of newly emerging influenza strain variants showing that China and Southeast Asia are the centers from which new variants that spread worldwide emerge.[50] This description has been refined with new data and improved methods that show new strains that spread globally can also originate from North America, but to a much lesser extent than China and Southeast Asia.[51]

Because vaccines are the focus of influenza control and the influenza virus is always changing to escape vaccine-induced immunity, understanding what drives the virus escape is currently a major focus of influenza phylodynamic studies using surveillance data. Despite decades of efforts to develop methods to predict influenza evolution, much remains unknown about what drives influenza antigenic variation. There are three major theories being explored. The first is that antigenic variation is driven by episodic selection, a theory that requires a strong selective pressure for a few key mutations.[52,53] Another theory, that clonal selection drives antigenic drift, requires a high rate of mutations affecting immunity but with weak selective effects acting on each mutation.[52,53] Finally, a more recent theory has been expressed in dynamic model terms.[54] It holds that avidity variation in the binding receptor of hemagglutinin to cells is the driver of antigenic drift with the drift being just a side effect of the binding receptor evolution. Experimental studies provide some support for each of these theories. But testing them must ultimately be done using surveillance data in the context of analytic phylodynamics where the competing models are fit to genetic, antigenic data, and general surveillance data.

Another use of analytic phylodynamics in influenza is to predict cross-species jumps and pandemic potential of different animal influenza outbreaks. A deep sequence approach to influenza virus surveillance across species has been proposed to serve this end.[55] This surveillance objective should also be pursued using analytic phylodynamic methods. Predicting the evolution of virulence after a species jump is an important part of predicting cross-species jumps. Indeed, recent analyses show that such evolution is necessary for cross-species infections to lead to epidemics in new species.[56] Finding genetic variants related to virulence is thus one step toward predicting cross-species jumps. Genetic variants of the virus causing the 2009 H1N1 influenza pandemic have been found that predict disease severity.[57] Other analyses demonstrate that deep sequence rather than just consensus sequencing will be necessary to detect and explain such transmission.[58] Complete sequences are now available for most human infections from animal strains. A variety of different source types of influenza strains are involved. Testing theories about cross-species jumps will require analytic phylodynamics methods. Again, once a strong theoretical base has been established by such studies, routine surveillance to predict cross-species jumps will continuously integrate analytic phylodynamic methods.

PUBLIC HEALTH AGENCY ORGANIZATION OF ANALYTIC EFFORTS

The power of population-level genetic patterns to inform public health decisions can be increased by each of the following: (1) analytical capacity available to the public health agency that encompasses both systems epidemiology and data mining, (2) the linkage of genetic surveillance data to the person, time, and place characteristics of individuals in the surveillance databases, (3) user-friendly software that makes analytic phylodynamics accessible to more epidemiologists, and (4) institutional relationships that enable public health leaders to guide analysis in directions that will most influence their disease control decisions. The importance of the first two points has been illustrated by our examples. The third point almost seems inevitable in our age of rapidly advancing computational systems. The last point, however, still represents a weak link. Perhaps the single most important thing that could be done to strengthen this link would be to organize a meeting between policy makers, modelers, and those organizing the genetic data that seek to establish the process of inference choice and inference robustness assessment presented in Chapter 25. Good communication between public health leaders, public policy makers, epidemiologists, and modeling and statistical experts is essential for creating the systems that will make a difference.

Because this field is changing so rapidly, the surveillance base for full use of ideal deep sequence data within an analytic phylodynamics approach cannot be immediately instituted. An initial foundation should be built first by instituting programs that advance typing analyses, then descriptive phylodynamics analyses, then transmission system model analyses that are not fit to genetic data, then finally to full analytical phylodynamics that fit transmission models to genetic sequence data. In setting up typing and descriptive phylodynamic analyses, however, decisions on how to sequence and how to handle and store sequence data should take into consideration their ultimate use for full analytical phylodynamics.

Analytic capacities in systems epidemiology and phylodynamics are mostly in academia and are currently rare in the public health system. A structure of collaboration must be established to eventually move these capacities into public health agencies. As that collaboration emerges and as the public health value of inferences made from systems epidemiology and data mining analyses becomes more evident, we can expect further increases in the generation and use of microbial sequence surveillance data.

There might be two types of modelers working with genetic data. One would have all of the functions and competencies suited to handling policy issues in Chapter 25. In that case, the functions and competencies of the genetic data analyst might be more constrained to the descriptive genetic analyses listed in Table 26-1 and the phylogeographic analyses under the analytic analyses in the second part of that table. More individuals will have the needed skills for these analyses. Fewer will be available to handle coalescent analyses and analytic phylodynamic analyses. The best option for many health departments will be to collaborate with academics. This type of genetic data analyst, along with academic phylodynamicists, could then help with the modeling skills needed to integrate genetic data into transmission models. That would be an efficient path to accomplish analytic phylodynamic analyses. A program manager having the functions and capacities listed for such a person in Chapter 25 will also be essential for the modeling team consisting of a modeler, a genetic data analyst, and academics to achieve public health goals.

CHALLENGES TO IMPLEMENTATION

There are several challenges to achieving the full integration of genetic information into public health surveillance. The infrastructure for collecting samples, sequencing them, and linking those samples to surveillance data needs improvement. The resulting genetic sequences linked to surveillance data are enormous data sets that require considerable investment to store and maintain them for current and future use. There are also bioinformatics challenges resulting from the continual evolution of sequencing platforms continue to evolve, with each sequencing technology producing different types of data, which requires the development of new analytic pipelines for data use and ways to either harmonize across data types or integrate the different types for surveillance. More appropriate analytic software with user-friendly interfaces is needed. Finally, descriptive data on the rates of diversity related to transmission within a population over time must be accumulated to strengthen inferences about new sequence patterns.

KEY SUMMARY POINTS

- In an age of genomic plenty, where massive amounts of sequence data on pathogens can be gathered inexpensively, surveillance of pathogen sequences is growing rapidly.
- Pathogen sequence data provide classification criteria that increase the power of traditional epidemiologic analyses and are replacing other typing methods.
- Phylodynamics assesses how genetic sequence patterns of pathogens relate to infection transmission system dynamics and pathogen evolution dynamics.
- Phylodynamic analyses use phylogenies as data inputs into models to detect individual traits associated with increased transmission in a way that routine surveillance cannot.
- Genetic sequences considerably increase the power of models to determine what drives the flow of infection through populations.
- Population genetic sequence patterns allow inferences about population transmission patterns because transmission represents a bottleneck in pathogen population patterns.
- Descriptions of genetic patterns in relationship to epidemiologic variables can help develop hypotheses about the infection transmission system and evolutionary phenomena that sustain pathogens.
- Fitting models of transmission systems to sequence patterns along with other surveillance data helps epidemiologists to make inferences about the potential effectiveness of control actions. New methods for such model fitting are developing rapidly.
- RNA viruses are the pathogens most readily analyzed by fitting models to genetic patterns. But new sequencing power means that all pathogens can be cost-effectively analyzed with these methods.
- Linking genetic sequence data to other surveillance variables adds considerable power for both traditional epidemiologic analyses and inferences from fitting models to data.
- Genetic surveillance systems are justified by the immediate benefits to traditional epidemiologic analyses and future potential to guide control decisions. Considering future applications as systems are built is essential, as the length of time with good surveillance adds power to the inferences that can be made from model fitting.

DISCUSSION QUESTIONS

Suppose you have a collection of consensus HIV sequence data from Sanger chemistry methods that has been gathered over the past 10 years to determine antiviral treatment resistance status. Each available sequence is linked to an individual whose gender, age group, principal risk behavior, date of diagnosis, geographical area of residence, and CD4 count are available.

1. Formulate a descriptive analysis of such sequences that groups sequences into different clusters and will be informative with regard to the groups where transmission is most active. Provide a blank table that could be filled in by your descriptive analysis. Discuss how different patterns in this table would influence decisions about HIV control actions.
2. Describe output that could be produced by a phylogeographic analysis that not only defines populations by geography but by major risk behavior as well. Outline a graphic or a table that could be produced by such a phylogeographic analysis. Discuss how different patterns in this graphic or table would influence decisions about HIV control actions.
3. Give the very broad outlines of how a phylodynamic analysis of this data would help determine the influence of risk behavior volatility (periods of high then low then high, etc., risk behavior) on infection levels in homosexual and heterosexual groups. To do this you must outline the broad characteristics of dynamic system models that would be fit to the data. Risk behavior volatility increases both the overall level of infection in a population and the fraction of transmissions that occur early in an infection.

Phylogeographic analyses are used to assign a region of origin for the source virus in all cases of polio anywhere in the world. In December 2012, a virus with an origin in Pakistan was discovered in Cairo, Egypt, sewage. There were no paralytic cases in Egypt. Then from March 2013 to March 2014 a highly related virus was found continuously in sewage in Israel. Again there were no paralytic cases in Israel. Two closely related but distinct strains were found during this time. Both Israel and Egypt have been without paralytic poliomyelitis cases for many years and they both have good acute flaccid paralysis surveillance and good vaccination programs. From 2005 to October 2013 only inactivated polio vaccine was used in Israel. It protects against paralytic polio but is less protective against asymptomatic infection. In late 2013, there was a large outbreak of paralytic poliomyelitis in Syria from a strain highly related to the Egypt and Israel strains. Vaccination had been interrupted in Syria due to the civil war. Note that paralytic poliomyelitis only occurs in individuals without immunity from either wild polio virus or oral polio vaccine virus.

4. What descriptive phylodynamics analyses comparing Israeli and Syrian phylogenetic patterns might be used to compare the overall number of transmissions and the rate of transmissions in these two countries? In Syria all the sequences come from patients and in Israel all the sequences come from sewage. The sewage sequences are from separate individual plaques on tissue culture plates from the sewage.
5. What would be the advantage of having done the sequencing of sewage using technology like the PacBio technology that gives long haplotype reads of different virus particles from the sewage?

Noroviruses are a major cause of nausea and vomiting in both higher income and lower or middle-income countries. They have caused major problems on cruise ships. They are classified into different strains and the nature of the illness produced varies a little from one strain to another. They are spread from feces and sometimes from vomit largely through direct skin contact or through water, although aerosols from vomit might also be involved. It is now possible to sequence noroviruses found in water and a recent study in Africa found a variety of strains in three different rivers.

6. How could norovirus sequences be used to guide control actions in high-income countries?
7. How might they be used cost-effectively to guide control of norovirus transmission in low- and middle-income countries?

REFERENCES

1. Definition provided by the chapter author.
2. Volz EM, Ionides E, Romero-Severson EO, Brandt MG, Mokotoff E, Koopman JS. HIV-1 transmission during early infection in men who have sex with men: a phylodynamic analysis. PLoS Med 2013;10(12):e1001568.
3. Volz EM, Koopman JS, Ward MJ, Brown AL, Frost SD. Simple epidemiological dynamics explain phylogenetic clustering of HIV from patients with recent infection. PLoS Comput Biol 2012;8(6):e1002552.
4. Koopman JS, Simon CP, Riolo CP. When to control endemic infections by focusing on high-risk groups. Epidemiology 2005;16(5):621–7.
5. Castro-Nallar E, Perez-Losada M, Burton GF, Crandall KA. The evolution of HIV: inferences using phylogenetics. Mol Phylogenet Evol 2012;62(2): 777–92.
6. Feil EJ, Li BC, Aanensen DM, Hanage WP, Spratt BG. eBURST: inferring patterns of evolutionary descent among clusters of related bacterial genotypes from multilocus sequence typing data. J Bacteriol 2004;186(5): 1518–30.
7. Odoom JK, Forrest L, Dunn G, Osei-Kwasi M, Obodai E, Arthur-Quarm J, et al. Interruption of poliovirus transmission in Ghana: molecular epidemiology of wild-type 1 poliovirus isolated from 1995 to 2008. J Infect Dis 2012;206(7):1111–20.
8. Duintjer Tebbens RJ, Pallansch MA, Kim J-H, Burns CC, Kew OM, Oberste MS, et al. Oral poliovirus vaccine evolution and insights relevant to modeling the risks of circulating vaccine-derived polioviruses (cVDPVs). Risk Analysis 2013;33(4):680–702.
9. Russell CA, Fonville JM, Brown AEX, Burke DF, Smith DL, James SL, et al. The potential for respiratory droplet–transmissible A/H5N1 influenza virus to evolve in a mammalian host. Science 2012;336(6088):1541–7.
10. Grenfell BT, Pybus OG, Gog JR, Wood JL, Daly JM, Mumford JA, et al. Unifying the epidemiological and evolutionary dynamics of pathogens. Science 2004;303(5656):327–32.
11. Pybus OG, Rambaut A. Evolutionary analysis of the dynamics of viral infectious disease. Nat Rev Genet 2009;10(8):540–50.
12. Volz EM, Koelle K, Bedford T. Viral phylodynamics. PLoS Comput Biol 2013;9(3):e1002947.
13. Croucher NJ, Harris SR, Grad YH, Hanage WP. Bacterial genomes in epidemiology—present and future. Philos Trans R Soc Lond B Biol Sci 2013; 368(1614):20120202.
14. Pybus OG, Fraser C, Rambaut A. Evolutionary epidemiology: preparing for an age of genomic plenty. Philos Trans R Soc Lond B Biol Sci 2013; 368(1614):20120193.
15. Orton RJ, Wright CF, Morelli MJ, Juleff N, Thebaud G, Knowles NJ, et al. Observing micro-evolutionary processes of viral populations at multiple scales. Philos Trans R Soc Lond B Biol Sci 2013;368(1614):20120203.
16. Wakeley J. Coalescent theory: an introduction. Greenwood Village, CO: Roberts and Company Publishers; 2008.
17. Frost SD, Volz EM. Viral phylodynamics and the search for an 'effective number of infections'. Philos Trans R Soc Lond B Biol Sci 2010;365(1548): 1879–90.
18. Pybus OG, Drummond AJ, Nakano T, Robertson BH, Rambaut A. The epidemiology and iatrogenic transmission of hepatitis C virus in Egypt: a Bayesian coalescent approach. Mol Biol Evol 2003;20(3):381–7.
19. Dearlove B, Wilson DJ. Coalescent inference for infectious disease: meta-analysis of hepatitis C. Philos Trans R Soc Lond B Biol Sci 2013; 368(1614):20120314.
20. Lemey P, Suchard M, Rambaut A. Reconstructing the initial global spread of a human influenza pandemic: a Bayesian spatial-temporal model for the global spread of H1N1pdm. PLoS Curr 2009;1:RRN1031.
21. Lemey P, Rambaut A, Drummond AJ, Suchard MA. Bayesian phylogeography finds its roots. PLoS Comput Biol 2009;5(9):e1000520.
22. Lemey P, Rambaut A, Welch JJ, Suchard MA. Phylogeography takes a relaxed random walk in continuous space and time. Mol Biol Evol 2010;27(8): 1877–85.
23. Bielejec F, Rambaut A, Suchard MA, Lemey P. SPREAD: spatial phylogenetic reconstruction of evolutionary dynamics. Bioinformatics 2011;27(20): 2910–2.
24. Volz EM. Complex population dynamics and the coalescent under neutrality. Genetics 2012;190(1):187–201.
25. Stadler T, Bonhoeffer S. Uncovering epidemiological dynamics in heterogeneous host populations using phylogenetic methods. Philos Trans R Soc Lond B Biol Sci 2013;368(1614):20120198.
26. Rasmussen D, Boni M, Koelle K. Reconciling phylodynamics with epidemiology: the case of dengue virus in Southern Vietnam. Mol Biol Evol 2014;31(2):258–71.
27. van Dijk EL, Jaszczyszyn Y, Thermes C. Library preparation methods for next-generation sequencing: tone down the bias. Exp Cell Res 2014; 322(1):12–20.
28. Poon AF, Swenson LC, Bunnik EM, Edo-Matas D, Schuitemaker H, van't Wout AB, et al. Reconstructing the dynamics of HIV evolution within hosts from serial deep sequence data. PLoS Comput Biol 2012;8(11):e1002753.
29. Zhang X, Zhong L, Romero-Severson E, Alam SJ, Henry CJ, Volz EM, et al. Episodic HIV risk behavior can greatly amplify HIV prevalence and the fraction of transmissions from acute HIV infection. Stat Commun Infect Dis 2012;4(1):1–21.
30. Sharp PM, Hahn BH. Origins of HIV and the AIDS pandemic. Cold Spring Harb Perspect Med 2011;1(1):a006841.
31. Caplinskas S, Loukachov VV, Gasich EL, Gilyazova AV, Caplinskiene I, Lukashov VV. Distinct HIV type 1 strains in different risk groups and the absence of new infections by drug-resistant strains in Lithuania. AIDS Res Hum Retroviruses 2013;29(4):732–7.
32. Li L, Han N, Lu J, Li T, Zhong X, Wu H, et al. Genetic characterization and transmitted drug resistance of the HIV type 1 epidemic in men who have sex with men in Beijing, China. AIDS Res Hum Retroviruses 2013;29(3): 633–7.
33. Li Z, He X, Wang Z, Xing H, Li F, Yang Y, et al. Tracing the origin and history of HIV-1 subtype B' epidemic by near full-length genome analyses. AIDS 2012;26(7):877–84.
34. Abecasis AB, Wensing AM, Paraskevis D, Vercauteren J, Theys K, Van de Vijver DA, et al. HIV-1 subtype distribution and its demographic determinants in newly diagnosed patients in Europe suggest highly compartmentalized epidemics. Retrovirology 2013;10:7.
35. Veras NM, Gray RR, Brigido LF, Rodrigues R, Salemi M. High-resolution phylogenetics and phylogeography of human immunodeficiency virus type 1 subtype C epidemic in South America. J Gen Virol 2011;92(Pt 7): 1698–709.
36. Lemoh C, Ryan CE, Sekawi Z, Hearps AC, Aleksic E, Chibo D, et al. Acquisition of HIV by African-born residents of Victoria, Australia: insights from molecular epidemiology. PLoS One 2013;8(12):e84008.
37. Pimentel VF, Morgado MG, Bello G, Guimaraes MD, Castilho EA, Veloso VG, et al. Temporal trends and molecular epidemiology of HIV type 1 infection in Rio de Janeiro, Brazil. AIDS Res Hum Retroviruses 2013;29(12):1553–61.
38. Wang Y, Rawi R, Hoffmann D, Sun B, Yang R. Inference of global HIV-1 sequence patterns and preliminary feature analysis. Virol Sin 2013;28(4): 228–38.
39. Brenner B, Wainberg MA, Roger M. Phylogenetic inferences on HIV-1 transmission: implications for the design of prevention and treatment interventions. AIDS 2013;27(7):1045–57.
40. Brenner BG, Roger M, Routy JP, Moisi D, Ntemgwa M, Matte C, et al. High rates of forward transmission events after acute/early HIV-1 infection. J Infect Dis 2007;195(7):951–9.
41. Brenner BG, Roger M, Stephens D, Moisi D, Hardy I, Weinberg J, et al. Transmission clustering drives the onward spread of the HIV epidemic among men who have sex with men in Quebec. J Infect Dis 2011;204(7):1115–9.
42. Brenner BG, Wainberg MA. Future of phylogeny in HIV prevention. J Acquir Immune Defic Syndr 2013;63(Suppl. 2):S248–54.

43. Chalmet K, Staelens D, Blot S, Dinakis S, Pelgrom J, Plum J, et al. Epidemiological study of phylogenetic transmission clusters in a local HIV-1 epidemic reveals distinct differences between subtype B and non-B infections. BMC Infect Dis 2010;10:262.
44. Lewis F, Hughes GJ, Rambaut A, Pozniak A, Leigh Brown AJ. Episodic sexual transmission of HIV revealed by molecular phylodynamics. PLoS Med 2008;5(3):e50.
45. Leigh Brown AJ, Lycett SJ, Weinert L, Hughes GJ, Fearnhill E, Dunn DT. Transmission network parameters estimated from HIV sequences for a nationwide epidemic. J Infect Dis 2011;204(9):1463–9.
46. Kapaata A, Lyagoba F, Ssemwanga D, Magambo B, Nanyonjo M, Levin J, et al. HIV-1 subtype distribution trends and evidence of transmission clusters among incident cases in a rural clinical cohort in southwest Uganda, 2004-2010. AIDS Res Hum Retroviruses 2013;29(3):520–7.
47. Wawer MJ, Gray RH, Sewankambo NK, Serwadda D, Li X, Laeyendecker O, et al. Rates of HIV-1 transmission per coital act, by stage of HIV-1 infection, in Rakai, Uganda. J Infect Dis 2005;191(9):1403–9.
48. Cohen MS, Shaw GM, McMichael AJ, Haynes BF. Acute HIV-1 infection. N Engl J Med 2011;364(20):1943–54.
49. Frost SD, Volz EM. Modelling tree shape and structure in viral phylodynamics. Philos Trans R Soc Lond B Biol Sci 2013;368(1614):20120208.
50. Russell CA, Jones TC, Barr IG, Cox NJ, Garten RJ, Gregory V, et al. The global circulation of seasonal influenza A (H3N2) viruses. Science 2008;320(5874):340–6.
51. Bedford T, Cobey S, Beerli P, Pascual M. Global migration dynamics underlie evolution and persistence of human influenza A (H3N2). PLoS Pathog 2010;6(5):e1000918.
52. Gillespie JH. The causes of molecular evolution. Oxford: Oxford University Press; 1991.
53. Sniegowski PD, Gerrish PJ. Beneficial mutations and the dynamics of adaptation in asexual populations. Philos Trans R Soc Lond B Biol Sci 2010;365(1544):1255–63.
54. Yuan HY, Koelle K. The evolutionary dynamics of receptor binding avidity in influenza A: a mathematical model for a new antigenic drift hypothesis. Philos Trans R Soc Lond B Biol Sci 2013;368(1614):20120204.
55. Chan JM, Rabadan R. Quantifying pathogen surveillance using temporal genomic data. MBio 2013;4(1):e00524–12.
56. Boni MF, Nguyen TD, de Jong MD, van Doorn HR. Virulence attenuation during an influenza A/H5N1 pandemic. Philos Trans R Soc Lond B Biol Sci 2013;368(1614):20120207.
57. Vazquez-Perez JA, Isa P, Kobasa D, Ormsby CE, Ramirez-Gonzalez JE, Romero-Rodriguez DP, et al. A (H1N1) pdm09 HA D222 variants associated with severity and mortality in patients during a second wave in Mexico. Virol J 2013;10:41.
58. Murcia PR, Baillie GJ, Daly J, Elton D, Jervis C, Mumford JA, et al. Intra- and interhost evolutionary dynamics of equine influenza virus. J Virol 2010;84(14):6943–54.

CHAPTER

27

Multifaceted Approaches and Emerging Trends in Public Health Analytics

Sanjay Zodpey, Habib Hasan

. . . the best time to plant a tree is always twenty years ago. If, for some reason, you did not plant it then, the next best time to plant a tree is now.

Carlos Acosta

KEY WORDS

Public health analytics
Predictive analytics
Prescriptive analytics
Data governance
Data acquisition
Data sharing
Data standardization
SNOMED CT
ICD-10-CM
Data integration
Biomedical Translational Research Information System (BTRIS)
National Institutes for Health (NIH)
Common Data Models (CDM)
Surveillance, Management, and Real-time Trends (SMaRT) system
Open Government Directive
Health Data Initiative (HDI)
Electronic Medical Record Support for Public Health (ESP)

INTRODUCTION

The emergence of novel pathogens like severe acute respiratory syndrome (SARS), avian influenza H5N1 infection, H1N1 influenza infection, and Middle East Respiratory Syndrome Coronavirus (MERS-CoV) has brought public health surveillance systems into the spotlight. The focus is now shifting from outbreak response to preparedness and planning, providing a unique opportunity to direct our resources and energy toward developing surveillance programs, which are robust in detecting outbreaks and in their ability to predict the "when" and "where" of emerging pathogens. Developing and deploying sophisticated analytics, which can link surveillance systems to cutting-edge research, may provide the best tools to harness information emanating from evolutionary biology. Moreover, the transformational leap in the computational abilities of processors has made possible the analysis of quantum data in real time through advanced analytics.

APPLICATIONS OF PUBLIC HEALTH ANALYTICS

Analytics involves the systematic use of data and related insights developed through applied analytical methods (e.g., statistical, contextual, quantitative, predictive, cognitive, and other [including emerging] models) to drive evidence-based decision-making for planning, management, measurement, and learning.[1] The application of these methods to public health is referred to as public health analytics. Public health analytics provide public health professionals with the necessary tools to readily audit, cleanse, analyze, and interpret multiformat data to enable immediate response to unanticipated questions and unexpected situations such as global outbreaks of infectious disease.

THE CHOICE OF ANALYTICS LEAVES MANY QUESTIONS TO BE ANSWERED

Public health analytics can be descriptive, predictive, or prescriptive. Though descriptive analytics are typically the most simple and frequently used approach, they provide a limited overview of the situation under consideration.[2] The models in descriptive analytics categorize, characterize, aggregate, and classify data, converting them into useful information for understanding and analyzing health care decisions, outcomes, and quality.[3] Such data summaries often take the form of meaningful charts and reports (e.g., distribution of disease in terms of time, person, and place; immunization coverage and drop out rates; and coverage of health services).

Predictive analytics allow for forecasting and planning.[2] Predictive analytics can anticipate risk and find relationships in health data, something descriptive analytics alone cannot achieve.[3] Advanced techniques like data mining give predictive analytics the power to detect hidden patterns in large quantities of data, allowing data to be segmented and grouped into coherent sets to predict behavior and detect trends.[3] For example, by looking at historical records of incidence of a vector-borne disease and its relationship with weather conditions like temperature, humidity, and rainfall, predictive analytics can predict changes in vector population and the potential of disease outbreaks under certain weather conditions.

Prescriptive analytics suggest possible interventions.[2] Prescriptive analytics utilize available data, information, and knowledge from several domains including public health, medicine, economics, management, and others to inform decision-making in situations of uncertainty. For example, in the event of an epidemic, prescriptive analytics can suggest whether immunizing the population at risk is a better approach than treating cases with antivirals when they seek care. This could provide guidance on whether to stockpile vaccines or antivirals and could send appropriate signals for connected events such as the decision to enhance production capacity of vaccines and/or antivirals.

EMERGING TRENDS

New analytics tools go beyond standard reporting and business intelligence; they include 3D graphing and visualization, interactive interfaces, animation, displays of multiple variables, and more.[4] Visual representations are able to highlight important features of the data, including commonalities and anomalies.[4] These connections are not easy to see when the only outputs are tables full of numbers.[4] Geovisual analytics that combine analytical reasoning facilitated by highly interactive visual interfaces offer an example that is especially relevant in public health where data with geographical references occur often and are directed toward development of new methods for analyzing complex data and communicating results for—and in—decision-making processes.[5]

In addition, techniques from artificial intelligence, machine learning, and data mining are now often employed for data analysis at the societal level to make sense of the massive quantity of data, to detect relevant patterns, and to assist public health decision-making. For example, current disease surveillance systems are relying more and more on massive quantities of data from nontraditional sources, ranging from internet search queries and user-generated web content, to detailed electronic medical records (EMR), to continuous data streams from sensor networks, cellular telephones, and other location aware devices.[6] Similarly, temporally and spatially compatible earth observation data sets (remote sensing data) are key elements to developing health early warning systems. These systems in turn enhance understanding of connections between the environment and health and improve the ability to make sound decisions to protect human health and the environment.[7] Further research is required to integrate climate science and health sciences to predict the impact of climate change on human risk exposure and disease burden.

THE BUILDING BLOCKS OF ANALYTICS

The reliability of the reports generated through any analytic approach is the product of the system's building blocks. These building blocks include data governance, data acquisition, data sharing, integration, standardization, and analytics.[4] **Data governance** is the specification of decision rights and an accountability framework to encourage desirable behavior in the valuation, creation, storage, use, archival, and deletion of data and information. It includes the processes, roles, standards, and metrics that ensure the effective and efficient use of data and information in enabling an organization to achieve its goals.[8]

Data acquisition practices ensure that data are captured in a usable form and include consistent documentation of metadata. In addition, standard taxonomies for demographic fields and medical codes should be used properly, and data should be de-identified to ensure privacy and security.[4]

Data sharing enables multiple applications and multiple users to access and work with the data at the same time to perform analysis and reporting. Data virtualization is one such technique. Cloud computing is also a related idea that makes it possible to migrate large amounts of data onto a temporary platform ("the cloud"), which users can log into and run high-powered analytic tools or reports.[4]

Data standardization is the adoption of common health vocabularies to facilitate the exchange and use of data in interoperable and integrated electronic information systems.[9]

The Public Health Data Standards Consortium (PHDSC) enables adherence to Common Data Models (CDM) so that data from disparate systems can be combined and compared. **Common Data Models** are codified standards to define the format and content of clinical observation data so that all software, devices, and protocols that implement the CDM standard can be utilized.[10] For example, the Biomedical Translational Research Information System (BTRIS) at the National Institutes for Health (NIH) translates data from different sources into a standard structure (e.g., Health Level 7) and language (e.g., ICD-9, SNOMED) so that the data can be managed and analyzed more easily, allowing researchers to query multiple data sources at once and get more comprehensive results.[8] **BTRIS** is a resource available to the NIH intramural community that brings together clinical research data from the Clinical Center and other NIH Institutes and Centers.[11] BTRIS provides clinical investigators with access to identifiable data for subjects on their own active protocols, while providing all NIH investigators with access to data (1976–present) without personal identifiers across all protocols.[11] **SNOMED CT** is a systematically organized, computer processable clinical health care terminology for electronic health records (EHR) and contains more than 311,000 active concepts with unique meanings and formal logic-based definitions organized into hierarchies.[12] **ICD-10-CM** is the standard diagnostic tool for epidemiology, health management and clinical purposes. It is used to monitor the incidence and prevalence of diseases and other health concerns, and to classify diseases and other health concerns recorded on many types of health and vital records including death certificates and health records.[13]

Data integration is the merger of data from internal and external data sources into an individual-centric data structure optimized for analysis. For example, an individual's demographics, disease conditions, diagnostics, drugs, and other observations from an EMR can be merged with geospatial data, contact patterns, movement patterns, and more to run analytics. Once all the building blocks are aligned—from governance to standardization—analytics provide the final payoff.

However, the robustness of these building blocks defines the type of analytics—descriptive, predictive, or prescriptive—that can be performed by a system. Analytical systems based on data with limited governance and quality assurance can only offer ad hoc and reactive analysis, whereas systems with a holistic model of data governance can provide continuous, real-time analytics alerts with drill down capabilities and rich analytics. CDMs are one such mechanism to create a holistic system of data governance and are often used for distributed research networks. Within a distributed network, the data partners maintain operational and physical control over their data but transform and then store the data in the common format. A CDM makes it possible to centralize query development and methodology testing. In the absence of a CDM, each data partner would be required to translate a study protocol for execution against its own data format.[14] One such model is Mini-Sentinel, a pilot program sponsored by the US Food and Drug Administration (FDA) intended to develop comprehensive approaches to facilitating the use of the data routinely collected and stored in EHR for the surveillance of the safety of marketed medical products. Currently more than 30 academic and private health care institutes are participating in this program as data partners who provide the data for the surveillance activity.[15] A detailed review and assessment of the best practices in the design, implementation, and use of collaborative data networks and recommendation regarding minimum standards for technical design, structural components, and organizational structure can be found elsewhere.[16,17]

AN ANALYTICS SYSTEM EXAMPLE

The Surveillance, Management, and Real-time Trends (SMaRT) system used by the state of Louisiana is an intelligent approach to data analytics for health outcomes and performance monitoring. This tool can create day-to-day data reports, measure trends, and complete performance monitoring and interactive work-board solutions for ad hoc and on-demand data analyses. In addition, it monitors performance toward goals, identifies trends in key performance indicators (KPIs), and provides interfaces for ad hoc data drill down and investigation.[18]

The SMaRT tool is a data visualization and outcome monitoring solution. There is recognition that a vast wealth of information exists but remains housed within disparate databases. (See Chapter 21 for more discussion of this topic.) Important trends, outcomes, and population health stories that remain hidden under layers of complicated data elements led to the implementation of SMaRT in Louisiana in 2013. The Louisiana Immunizations Program organized their SMaRT tool around five permeating themes: coverage rates, missed opportunities, vaccine inventory, vaccination safety, and quality of data submitted to the state immunization information system (IIS). An overview page containing an immunization strategy map and KPIs provide meaningful visualization of the major activities within the immunization program.[18] The SMaRT strategy map gives an at-a-glance snapshot of how the program is progressing toward its goals and objectives, whereas the KPIs provide further insight into specific statistics of programmatic importance. In addition, a geographic map provides ad hoc drill down into each county or parish ZIP codes to illustrate any geographic trends within the KPIs. Similarly, the immunization coverage page shows vaccination coverage rates by vaccine family, coverage over time, a drill-down geographic map, and nonmedical waivers by vaccine family. Furthermore, it offers select variables for slicing in terms of age, gender, race, provider, and time frame.[18]

OPPORTUNITIES PROVIDING A BIGGER ROLE FOR ANALYTICS

In February 2009, the US government launched an unprecedented effort, embodied in the Health Information Technology for Economic and Clinical Health (HITECH) Act, to transform the way the country collects, stores, and uses health information.[19] The **HITECH Act** would support the adoption and "Meaningful Use" (i.e., use intended to improve health and health care) of EHRs and other types of health information technology.[19]

The HITECH Act provided an opportunity for the creation of a nationwide, interoperable, private, and secure electronic health information system. The HITECH Act also created two new federal committees to advise the Department of Health and Human Services (HHS) for implementing the HITECH Act: the Health Information Technology Policy Committee (HITPC) provided general policy advice and Health Information Technology Standards Committee (HITSC) helped with developing standards, implementation specifications, and certification criteria for EHRs. It is reported that the HITECH Act spurred a rapid increase in the adoption of EHRs, an essential precondition to their meaningful use.[20] Furthermore, it facilitated development of standards for interoperability, protection of privacy and security.

Another significant thrust came from the Open Government Directive in 2009 and consequent actions of HHS under the Health Data Initiative (HDI). The **Open Government Directive** directs executive departments and agencies to take specific actions to implement the principles of transparency, participation, and collaboration.[21]

The **HDI** was originally launched by the IOM and the HHS as the Community Health Data Initiative, and is a public–private collaboration that encourages innovators to utilize health data to develop applications to raise awareness of health and health system performance and spark community action to improve health.[22]

The initiative would liberate significant public health data from agencies like the Centers for Medicare and Medicaid Services, the FDA, and the Centers for Disease Control and Prevention. Furthermore, it is expected that the value derived from the sharing and exchange of data will propel problem solving toward creative, cost-effective, and efficient solutions in areas such as data-driven decision-making in health care. It would also facilitate unleashing the power of private sector innovators and entrepreneurs to utilize HHS data in the creation of applications, products, and services that positively impact health and health care.[23]

In addition, the Affordable Care Act, enacted in March 2010, included a provision that authorizes HHS to release data that promotes transparency in the market for health care and health insurance.[24]

The implications of these reforms are far reaching. This integration of data across health care and federal systems has the potential to monitor individual as well as population health. For example, the patient code data emanating from EHRs could track lifetime disease, medication, and expenditure history of individuals. Similarly, genome-based data can enable health systems to facilitate presymptomatic diagnostics and personalized medicine. Furthermore, the development of implantable sensors that automatically report health data on real-time data streams could provide real-time decision support.[2]

The greatest public health benefits could be achieved in linking public health data to other types of health data, which would enable the development of deeper understanding of disease dynamics, transmission, and health systems responses. This opportunity could be leveraged to develop advanced public health analytics for real-time decision support. For example, a model EMR-based public health surveillance platform called **Electronic Medical Record Support for Public Health** (ESP), created by the Harvard Center of Excellence in Public Health Informatics in collaboration with the Massachusetts Department of Public Health, is operational in Massachusetts and Ohio.[25] This ESP platform uses software that loads EMR data from clinician-owned systems, analyzes these data for events of public health interest, and electronically communicates findings to public health agencies.[25] The ESP platform's surveillance modules automatically execute complex disease-detection algorithms to provide meaningful surveillance without requiring additional work by clinicians.[25] By reliably automating clinical analyses for selected outcomes, the ESP surveillance platform shifts the burden of reporting from clinicians to information systems. Current applications include notifiable disease case reporting, influenza-like-illness syndromic surveillance, and automated monitoring of diabetes risk factors, prevalence, care, and complications.[25]

CHALLENGES TO BE ADDRESSED

It is recognized that the amount of health data is increasing everyday. In order to effectively use it to improve, anticipate, and respond to public needs, public health entities need tools that allow them to quickly and easily collect and analyze multisource data in a range of formats.[26] Data come from a variety of heterogeneous sources including health insurance exchanges, EHRs, hospital admissions, patient histories, payers and providers, social media, clinical trials, prescriptions, demographic data, and others. Electronic health information systems thus seem a necessary foundation for realizing many other short-term and long-term health policy goals.[19]

The Institute of Medicine has repeatedly called for the increased use of health information technology in health care. However, barriers to dissemination and adoption of electronic information systems do exist. In the USA, at least four key barriers have been identified.[19] The most fundamental one is economic: the fee-for-service payment system in the USA does not financially reward the improved quality and efficiency that health information technology makes possible. Second, the adoption and use of health information technology is logistically and technically demanding especially in terms of installation, maintenance, and upgradation over time. Third, the ability to effectively transfer electronic health information between different information systems in various institutions and practices is underdeveloped and requires exchange solutions to make them work seamlessly. Finally, the concern about the privacy and security of digital health information is cited as an important barrier.[19] The growing personal health record industry, which is not currently regulated under the Health Insurance Portability and Accountability Act (HIPAA), emphasizes this concern. These barriers to the adoption of electronic health information systems are upstream events, which further lead to bottlenecks at the level of analytics.

USING CUTTING-EDGE ANALYTICS TO INFORM POLICY

In the context of public health surveillance, probably the best use of public health analytics was attempted during the H5N1 influenza pandemic in 2005 by infectious disease modelers to predict the spread of pandemic flu and identify appropriate interventions for prevention and control. An influenza prevention and containment strategy includes antiviral medication, vaccine, and nonpharmaceutical (case isolation, household quarantine, school or workplace closure, and restrictions on travel) measures.

Neil Ferguson[27] and colleagues developed and parameterized an individual-based simulation model of pandemic influenza transmission for Great Britain and the USA using high-resolution population density data, data on travel patterns, and realistic seeding of infection (via international travel) to explore the complex landscape of intervention strategies and quantifying the potential costs and benefits of different options. They reported that border restrictions and/or internal travel restrictions are unlikely to delay spread by more than 2–3 weeks, school closure during the peak of a pandemic can reduce peak attack rates by up to 40% but has little impact on overall attack rates, whereas case isolation or household quarantine could have a significant impact on overall attack rates (reduces cumulative attack rate from 34% to 27%). Furthermore, they reported that treatment of clinical cases can reduce transmission, but only if antivirals are given within a day of symptoms starting. Given enough drugs for half of the population, household-based prophylaxis coupled with reactive school closure could reduce clinical attack rates by 40–50%.[27]

The above-mentioned example highlights the culmination of best practices in surveillance, analytics, disease, and decision modeling that emerging surveillance systems should aspire for. In the future, public health surveillance should focus on creating new methods that can scale up to massive quantities of data and can integrate information from large numbers of data sources, especially richness and complexity of novel data sources at the societal scale.[6]

CONCLUSION

Public health analytics is emerging as cross-cutting domain, fostering application of information technology for evidence-based decision-making in public health practice. In addition, access to Big Data and quantum jump in the computational abilities of processors has made real-time analytics integral to surveillance systems. Although there are multiple challenges to developing CDM and shared distributed networks, an enabling environment has been created by regulatory bodies to foster cutting-edge research and innovation in public health analytics. This innovation-driven and shared resource model may lead to improved health security and health outcomes in future.

KEY SUMMARY POINTS

- Analytics is the systematic use of data and related insights developed through applied analytical disciplines to drive fact-based decision-making for planning, management, measurement, and learning.
- Public health analytics can be descriptive, predictive, or prescriptive. They offer public health professionals the necessary tools to respond to unexpected situations such as global outbreaks or infectious episodes.
- These building blocks of public health analytics include data governance, data acquisition, data sharing, integration, standardization, and analytics.
- The regulatory reforms initiated by the US government like the Health Information Technology for Economic and Clinical Health (HITECH) Act, the Health Data Initiative (HDI), and the Affordable Care Act have offered unprecedented opportunity to make best use of analytics to inform decision-making.
- There are economic and logistical barriers to disseminating and adopting electronic information systems with other concerns including the transferability of data and data privacy and security.
- The ultimate objective of any analytic approach should be to inform decision-making in the event of uncertainty with whatever limited information is available at that point of time. Predictive and prescriptive analytics can facilitate real time decision support and advice.

DISCUSSION QUESTIONS

1. Critically analyze the pros and cons of different types of public health analytics.
2. Explain in detail the different data layers that can be used to run advanced analytics.
3. Highlight key challenges in advancing the agenda of public health analytics.

4. Do you agree that investments in technologies that can perform predictive analytics are worth the cost? Why or why not?
5. Use an example to explain the limitations of descriptive analytics.
6. Prepare a case for establishing a data governance policy for the national surveillance center of your country.
7. Who are the different stakeholders involved in the development of a national public health analytics task force?

REFERENCES

1. Cortada J, Gordon D, Lenihan B. The value of analytics in healthcare: from insights to outcomes. 2012.
2. Crafts M. Application of integrated health analytics in a regulatory environment. 2012.
3. Raghupathi W, Raghupathi V. An overview of health analytics. J Health Med Informat 2013;4(132):1–11. doi:10.4172/2157-7420.1000132. [accessed on 5 January 2015].
4. Rhoads J, Ferrara L. Transforming healthcare through better use of data. Computer Sciences Corporation 2012; pg 1-7. <http://assets1.csc.com/health_services/downloads/CSC_Transforming_Healthcare_Through_Better_Use_of_Data.pdf>; [accessed on 5 January 2015].
5. Bohm K, Mehler-Bicher A, Fenchel D. GeoVisualAnalytics in the public health sector. Fuzhou: Spatial Data Mining and Geographical Knowledge Services (ICSDM), IEEE International Conference; 2011. June 29, 2011–July 1, 2011.
6. Neill DB. New directions in artificial intelligence for public health surveillance. IEEE Intell Syst 2012;27(1):56–9.
7. Wigbels L. Using earth observation data to improve health in the United States: accomplishments and future challenges. Center for Strategic and International Studies, Washington D.C.; 2011 <http://csis.org/files/publication/110927_Wigbels_UsingEarthObserHealth_WEB.pdf>; [accessed on 5 January 2015].
8. Sun H. Enterprise Information Management: Best Practices in Data Governance. Oracle Corporation, Redwood Shores, CA; 2011. <http://www.oracle.com/technetwork/articles/entarch/oea-best-practices-data-gov-400760.pdf>; [accessed on 5 January 2015].
9. PHDSC. Health information technology standards, <http://www.phdsc.org/standards/health-information/D_Standards.asp/>; [accessed on 5 January 2015].
10. Common Data Model. Observational medical outcomes partnership, <http://omop.org/CDM/>; 2015 [accessed on 5 January 2015].
11. Biomedical Translational Research Information System (BTRIS). National Institute of Health. <http://btris.nih.gov/index.html>; [accessed on 5 January 2015]
12. International Health Terminology Standards Development Organisation (IHTSDO). SNOMED CT, <http://www.ihtsdo.org/snomed-ct/>; 2015 [accessed on 5 January 2015].
13. WHO. International Classification of Diseases (ICD), <http://www.who.int/classifications/icd/en/>; 2014. [accessed May 30, 2015].
14. Curtis LH, Weiner MG, Boudreau DM, Cooper WO, Daniel GW, Nair VP, et al. Design considerations, architecture, and use of the Mini-Sentinel distributed data system. Pharmacoepidemiol Drug Saf 2012;21(Suppl. 1): 23–31.
15. McGraw D, Rosati K, Evans B. A policy framework for public health uses of electronic health data. Pharmacoepidemiol Drug Saf 2012;21(Suppl. 1): 18–22.
16. Kim K. Clinical data standards in health care: five case studies. Oakland: California HealthCare Foundation; 2005.
17. Ohno-Machado L, Day ME, El-Kareh R, Jiang X, Kim H, Meeker D, et al. Standards in the Use of Collaborative or Distributed Data Networks in Patient Centered Outcomes Research. 2012.
18. 2012 Public Health Annual Report. A Year of Innovation in Public Health Information and Technology. 2012.
19. Blumenthal D. Wiring the health system—origins and provisions of a new federal program. N Engl J Med 2011;365(24):2323–9.
20. Blumenthal D. Implementation of the federal health information technology initiative. N Engl J Med 2011;365(25):2426–31.
21. The United States Department of Justice. Open Government, <http://www.justice.gov/open/>; 2015 [accessed on 5 January 2015].
22. Definition provided by the chapter author.
23. Health Data Initiative. Strategy and Execution Plan, <https://docs.google.com/file/d/0B9hZC55hEGZUM19xczk2RTU2M2c/edit/>; 2013. [accessed on 5 January 2015].
24. Software I. Using analytics and collaboration to improve healthcare quality and outcomes. IBM Corporation Software Group, Somers, NY; 2012. <http://public.dhe.ibm.com/common/ssi/ecm/im/en/imw14650usen/IMW14650USEN.PDF>.
25. Klompas M, McVetta J, Lazarus R, Eggleston E, Haney G, Kruskal BA, et al. Integrating clinical practice and public health surveillance using electronic medical record systems. Am J Prev Med 2012;42(6 Suppl. 2): S154–62.
26. Actuate Corporation. Advanced and Predictive Analytics for Public Health Authorities, <http://www.actuate.com/download/whitepapers/BA-for-Public-Health-Authorities.pdf/>; 2015 [accessed on 5 January 2015].
27. Ferguson NM, Cummings DA, Fraser C, Cajka JC, Cooley PC, Burke DS. Strategies for mitigating an influenza pandemic. Nature 2006;442(7101): 448–52.

CHAPTER

28

Predictive Surveillance: An Outcome of Applied Interdisciplinary Translational Research in Public Health Surveillance

JP Chretien

A knotty puzzle may hold a scientist up for a century, when it may be that a colleague has the solution already and is not even aware of the puzzle that it might solve.

Isaac Asimov, The Robots of Dawn

KEY WORDS

Predictive surveillance
Prediction model
Input data
Static data
Dynamic data

INTERDISCIPLINARY COLLABORATION FOR PREDICTIVE SURVEILLANCE

Introduction to Predictive Surveillance

Practitioners of public health surveillance can draw on data and analytical tools that were unavailable just a few years ago. To exploit these opportunities, practitioners must expand their technical knowledge and collaborations beyond the boundaries that have traditionally defined public health practice domains. For example, in some current, innovative surveillance applications, surveillance practitioners are collaborating across disciplines, with:

- Veterinary health professionals, to integrate human and animal surveillance for pandemic influenza and other zoonotic diseases.
- Web programmers, to use social media to identify disease outbreaks, and to develop user-friendly websites for the public to access the surveillance information in near real time.
- Medical informaticians, to ensure the public health utility of new data and interoperability standards for electronic medical records in the USA.
- Computer scientists, to develop detailed simulation models of disease spread and public health interventions.
- Experts in database design and analysis methods for "big data" applications, to manage and make sense of large data sets from various sources that could enhance public health surveillance (e.g., genetic testing, environmental measurements, medical encounter data, and individual data recorded using mobile health devices, to name a few).

In this chapter, we focus on another area, "predictive surveillance", where public health researchers and practitioners are collaborating across domains to develop novel surveillance programs. Predictive surveillance is an emerging field, new enough to lack an agreed upon definition but involving use of surveillance data and models to make predictions about disease activity. **Predictive surveillance** is a type of surveillance that uses state-of-the-art computer models and algorithms to predict the presence or absence of a pathogen in a geographic area.[1]

Like traditional surveillance, predictive surveillance should produce information for action; it should assist decision-making (Table 28-1).

Predictive surveillance is not new; in the early 1900s, public health officials developed malaria early warning systems using climatic, social, and epidemiologic conditions. Malaria forecasting research and applications continued through today, throughout epidemic-prone regions, using diverse prediction methodologies.[2] Promising applications have encouraged hope that climate data could help predict outbreaks of other infectious diseases.[3]

But predictive surveillance today is different from the applications of nearly 100 years ago, and interdisciplinary collaboration in this field is more important than ever. Reasons for this include:

- Surveillance data may be available in near real time, enabling near-real-time updates of epidemiologic forecasts using appropriate information technology and statistical methods.
- Surveillance data sets are larger and include data on a wide range of potential predictors not used extensively in public health analyses previously (e.g., climate data from satellites, global air travel networks, and internet search queries).
- Understanding of within-individual and between-individual disease dynamics is better, facilitating development of epidemiologic models that may improve predictions if used appropriately.
- Many sophisticated analytical tools are available, beyond the statistical tools used traditionally in public health surveillance. Current predictive surveillance applications use Bayesian methods, machine-learning approaches, data assimilation, individual-based modeling, and other methods that require computational capabilities not available until recently.

Predictive Surveillance Data, Models, and Predictions

Before considering current and possible future predictive surveillance applications, it may be useful to propose a basic framework for describing these applications. A standard approach for describing public health surveillance systems[4] applies to predictive surveillance as well, and includes:

- The system's purpose
- Planned use of the system's data
- Health-related event under surveillance
- Any legal authority for data collection
- Organizational context
- Integration with other systems
- Data flow
- System components (e.g., population under surveillance, type of data collected and collection method, reporting sources, data management and analysis)

TABLE 28-1 Decisions that Predictive Surveillance Systems May Support

DECISION-MAKER	DECISION	EXAMPLE PREDICTIVE SURVEILLANCE SYSTEM
Public health officials	What epidemic/epizootic interventions to initiate during an outbreak?	Forecasting foot-and-mouth disease spread during an outbreak[19]
Medical facility staff	How to allocate staff and resources during high-volume periods?	Forecasting near-term hospital admissions for respiratory illness[20]
Employers	What types of health-related services to develop?	State-level forecasts of diabetes prevalence[21]
General public	When to heighten alertness or seek medical care for symptoms?	Population-based forecasts of influenza-like illness[22]

For predictive surveillance, the central additional feature compared to traditional public health surveillance is the *prediction model*, which may comprise several models and takes various *input data*, including public health surveillance data, and produces various outputs, including the *predictions* of interest. Predictive surveillance systems may have a relatively simple structure, e.g., predicting future epidemiological patterns based on previous patterns. Some are considerably more complex, incorporating various external predictors and statistical models (Fig. 28-1). Next, we describe three important components of predictive surveillance systems—input data, prediction model, and predictions—in more detail.

Input Data

A predictive surveillance system may use static or dynamic input data (e.g., baseline data), or both types of data, to make predictions. **Static data** are the data the system captures once to help generate predictions, while **dynamic data** are the data the system captures periodically to update predictions.[1] For example, a predictive surveillance system for an infectious respiratory disease might use demographic data for a population, collected recently enough to remain accurate, to develop age-specific models of population mixing needed for the prediction model. This system might also use monthly disease surveillance data. Each month, the system predicts future disease activity by feeding the (static) demographic data and most recent (dynamic) incidence data into its prediction model.

Other examples of static data that predictive surveillance systems commonly use are location, transportation, socioeconomic, and comorbidity or immunity data. The surveillance data the system uses might also be static if, for example, it uses the previous year's surveillance data to predict disease activity over the next year. Other examples of dynamic input data are meteorological data and health-related behavioral data, such as drug or medical product purchases or internet search queries.

Prediction Model

The system may use one or more models to predict disease activity. A relatively simple system might use a single model to extrapolate an epidemic curve based on recent surveillance data (Fig. 28-1b). A more complex system might

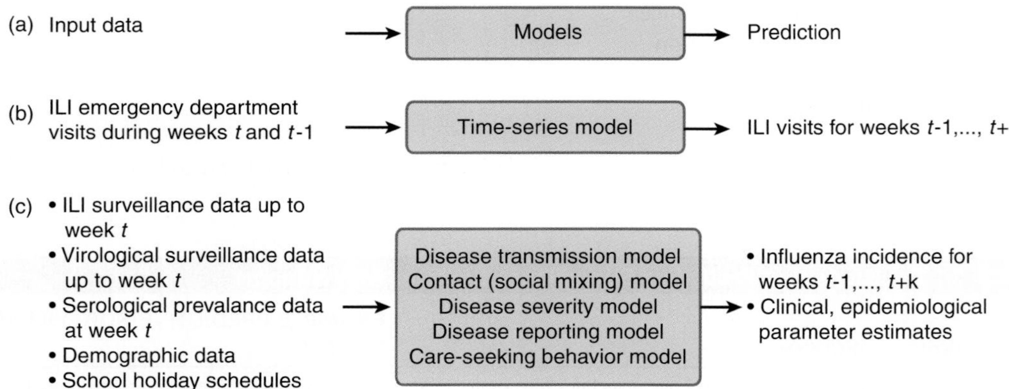

FIG. 28-1 Data, models, and predictions in predictive surveillance systems. (a) Generic representation of these system components. (b) Example of a predictive surveillance system with relatively simple structure, developed for use in a hospital.[23] A time-series model incorporates the number of ILI presentations to the facility during the previous 2 weeks, and predicts the number of admissions each week into the future. (c) Example of a predictive surveillance system with relatively complex structure, developed using data from the 2009 influenza A/H1N1 pandemic.[24] Several models incorporate various surveillance and other data, and predict influenza incidence each week into the future as well as values for key model parameters.

use several linked models, requiring additional data sources (Fig. 28-1c). Besides identifying the specific models in a predictive surveillance system, it is useful to make a basic distinction between two general modeling approaches these systems use: ones that explicitly represent the underlying epidemiologic or biological processes that contribute to observed input data, and ones that do not (Table 28-2).

The former models (sometimes called "dynamic[al]" models) demand some knowledge of disease characteristics within individuals and how the disease spreads through populations, which may come from previous clinical and epidemiologic studies and views of experts. The latter models (sometimes called "statistical" or "association" models), in contrast, relate input data to predictions using mathematical approaches that do not include biological or epidemiologic parameters.

While dynamic models require assumptions about biological and epidemiologic processes that association models do not, they offer key advantages when these assumptions are appropriate. By providing estimates of important parameters (e.g., the basic reproduction number [R_0] for an infectious disease, the number of additional cases generated by each case), they more directly yield insight into the epidemiology of the disease and they allow users to test the effects of modifying key parameter values to evaluate the impact of mitigation measures, or to assess prediction sensitivity to epidemiologic assumptions.

Prediction models that take dynamic input data use different methods for producing the next set of predictions. In general, we may distinguish between two approaches. The simplest approach, often used in association models (Table 28-2), is to set parameter values before the first prediction (e.g., based on model development using historical data) and keep the parameter values fixed at those values as the system makes predictions using dynamic surveillance input data. For example, Soebiyanto et al.[5] developed time series (autoregressive integrated moving average) models to predict influenza incidence based on previous monthly incidence and monthly environmental data from 2005–2007 in Hong Kong. They fixed the parameter values to those estimated using 2005–2007 data, and applied the models using monthly inputs during 2008 to test its performance.

TABLE 28-2 Models Used in Predictive Surveillance Systems

GENERAL TYPE OF MODEL	EXAMPLE MODEL	MODELING APPROACH	EXAMPLE APPLICATION
Dynamic	Compartmental models	Model dynamic change of population numbers in each compartment	SIR model with modification for environmental transmission) to predict avian influenza outbreaks in duck populations[25]
	Individual-based (or agent-based) models	Simulate behavior and interactions at the level of the individual	Individual-level simulation of large metropolitan area to predict seasonal influenza peaks based on internet search queries (Google Flu Trends)[26]
Association	Regression models	User generalized linear models to predict future disease activity based on previous activity, other predictors	Linear regression to predict malaria case counts based on previous counts, meteorological data[27]
	Time-series regression models	As for regression models, but account for internal data structure (especially serial autocorrelation)	Seasonal autoregressive integrated moving average to predict asthma hospitalizations based on previous counts, influenza incidence[28]
	Machine learning (e.g., support vector machines, Bayesian networks, association rule-mining)	Various algorithms find relationships between previous disease activity, other predictors and future activity	Fuzzy association rule mining to predict high dengue incidence periods based on previous incidence, meteorological and socioeconomic data[29]

This approach can be simple for users of established models to implement, but an important limitation is that it cannot adapt to new patterns in the input data. For example, if a model was developed using seasonal influenza data but applied during an influenza pandemic, where immunity is much lower and transmissibility and clinical severity may differ, it cannot set key parameters to more appropriate values. Predictions using the parameter values established during seasonal epidemics may be highly inaccurate.

An alternative is to re-estimate model parameters as the system incorporates new dynamic input data. One way to do this is to incorporate the latest input data into the data set, re-estimate parameters using that expanded data set, and make predictions using those new parameter values. For example, Hall et al.[6] developed a pandemic influenza prediction model, based on a modified Susceptible–Infectious–Removed (SIR) model, using data from pandemics beginning in 1918, 1957, and 1968. Their approach fixes values for disease kinetics parameters at the beginning of the pandemic, but re-estimates the reproductive number and proportion of cases captured by surveillance as new surveillance data are incorporated. Similarly, Hyder et al.,[7] using an individual-based model (IBM) to predict influenza transmission in Montreal, set values for key parameters using historical data but re-estimate case capture with each new surveillance report.

Recently, developers of predictive surveillance models have adapted methods used in other fields, such as weather prediction, for re-estimating parameters using dynamic input data. One method, data assimilation, uses the most recent surveillance data and estimates of the error associated with those data to adjust the previous parameter estimates (a technical description is beyond the scope of this chapter, but, intuitively, data assimilation seeks to balance errors in the observed data against model error when updating estimates).

Examples include use of Kalman[8] and particle[9] filtering, in conjunction with modified SIR models, to predict influenza incidence. Nsoesie et al.,[10] also proposing a predictive surveillance method for influenza, used a related optimization approach in conjunction with an IBM simulation. These methods generally require more computational resources and expertise than other approaches. They have not yet found wide application in predictive surveillance, but many researchers and practitioners in predictive surveillance and related areas view them as promising for this application.

Predictions

Important considerations in describing the predictions a predictive surveillance system makes include:

- *What is predicted*: Epidemiologic variables that systems predict include incidence, prevalence, the timing of an epidemic peak, and epidemic duration, among others.
- *What is the dimensionality of predictions*: Depending on the input data and prediction model used, systems may make spatial as well as temporal forecasts, and make separate predictions for subpopulations based on demographic, clinical, or other factors.
- *How often predictions are made*: Systems may make predictions at regular intervals, such as weekly using new surveillance data from the previous week, or predict just once based on previous surveillance data.
- *How far into the future predictions are made*: Prediction models typically allow prediction to arbitrary future times, though determination of the appropriate time horizon for prediction depends on the purpose of the system (i.e., the decisions it supports) and its predictive accuracy at various time horizons.
- *What, if any, measures of variability or uncertainty accompany the predictions*: Measures such as confidence intervals or credible intervals (for Bayesian methods) are important for decision-makers who must determine what actions to take based on the predictions.

Before practitioners use a predictive surveillance system in a real-world setting, the prediction model must be validated. Ideally, validation involves comparison of predictions made using out-of-sample surveillance data (i.e., data that was not used to develop the model) to observed values. Use of independent data for validation is important because, in real-world applications, the system will not have "seen" the surveillance data before; testing the model against the same data used to develop the model produces (optimistically) biased estimates of prediction accuracy.[11]

A common approach to validating models for predictive surveillance is the holdout method, where the data are divided into a training set for model development and a test set for assessing prediction accuracy. Another approach is cross-validation, where the data are divided into several sets, and the model sequentially trained using all but one of the sets and tested against the remaining set; an overall accuracy measure aggregates the accuracy across all of the testing applications.

Various statistics are used to measure the accuracy of predictive surveillance models using out-of-sample data. A simple and common approach is the prediction error at time t, or $e_t = Y_t - P_t$, where Y_t and P_t are the observed and predicted values, respectively, at time t. For example e_t could measure the difference in days between the observed and predicted epidemic peak, or the difference in counts or incidence between the observed and predicted values at time t. A validation study may report the prediction error for a specific time t of particular interest, or some summary measure of the prediction error or related statistic across multiple prediction times (Table 28-3).

When considering different predictive surveillance approaches, a practitioner may wish to compare validation studies for various prediction models using various data sets.[12] Many common measures of prediction accuracy (Table 28-3) do not facilitate such a comparison. Measures based on absolute error depend on the scale of the data, which may differ across studies. Measures based on percentage error avoid the scale-dependence problem, but are undefined when the observed value is zero (as may occur in surveillance data with small counts). Measures based on relative error have statistical distributional problems, and they and relative measures both require application of different prediction models to the same data set. Unfortunately, validation studies for predictive surveillance models rarely do this.

In addition to undergoing validation, following best practices in epidemiologic modeling,[13] models used in predictive surveillance should also be subject to sensitivity analysis. At many steps of model development, modelers may make assumption—for example, in predictive surveillance, about the transmissibility of the disease, or the accuracy of surveillance data used in modeling, or the behavior of people affected by the disease. In many cases, and especially for new or rare diseases, where predictive surveillance could be especially helpful, such assumptions are made on the basis of very limited data. In sensitivity analysis, the modeler modifies the assumptions within a plausible range of possibilities, and assesses the sensitivity of model outputs to each assumption. One would have more confidence in results that change little despite assumed values for disease transmissibility or other parameters, and might attempt to identify additional data to refine assumptions for parameters that exert substantial influence on the results.

TABLE 28-3 Some Measures of Prediction Accuracy for Predictive Surveillance Systems

TYPE OF MEASURE	STATISTIC[a]	DEFINITION[a]
Based on absolute error	Mean Square Error (MSE)	mean(e_t^2)
	Root Mean Square Error (RMSE)	sqrt(MSE)
	Mean Absolute Error (MAE)	mean($\|e_t\|$)
	Median Absolute Error (MdAE)	median($\|e_t\|$)
Based on percentage error	Mean Absolute Percentage Error (MAPE)	mean($\|p_t\|$)
	Median Absolute Percentage Error (MdAPE)	median($\|p_t\|$)
	Root Mean Square Percentage Error (RMSPE)	sqrt(mean(p_t^2))
	Root Median Square Percentage Error (RMdSPE)	sqrt(median(p_t^2))
Based on relative error	Mean Relative Absolute Error (MRAE)	mean($\|r_t\|$)
	Median Relative Absolute Error (MdRAE)	median($\|r_t\|$)
Relative measures	e.g., RelMAE	MAE/MAE*

[a] p_t is the percentage error at time $t = 100\ e_t / y_t$. r_t is the error relative to a comparison prediction model $= e_t / e^*_t$, where e^*_t is the error with the comparison model.

Note: MAE* is the MAE obtained with a comparison prediction model.

VISION FOR PREDICTIVE SURVEILLANCE

A near-term goal for the emerging field of predictive surveillance is to identify, through research efforts, the public health challenges and questions for which predictive surveillance might be useful. Could predictive surveillance provide sufficiently timely and accurate predictions to help in responding to an emerging infectious disease outbreak? How about for endemic, seasonal infections, such as dengue? Or noncommunicable diseases, such as diabetes and cancer? There are exciting opportunities now to undertake a broad range of predictive surveillance research applications, with unprecedented epidemiologic, sociodemographic, climatological, and other data resources; and with ever-advancing computational resources to manage and analyze such data.

In the longer term, if areas of public health practice are identified where predictive surveillance can be useful, predictive surveillance might be incorporated into the routine functions of health departments and organizations. One might imagine a subnational or national health department issuing seasonal or weekly forecasts for certain infectious diseases (as a weather service would for meteorological conditions), or predictions of global spread and severity for a newly emerged pathogen. Important impediments to achieving this vision include the computational and organizational challenges in integrating the diverse data sets that may be required for useful predictions, and the quality of surveillance data essential for initiating and validating models (please see below for additional discussion of impediments).

PREDICTIVE SURVEILLANCE EXAMPLE: 2009 H1N1

In 2009, a novel influenza strain, later named influenza A (H1N1), emerged in Mexico and spread to countries around the world. In April, the World Health Organization (WHO) declared the situation a public health emergency of international concern (PHEIC) under the International Health Regulations, and in June labeled it a pandemic. Researchers with the US Centers for Disease Control and Prevention and collaborators estimated that between 151,700 and 575,400 people worldwide died because of influenza A (H1N1) infection during the first 12 months of the pandemic.[14] WHO announced an end to the pandemic in August 2010.

As air travel by people infected with the virus was the dominant means of international spread,[15] several efforts attempted to predict the regional or global dynamics of influenza A (H1N1), using international air travel data and other potential predictors. While these studies were not performed in real time during the early days of the pandemic, they did use appropriate methods to validate their (retrospective) predictions.

Tizzoni et al.[16] integrated a compartmental disease transmission model with global population data and a mobility model, which included international air travel and daily commuting models. They initiated the model near La Gloria, Mexico, where the outbreak is thought to have begun, in February 2009, and ran the model forward in time to predict the peak incidence week in 48 countries around the world. They compared model predictions to surveillance data reported by these countries. The model peak week predictions showed statistically significant correlation with the observed peak weeks (Spearman correlation coefficient = 0.48; p = 0.0001), with an error of 2 weeks or less for 90% of the countries.

Merler et al.[17] focused on spread of influenza A (H1N1) in Europe. Like Tizzoni et al.,[16] they used population and transportation (air and railway) data to predict the week of peak incidence. Additionally, they used an IBM for mixing and transmission within households, schools, and workplaces; and incorporated country-specific data (reported by WHO) from the early days of the pandemic in Europe to help guide model predictions. This study also reported a statistically significant correlation with country peak week based on reported surveillance data (Spearman correlation coefficient = 0.53; p = 0.006), with an error of 2.5 weeks or less for 50% of the countries. Notably, Merler et al. compared their approach with a simpler model: one that retained all aspects of the original model except for the individual-level modeling, which they replaced with a simpler, homogenous mixing model. Qualitative assessments suggested that the more complex model generated predictions more similar to the observed incidence data.

In contrast to Tizzoni et al.[16] and Merler et al.,[17] who used dynamic models (compartmental and individual-based, respectively), Hosseini et al.[18] used an association model—survival analysis—to predict arrival of influenza A (H1N1) to countries reporting initial cases early in the pandemic (model fitting using the 39 countries that reported a first case before May 8, 2009; validation using the 14 countries reporting a first case between May 9 and May 19, 2009). They also incorporated country-level economic data as a possible predictor of health-care-seeking behavior, or outbreak detection or reporting capacity. Like Tizzoni et al.[16] and Merler et al.,[17] they modeled international air travel, but they did not use detailed models of population location or mixing. The correlation between model predictions and observed reporting date for the first case was 0.62.

These three examples of predictive surveillance to forecast regional or global spread of influenza A (H1N1), though they did not generate predictions in real time during the pandemic, offer a glimpse of how such methods could be used as future emerging infection epidemics unfold. With the modeling infrastructure established, modelers could use initial surveillance data to set key epidemiological parameters, and provide near-real-time predictions of global disease dynamics to guide public health planning.

There are a few important obstacles to performing such applications in real time today, though. First, two of the examples described above[16, 17] used models requiring substantial computational capabilities. Few groups may have the resources to run such models, though with additional funding for high-performing modeling teams lacking the computational resources, more widespread application (enabling teams to address a greater diversity of public health questions, and a broader set of results for comparison).

Second, accurate surveillance data are critical for such models. They use data from early in the outbreak to initiate the models, but early-outbreak data—especially if obtained in low-resource areas—may be highly inaccurate. This was the case with influenza A (H1N1), where initially high estimates of the case fatality rate subsequently were attributed to failure to identify many more, less-severe infections. Surveillance data would be essential for validating model predictions as the epidemic progresses. In areas where surveillance capabilities are limited, important opportunities for model assessment and improvement would be lost.

KEY SUMMARY POINTS

- Predictive surveillance is an emerging field that uses surveillance data and models to make predictions about disease activity that can guide public health preparedness.
- Predictive surveillance is mostly a research area, with few operational applications. However, unprecedented computational and data resources provide exciting new opportunities to define whether, and where, predictive surveillance could be useful in public health practice.
- All predictive surveillance models should undergo validation and sensitivity analysis, using accepted best practices in epidemiologic modeling, before operational application.
- Several modeling teams used predictive surveillance approaches to forecast the regional or global spread of influenza A (H1N1). While these efforts did not generate real-time predictions to guide public health preparedness, they do provide a vision of how predictive surveillance might be useful as future emerging infection outbreaks unfold.

DISCUSSION QUESTIONS

1. What is a possible application of predictive surveillance? Consider the specific public health problem, planning, and policy questions that predictive surveillance could inform, and possible data sources that could be used.
2. Identify a published study that used epidemiologic modeling to link health-related outcomes with predictors. Would it be appropriate to "operationalize" this approach as a predictive surveillance program? In assessing why or why not, consider whether and how model validation and sensitivity analysis were performed, among other issues?
3. What are some potential challenges in promoting the use of predictive surveillance modeling results among policy makers and other decision-makers?

REFERENCES

1. Definition provided by the chapter author.
2. Zinszer K, Verma AD, Charland K, Brewer TF, Brownstein JS, Sun Z, et al. A scoping review of malaria forecasting: past work and future directions. BMJ Open 2012;2(6): e001992.
3. World Health Organization. Using climate to predict infectious disease outbreaks: a review. Geneva; 2004.
4. German RR, Lee LM, Horan JM, Milstein RL, Pertowski CA, Waller MN, et al. Updated guidelines for evaluating public health surveillance systems: recommendations from the Guidelines Working Group. MMWR Recomm Rep 2001;50(RR–13):1–35.
5. Soebiyanto RP, Adimi F, Kiang RK. Modeling and predicting seasonal influenza transmission in warm regions using climatological parameters. PLoS One 2010;5(3):e9450.
6. Hall IM, Gani R, Hughes HE, Leach S. Real-time epidemic forecasting for pandemic influenza. Epidemiol Infect 2007;135(3):372–85.
7. Hyder A, Buckeridge DL, Leung B. Predictive validation of an influenza spread model. PLoS One 2013;8(6):e65459.
8. Shaman J, Karspeck A. Forecasting seasonal outbreaks of influenza. Proc Natl Acad Sci U S A 2012;109(50):20425–30.
9. Ong JB, Chen MI, Cook AR, Lee HC, Lee VJ, Lin RT, et al. Real-time epidemic monitoring and forecasting of H1N1-2009 using influenza-like illness from general practice and family doctor clinics in Singapore. PLoS One 2010;5(4):e10036.
10. Nsoesie EO, Beckman RJ, Shashaani S, Nagaraj KS, Marathe MV. A simulation optimization approach to epidemic forecasting. PLoS One 2013;8(6):e67164.
11. Trevor Hastie, Jerome H. Friedman, Robert Tibshirani. The elements of statistical learning: data mining, inference, and prediction. 2nd ed. New York: Springer; 2009.
12. Hyndman RJ, Anne B. Another look at measures of forecast accuracy. Int J Forecasting 2006;22:679–88.
13. Woolhouse M, Fèvre EM, Handel I, Heller J, Tildesley MJ, Parkin T, et al. Guide to good practice for quantitative veterinary epidemiology. EERA; 2011.
14. Dawood FS, Iuliano AD, Reed C, Meltzer MI, Shay DK, Cheng PY, et al. Estimated global mortality associated with the first 12 months of 2009 pandemic influenza A H1N1 virus circulation: a modelling study. Lancet Infect Dis 2012;12(9):687–95.
15. Khan K, Arino J, Hu W, Raposo P, Sears J, Calderon F, et al. Spread of a novel influenza A (H1N1) virus via global airline transportation. N Engl J Med 2009; 361:212–4.
16. Tizzoni M, Bajardi P, Poletto C, Ramasco JJ, Balcan D, Gonçalves B, et al. Real-time numerical forecast of global epidemic spreading: case study of 2009 A/H1N1pdm. BMC Med 2012;10:165.
17. Merler S, Ajelli M, Pugliese A, Ferguson NM. Determinants of the spatio-temporal dynamics of the 2009 H1N1 pandemic in Europe: implications for real-time modelling. PLoS Comput Biol 2011;7(9):e1002205.
18. Hosseini P, Sokolow SH, Vandegrift KJ, Kilpatrick AM, Daszak P. Predictive power of air travel and socio-economic data for early pandemic spread. PLoS One 2010;5(9):e12763.
19. Ferguson NM, Donnelly CA, Anderson RM. The foot-and-mouth epidemic in Great Britain: pattern of spread and impact of interventions. Science 2001;292:1155–1160.
20. Spaeder MC, Fackler JC. Time series model to predict burden of viral respiratory illness on a pediatric intensive care unit. Med Decis Mak Int J Soc Med Decis Mak 2011;31:494–499.
21. Shi L, van Meijgaard J, Fielding J. Forecasting diabetes prevalence in California: a microsimulation. Prev Chronic Dis 2011;8:A80.
22. Shaman J, Karspeck A, Yang W, Tamerius J, Lipsitch M. Real-time influenza forecasts during the 2012-2013 season. Nat Commun 2013;4:2837.
23. Moriña D, Puig P, Ríos J, Vilella A, Trilla A. A statistical model for hospital admissions caused by seasonal diseases. Stat Med 2011;30:3125–3136.
24. Birrell PJ, Ketsetzis G, Gay NJ, Cooper BS, Presanis AM, et al. Bayesian modeling to unmask and predict influenza A/H1N1pdm dynamics in London. Proc Natl Acad Sci USA 2011;108:18238–18243.
25. Wang R-H, Jin Z, Liu Q-X, van de Koppel J, Alonso D. A simple stochastic model with environmental transmission explains multi-year periodicity in outbreaks of avian flu. PloS One 2012;7:e28873.
26. Nsoesie E, Mararthe M, Brownstein J. Forecasting peaks of seasonal influenza epidemics. PLoS Curr 2013;5. doi:10.1371/currents.outbreaks.bb1e879a23137022ea79a8c508b030bc.
27. Adimi F, Soebiyanto RP, Safi N, Kiang R. Towards malaria risk prediction in Afghanistan using remote sensing. Malar J 2010;9:125.
28. Gerke AK, Yang M, Tang F, Foster ED, Cavanaugh JE, et al. Association of hospitalizations for asthma with seasonal and pandemic influenza. Respirol Carlton Vic 2014;19:116–121.
29. Buczak AL, Koshute PT, Babin SM, Feighner BH, Lewis SH. A data-driven epidemiological prediction method for dengue outbreaks using local and remote sensing data. BMC Med Inform Decis Mak 2012;12:124.

6 SECTION

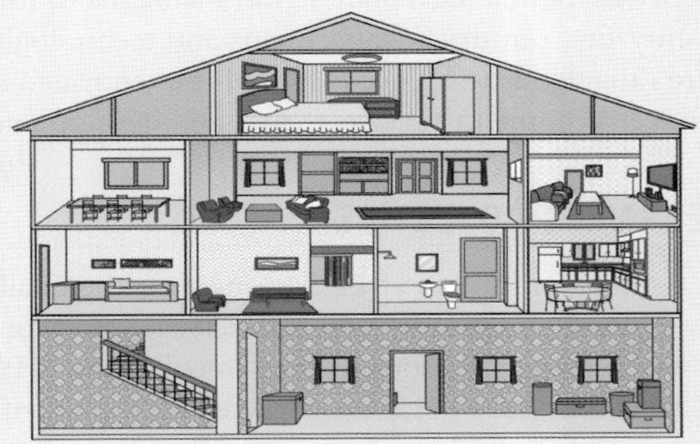

Impacts of Transformed Public Health Surveillance

Vivek Singh

Section Outline

The purpose of any PHS system is unfulfilled until it is linked to public health action. PHS systems can ensure a positive impact on population health only by ensuring that the right information is available at the right time, and in the right place, to inform public health decisions and actions. The public health actions should lead to equitable access to quality health care. PHS systems can ensure that every individual "counts" in a similar way to ensure that the actions are equitable. PHS information may also be used to guide health systems' improvement efforts, inform health service delivery, and measure progress toward health-related development goals.

The Millennium Development Goals (MDGs) as a roadmap to address poverty was arguably the most politically important pact ever made for international development. As the end line for the MDGs draws close, the lessons from measuring outcomes of health will provide the opportunity to strengthen capacity for PHS for the post-2015 agenda in the twenty-first century. The world is facing unique challenges to global health security in the twenty-first century, and, at the same time, advancements in technology and our understanding of determinants of health also offer immense opportunities for surveillance systems to find innovative ways to inform and guide the public health actions to tackle these challenges. PHS-related research will have to focus particularly on strengthening the evidence base for health policies and public health interventions that foster resilience, promote equity, and lead to sustainable development.

Achieving the ideal-state PHS (analogous to fully renovated smart home) will help unlock the potential of new twenty-first century advancements and technologies and leads to equitable access to quality and sustainable health care (analogous to all occupants of the renovated smart home are able to equally access all modern facilities in the renovated home to survive, thrive, and develop and the smart home will stand to last longer).

LEARNING OBJECTIVES

- Explain the use of PHS to monitor the quality and capacity of health services, identify underserved populations, and inform new research priorities for ensuring health equity.
- Discuss the lessons learned in collecting PHS data for monitoring MDGs.
- Discuss how PHS data collected for monitoring MDGs could be potentially used to improve inequalities within and between countries in health.
- Describe the limitations to the indicator data collected to measure a country's progression toward the MDGs.
- Explain the reporting issues and challenges that have arisen since global health initiatives have proliferated in LMICs.
- Identify the importance of qualitative research in PHS.
- Discuss establishment a common platform to bring together meaningful data from multiple sources at all levels of the health system to monitor post-2015 development goals.
- Describe the future challenges that need to be addressed for continued success in the transformation of PHS.
- Explain how research and innovation have and will continue to shape public health surveillance.
- Explain the importance of "counting" marginalized populations in surveillance, disease control, and elimination efforts.
- Identify how stigma and fear of discrimination impact PHS practice. Describe the lessons learned from the polio eradication campaign and the smallpox eradication campaign for transforming PHS as a toll to ensure health equity.
- Describe the technical and policy solutions that can be developed to transform PHS with an equity focus to strengthen efforts for global disease control, elimination, and eradication, which leads to sustainable development.

CHAPTER

29

Tracking Progress toward Health and Equity through the Millennium Development Goals—Lessons for Public Health Surveillance

Mahomed Said Patel, Kaosar Afsana, Christine Phillips

Without a system of public health surveillance and communication, public reason will be incomplete...[T]he duties of assistance between countries can only be realized if health issues that matter to the poorest nations of the world are accurately reported in those countries that have the greatest responsibility for providing assistance.

Richard Horton

KEY WORDS

Health equity
Social determinants of health
Health outcomes
Millennium Development Goals (MDGs)
Gender equality
Health Metrics Network (HMN)

THE OPPORTUNITY TO TRANSFORM PUBLIC HEALTH SURVEILLANCE

Why are there differences within and between countries in rates of morbidity and mortality for the same diseases? How can public health surveillance (PHS) help us elucidate the connections and barriers between poverty and sickness? The methods and technologies of PHS are becoming increasingly sophisticated. If we fail, however, to expand surveillance to capture the "causes of causes" for differences in health outcomes, then in McMichael's memorable phrase, we are simply counting the numbers of corks bobbing on the surface of an ocean, while ignoring the ocean flows that determine the direction of the current.[1]

The purpose of PHS is not only to monitor patterns and trends in diseases but also to monitor the quality and capacity of health services, identify underserved populations, and inform new research priorities.[2] The data that will assist us to do this must extend beyond the data that public health institutions themselves produce. Relevant data sources may include registries of vital events (e.g., births and deaths), censuses, population surveys, disease registers, health service and health resource records, and results of health research.[2-4] We should also incorporate qualitative data on how health is delivered, how people understand health, and more generally, on the social determinants of health.[5,6] These come from the fields of monitoring and evaluation, and may very often reflect resources and processes rather than outputs and outcomes.[7]

The health-related Millennium Development Goals (MDGs) use health data to report on outcomes and access to quality interventions for the 191 member states of the United Nations (UN). **MDGs** cover eight goals that all 191 UN member states are working to reach by the year 2015.[8] The United Nations Millennium Declaration, signed in September 2000, commits world leaders to battle poverty, hunger, disease, illiteracy, environmental degradation, and discrimination against women.[8] The MDGs come from this Declaration, and all have specific targets and indicators.[8] Few global ventures have been the subject of so much reportage and review as the MDGs, with debates about the capacity of countries to meet these goals or to collect PHS data appropriate for tracking progress toward the goals. There has been little debate on the next element of the discussion: can countries describe what enabled them to meet their targets, or prevented them from doing so? This is a question that could be answered through PHS using a rigorous monitoring framework.

In this chapter we explore the example of the health-related MDGs to draw out lessons about collecting PHS data, and the potential for the data to be used to improve inequalities within and between countries in health. We use the example of Bangladesh to tease out the reasons for a resource-poor country managing to achieve many of the targets set for the MDGs. Finally, we discuss a framework for transforming PHS, drawing on the common framework for monitoring, evaluating, and reviewing national plans and strategies.

THE MILLENNIUM DEVELOPMENT GOALS

In 2000, the 191 States of the UN made an unprecedented commitment, arguably the most politically important pact ever made for international development: together they would develop a roadmap to address poverty.[9-12] Member states agreed to prioritize efforts in eight areas, termed the Millennium Development Goals: to increase incomes and reduce hunger (MDG 1); to achieve universal primary education (MDG 2); to eliminate gender inequality (MDG 3); to reduce child mortality (MDG 4); to improve maternal health (MDG 5); to reverse the spread of HIV/AIDS, tuberculosis (TB), and malaria (MDG 6); to reverse the loss of natural resources and biodiversity, and to improve access to water, sanitation, and good housing (MDG 7); and to establish effective global partnerships to support development (MDG 8). MDGs 4, 5, and 6 are referred to as the "health-related MDGs" because they define specific health outcomes to monitor progress in achieving these goals. A **health outcome** is a change in the *health status* of an individual, group, or population, which is attributable to a planned intervention or series of interventions, regardless of whether such an intervention was intended to change *health status*.[13]

What set the health-related MDGs apart from other international declarations of good intent was the identification of outcome indicators that member states would report against to track progress toward the goals and targets.[14] The challenge this posed for low- and middle-income countries (LMICs) was substantial. Many had fragile data collection systems, with perfunctory reporting systems and few mechanisms for analyzing and interpreting the data to provide an evidence base that could inform policies and actions. [4,7,12,15] Yet, the requirement to report on the outcome indicators also offered an opportunity for LMICs to improve their capacity for PHS.

Developing the Millennium Development Goals and Targets

The UN Millennium Declaration reflected decisions taken at a series of world summits and conferences in the latter part of the last century addressing human rights, education, children, population, social development, women's rights, human settlement, and food. Each of these summits led to the definition of a set of sector-specific targets.[9,11,12] Of these, 18 targets were structured into the freestanding categories of the eight MDGs.[9,11,12]

The targets were to be achieved at the global level, and countries were expected to adapt these according to national priorities and aspirations. Countries also had to develop their own strategies and pathways for achieving their targets, and their own approach to monitoring and evaluation because it was considered inappropriate to recommend a uniform, "one-size-fits-all" approach toward the goals.[11,12] The global targets were formulated through observations and experience before 1990, taking into consideration anticipated developments in social, economic, and technological fields in the upcoming 25 years.[9,11,12]

The global-level goals, targets, indicators, and data sources for monitoring national progress toward the health-related MDGs (updated in 2012) are listed in Table 29-1.[14] The targets were framed around known packages of effective, high-impact, and generally low-cost interventions to impact on child mortality, maternal health, and the morbidity and mortality associated with malaria, HIV, and TB.[9,11] These interventions offered potential "huge quick

TABLE 29-1 **Goals, Targets, Indicators, and Data Sources for Monitoring Progress Toward the Health-Related MDGs**[14]

	INDICATOR	DATA SOURCES
Goal 4: Reduce Child Mortality		
Target 4.A: Reduce by two thirds, between 1990 and 2015, the under-five mortality rate	4.1 Under-five mortality rate 4.2 Infant mortality rate 4.3 Proportion of 1-year-old children immunized against measles	4.1 and 4.2: Vital registration systems, national population censuses, household surveys 4.3: Administrative data and household surveys
Goal 5: Improve Maternal Health		
Target 5.A: Reduce by three quarters, between 1990 and 2015, the maternal mortality ratio	5.1 Maternal mortality ratio	5.1 Vital registration systems, household surveys, mortality studies, special studies
	5.2 Proportion of births attended by skilled health personnel	5.2 Household surveys
Target 5.B: Achieve, by 2015, universal access to reproductive health	5.3 Contraceptive prevalence rate	5.3 Representative population-based surveys
	5.4 Adolescent birth rate	5.4 Data on births by age of mother from civil registration systems, census, or survey estimates
	5.5 Antenatal care coverage (at least one visit and at least four visits)	5.5 Household surveys
	5.6 Unmet need for family planning	5.6 Household surveys
Goal 6: Combat HIV/AIDS, Malaria, and Other Diseases		
Target 6.A: Have halted by 2015 and begun to reverse the spread of HIV/AIDS	6.1 HIV prevalence among population aged 15–24 years	6.1 Antenatal clinic attendees, population-based surveys, focus on populations with high-risk behaviors
	6.2 Condom use at last high-risk sex	6.2 Household surveys, representative population-based surveys
	6.3 Proportion of population aged 15–24 years with comprehensive correct knowledge of HIV/AIDS	6.3 Household surveys, other nationally representative household surveys
	6.4 Ratio of school attendance of orphans to school attendance of nonorphans aged 10–14 years	6.4 Household surveys, other nationally representative household surveys
Target 6.B: Achieve, by 2010, universal access to treatment for HIV/AIDS for all those who need it	6.5 Proportion of population with advanced HIV infection with access to antiretroviral drugs	6.5 National program reporting systems, aggregated from health facilities or other service delivery sites
Target 6.C: Have halted by 2015 and begun to reverse the incidence of malaria and other major diseases	6.6 Incidence and death rates associated with malaria	6.6 Data collected by national administrations of health services.
	6.7 Proportion of children under 5 sleeping under insecticide-treated bed nets	6.7 National-level household surveys
	6.8 Proportion of children under five with fever who are treated with appropriate antimalarial drugs	6.8 Household surveys
	6.9 Incidence, prevalence, and death rates associated with tuberculosis	6.9 Case notifications and death records from routine surveillance and vital registration. Prevalence data from population-based surveys.
	6.10 Proportion of tuberculosis cases detected and cured under directly observed treatment short course	6.10 National TB programs

wins" even without breakthroughs in public management or major expansions of human resources for health or infrastructure.[9] The diverse sources for collecting data on the indicators listed in Table 29-1 encompass those recommended for PHS by Thacker et al.[3] and Hall et al.[2]

THE CHALLENGES OF DATA COLLECTION FOR INDICATORS

It was acknowledged from the outset that collecting data for the 21 indicators (Table 29-1) might be demanding for many countries.[16] The handbook on "Indicators for Monitoring the MDGs" provided guidance on collecting data, the definition, rationale for selection, data sources, disaggregation, and gender equity issues for each indicator.[14,16] It acknowledged potential limitations in collecting and interpreting the data in terms of their validity (the extent to which a measurement is capturing what it is intended to measure), reliability (the repeatability or consistency of a set of measurements or measuring instrument), and comparability (the possibility that the same value can mean the same thing in comparison settings).[15]

In an examination of MDG indicator data submitted by countries, Murray[15] confirmed these limitations. Overall, data availability was below 50%, crude data were often presented without adjusting for potential biases, and because data for many indicators were not available, these had to be estimated with predictive modeling techniques.[15] An additional factor threatening the validity of the data was the uncritical acceptance of national data as an act of respect for national sovereignty.[15] Thus, difficulties existed at the levels of data collection (incomplete data sets or lack of data), quality (validity, reliability, and comparability), and analysis and interpretation (failure to take into consideration the first two limitations or to adjust data as needed). Murray concluded that the set of indicators, measurement strategies, and their implementation was "very poor" and not a reasonable basis for monitoring progress toward the MDGs.[15]

These challenges in collecting and using quality data have been attributed to weak and fragmented health systems.[4,7,15,17–19] As an example, a series of global consultations and workshops that focused on reducing childhood deaths from pneumonia and diarrhea identified weak health systems and health information systems (HIS), including PHS, among the key bottlenecks and barriers to achieving MDG 4.[20] Poor PHS undermined health system performance because the data that would enable countries to monitor and improve programs were not available; and at the same time, failures of coordination led to workers devoting time to the production of duplicate or redundant data. In other words, in weak health systems, PHS activities are compromised and can contribute in their own right to compromising those systems. The recommendations for improving PHS were to harmonize data collection across agencies using a common set of key metrics, invest in data collection systems that are user friendly, robust, and can be aggregated at different levels in the health system, and involve stakeholders across the health system "since those who collect the data should be informed about the results of their efforts."[20] The merits of these recommendations will be demonstrated later in this chapter when we consider the case of Bangladesh.

What Have We Learned from the Experience of Public Health Surveillance for the MDGs?

Despite limitations in the collection and interpretation of PHS data, the MDG framework provided a distinctive approach; it revealed how it was possible for nations to reach political consensus on aspirational goals and to attract global investments for these initiatives, as well as to collect and share PHS data for monitoring progress toward the goals.[4,9,15,17,21] In this way, the MDGs provided a focus for advocacy and galvanized political leaders, civil society, the private sector, media, and the development sector and improved the targeting and flow of aid.[9,11,12,22]

In addition, the challenges and successes for assessing progress yielded invaluable lessons to help scale up high-impact health interventions.[4,9,15,17,21,22] Of particular importance is that they stimulated a culture of assessment and increased investments to strengthen HIS encompassing PHS and systems for monitoring and evaluating health plans, strategies and targeted interventions.[4,7,12,15]

Where the MDG indicator data were considered valid, reliable, and comparable, it was possible to assess whether progress was consistent with, lagged behind, or exceeded national targets. However, because the data were all outcome indicators (i.e., reflecting morbidity, mortality, and levels of coverage by health services), they can tell us little about the contributions or shortcomings of the range of initiatives intended to accelerate progress toward the MDGs.

Establishing a Common Platform to Bring Together Meaningful Data from Multiple Sources at All Levels of the Health System

Collecting and using only outcome data to help drive change is analogous to Olympic sport coaches trying to drive improvements based on results of performance in previous Olympic Games. The coaches can make the outcome data as accurate and sensitive as possible and invest in state-of-the-art technology to record and review each race from start to finish in slow motion and from multiple vantage points. But this would not offer a clear picture of why the team performed the way it did. For this, they need other data such as the background attributes of the athletes, the context in which they were trained, the resources invested in training, the nature, quality, and intensity of support from their coaches, and their social world of other commitments and obligations. With all these data they should be in a better position to understand why the team achieves its results and how to help improve performance.

At the end of each Olympic Games, a league table ranks countries by the numbers of gold, silver, and bronze medals achieved. These are, of course, a little specious; richer countries, which devote more resources to training, tend to come out on top. A table of which countries are and are not on track to achieve their MDG targets is subject to similar criticisms, but this is against the spirit of the Millennium Declaration. The targets were not intended to stigmatize "failing" countries but, rather, to point to areas that need improvement and to engage the global community in that enterprise.

It is clear that there are limitations in the MDG outcomes-based framework.[12,15] The targets and indicators were meant to be indicative of progress and never to measure all progress against a complex goal. Because of the need for parsimony, the PHS data are not able to capture the complexity of the targets and the national context and priorities, nor the scope and intensity of the effort required for developing the health system or for addressing the social determinants of health.[4,7,11,12,17] To capture these complexities and monitor, evaluate, and review overall health plans and strategies, including program-specific priorities, countries need to establish a common platform that can bring together meaningful data from multiple sources at all levels of the health system.[2–4,7] General guidance for developing and adapting such a platform has been published recently by the IHP+[7,17] as discussed below, following the case study from Bangladesh.

The latter study shows the utility of outcome indicators for monitoring progress. It illustrates how Bangladesh analyzed and synthesized PHS data with other quantitative as well as with qualitative data on the social determinants of health and on the health system more generally to explain progress and to identify gaps in the indicators and in public health actions.

GOOD HEALTH OUTCOMES IN THE FRAGILE POLITICAL ECONOMY OF BANGLADESH

Despite being one of the world's poorest countries, Bangladesh is on track to meet almost all of the MDGs.[23] The under-five mortality rate (MDG 4) dropped from 133 per 1000 live births in 1990 to 53 per 1000 live births in 2011,[24] achieving the target 4 years ahead of time. Furthermore, the gains were experienced disproportionately in the most disadvantaged populations.[24] MDG 6 targets for TB detection and cure were also achieved ahead of time, and Bangladesh has made significant reductions in the prevalence of and mortality from malaria.[23] The target for MDG 5 (improving maternal health) has proven the most difficult health-related target to achieve for most countries.[23] Nonetheless, by 2011, Bangladesh had attained a reduction of around two thirds from the baseline of 574 deaths per 100,000 live births. How has this happened in a country that is still one of the poorest in Asia, with rapid population growth and lackluster improvement in poverty and income inequalities?[24] Can countrywide indicators capture differences within a country, especially one as populous and diverse as Bangladesh?

The Context and Input Explanations for Good Health at Low Cost

Social determinants are defined as "the circumstances in which people grow, live, work, and age, and the systems put in place to deal with illness."[25] A salutary example of using a social determinants of health framework to capture contextual and process data for explaining outcomes—and of the importance of indicator data to demonstrate the successes of countries—is provided by the case of Bangladesh.

To understand the underpinnings of the "Bangladesh paradox,"[26] we need to understand the context and the human, system, and material resources used to construct health responses. Using a social determinants of health approach to explain health outcomes, Chowdhury et al.[26] demonstrated that at least some of the reasons lie in contextual and input factors such as a pluralistic health system that includes long-term collaborative work with the nongovernmental sector, targeted health interventions, and a sustained focus on gender equity. **Gender equality** is the absence of discrimination—on the basis of a person's sex—in providing opportunities, in allocating resources and benefits or in access to services.[27] Let us start by looking at data collection itself, a basic building block for effective PHS. In contrast to many LMIC Bangladesh has a functional system of collecting data through household surveys, delivered through a number of research institutes, a culture of collecting and using monitoring data, and a harmonized set of priorities for data collection between donors and country.[26,28] Public–private partnerships that connect the surveillance process with action strengthen this system.

Gender equity functions as both an MDG outcome and a human resource to improve capacity to meet other MDG targets. Gender parity in primary and secondary education, the indicator for MDG 3, was achieved in Bangladesh by 2005. At the 2008 national election, 20% of seats were won by women, making Bangladesh roughly equivalent with the international rate of female representation in parliament, and almost double that of the USA.[26] Focusing on women's education and civic participation and on family planning reinforces maternal health initiatives[29] and the chances of success of child health initiatives.

A critical contextual factor, which also both reflects and drives gender equity, is the plurality of the health system and its entrenched focus on maternal and child health. The government provides hospitals at the district level and subdistrict level and frontline workers at the village and union level. The public health service has two wings that focus on health services and family planning. Maternal health care is shared by these two wings of the Ministry of Health & Family Welfare. This is mirrored by a vibrant and long-standing nongovernmental organization (NGO) sector, which provides health care services to villages and cities focusing on maternal and child health, and family planning. These public–private partnerships provide flexibility and some intrinsic system redundancy in the health worker supply and deployment; in systems engineering terms, this is a failsafe mechanism to improve the resilience of health worker supply and deployment. Bangladesh has a severe undersupply of trained health personnel such as doctors and nurses.[30] Nevertheless, it has been able to develop, through this pluralist system focusing on maternal and child health and reproductive health, a cadre of female frontline health workers (from government and NGOs) who have fanned out to deliver targeted services across the country.

Many of the world's most prominent NGOs were developed in Bangladesh, by Bangladeshis, after the liberation war in 1971, with a specific focus on poverty alleviation. BRAC (known previously as the Bangladesh Rural Advancement Committee) is now the largest NGO in the world, reaching over 135 million people in 10 countries. The contributions by BRAC to Bangladesh's development are substantial: it has a university, runs primary schools that educate at least 1 in 10 of Bangladesh's children, pioneered microcredit for the poor, and has instituted many door-to-door health services for the poor. BRAC is not the only flourishing NGO in Bangladesh. The Grameen Bank, whose founder Mohammed Yunus won the Nobel Peace Prize, has also fostered microcredit for the poor. Gonoshasthaya Kendra (People's Health Centre) was at the forefront of moves to demonstrate the viability of paraprofessionals as deliverers of health services, including maternal health services.[31] Part of the vibrancy of the NGO sector arises from the Bangladesh government's willingness to provide an open environment in which the NGOs can develop innovative responses. We can identify these factors, all important contributors to Bangladesh's success in meeting the health-related MDGs, through rich qualitative accounts, and by the community research conducted through the NGO sector. None of these important contributors to Bangladesh's success is captured by the MDG indicators.

How Effective Are the MDG Indicators at Uncovering Inequity in Bangladesh?

One of the criticisms levied at MDGs, and seen in Bangladesh, is that the targets focus on averages and obscure the fact that improvements in health are unequally distributed. Bangladesh has established an infrastructure for large-scale household surveys and is able to demonstrate, through these surveys, differences in rural versus urban settings and across the socioeconomic strata in the outcome indicators. For example, the proportion of pregnant women who have four or more antenatal visits has improved from 15.9% in 2004 to 25.5% in 2011; however, urban women are now twice as likely (44.7%) as rural women (19.8%) to have this degree of antenatal care. Women in the richest quintile are far more likely (87%) to have antenatal care provided by a medically trained provider than women in the poorest quintile (30%). The national mean of 55% for skilled antenatal care obscures these wide gaps between poor and rich women and between urban and rural populations.[23]

Future Indicators and Equity in Bangladesh

Bangladesh has proposed that the Post-2015 Development Agenda focus more specifically on equity, with suggested indicators in health stratified by geography, gender, and wealth quintiles.[23] These changes will enable countries to track for themselves the degree to which each section of its population is benefiting from health gains. They will also serve to identify underserved populations, and demonstrate where resources should be funneled for health improvement.

The indicators proposed by Bangladesh may be insufficient for the needs of a rapidly urbanizing population. Bangladesh, in common with most poor countries, has experienced a marked population shift from rural to urban; 45 million people (28% of the population) now live in urban settings.[32] As this population grows, the existing health and environmental infrastructure is being overwhelmed, and large-scale slums, located in low-lying areas prone to flooding and other natural disasters, become permanent communities of disadvantage.[33] In the future, the urban slum/urban nonslum differential may be more important in signaling internal disadvantage than the contemporary urban/rural differential.

LESSONS FROM BANGLADESH

This case study from Bangladesh shows how the outcome indicators revealed accelerated progress toward the MDGs. When synthesized with quantitative and qualitative data on changes in other social determinants of health, including the health system, they provide insights into reasons for the success. However, such a synthesis was only possible because of Bangladesh's culture of research, its well-described and elaborated health sector, and its focus on both qualitative and quantitative data. The current MDG indicators do not themselves enable us to develop such a synthesis. Integrating outcome-specific PHS data with contextual data offers important lessons for the global community on how it is possible to achieve "good health at low cost."

TRANSFORMING PUBLIC HEALTH SURVEILLANCE

How can we transform PHS so that the data can be used not only to track the performance of health programs more effectively but also to identify and explore the enablers and barriers to good performance? To plan for the future we have to have some understanding of the historical role of surveillance in the public health lexicon, and to recognize that surveillance is now positioned as a key component of monitoring and evaluation (M&E) systems, rather than being a conceptually and operationally separate activity. In the following section, we describe these transitions in the understanding and application of PHS from a systems perspective. We then outline the common M&E framework that was developed recently by the IHP+ as part of the country-led platform for monitoring, evaluation, and review of national health plans and strategies as an area in which PHS can support health systems to improve health outcomes and drive equity.[7,17,21]

Expanding the Scope of Public Health Surveillance from Outcomes to Health Systems and Social Determinants

PHS is defined as the "ongoing, systematic collection, analysis, and interpretation of health data essential to the planning, implementation, and evaluation of public health practice, closely integrated with the timely dissemination of these data to those who need to know."[34] This definition separates responsibilities for the "analysis and interpretation of health data" to generate health intelligence from the requirement to respond to these data by "those who need to know." This reflects the conceptual—and sometimes physical—separation that has existed between PHS and public health actions in the developed world. For much of the developing world, this distinction is artificial. The practitioners responsible for analyzing and interpreting PHS data are also responsible for transforming the results into public health actions.

Outcome-specific surveillance data are necessary but not sufficient to provide the evidence essential for informing policy and for planning, implementing, and evaluating public health actions. Two other processes are needed to transform intelligence from PHS data into decisions. First, outcome data need to be synthesized and triangulated with other types of data for deeper analysis and comparison, particularly data on trends in the social determinants of health including health system operations.[4,7,17,21] This process of integration and synthesis is essential to generate the context-specific evidence needed for decision-making. Even in rich countries, systems for collecting and integrating health data from multiple sources are only starting to be developed.[4,7] For LMICs, the task of collecting data on morbidity and mortality is challenging enough,[4,15] let alone collecting data on health system operations and other health determinants. The widespread uptake of mobile phone technology in LMICs offers us the possibility for the first time of simple collection and transmission of surveillance data, including those on health system processes. To date, much of the discussion about the potential of mobile telephones or smartphone apps has stressed existing models of PHS (emerging infections and burden of disease).[35-37] As the capacity of mobile phone technology in PHS is explored further, it is important that applications to capture the contextual determinants of health outcomes are also developed.

Second, the evidence then needs to be considered in the context of competing needs and priorities for allocating limited resources so that it can be transformed into compelling and actionable knowledge. This process requires strategic packaging of evidence into presentation formats that will influence senior decision-makers who usually oversee both the intelligence and action arms of public health. Activities synthesizing intelligence into evidence and transforming evidence into actionable knowledge are part of a continuum; these activities therefore require ongoing collaborations by the practitioners assigned these responsibilities.

The demands of the twenty-first century, resulting from changes in health information needs, accessibility to an expanding range of data sets, and changing expectations of decision-makers and the community, call for a flexible and broader interpretation of the current definition of PHS.[2] New areas of public health inquiry can be established using innovative data sources, methods of data collection and analysis, and their application to emerging public health concerns. Among the emerging concerns Hall et al. identified were monitoring health care reform implementation, quality of care and performance accountability, and assessments of the comparative effectiveness of health interventions.[2]

How can PHS —focused on outcomes and risk factors—be integrated with the collection, analysis, and interpretation of contextual data essential for informing policy, and for planning, implementing, and evaluating public health actions? A health system consists of all the organizations, institutions, resources, and people whose primary purpose is to improve health and influence the determinants of health.[21] An HIS (encompassing PHS) is one of the six interrelated building blocks of a health system that provides the foundation for decision-making across the other five building blocks: service delivery, health workforce, access to essential medicines, financing, and leadership and governance.[21] A well-functioning HIS should provide reliable information on three key indicators: the health status of the population, activities and performance of the health system, and trends in the other social determinants of health.[4] The collection, analysis, and synthesis of data for these indicators reflect a system's approach to population health needed to shift us from a linear, reductionist focus on individual components (e.g., on PHS of disease outcomes) to a consideration of the dynamic interrelationships across components of the health system and other health determinants.[38] It enables the shift from "tree-by-tree thinking" (focusing on the details of each individual component) to "forest thinking" (understanding the context of the relationships between the components).

Toward a Uniform Framework for Informing and Evaluating Public Health Programs

Measuring health from a systems perspective is conceptually and technically complex. National HIS evolved in a haphazard and fragmented way as a result of administrative, economic, legal, and donor pressures. It therefore became necessary to enhance the entire information and statistical systems rather than focusing only upon specific diseases.[4,15,18] The **Health Metrics Network (HMN)** was launched in 2005 as a network of global, regional, and country partners dedicated to strengthening national HIS and harmonizing approaches to collect, collate, analyze, and use health data to inform decisions and programming.[4] Six major data sources were identified for this purpose from two domains: data from populations (census, civil registration, and population surveys) and data from institutions (individual health records such as for notifiable diseases and disease registers, health service records, and health resource records).[4] Thacker[3] also included these six sources as contributing to PHS. It is therefore necessary to reconcile operations of PHS focused on disease outcomes and risk factors with the broader HIS, which generates data on inputs, processes, outputs, and outcomes to inform decisions on policies and programming for the overall health system. The HMN has acknowledged "that the appropriate reconnection of the surveillance community with broader HIS has much to offer to each" and recommended that "standardization and integration of surveillance across diseases could become a model for the much broader standardization and integration of health information across data sources."[4]

As global health initiatives to support health development in LMICs proliferated, so did the burden of reporting on a broad range of program indicators to track progress and performance.[4,7,17,18] Furthermore, development agencies at times used different definitions for the same indicators and required different levels of disaggregation and reporting formats, thus exaggerating the disconnect between national strategic plans and disease-specific plans in terms of indicators and definitions, and data collection systems. A broad consensus therefore emerged on the need for a common M&E framework that incorporated data from HIS of all major health programs.[4,7,17,18] Such a framework would reduce demands for more data, increase efficiencies, minimize the apparent dichotomy between systemic and disease focused approaches, and allow countries to focus on data aimed primarily at informing national decision-making and programming. Importantly, this framework would also streamline global reporting with country plans and review cycles in terms of timing, methods, and content.[7]

The common M&E framework, adapted in Table 29-2, was developed through the IHP+ as one component of the country-led platform for monitoring, evaluation, and review of national health plans and strategies, and was aimed at putting the principles of the Paris Declaration on Aid Effectiveness into practice.[7,17,39] (Interestingly, in its earlier incarnation, this platform was referred to as the "country health systems surveillance" [CHeSS] platform.[17,40]) The platform brings together all the elements relating to M&E including the processes by which M&E is developed; the country coordination mechanisms and institutional capacity; the common M&E framework including the technical elements such as indicator selection, data sources, analysis and synthesis practices, data quality assessment and data dissemination; and the country review processes for planning and decision-making. The common M&E framework has been adapted for disease-specific programs such as for TB, HIV/AIDS, and malaria,[19] initiatives to promote maternal and child health,[6,41] and for cross-cutting efforts across health systems such as for tracking human resources, logistics, and procurement by health services.[5,21] The framework can be used not only for M&E but also as a guide for program planning, as a basis for designing prospective program evaluations, as a road map for program-relevant research, and for cross-site and global learning.[5,6,41]

The common M&E framework is based on a conceptual model[7,17] that specifies the pathways and results chain through which program inputs (e.g., policies and resources) and processes (e.g., implementation of plans) are reflected in outputs (e.g., access to health services) and eventual outcomes (e.g., intervention coverage) and impacts (e.g., improved health outcomes and equity). The inputs, processes, and outputs reflect health system capacity

TABLE 29-2 **Common Framework for Monitoring, Evaluating, and Reviewing National Plans and Strategies (Adapted from Refs[5–7,17])**

	INPUTS	PROCESSES	OUTPUTS	OUTCOMES	IMPACTS
Indicator domains	**Policies** Disease control Disease treatment and care Access fees **Plans** Coherent, prioritized, and funded **Human resources** **Financing** Domestic sources International sources **Infrastructure**	**Implementation of plans** Strengthening health systems Scale-up of priority interventions **Capacity building** Organizational relationships, infrastructure, staff competencies **Accountability** Performance monitoring **Harmonization** Well-coordinated and harmonized support across partnerships	Access to services and interventions Intervention quality and safety	Effective coverage and utilization of interventions Prevalence of risk behaviors and factors	Reduced morbidity and mortality Improved health outcomes and equity Social and financial risk protection Responsiveness
Data collection	**Administrative sources** Track resources and implementation		**Facility assessments** Quality, coverage Facility reporting systems Operational and implementation research	**Population-based sources:** Census, vital registrations, population and health surveys, effective coverage of services, health status, equity **Institution-based sources**: Health Information Systems (including surveillance)	
Analysis and synthesis	Data quality assessment. Estimates and projections. In-depth studies. Use of research results. Assessment of progress and performance and efficiency of health systems.				
Communication and use	Targeted and comprehensive reporting. Regular review processes. Global reporting.				

Note: Indicator data should be stratified by gender, socioeconomic status, ethnic group, and geographical location to capture potential health inequities.
Contextual factors (health determinants) include political, economic, social, technological, legal, and environmental factors.

whereas the outputs, outcomes, and impacts are the results of investments reflecting performance of the health system. The framework addresses selection of indicators for each step in the results chain, data collection methods, analysis and synthesis, and communication and use of the results (Table 29-2). Capacity and performance indicators are important because they drive policy attention, resource allocation, and implementation.[4,11,12,18] Murray[15] has detailed the criteria for selecting a small number of priority indicators to minimize the burden of data collection on LMICs:

- Specify what each indicator is intended to measure
- Identify the public health significance of each indicator
- Ensure a practical measurement strategy is available

- Ensure the indicator measures the quantity of interest
- Ensure its value is readily interpretable

Albert Einstein kept a sign on his wall that said: "Not everything that counts can be counted; not everything that can be counted counts." Quantitative indicators are intended to be indicative of reality and cannot capture all the elements, interactions, and products of complex adaptive systems such as health systems.[7,12,17,18,41] They need to be supplemented with qualitative assessments of inputs and implementation efforts and analysis of the social determinants of health that impact population health as well as health systems operations.[25]

Indicator data collected prospectively using this type of common framework for the Bangladesh case study would have been able to tell us more about reasons for the noted achievements. This information would have assisted other countries and development partners to see if lessons were relevant for their own countries, and enabled Bangladesh to rapidly detect and respond to areas that needed improvement.

In 2013, Bryce et al.[5] described an interesting adaptation of the common framework to monitor, evaluate, and enable cross-site learning from an initiative to strengthen health systems across five countries. In particular, they elaborated on the qualitative methods to be used for assessing the contextual factors (baseline and ongoing) (Note, Table 29-2) needed to identify positive and negative confounders that may affect the internal validity of the evaluation results, and potential effect modifiers that may enhance or diminish program implementation efforts, which can affect the generalizability of the evaluation results. The global community keenly awaits the realized value of the approach. Integrating the collection, analysis, and use of outcome-specific PHS data with the common M&E framework of the country-led platform will enable a deeper and more meaningful analysis of, and triangulation with, data on the concurrent activities and performance of the health system, and trends in the social determinants of health. This systems-based approach is needed to explore and unravel the dynamic interrelationships across components of the health system and other health determinants to generate the context-specific evidence needed for decision-making.

CONCLUSIONS

The MDGs have shown us that global health goals and targets are powerful tools for driving national development. While data on outcome indicators can be used to assess progress, they cannot explain the level of progress, nor can they, on their own, generate the evidence needed to inform decisions and actions for achieving the targets. To use them meaningfully for these purposes, outcome data need to be synthesized and triangulated with contextual data, taking into consideration changes in the social determinants of health that include access to, and the quality and utilization of, health services.

The case study from Bangladesh demonstrates that outcome indicators can reveal accelerated progress toward the MDGs. However, quantitative data alone cannot capture the intensity of efforts or the interactions between actors within the health sector and across other sectors to explain the success and identify gaps. The synthesis of outcome data with trends in the social determinants of health, including the health system, provides insights into reasons for the success of, as well as the gaps in, indicators and public health actions, particularly to address health equity. **Health equity** is the attainment of the highest level of health for all people.[42] Achieving health equity requires valuing everyone equally with focused and ongoing societal efforts to address avoidable inequalities, historical and contemporary injustices, and the elimination of health and health care disparities.

Integrating outcome-specific PHS data with contextual data offers important lessons for the global community on how it is possible to achieve "good health at low cost."

Mature PHS systems that wish to capitalize on the opportunities for improving population health and identifying and addressing health equity effectively will build a broader range of indicators into their frameworks, aiming for seamless integration of PHS with a common M&E framework housed within a country-led platform for monitoring, evaluation, and review of national health plans and strategies.[7]

KEY SUMMARY POINTS

- The purpose of PHS is not only to monitor patterns and trends in diseases but also to monitor the quality and capacity of health services, identify underserved populations, and inform new research priorities.
- By failing to expand surveillance for capturing data on the "causes of causes," we are simply counting the numbers of corks bobbing on the surface of an ocean, while ignoring the ocean flows that determine the direction of the current.
- The health-related Millennium Development Goals (MDGs) is a unique global venture that has provoked debates about the capacity of countries to meet the goals or to collect PHS data appropriate to track progress toward these goals.
- Three of the eight MDGs defined specific health targets; the 21 associated outcome indicators to monitor progress are quantitative variables selected to measure the impacts of known effective and low-cost interventions that could deliver "huge quick wins" to reduce child mortality, improve maternal health, and combat selected communicable diseases (MDGs 4, 5, and 6, respectively).
- Measuring outcomes of health interventions is conceptually and technically complex. The requirement for low- and middle-income countries (LMICs) to report on them proved a challenge—yet provided the opportunity to strengthen capacity for public health surveillance.
- Outcome-specific public health surveillance data cannot, on their own, explain success or lags in progress toward goals and targets or provide the evidence needed to inform ongoing decisions and programming.
- The case study from Bangladesh shows how the outcome indicators can reveal accelerated progress toward the MDGs. However, these data have to be interpreted in the context of changes in the social determinants of health (that affect both the health of the population and access to, and quality and utilization of, health services) that revealed reasons for the success as well as gaps in the indicators, particularly for addressing health equity.
- Integrating the collection, analysis, and use of outcome-specific public health surveillance data with the recently proposed common country-led platform to monitor, evaluate, and review progress in national health strategies and plans will enable a deeper and more meaningful analysis of, and triangulation with, data on the concurrent activities and performance of the health system, and trends in the social determinants of health.
- This systems-based approach is needed to explore and unravel the dynamic interrelationships across components of the health system and other health determinants to generate the context-specific evidence needed for decision-making.

DISCUSSION QUESTIONS

1. Compare the relative roles of the three health-related MDGs and the other five MDGs in contributing toward achievement of the health goals and targets.
2. Outcome-specific surveillance data are necessary but not sufficient for providing evidence to inform decisions and programming. How would you defend or refute this assertion?
3. To what extent do the indicators listed in Table 29-1 meet the criteria recommended by Murray[15] for selecting priority indicators?
4. Discuss potential measurement and selection biases in collecting and interpreting the MDG indicator data from the sources listed in Table 29-1.
5. List and elaborate on the indicators useful for identifying and addressing health equity.
6. How might a country's focus on the MDGs add to, and potentially compromise, other efforts for strengthening health systems?
7. Discuss the benefits and drawbacks of separating responsibilities for surveillance of outcome-specific data from decision-making, planning, and implementation.
8. PHS should be defined by the type of data or system used to collect the data. Make arguments for and against this statement.
9. How do you interpret the scope of the term "health data" in the current definition of public health surveillance found under the section on "Expanding the scope of public health surveillance from outcomes to health systems and social determinants"? Explain the reasoning for your interpretation.
10. What lessons do you draw from the Bangladesh case study about the use of surveillance and other data in LMICs and in rich countries?

REFERENCES

1. McMichael AJ. The health of persons, populations, and planets: epidemiology comes full circle. Epidemiology 1995;6(6):633–6.
2. Hall HI, Correa A, Yoon PW, Braden CR, Centers for Disease C, Prevention. Lexicon, definitions, and conceptual framework for public health surveillance. Morbidity and mortality weekly report. Surveillance Summaries 2012;61(Suppl.):10–14.
3. Thacker SB, Qualters JR, Lee LM, Centers for Disease C, Prevention. Public health surveillance in the United States: evolution and challenges. Morbidity and mortality weekly report. Surveillance Summaries 2012;61(Suppl.):3–9.
4. Health Metrics Network. Framework and standards for country health information systems. 2nd ed. Geneva: WHO; 2008.
5. Bryce J, Requejo JH, Moulton LH, Ram M, Black RE. A common evaluation framework for the African Health Initiative. BMC Health Serv Res 2013;13(Suppl. 2):S10.
6. Bryce J, Victora CG, Boerma T, Peters DH, Black RE. Evaluating the scale-up for maternal and child survival: a common framework. Int Health 2011; 3(3):139–146.
7. IHP+, WHO. Monitoring, evaluation and review of national health strategies: a country-led platform for information and accountability. Geneva: WHO; 2011.
8. WHO. Millennium Development Goals (MDGs). 2014, <http://www.who.int/topics/millennium_development_goals/en/>; 2015.
9. Sachs JD, McArthur JW. The Millennium Project: a plan for meeting the Millennium Development Goals. Lancet 2005;365(9456):347–53.
10. United Nations Development Program. Human Development Report 2003. Millennium Development Goals: a compact among nations to end poverty. Oxford: Oxford University Press; 2003.
11. Vandemoortele J. The MDG story: intention denied. Devel Change 2011;42(1):1–21.
12. Waage J, Banerji R, Campbell O, Chirwa E, Collender G, Dieltiens V, et al. The Millennium development goals: a cross-sectoral analysis and principles for goal setting after 2015 Lancet and London International Development Centre Commission. Lancet 2010;376(9745):991–1023.
13. Health Promotion Glossary. Geneva: World Health Organization; 1998.
14. United Nations Development Group. Indicators for monitoring the millennium development goals. Definitions, rationale, concepts, and sources. New York: United Nations, <http://mdgs.un.org/unsd/mi/wiki/MainPage.ashx/>; 2012. [accessed 20.12.2013].
15. Murray CJ. Towards good practice for health statistics: lessons from the millennium development goal health indicators. Lancet 2007;369(9564):862–73.
16. United Nations Development Group. Indicators for monitoring the millennium development goals. Definitions, rationale, concepts, and sources. New York: United Nations; 2003.
17. Boerma T, Abou-Zahr C, Bos E, Hansen P, Addai E, Low-Beer D. Monitoring and evaluation of health systems strengthening. An operational framework. Geneva: WHO; 2010.
18. Murray CJ, Frenk J. Health metrics and evaluation: strengthening the science. Lancet 2008;371(9619):1191–99.
19. The Global Fund. Monitoring and evaluation toolkit HIV, tuberculosis, malaria and health and community systems strengthening. 4th ed. 2011.
20. Gill CJ, Young M, Schroder K, Carvajal-Velez L, McNabb M, Aboubaker S, et al. Bottlenecks, barriers, and solutions: results from multicountry consultations focused on reduction of childhood pneumonia and diarrhoea deaths. Lancet 2013;381(9876):1487–98.
21. WHO. Monitoring the building blocks of health systems: a handbook of indicators and their measurement strategies. Geneva: WHO; 2010.
22. Manning R, Harland Scott C, Haddad L. Whose goals count? Lessons for setting the next development goals. IDS Bull 2013;44(5–6):1–9.
23. Government of the People's Republic of Bangladesh. Bangladesh Planning Commission GED. The millennium development goals. Bangladesh Progress Report 2012. June 2013.
24. Adams AM, Rabbani A, Ahmed S, Mahmood SS, Al-Sabir A, Rashid SF, et al. Explaining equity gains in child survival in Bangladesh: scale, speed, and selectivity in health and development. Lancet 2013;382(9909):2027–37.
25. WHO. Closing the gap in a generation: health equity through action on the social determinants of health. Final report of the commission on social determinants of health. Geneva: World Health Organization; 2008.
26. Chowdhury AM, Bhuiya A, Chowdhury ME, Rasheed S, Hussain Z, Chen LC. The Bangladesh paradox: exceptional health achievement despite economic poverty. Lancet 2013;382(9906):1734–45.
27. WHO. Gender, equity, and human rights, <http://www.who.int/gender-equity-rights/en/>; 2015.
28. Bhuiya A, Datta PG, Chowhdury AMR. Health progress and research culture in Bangladesh. Lancet 2013;382(9906):1699.
29. Dreze J, Sen A. An uncertain glory; India and its contradictions. London: Penguin Group, Books Ltd; 2013.
30. Ahmed SM, Hossain MA, Rajachowdhury AM, Bhuiya AU. The health workforce crisis in Bangladesh: shortage, inappropriate skill-mix and inequitable distribution. Hum Resour Health 2011;9:3.
31. Potts M, Henderson C. Global warming and reproductive health. Int J Gynecol Obstet 2012;119(Suppl. 1):S64–7.
32. Afsana K, Wahid SS. Health care for poor people in the urban slums of Bangladesh. Lancet 2013;382(9910):2049–51.
33. Rashid SF. Strategies to reduce exclusion among populations living in urban slum settlements in Bangladesh. J Health Popul Nutr 2009;27(4):574–86.
34. Thacker SB, Berkelman RL. Public health surveillance in the United States. Epidemiol Rev 1988;10(1):164–190.
35. Freifeld CC, Chunara R, Mekaru S, Chan EH, Kass-Hout T, Ayala Iacucci A, et al. Participatory epidemiology: use of mobile phones for community-based health reporting. PLoS Med 2010;7(12):e1000376.
36. Pascoe L, Lungo J, Kaasboll J, Kolelini I. Collecting integrated disease surveillance and response data through mobile phones. IST-Africa 2012 Conference Proceedings; 2012:1–6. [accessed 19.08.2014].
37. St Louis M. Global health surveillance. MMWR 2012;61(Suppl.):15–19.
38. Adam T, de Savigny D. Systems thinking for strengthening health systems in LMICs: need for a paradigm shift. Health Policy Plan 2012;27(Suppl. 4): iv1–3.
39. OECD. The Paris declaration on aid effectiveness and the Accra Agenda for Action. 2005.
40. Report of Technical Meeting. Global initiative to strengthen Country Health Systems Surveillance (CHeSS): summary report of a technical meeting and action plan. Italy: Bellagio Rockefeller Centre; October 28–30, 2008.
41. Bryce J, Arnold F, Blanc A, Hancioglu A, Newby H, Requejo J, et al. Measuring coverage in MNCH: new findings, new strategies, and recommendations for action. PLoS Med 2013;10(5):e1001423.
42. HHS. Health Equity & Disparities, <http://www.minorityhealth.hhs.gov/npa/templates/browse.aspx?lvl=1&lvlid=34; 2015/>.

CHAPTER

30

Research and Innovations Guiding Public Health Surveillance in the Twenty-first Century

Thomas Krafft, Eva Pilot, Bidyut K Sarkar, Paige Ryland, Lauren Reeves, Vivek Singh

If you think research is expensive, try disease.

Mary Lasker

KEY WORDS

Big Data
GIS
Point-of-care diagnostics
System for Early warning based on Emergency Data (SEED)

INTRODUCTION

All countries need effective disease surveillance systems for early outbreak detection, reporting, and evidence-based decision-making. Public health surveillance has an increasingly crucial role in assessing public health status, defining and focusing public health priorities, evaluating interventions and programs, and providing early detection and warning of outbreaks and pandemics. These important roles will stimulate further research to improve surveillance methods, techniques, and concepts, and to strengthen the multidisciplinary nature of public health surveillance.

The Global Burden of Disease Study 2010, published in 2012, triggered an intense debate on how to provide the right evidence base for public health interventions and international health programs.[1,2] The recent publication of the manifesto From Public to Planetary Health in *The Lancet* is but another call for a more comprehensive and integrative public health approach that is already reflected in the conceptual debates on global health and One Health and in earlier debates on health determinants and health equity.[3] Notwithstanding the distinct differences and originality of each of these approaches, they have in common a vision of public health rooted in the values of social justice and fairness. This common vision keeps a focus on the collective actions of interdependent and empowered populations and their communities.[3] Public health surveillance will have to incorporate this integrative view to contribute to health protection and well-being, and to sustainable development. Public health surveillance-related research will have to focus particularly on strengthening the evidence base for health policies and public health interventions and on fostering resilience and adaptation.

Research and innovations are the driving influences of the practice of public health surveillance and both are guided by current capabilities, future possibilities, and the health challenges shaping our world. They influence the current transformation of public health surveillance described in this book and will power the inevitable transformations of the future necessary for meeting the health needs of a population. This chapter will critique how research and innovation are shaping public health surveillance in the twenty-first century, while also highlighting the role public health surveillance plays in driving cutting edge research and innovation in public health to inform policy and practice. Examples of current public health surveillance best practices in India are offered to illustrate research and innovations shaping public health surveillance. India, an LMIC country, which has been operationalized even in low resource settings.

EMERGING TRENDS IN PUBLIC HEALTH SURVEILLANCE

The following stand out as important fields of innovative public health surveillance that will continue to grow in the coming years. These trends will influence and shape public health surveillance at a global scale in the foreseeable future and illustrate the need for further research and innovation. Still the selection of emerging trends presented hereafter is neither complete nor comprehensive due to space limits in this chapter and also because public health surveillance continues to evolve along a continuum of transformation.

One Health

One Health (see Chapter 14) recognizes inextricable linkages among human health, animal health, and ecosystem health that will change approaches to public health surveillance and extend the scientific knowledge base.[4] Multilateral environmental agreements, among other One Health-related processes, necessitate finding new synergies and quickly expanding the scope of public health surveillance to be able to assess the effects of animal health and the ecosystem on human health. Public health surveillance has already started to develop synergies between human and animal health surveillance. Veterinary surveillance complements human health surveillance by monitoring zoonotic pathogens; by seeking early detection via sentinel animals (e.g., West Nile virus surveillance); by using similar epidemiologic and statistical tools; and by helping to interpret alarms from human surveillance systems.[5,6] Sharing knowledge will further improve syndromic surveillance system performance for human and animal diseases in terms of timeliness, sensitivity, and awareness. Concurrent alerts from both human and animal systems may indicate a signal and the presence of a health threat.[7]

Strengthening the links between human health, animal health, and the environment can strengthen all of these sectors, as no sector alone has enough knowledge and resources to detect or prevent the emergence or resurgence of diseases in a highly interconnected world. Seven veterinary systems in Europe already share their outputs with human-health institutes, and three more systems plan to do so in the near future.[7] The human health, animal health, and environmental fields, together, need to develop nonspecific alarms that result from the observed aberration from predicted values (e.g., call volumes, emergency room visits, internet searches, and use of pharmaceuticals in animal husbandry). Thus, moving the One Health concept forward toward a useful public health surveillance approach will also further encourage the necessary capacity building and training of the respective workforce.

Public Health Genomics

Future progress in public health genomics will allow for including host-specific factors in the identification of risk factors. Infectious disease surveillance will expand to include host genetic factors that influence disease susceptibility or severity and that affect responsiveness to vaccines and therapies. As discussed in Chapter 26, phylogenetic analyses are already replacing older genotyping technologies. This type of surveillance allows for a more detailed level of classification leading to a clearer understanding of disease etiology and routes of transmission.

This innovation is expected to lead to a more comprehensive understanding of the biological mechanisms of disease, to new avenues for prevention and treatment, and to new insights for continuing public health efforts to control disease. The incorporation of public health genomics in public health surveillance and the degree of public acceptance depend on how convincingly the extensive ethical concerns about nondiscriminatory use, confidentiality, and privacy will be addressed. Public health research will have to identify and analyze the implications of these concerns and to provide the foundation for developing effective policies about the appropriate use of genetic and other health information. Also, the rapid evolution of more comprehensive sequencing techniques and platforms will require further harmonizing and integration of data to allow for continuous use of data and time sequence analysis.

THE ROLE OF TECHNOLOGY AS AN INNOVATOR IN RESHAPING PUBLIC HEALTH SURVEILLANCE

In the last decade, new technology, in combination with established data sources, has been reshaping public health surveillance. Technology and social media are increasingly important players in public health surveillance. Compared to the basic methods used for public health surveillance in the past, these technologies and data sources are very innovative. As such, they require caution as well as policies and safeguards, as discussed in Section 3 of this book. This section discusses several examples of the innovative technologies reshaping public health surveillance.

Big Data

Huge and complex digital data sets that usually require nonstandard computational infrastructure for storage, management, and analysis have been labeled as Big Data.

Big Data are now available from many new sources, including electronic health records, telemedicine, and e-health. These data, originate from health care systems, from the private sector, from such diverse sources as mobile phone records or supermarket loyalty cards or data mining of online activities including Facebook and Twitter, and geolocation or tracking systems. Big Data have enormous potential, but the use for and the integration into public health surveillance has to be viewed with caution and requires further research.[8,9] Elsevier currently publishes a *Big Data Research*[10] journal dedicated to promoting and communicating advances in Big Data research so they may be adopted quickly and extensively by appropriate stakeholders. Big Data technology provides access to an ever-growing list of types of data.[11] The increasing adaption and inclusion of communications technology, digital records, and social media open additional information pathways that will demand new analysis tools and concepts to ensure that data are interoperable and accessible across platforms and users. Furthermore, while recognizing data as socially constructed a clear understanding of where the data come from including context and the pathways of collation, aggregation, and analysis are essential for deriving informed public health decisions.

Geographical Information Systems

Spatial data are getting new attention with the improved understanding of the effect of time and space on health. These data are considered to be very important for the future of public health surveillance.[12,13] In recognition of the potential of spatial data in mitigating and controlling the spread of disease, user-friendly geographical information systems (GIS) have been developed to perform daily outbreak analyses and to monitor the spread of disease.[14] The goal of using GIS is to strengthen the capacity of local, national, and international public health programs to manipulate and analyze data in different visual ways. This geographic approach adds benefit and can lead to innovative public health surveillance solutions. With these obvious advantages, research suggests that among public health professionals GIS is viewed as a useful tool to inform and support decision-making but still remains underused. This has been attributed to concerns that GIS outputs can potentially be misinterpreted or used erroneously due to insufficient training and experience. Applying GIS in multidisciplinary collaboration and adding GIS training to the standard public health curricula will facilitate a more effective use and wider acceptance. High-resolution satellite data and global mapping programs that are available for literally almost any place have already helped to overcome the issue of finding the basic geographic information. Cross-border analysis is still hampered by limited interoperability of health system data and reporting, but might improve with the IHR requirements coming into place. The further use of advanced GIS that integrates data from remote sensing, satellite data and telecommunication will improve the use and future development of *Predictive Surveillance* (see Chapter 3). The rapid advances in operations research and in autonomous agents or multiagents (modeling) research will further support and even drive this development.

Internet-Based Surveillance

The public's access to internet-based health information has been used increasingly as a source of data for public health surveillance and research. Systematic monitoring of web searches within medical websites provides insight to individuals who may be experiencing symptoms but are not yet seeking medical care. Hulth et al.[15] have shown that searches on influenza and influenza-like illness using dedicated health web services provide a basis for estimating the timing of the peak and the intensity of the annual influenza outbreaks with similar accuracy as existing laboratory and sentinel surveillance. "Google Flu Trends" (GFT) remains controversial. Having been viewed as a useful supporting tool by some authors,[16] it has received more critical evaluations continuously for the 2011–2012, 2012–2013, and 2013–2014 flu seasons. The scientific debate on GFT has highlighted the need for further research on algorithms that can adjust for sudden intense media coverage of health issues, but it has also and even more so highlighted the problems resulting from an in-transparent way of setting and adjusting algorithms by a global company that prioritize the protection of its competitive advantage. In another example for regions where traditional data for emerging and re-emerging diseases like dengue are often not available or only with substantial delay, web search query data were found to be capable of tracking dengue activity in Bolivia, Brazil, India, Indonesia, and Singapore.[17] These data represent a valuable complement to assist with traditional forms of surveillance. In North America (Argus, GPHIN, EpiSPIDER, etc.) and Europe (EWRS, MedISys, etc.), several event-based surveillance systems have been established that continuously screen data from all possible media sources and short message services. Currently the information generated by these systems, whether they run automatically or moderated, need careful and elaborate analysis and interpretation by epidemiologists and public health professionals resulting in a reluctance of health agencies to fully incorporate data from these systems into their working routine. Future research to improve the technologies and to overcome the limitations will determine whether these approaches can eventually have a more prominent role in public health surveillance.

Social Media

The rapid development and wide acceptance of social media sites, such as Facebook and Twitter, have introduced innovative surveillance methods to the public health practitioner's toolbox, including text mining, aggregation, and analysis of short online text messages in real time. Terms like "infoveillance" and "infodemiology" have been coined to describe these new approaches.[18] In addition to quantitative analysis, these methods permit qualitative analysis to identify changes in opinions, risk behavior, and responses by populations to public health threats and interventions. Interventions to change responses generate critical questions about the ethical nature of whether social media posts are considered public or private and social media users' right to anonymity.[19] There is still limited scientific evidence proving the added value to traditional surveillance methods, but research has just begun to discover the potential of social media monitoring. Firsthand observation by users could benefit epidemiological analysis and social media could provide primary data on how alerts and public health warnings have been perceived, understood, and followed. The increased research on social and behavioral aspects of social media content and interaction will provide more evidence to assess the new systems.

Smartphones and Wearable Diagnostics

The smartphones are getting smarter and will soon be powering a revolution in health care that will allow health care providers to spot problems—and intervene—no matter where the person is in the world. Scientists at the University of Southern California have been working on wearable and implanted device to monitor from a distance their cardiovascular disease patients. Networked gadgets, such as an iPhone fitted with a heart rate monitor, could be the start of a revolution in health care that will allow health care providers to spot problems—and intervene—even if they are thousands of miles away.[20]

Using wearable wireless sensors, people can use their smartphone to generate their own medical data, including measuring blood-oxygen and glucose levels, blood pressure, and heart rhythm. These innovations have started and can soon transform monitoring of individual risk factors for diseases and not only prehospital care of individuals but also trends of diseases in populations.[21]

Internet of Things

Internet of Things (IoT) is a computing concept that describes a future where everyday physical objects will be connected to the internet and be able to identify themselves to other devices.[22] IoT will be increasingly used to improve the quality of life of people through measures that promote an eco-friendly, sustainable environment. Big Data that are continuously generated by IoT sensors, devices, systems, and services are geotagged or geolocated and with robust, intelligent geospatial analytics systems in place, offer opportunities for monitoring and improving population health. The WHO Healthy Cities Network and associated national networks have hundreds of member cities around the world where IoT could be used in positive ways to contribute to the health of the people.[23,24] IoT can be used for monitoring environmental hazards, for example, measurement of UV sunrays to warn people not to be exposed in certain hours. IoT offer opportunities for increased used in infection prevention and control by using monitoring system of wrist bands in combination of Bluetooth tags on a patient's doorway controlling hand hygiene in hospitals by sending vibration notifications to inform about time for handwashing. The data collected from these loggers produce analytics, which can be used to potentially trace patient infections to particular health care workers and institute corrective actions.[16]

CHALLENGES TO BE LEVERAGED FOR PUBLIC HEALTH SURVEILLANCE RESEARCH AND INNOVATION

Global public health surveillance, under the revised International Health Regulations (2005) (IHR - 2005) framework will significantly shape the future development of public health surveillance through international collaboration, standardization, and dedicated funding streams.[25]

Informatics and Interoperability

Global health security concerns are rising with the increasing pace of population movement in the twenty-first century; diseases are emerging and re-emerging at rates higher than ever before, as is the threat for deliberate use of biological weapons. There is an increasing need to strengthen national and global health surveillance networks to meet and tackle these concerns. Guidance documents like the IHR (2005) drive the strengthening of surveillance networks but a lack of interoperability between information systems remains a big challenge (see Chapter 20). There is need for further research and innovation in establishing detailed informatics standards for surveillance at the global level that would provide all levels of surveillance (local, national, regional) with the opportunity to contribute toward global health security and also to adapt those standards to their specific epidemiology, disease control, and health promotion priorities.[26,27]

Point-of-Care Diagnostics

Point-of-care diagnostics (POC) refers to when patient specimens assayed at or near the patient with the assumption that test results will be available instantly or in a very short time frame to assist caregivers with immediate diagnosis and/or clinical intervention.[28] One of the challenges in disease detection is the limited availability of POC, rapid, and cost-effective diagnostics. Point-of-care data are important for matching the speed of disease occurrence and spread, and for minimizing morbidity and mortality, especially in resource-limited settings. Studies have shown that POC diagnostics may result in increased acceptance and volume of HIV testing.[29] There are promising results from field tests on the possibility of POC diagnostics enhancing dengue diagnosis in an endemic setting. These POC diagnostics also have the potential to markedly improve clinical management of dengue in the field but further research is required.[30] Research is also required in POC diagnostics in noncommunicable diseases (NCDs) that could connect laboratory results and the patient's electronic health records with the physician's clinic in future.[31]

Public Health Workforce

Population health problems are increasingly known to have multiple and complex determinants. How to equip the public health surveillance workforce of the twenty-first century to be able to deal with the many and varied aspects required for measuring and responding to these health problems remains a challenge.[32] Data from across the globe highlight a shortage of public health professionals capable of performing surveillance and response functions.[26,32] Moreover, health systems lack the capacity to systematically and dynamically quantify their own workforce shortages and assess the core competencies needed to perform essential public health functions. Maintaining a trained health workforce and ensuring up-to-date knowledge of current challenges, concepts, and solutions is also a challenge. In a study to estimate the knowledge of zoonoses among medical students and recent graduates, used to understand critical gaps in medical education with respect to zoonoses in India, it was found that, on average, subjects knew only 40–60% of what is deemed necessary to diagnose, treat, and report zoonotic diseases effectively.[33] This finding highlights the need for the current medical curriculum to be revised to keep pace with emerging and re-emerging disease challenges like zoonoses. While this particular study refers to India, it is likely that other countries will require similar revisions to their training programs. Research and innovation is required to find pedagogies that will quickly reach and continuously update a large public health workforce to meet current and future challenges. The still emerging field of Global Health with new educational programs developing among the leading medical and public health schools around the world.

Funding Limitations

The underfunding of public health surveillance and limited public health resources were seen as a main concerns in a recent stakeholder analysis that involved public health surveillance experts from 24 EU countries.[34] Most experts stated that the austerity measures enacted in many countries in reaction to the recent economic crisis have exacerbated this situation. The CDC highlights a shortage of funding as one of the contributing factors to the public health workforce shortage.[35] Therefore, priorities have to be made when developing new surveillance systems and other surveillance initiatives to account for components that may not be optimally available.

With dedicated funding sources, public health surveillance progress can continue uninterrupted. Microbiological methods are rapidly improving, and the implementation of new rapid diagnostic assays reduces the delay from suspicion of an illness to confirmation. With the development of more comprehensive systems for molecular surveillance, there will be very specific systems in place for outbreak detection. Of course, the development, implementation, and maintenance of these improvements do not come cheaply. To sustain these innovations, funding should be considered from the very beginning planning stages and included in discussions through all phases of project implementation.

EXAMPLES OF CURRENT BEST PRACTICES IN INDIA

Influenza outbreaks, like SARS in 2003, avian influenza in 2005, and H1N1 in 2009, highlighted the need for effective disease surveillance systems for early outbreak detection and rapid reporting.[36] With increasing globalization and economic growth, more travelers intensify the risk of rapid disease transmission, and thus, early case detection, and harmonized and rapid response are needed to effectively control disease outbreaks. Global public health surveillance under IHR has been reshaped, highlighting the need for improved international communication and focusing on alternative data sources for timely response.[37] Effective public health surveillance is a core function during pandemics and large outbreaks that improve the public health system's capacity to respond to the outbreak. When pandemic outbreaks occur, rapid detection and timely information sharing are essential, yet also a key challenge. Key questions during disease outbreaks and questions for public health surveillance include: How can different regional, national, and international systems communicate with each other to integrate information for timely and coordinated response? Can integrated information lead to more effective decision-making?

Outbreak detection is crucial for quickly detecting and containing initial outbreaks so that broader spread of communicable disease can be prevented. Health data sources are left untapped or are not utilized to their fullest potential. In particular, in low- and middle-income countries, where health information systems are not fully operational, alternative health data sources are critical for outbreak detection and control. Siloed surveillance systems based on specific vectors or diseases can be costly and need extensive manpower to be maintained.[38] The prediagnostic observation approach of syndromic surveillance based on existing data sources proved useful for emerging and re-emerging infectious disease surveillance and earlier outbreak detection.[39] Further research needs to focus on innovative public health surveillance solutions for countries with limited resources and less than optimal surveillance systems.

This section will highlight two best practices of public health surveillance in India. The first example emphasizes the challenge of conducting surveillance and the incentive of international collaboration in research. It will demonstrate a research initiative to overcome the challenge of early warning. The second example focuses on polio surveillance in India and its success using a central health program.

System for Early Warning Based on Emergency Data

In the fragmented health care systems of India, reporting timely and reliable health data for influenza surveillance purposes is a huge challenge. Different surveillance systems are used depending on the level of collection, which results in a lengthy period of data processing that means data cannot be used in real time.[40] Centralized programs have been implemented to overcome these reporting challenges, but public health still struggles to receive timely and reliable health information.[41] During pandemics, when disease spreads quickly around the globe, innovation and research are particularly needed to overcome these struggles. International joint research activities can build on collaboration to bridge knowledge and experience to improve communication and data quality and timeliness. This type of research was demonstrated by the **System for Early warning based on Emergency Data (SEED)**[40] using emergency medical services (EMS) data related to fever in Andhra Pradesh, India. SEED was a collaborative project of the GVK Emergency Management and Research Institute (EMRI), India, and GEOMED Research, Germany, funded by the German Federal Ministry of Education and Research (BMBF) and Indian Council of Medical Research (ICMR) to systematically explore the use of emergency data for syndromic surveillance in India. German and Indian researchers working together on SEED used real-time data for surveillance results for the first time in India to supplement existing surveillance systems and provide early warning for disease outbreak where the primary symptom is fever.[40] SEED was set up as a pilot research project to systematically test and evaluate the applicability of routinely collected EMS data in India for the use of syndromic surveillance.[42-44] The research project is a combination of a database and corresponding algorithm, and GIS tools, which can aid in the early detection of health threats. EMS data are collected through a surveillance system set up in 15 Indian states and 2 union territories based on emergency data and symptoms. EMS data are generated and captured automatically at the state dispatch center in Hyderabad.

The system serves as an early warning system for disease outbreaks through automatic comparisons of real-time data and predetermined alert thresholds. Local spatial temporal baselines and thresholds for syndromes are calculated and periodically updated within **SEED** using historical data. Routinely collected data are automatically transferred to **SEED** in near real time and then analyzed for temporal and spatial aberrations. The system compares the actual demand for EMS with the expected (forecasted) demand for a certain time and region (baseline). An alert is issued from the system if the predefined threshold is exceeded. **SEED** was tested using the symptom of fever, continuously monitoring the demand for EMS based on patients with fever.[40] The system was enacted during a dengue fever outbreak in 2010 and showed the capability of emergency data for early detection and monitoring of an infectious disease outbreak.[42]

The **SEED** project was the first attempt in India to systematically develop a surveillance system based on real-time data. The **SEED** concept does not replace but rather supplements and enhances existing surveillance systems in India. The concept can be applied to other disease syndromes and can be transferred to other districts or states in India served by the same EMS dispatch centers collecting routine data. This example demonstrates one way that India is using alternative data sources to supplement public health surveillance.

Polio Surveillance in India

India successfully prioritized polio eradication and achieved immense success, despite the public health surveillance constraints that presented challenges to the eradication initiative.[45] Polio was prioritized as a disease for active, case-based surveillance in India as a World Health Organization (WHO) target disease for eradication.[45,46] In contrast to smallpox, the last disease to be eradicated in India, with its characteristic rash, polio is difficult to detect; diagnosing polio is a clinical challenge, as paralysis could be due to numerous causes. In polio, paralysis is an unusual manifestation of infection, and hence most infections are not detected. The epidemiology of poliovirus presents a special challenge to detection due to the very high ratio of subclinical to clinical infection. A single case of poliomyelitis is considered to be an epidemic of polio, warranting quick action and focused immunization activity.

India's acute flaccid paralysis (AFP) surveillance system for detecting poliovirus transmission is considered to be one of the most sensitive surveillance systems in the world.[47] The surveillance network includes reporting sites from both public and private sector and even non-allopathic healthcare providers and traditional healers, who immediately give a call on mobile phone to a designated surveillance/immunization officer who ensures sample collection for lab diagnosis. India not only met but also surpassed all of the WHO AFP surveillance global performance indicators over 10 years before being certified polio-free in 2014. The development of surveillance performance indicators is unique to AFP surveillance for polio and is an innovation worth applying to other diseases' surveillance to ensure accurate data are being collected. The AFP surveillance system in India provides evidence of operational feasibility and a roadmap for global quality surveillance in low- and middle-income countries. The WHO Director General, Dr Margaret Chan, while addressing the "India celebrates triumph over polio" event in New Delhi, India, on February 11, 2014, said, "India, arguably facing the toughest challenges of any polio-endemic country, met each problem with creativity and innovation. In so doing, this country pioneered key operational and technical strategies as lessons for other countries."[48] India was innovative in its health systems response by engaging all possible stakeholders for surveillance and response; using unique financing mechanisms; garnering and coordinating global support for the polio-eradication efforts through effective governance; inclusive and sustained social mobilization efforts, and meticulous microplanning to ensure universal coverage of vaccines.[48,49]

CONCLUSION

Scientists and managers of health systems must continuously adapt and transform surveillance systems to meet the public health requirements of tomorrow. Research and innovation have a reciprocal relationship with public health surveillance: public health surveillance needs drive research and innovation while research and innovation result in the constant transformation of public health surveillance. These processes do not happen easily; they require a well-coordinated environment with technology that is effective and interoperable, a trained workforce capable of applying the research and innovation in the field of public health surveillance, and dedicated funding to sustain the changing needs of the field.

KEY SUMMARY POINTS

- Public health surveillance is an ever-evolving field.
- Research and innovation shape the transformative nature of public health surveillance.
- A One Health approach calls for strengthening the links between human health, animal health, and the environment to strengthen all of these sectors.
- Existing and emerging technologies provide the opportunity and pathway for public health surveillance transformation.
- The crucial challenges of interoperability, evolving diagnostics, workforce, and funding will need to be addressed for continued success in the transformation of public health surveillance.

DISCUSSION QUESTIONS

1. What are key research questions for public health surveillance?
2. What is the role of research in public health surveillance?
3. Describe the connections between research and innovation and public health surveillance.
4. What global health security challenges drive research and innovations in public health surveillance?
5. What are the opportunities for advancing research and innovations in public health surveillance in the twenty-first century?

REFERENCE

1. Horton R. GBD 2010: understanding disease, injury, and risk. Lancet 2012;380(9859):2053–54.
2. Murray CJ, Ezzati M, Flaxman AD, Lim S, Lozano R, Michaud C, et al. GBD 2010: a multi-investigator collaboration for global comparative descriptive epidemiology. Lancet 2012;380(9859):2055–58.
3. Horton R, Beaglehole R, Bonita R, Raeburn J, McKee M, Wall S. From public to planetary health: a manifesto. Lancet 2014;383(9920):847.
4. Wurapa F, Afari E, Ohuabunwo C, Sackey S, Clerk C, Kwadje S, et al. One Health concept for strengthening public health surveillance and response through Field Epidemiology and Laboratory Training in Ghana. Pan Afr Med J 2011;10(Suppl. 1):6.
5. Mariner JC, Hendrickx S, Pfeiffer DU, Costard S, Knopf L, Okuthe S, et al. Integration of participatory approaches into surveillance systems. Rev Sci Tech 2011;30(3):653–9.
6. Gubernot DM, Boyer BL, Moses MS. Animals as early detectors of bioevents: veterinary tools and a framework for animal-human integrated zoonotic disease surveillance. Public Health Rep 2008;123(3):300–15.
7. Dupuy C, Perrin JB, Bronner A, Calavas D, Hendrikx P, Fouillet A. Synergies between human and animal health syndromic surveillance: triple-S Outputs. Online J Public Health Inform 2013;5(1).
8. Hoffman S, Podgurski A. Big bad data: law, public health, and biomedical databases. J Law Med Ethics 2013;41(Suppl. 1):56–60.
9. Pope C, Halford S, Tinati R, Weal M. What's the big fuss about 'big data'? J Health Serv Res Policy 2014;19:67–8.
10. Big Data Research, <http://www.journals.elsevier.com/big-data-research/>; October 2014.
11. Marr B. Big data: the 5 Vs everyone must know. Linkedin.com; 2014.
12. Jerrett M, Gale S, Kontgis C. Spatial modeling in environmental and public health research. Int J Environ Res Public Health 2010;7(4):1302–29.
13. Wiafe S, Davenhall B. Extending disease surveillance with GIS, <http://www.esri.com/news/arcuser/0405/disease_surveil1of2.html/>; October 2014.
14. Hossain I, Firdausy TP, Behr FJ. WHO's public health mapping and GIS programme. In: Behr FJ, Pradeepkumar AP, Castaepkumar editors; 2010.
15. Hulth A, Rydevik G, Linde A. Web queries as a source for syndromic surveillance. PLoS One 2009;4(2):e4378.
16. Internet of Things - From Research and Innovation to Market Deployment; 2014.
17. Chan EH, Sahai V, Conrad C, Brownstein JS. Using web search query data to monitor dengue epidemics: a new model for neglected tropical disease surveillance. PLoS Negl Trop Dis 2011;5(5):e1206.
18. Eysenbach G. Infodemiology and infoveillance: framework for an emerging set of public health informatics methods to analyze search, communication and publication behavior on the Internet. J Med Internet Res 2009;11:e11.
19. Chew C, Eysenbach G. Pandemics in the age of Twitter: content analysis of tweets during the 2009 H1N1 outbreak. PLoS One 2010;5(11):e14118.
20. Will mobile sensors revolutionise healthcare? bbc.com: BBC; 2012.
21. Topol EJ. The future of medicine is in your smartphone. WSJ 2015.
22. Internet of things (IoT). 2010, <http://www.techopedia.com/definition/28247/internet-of-things-iot/>; October 2014.
23. Kamel Boulos MN, Al-Shorbaji NM. On the Internet of Things, smart cities and the WHO Healthy Cities. Int J Health Geogr 2014;13:10.
24. WHO European Healthy Cities Network, <http://www.euro.who.int/en/health-topics/environment-and-health/urban-health/activities/healthy-cities/who-european-healthy-cities-network/>; October 2014.
25. Nuttall I. International Health Regulations (2005): taking stock. Bull World Health Organ 2014;92(5):310.
26. Buehler JW. CDC's vision for public health surveillance in the 21st century. Introduction. MMWR Surveill Summ 2012;61(Suppl.):1–2.
27. Stansfield S. Structuring information and incentives to improve health. Bull World Health Organ 2005;83:562.
28. Ehrmeyer SS, Laessig RH. Point-of-care testing, medical error, and patient safety: a 2007 assessment. Clin Chem Lab Med 2007;45(6):766–73.
29. Gilbert M. Impact and use of point of care HIV testing: a public health evidence paper. STI/HIV Prevention and Control. BC Centre for Disease Control; 2010.
30. Gan VC, Tan LK, Lye DC, Pok KY, Mok SQ, Chua RC, et al. Diagnosing dengue at the point-of-care: utility of a rapid combined diagnostic kit in Singapore. PLoS One 2014;9(3):e90037.
31. Warren AD, Kwong GA, Wood DK, Lin KY, Bhatia SN. Point-of-care diagnostics for noncommunicable diseases using synthetic urinary biomarkers and paper microfluidics. Proc Natl Acad Sci USA 2014;111(10):3671–6.

32. Lee L, Teutsch S, Thacker S. Principles and practice of public health surveillance. St. Louis M: Oxford University Press; 2010.
33. Kakkar M, Ramani S, Menon G, Sankhe L, Gaidhane A, Krishnan S. 'Zoonoses? Not sure what that is...' An assessment of knowledge of zoonoses among medical students in India. Trans R Soc Trop Med Hyg 2011;105(5):254–61.
34. Triple S Project. Assessment of syndromic surveillance in Europe. Lancet 2011;378(9806):1833–4.
35. Drehobl PA, Roush SW, Stover BH, Koo D. Public health surveillance workforce of the future. MMWR Surveill Summ 2012;61(Suppl.):25–9.
36. St. Louis M. Global Health Surveillance. MMWR Morb Mortal Wkly Rep 2012;61(3):15–9.
37. World Health Organization. International Health Regulations (2005). Geneva: WHO; 2008.
38. Atun R, Bennett S, Duran A. When do vertical (stand-alone) programmes have a place in health systems? Copenhagen, Denmark: World Health Organization; 2008.
39. Lemon S, Hamburg M, Sparling P, Choffnes E, Mack A. Global infectious disease surveillance and detection: assessing the challenges—finding solutions. Washington, DC: Institute of Medicine; 2007.
40. Institute GEMaR, mbH GRF. System for Early warning based on Emergency Data (SEED), <http://www.geomed-research.eu/GVK EMRI-Geomed_Leaflet.pdf/>; October 2014.
41. Kant L, Krishnan SK. Information and communication technology in disease surveillance, India: a case study. BMC Public Health 2010;10(Suppl. 1):S11.
42. Jena B, Prasad M, Murthy S, Ramanarao G. Demand pattern of medical emergency services for infectious diseases in Andhra Pradesh- a geo-spatial temporal analysis of fever cases. Indian Emerg J 2010;5(1):5–8.
43. Pilot E, Jena B, Kauhl B, Rao R, Pardeschi RR, Ziemann A, Krafft T.. Disease Surveillance and Early Outbreak Detection in India. Salute e Solidarieta Decimo Seminario Internazionale di Geografia Medica 2012:287–92.
44. Pilot E, Jena B, Krafft T, Ziemann A, Rao R, Kauhl B, et al. New approaches to disease surveillance and early outbreak detection in India. In New Delhi, India: Proceedings of the Fourth International Conference on Health GIS, 5-6 August 2011. p. 240–7.
45. John TJ, Vashishtha VM. Eradicating poliomyelitis: India's journey from hyperendemic to polio-free status. Indian J Med Res 2013;137(5):881–94.
46. Field guide surveillance of acute flaccid paralysis. 3rd ed. New Delhi: Ministry of Health & Family Welfare; 2005.
47. Heymann D, Ahmed Q. The polio eradication end game: what it means for Europe. Euro Surveill 2014;19(7):20702.
48. WHO. WHO Director-General celebrates polio-free India, <http://www.who.int/dg/speeches/2014/india-polio-free/en/>; October 2014.
49. Sheldrick M. India is polio-free: what can Pakistan, Afghanistan and Nigeria learn? The Guardian, <http://www.theguardian.com/global-development-professionals-network/2014/jan/13/lessons-india-polio-free-landmark/>; October 2014.

CHAPTER

31

Improving Health Equity and Sustainability by Transforming Public Health Surveillance

Ann Marie Kimball, Beth E Rivin

Injustice anywhere is a threat to justice everywhere.

Martin Luther King, Jr

KEY WORDS

Health equity
Expanded Program of Immunizations (EPI)
Disease eradication
Human rights
Strengthening Health Delivery Systems (SHDS)
Vital registration (VR) systems

THE OPPORTUNITY: PROMOTING EQUITY THROUGH ENHANCING DISEASE SURVEILLANCE; MAKING EVERYONE COUNT

Equity suggests that every individual "counts" in a similar way. Each individual has access to food, shelter, and services in an equitable way. This chapter explores how this basic concept of equity figures in the area of disease surveillance. Clearly if one is not counted one "does not count." The majority of the poorest of the poor in the world are not counted by their governments.[1,2] This is reflected in weak civil registration and vital statistics systems in most poor countries. Some surveillance activities promote counting, and therein potentially enfranchisement of the poor. They are discussed herein.

Eradication: Counting Every Case

The goal of **disease eradication**—the permanent reduction of new infection to zero, with interventions no longer needed—presents an opportunity to ensure everyone is counted in disease surveillance.[3] In practice, sustaining the surveillance infrastructure and its supporting resources proves much more difficult. In fact, Dowldle[4] has asserted that eradication represents the ultimate disease equity. The thinking is clear: targets of eradication (e.g., smallpox, polio, and guinea worm) disproportionately affect poor populations. Thus, their eradication brings a direct benefit in lack of illness in the population. Indirectly, populations benefit from the absence of control program expenditure over time. This theoretically creates a "bonus" allowing resources to be redirected into other health priorities after eradication to the benefit of poor populations. What is essential to the success of eradication is that every single case (i.e., individual) is counted and there is a rapid and definitive response. Response is vaccination of potential susceptible cases to prevent further transmission. If vaccines are not available, such as in lymphatic filariasis, response is vector control and case treatment.

More specifically, recent analytic and modeling efforts have extended the paradigm of polio eradication. As the dynamism of polio circulation and spectrum of infection is increasingly appreciated, the focus has centered on the management of population immunity levels. Managing population immunity requires consideration of all individuals in the population because vaccinated individuals potentially can become reinfected and participate in the spread of infection without being symptomatic.[5]

In May 1980, the World Health Assembly declared the global eradication of smallpox, 22 years after its initial eradication resolution. Smallpox was endemic in more than 30 countries worldwide, as late as 1967.[6] Specifically, approximately 1 billion people in 31 countries were considered at risk for smallpox. Innovations in technology, surveillance, and monitoring strategy, and a significant mobilization of financial, human, and political resources attributed to this still unrepeated historic achievement.

The surveillance strategy evolved over the course of the eradication campaign, from one focused solely on mass vaccination to one that also employed an alternative surveillance containment strategy. The successful containment of a 1966 outbreak in Nigeria's Ogoja province by identifying and vaccinating only people likely exposed and infected by smallpox when faced with a local vaccine shortage supply demonstrated the effectiveness of the containment approach.[7] Gradually, the World Health Organization (WHO) and national eradication efforts would endorse the surveillance/containment approach as a part of eradication efforts in endemic areas.

This surveillance approach of search and contain required the mobilization of an army of health workers. In India, a typical search would last 6 days and employ all available health workers, including workers borrowed from other health programs, such as malaria, to help find cases of smallpox. As surveillance evolved, secondary and tertiary search techniques would send workers to crowds and groups at the fringes of society.[7] The distinctive smallpox rash, starting on the face and then moving to the hands, forearms, and trunk, made identification possible. Containment teams complemented search operations and, armed with improved vaccination technology, including first the Ped-O-Jet and then the bifurcated needle, the speed of vaccination and uptake rates improved.

Not surprisingly, the active surveillance/containment approach detected significantly more cases than the previous passive surveillance regime. For example, in September 1973, 437 cases of smallpox were reported using the existing reporting system, but in October, the searches had identified 5989 new cases.[7] This trend of increasing cases would continue as the surveillance improved, which at times would also generate negative national and international publicity.

The overall costs and benefits of the smallpox campaign have been well documented.[8,9] Certainly the direct impact of the campaign on population health was transformative. Eradicating the scourge of a disfiguring and potentially fatal disease was a signal achievement. Perhaps the greatest benefit was the creation of a network of smallpox warriors: workers from all different countries of the globe working toward a common goal. The achievement was emboldening to global public health. It ushered in the **Expanded program of immunizations (EPI)** into the populations of sub-Saharan Africa.[10] EPI is a WHO program with the goal of universal access to all relevant vaccines for all at risk. The program aims to expand the targeted groups to include older children, adolescents, and adults and work in synergy with other public health programs in order to control disease and achieve better health for all populations, particularly the underserved populations. The campaign made the infectious disease burden of poor countries look vulnerable to modern interventions. Thus, from an equity point of view, the obligation of health systems in poor economies to deliver services to their citizens became more achievable.

Polio: A Work in Progress

In contrast to smallpox, polio eradication has proven more complex. The global effort is much larger in scale, with 4.5 billion individuals in 125 countries at risk of disease at the outset of the global campaign. The World Health Assembly made the declaration for eradication in 1988 following successful regional eradication in the Americas. As today's molecular technologies were not available in the era of smallpox that ended in the late 1970s, it is difficult to compare the results of the smallpox and polio campaigns on a molecular level.

Polio differs from smallpox in several fundamental ways. First, polio infection is usually announced by acute flaccid paralysis (AFP) but the syndrome is not pathognomonic; the syndrome may be caused by several other enteroviruses. Infection may also be asymptomatic. This contrasts with smallpox, which was absolutely recognizable with its highly characteristic rashes. Second, there are carriers of polio who are not impacted. Sewage studies suggest that even in the absence of apparent disease, there may be carriage of the virus. Third, intimate knowledge of populations—down to the smallest population level—on a continuing basis seems to be necessary for successful polio campaigns. With smallpox, this was less the case; once the evident disease was eradicated, there was less need for continued vigilance than with polio. Fourth, the world's politics are very different.

In traditional societies today, there is increasing mistrust of modernity. Whereas in the 1970s, it seemed the modern world brought a miraculous vaccine, which ended a disfiguring illness (smallpox), the polio vaccine is under suspicion today. In fact, polio vaccinators have been attacked and killed simply for bringing the vaccine into traditional Islamist areas. The "street" rumors alleging that the vaccine is bringing infertility to Islamist communities have gained alarming traction, despite earnest efforts by WHO and other international bodies to work with Islamist religious leaders in issuing *fatwas* and trying to convince the faithful that the lies are just that—lies. The world has changed, and polio eradication lies in the balance.

Worldwide polio eradication campaigns with the live attenuated Sabin vaccine have been intense, especially in the endemic areas of the world. As the polio campaign approaches eradication, there have been concentrated efforts of multiple vaccine campaign rounds requiring extra resources and manpower to vaccinate every child in every district. As coverage in countries increased, there has been a reduction in diversity of the wild-type polioviruses. Circulation of Wild Poliovirus (WPV) type 2 has ceased since 2000. However, WPV types 1 and 3 have continued to circulate in some geographic areas, and international spread from these areas has been demonstrated.[11]

Legacies from Eradication: Is the Dividend Real for Poor People?

So, at the end of the day, does polio eradication with its opportunity costs to health systems in poor countries actually contribute to economic development and prosperity? Common sense says "of course," but the evidence is only now being systematically reviewed. It is hard to imagine how an economy can prosper with a preventable cause of lifelong lameness still at large. A key question with polio eradication will be about the legacy left behind. Polio expenditure globally has included major investments in surveillance, case finding (rapid response teams), sample collection, and laboratory. In fact, the Global Polio Eradication Initiative has established these systems in every WHO Member State. Will this vertical move strengthen overall surveillance at the country level? Will the polio laboratories in each WHO Member State be repurposed to meet new challenges? How will the rapid response teams within the Ministries in the public sector be utilized going forward? Will the poor in poor countries have a lasting "polio dividend" which is palpable and real?

Polio is a disabling disease. In the early 1980s in West Africa, each street corner of modern capitals like Abidjan, Dakar, and Ouagadougou were home to the "crawlers." Individuals with a begging bowl, crawling in the dust from car to car for a handout. Clearly a whole generation of Africans had been lost to the physical disability of polio. This has fundamentally changed. With release operations (operations to release key muscle groups and allow the straightening of paralyzed limbs), those who were once beggars can now stand up and walk. With immunization, prevalence has diminished such that street corners in these capitals are now empty of polio victims. The burden of losing so much intellect and vibrancy to polio is clearly an obstacle to economic development.

Eradication efforts, such as those for smallpox and polio, have potential legacy benefits for resource poor settings and their populations.[12] After the global eradication of smallpox, scores of trained personnel were present in countries where public health training had previously been unknown. A network of smallpox workers existed informally, linking individuals across the globe. In Africa, the EPI was launched at the end of the 1970s at the request of African governments that had seen the impact of immunizations through the smallpox campaign. The first EPI demonstration zones in Ivory Coast, Cameroon, and the Gambia were well established by 1980 through the regional Strengthening Health Delivery Systems (SHDS) project of the United States Agency for International Development (USAID) working with WHO.[13]

The legacy of polio promises to be even more profound. However, until global eradication is achieved, there is reluctance to "stand down" the current vertically oriented resources of personnel, laboratories, and other systems.

India provides some clues: after passing a full year with no new cases in 2012, the government has been able to devote additional resources to a renewed effort against measles, including enhancing their routine EPI delivery.

A less tangible scientific benefit of polio, the increasing centrality of management of population immunity for success, promises to shift the policy paradigm for vaccine preventable diseases (VPDs). This core concept will be further explored later in this chapter.

SURVEILLANCE OF INFECTIOUS DISEASES: BURDEN OF THE POOR

The global policy agenda is increasingly focusing on eradicating extreme poverty and promoting the health of vulnerable groups. The Millennium Development Goals[14] adopted by 191 countries in 2000 embody these priority concerns (see Chapter 29). Nonetheless, the burden of infections continues to concentrate among the poorest of the poor. In this section we review (1) the disproportionate burden of infectious diseases in low and middle income countries and poor populations; (2) the accompanying paucity of data from the poorest populations in the world; (3) the impact of stigma and discrimination (human rights violations) on "counting"; and (4) the lack of "counting" systems in many poor countries in terms of civil registration and vital statistics. While our earlier discussion focused on vaccine preventable eradication targets, this discussion will expand the scope to include the larger spectrum of infectious disease threats to the global poor and vulnerable.

Disproportionate Burden for the Poor

Globally, noncommunicable diseases now account for the majority of disease burden, but many people in resource poor settings continue to suffer a disproportionate burden of preventable and treatable infectious disease. In 2010, global communicable, maternal, neonatal, and nutrition-related causes of death accounted for 13.2 million deaths, down from 15.9 million in 1990. In contrast, noncommunicable diseases increased from 26.6 million deaths in 1990 to 34.5 million—65.5% of all deaths—in 2010. This transition toward noncommunicable diseases is not seen uniformly across regions of the world. In the developed world in 2010, communicable, maternal, neonatal, and nutrition causes accounted for 5.87% of total deaths, whereas in developing countries they accounted for 31.14% of total deaths. The treatable diseases of lower respiratory infections, diarrheal diseases, and malaria alone account for 4.9 million deaths in the developing world. 15 Trends in global and regional morbidity present a similar picture. In high-income North America, communicable, maternal, neonatal, and nutrition disorders comprise 5.36% of total disability-adjusted life years (DALYs), but equal 42.97% in South Asia and 68.46% in sub-Saharan Africa.[16]

Historical "Undercount" and Imprecision

Vital registration (VR) is defined by the United Nations "as the total process of (a) collecting information by civil registration or enumeration on the frequency or occurrence of specified and defined vital events, as well as relevant characteristics of the events themselves and the person or persons concerned, and (b) compiling, processing, analyzing, evaluating, presenting, and disseminating these data in statistical form."[17] VR systems are a key source of population and demographic data, but their coverage is limited.

In 2005, 100 countries reported deaths from VR systems; these systems captured 18.8 million deaths out of an estimated total of 51.7 million.[15] In other words, less than half of the deaths that occurred were covered by VR systems. In the absence of VR data, verbal autopsy (VA) is a means of gathering cause of death data through structured interviews of a deceased's next of kin. VA data are gathered from multiple sources, such as demographic surveillance systems or surveys, and are heterogeneous in nature, using differing methods to gather data and assign cause of death. For the Global Burden of Disease Study 2010, the authors note that VA data were extensively used in estimating mortality in low-income settings.[15]

In the same study, poor countries had few data points. Thus, many of the estimates for their disease burden were derived from modeled rather than empirical data. In sub-Saharan Africa, for example, the 10 countries with the fewest data points were South Sudan, Equatorial Guinea, Somalia, Djibouti, Eritrea, Angola, Gabon, Guinea-Bissau, Central African Republic, and Comoros.[18] With the exception of Equatorial Guinea (an outlier due to its extraction industry wealth), the World Bank 2010 GDP per capita data place most of these countries as low or lower middle income. In fact, this indicator is not available for 4 of the 10 countries, perhaps because of their impoverished national information systems. Only Gabon is ranked as upper middle income. Thus, lack of empirical data and the broader uncertainties of modeled DALYs seem correlated with poverty.

What is Counted: Undercounting and Poor Access to Diagnostics

Central to disease surveillance is defining what is counted. What, exactly, is a "case?" As noted in the previous sections, the very design of current information systems may contribute to this problem. Lack of counting through VR effectively eliminates the ability to assure population coverage of health services. Coincidentally, lack of access to diagnostics that aid in accurate case definitions can further disenfranchise those living in low-resource settings.

It is accurate to say that sensitive diagnostics are less available to marginalized populations. Therein, case definitions for surveillance of infections are apt to be less sensitive as well. As shown with HIV, this is particularly acute for new infections where diagnostics must be invented, tested, and distributed. Often such diagnostics are more costly, or dependent on other systems that do not exist in resource poor settings.

The Undercount: Poor Case Definitions for Poor People

The HIV/AIDS epidemic highlighted the differences between "counting a case" in resource-poor and resourced settings. HIV testing was commonplace after 1985 but was not available in resource-poor settings. Thus, the "Bangui Definition"[19] of AIDS in Africa did not require HIV testing, whereas the "Caracas Definition"[20] of AIDS in Latin America did. The coexistent US Centers for Disease Control and Prevention (CDC) definition required not only HIV testing but also confirmed pathologic diagnostics for opportunistic infections. There was no effective treatment for HIV until a full decade later. Had there been the 60% sensitivity for AIDS as defined in Africa,[19] the use of this definition would have left many untreated. Certainly it led to a profound undercount of the grave epidemic in Africa. In that sense, the design of a core component of surveillance, the case definition, may have disenfranchised the poorest populations affected.

A provisional clinical case definition for AIDS, developed by WHO for use in Africa, was tested on 174 inpatients at Mama Yemo Hospital in Kinshasa, Zaire. In this hospital population with a 34% infection rate of HIV, the clinical case definition's specificity was 90%, sensitivity was 59%, and predictive value was 74% for HIV seropositivity. These results support the use of the WHO clinical case definition for AIDS in Africa. However, since HIV prevalence and disease expression vary, similar evaluations should be carried out in different regions.

Human Rights Perspective: Counting and Access to Diagnostics

Accurate counting is not only affected by diagnostic availability; it is also affected by fear of stigmatization and discrimination. When people fear that their individual rights will be violated by stigmatization and discrimination if they test positive for a disease, they will often decide against testing, even if treatment is available. This has been documented in HIV voluntary counseling and testing in a black township in Cape Town, South Africa.[21]

In the case of another disease, leprosy, stigma and fear of discrimination have interfered with early diagnosis and treatment, resulting in "disease pockets."[22-24] Although a new, rapid serological test for the detection of early infection with *Mycobacterium leprae* has recently been developed, the most vulnerable populations may not submit to being tested due to fear of stigmatization and discrimination.[25] In 2012, WHO stated in a weekly EPI record[26] that "the reduction in leprosy burden needs to be accompanied by a reduction, if not elimination of the socioeconomic challenges related to the disease. National programmes, with the support of governments and partners, have an obligation to put into practice the principles of the United Nations Resolution on the elimination of stigma and discrimination against persons affected by leprosy and their families."[27]

Who or what entity has the responsibility to create an environment free from discrimination, allowing greater access to diagnostics for all? Access to health services, including prevention and diagnostic disease testing, is fundamental to the right to health. The human right to health is understood as an economic, social, and cultural right and inextricably linked to all other **human rights**—the rights inherent to all human beings, whatever our nationality, place of residence, sex, national or ethnic origin, color, religion, language, or any other status.[28] We are all equally entitled to our human rights without discrimination. These rights are all interrelated, interdependent and indivisible. The specific human rights language in the 1966 International Covenant on Economic, Social, and Cultural Rights is "the enjoyment of the highest attainable standard of health."[29] International human rights treaty law and United Nations documents in the form of "Comments" inform us about States' (country) obligations to respect, protect, and fulfill the human right to health.[29,30]

How does this relate to disease surveillance? The right to health includes preventive and curative health services and the determinants of health. The States that are obligated under international treaty law must take steps toward realizing the right to health for all. Although weak, accountability mechanisms exist, and public health professionals should collaborate with legal and other professionals in civil society to hold governments accountable for their human rights commitments. Moreover, public health professionals are critical in the process of developing indicators to measure the components of the right to health, which include availability, accessibility, acceptability, and quality. These aspects of the right to health are articulated in human rights documents and are important in assessing governments' progressive realization of the right to health.

Human rights law provides guidance on access to technologies that are useful in surveillance and disease control and/or eradication. The human rights perspective on "access" is broad. It has four dimensions including physical access, information access, nondiscrimination, and economic access or affordability. In addition to an expanded definition of access, human rights provide a fundamental understanding about the most needy and marginalized in society, such as the poor. Poor and vulnerable populations should be preferentially targeted for health interventions when resources are limited.

As the world increasingly focuses on technological advances to solve public health problems, including new diagnostic testing for disease surveillance, questions arise about government obligations to marginalized populations. Human rights address the right to enjoy the benefits of scientific progress.[29] Scholars are probing the practical aspects of this right when asking who or what entity makes the policy decision about access, which communities benefit and what are the obligations of multinational corporations? [31]

Human rights law states that every human being has dignity and rights. Discriminating against the poor in terms of unequal access to newly developed diagnostics for disease testing—discrimination based on socioeconomic status—is a violation of human rights. If poor populations are less likely to be counted, less likely to have access to diagnostics and treatment, and more likely to be disabled or die from preventable diseases, then their human rights are being violated. According to human rights law, governments are obligated to progressively realize nondiscriminatory access to preventive health services and the international community has a responsibility to assist governments in fulfilling their right to health obligations.[29,30,32] Addressing the rights of poor populations within and among countries are supported by international human rights law, and it is at the core of surveillance, disease control, and eradication.

PANDEMIC RISK AND THE POOR

Over the past 5 years, the world has been gripped by fear of a pandemic; rightly so given the history of Severe Acute Respiratory Syndrome (SARS) in 2003. Based on the influenza pandemic of 1918, the Institute for Health Metrics and Evaluation has estimated that in the event of a pandemic of avian influenza "most deaths will occur in poor countries—i.e., in societies whose scarce health resources are already stretched by existing health priorities."[12] However, even more profoundly, an editorial on this article notes: "History tells us poor populations always endure a disproportionate burden of disease and death from Infectious Diseases."[33] Given these assertions we must consider how the pandemic threat factors into the surveillance agenda for poor societies and whether that threat will bring us to counting the poor more carefully.

There has been a great deal of emphasis in the discourse on whether the AIDS epidemic could have been averted or more carefully controlled if the initial shift in clinical syndromes in Uganda and elsewhere had been recognized. However, the discussion above about the low sensitivity of the Bangui definition suggests that without diagnostics, 40% of the burden would not have been counted as AIDS. Thus, the key to sharpening our watch for pandemics and accurate global burden of disease seems to be getting good diagnostics to high-risk geographic areas before a pandemic event.

Of all the WHO networks, FluNet for monitoring global influenza has been one of the most functional. Nonetheless, it has been plagued with issues of data and specimen sovereignty. For example, the evolution and resolution of the challenges for data and specimen sovereignty involving avian influenza A highly pathogenic (H5N1) virus are illustrative. The Asian context within which H5N1 was identified is significant. Asia had introduced intensive poultry agriculture in the late 1970s and the risk for a new avian infection had been intensifying.[34] During the Indonesia outbreak of avian influenza (H5N1), the government decided to withhold viral samples from WHO, causing a crisis in global health diplomacy and disease surveillance.[35] The existing global framework for data and sample sharing was undermined by Indonesia's actions in 2006.[35] Negotiations between Indonesia and WHO for fair access to influenza vaccines were not smooth. They highlighted the fundamental issue of equity that was underpinning the controversy about sharing data and specimens. Since the H5N1 viral sample controversy, new influenza threats have emerged. However, by 2011 a more equitable global public health framework was developed that placed equity at its core.[36] The framework is a milestone for pandemic preparedness and represents the first international agreement on influenza and benefit sharing. While not legally binding for WHO member states, it encourages states to share viruses and enhances equitable access to benefits for developing countries, such as vaccines, antiviral drugs, and scientific information.[36,37]

The new framework is intended to provide diagnostics in the most needed areas to prepare for a pandemic.[36] Unfortunately, the framework does not make specific demands on wealthy countries to contribute to low and middle income countries' influenza pandemic preparedness.[37] Since pandemics are known to disproportionately affect poor people in poor countries, it will indeed be essential to place diagnostics, early warning systems, vaccines, and antivirals in the most vulnerable geographies, not only for reasons of equity but also for influenza pandemic control.

CONCLUSION

We have outlined the following dynamic realities in the above discourse. (1) A paradigm of monitoring population immunity that requires all individuals (even the economic and politically marginalized) to be included has evolved from the global eradication campaigns for smallpox and polio. This expands the imperative to include hard-to-reach populations into health systems. (2) Systems for routine VR and determination of cause of death are minimal in the very poorest nations. The potential for distortion of the "real" burden of disease is great, risking misdirected public health prevention and intervention efforts. (3) The burden of infectious diseases has always been disproportionate in poor and marginalized populations. (4) Pandemic risk, which is a high political and economical priority for the developed world, is similarly likely to disproportionately affect the poor in both mortality and economic effects.

THE WAY FORWARD: RELATION TO FINAL SCENARIOS IN THIS WORK

The scenario of "The Emergence of the Superbug" is relevant to considering the success of eradication and population immunity.

Microbes vary in their "targets." For polio, for example, vaccine associated strains from oral polio vaccine (OPV) can cause paralysis. These are known as vaccine-derived polioviruses (VDPVs), and there is some evidence that such strains can genetically revert to near wild type.[38] This tendency to reversion is similar to the response to antimicrobial pressure demonstrated in the public health scenario on the super bug [see Superbug Scenario]. This dynamic ability of viruses and microbes to adopt genetic abilities that allow them to continue replication in the face of vaccines or medicines is not confined to the polio initiative. In fact, active surveillance of serotype replacement is critical to assuring the stability of population immunity gains for meningitis A, pneumococcal disease, and other conjugate vaccines that include only some, but not all, of the potentially pathogenic types of agents. It is crucial for poor countries to assure their investment in vaccines is stable and that there will not simply be another pathogen that infects, sickens, and kills the population when known pathogens achieve high population immunity.

While it is clear that monitoring population immunity is central to eradication success, there are two large streams of misaligned policy discourse at play in the global community. First is the discussion of inclusion and the technical, political, and logistical barriers outlined above in the very concrete empirical space of data and evidence. Second is the entire area of "human rights"-based imperatives for population coverage. Few authors have attempted to merge these two lines of discussion. However, it is clear from the evolution of technical thinking about population-based immunity coming forward in the polio effort that such rethinking is due.

The development of systems to monitor the population's health is crucial for broader economic development; VR and cause of death systems will be developed incrementally as the first step in this process.[1,2] As these services are more widely available, the government's ability to understand their populations becomes more important; while there is a global call for such expansion, the responsibility relies on individual national governments. Polio eradication, prospective malaria eradication, and control of VPDs have brought new technologies forward that give "technical" fixes to the challenge of counting the undercounted, such as using satellite imagery in hard to reach areas to document target populations, combining immune markers with household survey work, bringing mobile telephone platforms into point-of-care diagnostics, and data reporting and consolidation in the field. Many of these innovations are covered elsewhere in this volume. These systems will develop incrementally, as the ability to assure population coverage can only extend as the available resources allow.

Fusing the important policy considerations of human rights and technical success in control and eradication is underway. Increasingly, proponents of universal coverage of health services from a human rights perspective are meeting others from the technical space in discourse. Leveraging these two powerful lines of argument will be important in realizing the scope of health interventions necessary for successful eradication and ongoing well-being of poor populations.

KEY SUMMARY POINTS

- Eradication efforts have been called the ultimate expression of global health equity.
- Such efforts mandate that every person counts and tools for prevention are put in the hands of governments.
- Disease burden remains disproportionate: poor populations suffer the highest burden.
- Poor populations are also likely to be the least effectively counted in surveillance systems.
- Motivation to "count" disease occurrence is directly linked to the capacity to intervene and mitigate disease occurrence.
- Poor diagnostics also conspire to undercount disease in poor populations.
- Successful surveillance, disease control and elimination efforts require concomitant efforts to respect, protect, and fulfill the right to health. This includes interventions to reduce stigma and discrimination of marginalized populations, particularly the poor.
- The true test of eradication as a tool for enhancing equity is in the legacy of eradication—whether poor populations enjoy an "eradication bonus" and actually benefit from the health system's ability to address population needs once disease is eradicated.

DISCUSSION QUESTIONS

1. What populations/population groups suffer the highest disease burden?
2. Describe how "counting" poor and marginalized populations matter in surveillance, disease control, and elimination efforts?
3. How and why did the successful smallpox eradication strategy evolve?
4. How is the current polio eradication campaign similar to or different from the smallpox eradication campaign?

5. Explain what is meant by a legacy benefit of smallpox and polio eradication in resource poor settings.
6. In what ways do human rights support the legal rights of poor people to be counted?
7. How do stigma and fear of discrimination affect disease surveillance?
8. In the event of a pandemic of avian influenza, what populations/population groups will bear the greatest disease burden?
9. What technical and policy solutions can be developed to improve surveillance, disease control, and eradication efforts while simultaneously improving human rights?

REFERENCES

1. Setel PW, Macfarlane SB, Szreter S, Mikkelsen L, Jha P, Stout S, et al. A scandal of invisibility: making everyone count by counting everyone. Lancet 2007;370(9598):1569–77.
2. AbouZahr C, Cleland J, Coullare F, Macfarlane SB, Notzon FC, Setel P, et al. The way forward. Lancet 2007;370(9601):1791–9.
3. Definition provided by the chapter author.
4. Dowdle WR, Cochi SL. The principles and feasibility of disease eradication. Vaccine 2011;29(Suppl. 4):D70–3.
5. Thompson KM. Modeling poliovirus risks and the legacy of polio eradication. Risk Analysis 2013;33(4):505–15.
6. The Smallpox Eradication Programme - SEP (1966–1980). World Health Organization, <http://www.who.int/features/2010/smallpox/en/>. [cited 2014].
7. Foege WH. House on fire: the fight to eradicate smallpox. Berkeley and Los Angeles, California: University of California Press; 2011. p. 240.
8. Tomori O. From smallpox eradication to the future of global health: innovations, application and lessons for future eradication and control initiatives. Vaccine 2011;29(Suppl. 4):D145–8.
9. Henderson DA. The eradication of smallpox—an overview of the past, present, and future. Vaccine 2011;29(Suppl. 4):D7–9.
10. WHO | The Expanded Programme on Immunization. World Health Organization, <http://www.who.int/immunization/programmes_systems/supply_chain/benefits_of_immunization/en/>; 2013. [updated December 1, 2013; cited 2015].
11. Kew O. Reaching the last one per cent: progress and challenges in global polio eradication. Curr Opin Virol 2012;2(2):188–98.
12. Murray CJ, Lopez AD, Chin B, Feehan D, Hill KH. Estimation of potential global pandemic influenza mortality on the basis of vital registry data from the 1918–20 pandemic: a quantitative analysis. Lancet 2006;368(9554):2211–8.
13. Brownlee A, French DM, Neuhauser L. Project for Strengthening Health Delivery Systems (SHDS) in Central and West Africa: applied research program. Public Health Rev 1984;12(3–4):297–300.
14. United Nations Millennium Development Goals. United Nations, <http://www.un.org/millenniumgoals/>.
15. Lozano R, Naghavi M, Foreman K, Lim S, Shibuya K, Aboyans V, et al. Global and regional mortality from 235 causes of death for 20 age groups in 1990 and 2010: a systematic analysis for the Global Burden of Disease Study 2010. Lancet 2012;380:2095–128.
16. Murray CJL, Vos T, Lozano R, Naghavi M, Flaxman AD, Michaud C, et al. Disability-adjusted life years (DALYs) for 291 diseases and injuries in 21 regions, 1990?2010: a systematic analysis for the Global Burden of Disease Study 2010. Lancet 2012;380(9859):2197–223.
17. Castellanos PL. On the concept of health and disease. Description and explanation of the health situation. Epidemiol Bull 1990;10(4):1-8.
18. Kimball A. Personal Communication. 2013.
19. Belec L, Mbopi Keou FX, Cancre N, Gresenguet G, Georges AJ. [The WHO/Bangui clinical case definition of AIDS in Black Africa. Status of 1986–1991]. Ann Med Interne (Paris) 1992;143(3):204–13.
20. Pan American Health Organization. On the concept of health and disease: description and explanation of the health situation. Pan American Health Organization; 1989.
21. Kalichman SC, Simbayi LC. HIV testing attitudes, AIDS stigma, and voluntary HIV counselling and testing in a black township in Cape Town, South Africa. Sex Transm Infect 2003;79(6):442–7.
22. Nicholls PG, Wiens C, Smith WC. Delay in presentation in the context of local knowledge and attitude towards leprosy—the results of qualitative fieldwork in Paraguay. Int J Lepr Other Mycobact Dis 2003;71(3):198–209.
23. Bainson KA, Van den Borne B. Dimensions and process of stigmatization in leprosy. Lepr Rev 1998;69(4):341–50.
24. World Health Organization. Leprosy, <http://www.who.int/mediacentre/factsheets/fs101/en/>. [cited March 19, 2014].
25. Duthie MS, Balagon MF, Maghanoy A, Orcullo FM, Cang M, Dias RF, et al. Rapid quantitative serological test for detection of infection with Mycobacterium leprae, the causative agent of leprosy. J Clin Microbiol 2014;52(2):613–9.
26. World Health Organization. Global leprosy situation, 2012. Geneva; 2012. Weekly Epidemiological Record 24 August 2012;87(34):317–328.
27. UN Human Rights Council. Resolution 8/13: Elimination of discrimination against persons affected by leprosy and their family members. 2008.
28. UNHR. What are Human Rights? <http://www.ohchr.org/en/issues/pages/whatarehumanrights.aspx/>. [cited 2015].
29. UN General Assembly. International Covenant on Economic, Social and Cultural Rights, 16 December 1966, United Nations, Treaty Series, vol. 993, p. 3. <http://www.refworld.org/docid/3ae6b36c0.html>; 30 September 2015.
30. UN Economic and Social Council. Committee on Economic, Social and Cultural Rights: Report on the Twenty-Second, Twenty-Third and Twenty-Fourth Sessions. New York and Geneva: United Nations; 2000. <http://www.un.org/documents/ecosoc/docs/2001/e2001-22.pdf>; 29 September 2015.
31. Donders Y. The right to enjoy the benefits of scientific progress: in search of state obligations in relation to health. Med Health Care and Philos 2011; 14(4):371–81.
32. UN Committee on Economic, Social and Cultural Rights (CESCR). General Comment No. 3: The Nature of States Parties' Obligations (Art. 2, Para. 1, of the Covenant), 14 December 1990, E/1991/23. <http://www.refworld.org/docid/4538838e10.html>; 30 September 2015.
33. Ferguson N. Poverty, death, and a future influenza pandemic. Lancet 2006; 368(9554):2187–8.
34. Kimball A. Risky trade: Infectious disease in the era of global trade. Aldershot: Ashgate Publishing; 2006. p. 212.
35. Fidler DP. Influenza virus samples, international law, and global health diplomacy. Emerg Infect Dis 2008;14(1):88–94.
36. World Health Organization. Landmark agreement improves global preparedness for influenza pandemics. Geneva; 2011. <http://www.who.int/mediacentre/news/releases/2011/pandemic_influenza_prep_20110417/en/>; 29 September 2015.
37. Fidler DP, Gostin LO. The WHO pandemic influenza preparedness framework: a milestone in global governance for health. JAMA 2011;306(2):200–1.
38. Sharif S, Abbasi BH, Khurshid A, Alam MM, Shaukat S, Angez M, et al. Evolution and circulation of type-2 vaccine-derived polioviruses in Nad Ali district of Southern Afghanistan during June 2009–February 2011. PLoS One 2014;9(2):e88442.

INTRODUCTION

Public Health Surveillance Strengthening is the process of transitioning the current antiquated governance structures and practices, collaborations, policies, and standards in PHS to an enhanced structure and platform that supports and bolsters these new opportunities in technology, analytics, and informatics, and is needed to advance PHS in the twenty-first century.[1]

Public health surveillance is the continuous, systematic collection, analysis and interpretation of health-related data needed for the planning, implementation, and evaluation of public health practice.[1]

e-Surveillance is the use of information and communication technology (ICT) to empower and enable efficient and effective PHS workflow processes with functions designed to prevent, predict, detect and respond.[1]

One Health is a holistic approach to PHS that considers the interconnectivity of animals, humans, and their surrounding environment.[1]

CHAPTER 1

Surveillance system is the ongoing systematic collection and analysis of data. The data may lead to actions taken to prevent and control an infectious disease.[2]

Data management is an administrative process by which the required data are acquired, validated, stored, protected, and processed, and by which their accessibility, reliability, and timeliness is ensured to satisfy the needs of the data users.[3]

Data analysis is a process systematically applying statistical and/or logical techniques to describe and illustrate, condense and recap, and evaluate data.[4]

Notifiable disease is one for which regular, frequent, and timely information regarding individual cases is considered necessary for the prevention and control of the disease.[5]

CHAPTER 2

CDC Surveillance Strategy is the US CDC's strategy that guides efforts to make essential surveillance systems more adaptable to the rapidly changing technology landscape, more versatile in meeting demands for expanding knowledge about evolving threats to health, and more able to meet the demands for timely and population-specific and geographically specific surveillance information. The Strategy will also facilitate work to consolidate systems, eliminate unnecessary redundancies in reporting, and reduce reporting burden.[6]

Informatics is the science concerned with gathering, manipulating, storing, retrieving, and classifying recorded information.[7]

Electronic laboratory reporting is the electronic transmission from laboratories to public health of laboratory reports, which identify reportable conditions. ELR has many benefits, including improved timeliness, reduction of manual data entry errors, and reports that are more complete.[8]

Morbidity and Mortality Weekly Report (MMWR) is a publication series prepared by the US Centers for Disease Control and Prevention (CDC). Often called "the voice of CDC," the MMWR series is the agency's primary vehicle for scientific publication of timely, reliable, authoritative, accurate, objective, and useful public health information and recommendations.[9]

Health Information Technology for Economic and Clinical Health (HITECH) Act was enacted as part of the American Recovery and Reinvestment Act of 2009 and was signed into law on February 17, 2009, to promote the adoption and meaningful use of health information technology.[10]

National Notifiable Diseases Surveillance System (NNDSS) is USA's public system for monitoring the occurrence and spread of the diseases and conditions that STLT agencies have agreed to report voluntarily to CDC. Currently, there are over 70 reportable diseases and conditions. This complex system is supported and used by numerous stakeholders and is expected to provide accurate, timely, and sufficient information for surveillance and response on notifiable conditions.[11]

CDC Health Information Innovation Consortium (CHIIC) is described in Goal 1 of the CDC Surveillance Strategy to be established in order to foster and promote creative solutions to surveillance challenges implemented through innovative projects in CDC programs and STLT agencies.[6]

BioSense was established in 2003 after 9/11 and the subsequent anthrax attacks, and is a syndromic surveillance system that provides data necessary for public health officials to monitor and respond to possible disease or hazardous conditions. It is an electronic health information system with standardized tools and procedures for rapidly collecting, sharing, and evaluating information about emergency department visits and other health-related data from health care sources and clinical care facilities.[12]

National Vital Statistics System is the oldest and most successful example of intergovernmental data sharing in US Public Health and the shared relationships, standards, and procedures form the mechanism by which NCHS collects and disseminates the Nation's official vital statistics. These data are provided through contracts between NCHS and vital registration systems operated in the various jurisdictions legally responsible for the registration of vital events—births, deaths, marriages, divorces, and fetal deaths.[13]

US Centers for Disease Control (CDC) is one of the major operating components of the Department of Health and Human Serves and is recognized as the nation's premiere health promotion, prevention, and preparedness agencies. CDC focuses in five strategic areas: supporting state and local health departments, improving global health, implementing measures to decrease leading causes of death, strengthening surveillance and epidemiology, and reforming health policies.[14]

CHAPTER 3

Passive surveillance is a type of surveillance that relies on regular reporting of disease data by all institutions that see patients (or test specimens) and are part of a reporting network. In passive surveillance there is no active search for cases; rather, it involves passive notification by reports generated by the local level.[15]

Sentinel surveillance is a type of surveillance that relies on data from selected reporting units with a high probability of seeing cases of the disease in question, good laboratory facilities and well-qualified staff. Sentinel surveillance is used when high-quality data are needed about a particular disease that cannot be obtained through a passive system.[16]

One Health Approach is a holistic approach to zoonotic disease surveillance. In the broadest sense, One Health integrates the relationships among vectors, animals (domestic and wildlife), plants, and humans to develop surveillance systems that are attuned to real-world models of disease transmission.[17]

Community-based surveillance is a type of surveillance that uses community volunteers or leaders to actively participate in discovery and reporting of cases. This type of surveillance puts public health and health officials in direct contact with suspected, probable, and confirmed cases of disease and allows for rapid, if not immediate, medical response and quarantine. Community-based surveillance is the most effective type of surveillance to monitor diseases nearing eradication.[18]

Digital surveillance entails data collection via web-based protocols and is increasingly critical in improving the timeliness of surveillance and response.[1]

Syndromic surveillance is a type of surveillance that uses existing health data in real time to provide immediate analysis and feedback to those charges with investigation and follow-up of potential outbreaks. Syndromic surveillance has been used for early detection of outbreaks, to follow the size, spread, and tempo of outbreaks, to monitor disease trends, and to provide reassurance that an outbreak has not occurred.[19]

Event-based surveillance is the "organized rapid capture of information about events that are a risk to public health, and is complementary to IBS, particularly during the course of an outbreak."[20]

Population-based surveillance is a type of surveillance that "involves identifying all new cases of the disease under surveillance in a defined population" using community-based cohort studies and active surveillance of households to determine attack rates and disease burden.[21, 22]

Indicator-based surveillance is a type of surveillance that involves routine reporting of disease, conditions and events through notifiable disease surveillance systems, including sentinel surveillance channels and laboratory-based surveillance.[20]

Predictive surveillance utilizes state-of-the-art computer models and algorithms to simulate interrelated and, at times, interdependent pathogen, vector (arthropod), and host (animal and human) behaviors and to forecast disease outbreaks.[23]

Participatory surveillance uses direct engagement with community members at large to collect data and improve public health understanding of disease patterns and population health.[24] It is predicated on traditional concepts of epidemiology but recognizes the value of collective intelligence and awareness.[25] It uses community knowledge to develop epidemic intelligence in a participatory manner and complements these data with secondary information sources, observations, and laboratory diagnostics.[24]

Active surveillance is a type of surveillance that is dynamically seeking data from participants in the surveillance system on a regular basis.[26]

Laboratory-based surveillance is a type of surveillance that uses laboratory data to detect trends and outbreaks, estimate burden of illness, and allow subtyping of pathogens, which is critical for linking illness to vehicles and reservoirs.[27]

Genetic surveillance is a specialized branch of laboratory-based surveillance focusing on molecular subtyping to identify pathogens and genetic markers for heritable diseases or increased susceptibility to risk factors.[28–31]

CHAPTER 4

Integrated surveillance is a type of surveillance that uses a common approach to provide a universal surveillance service using similar structures and techniques.[26]

Vertical surveillance is a type of surveillance that focuses on a single disease or injury. Information is collected and fed back into the specific disease control program.[26]

Integrated Disease Surveillance and Response (IDSR) is a comprehensive regional framework for strengthening national public health surveillance and response systems in Africa. In 2006, WHO/AFRO member states recommended that the International Health Regulations (IHR 2005) be implemented using the IDSR framework, especially for strengthening core capacities for surveillance and response. The IDSR framework illustrates the functions, activities, and skills required to implement an integrated, coordinated, comprehensive surveillance and response system.[32]

CHAPTER 5

Reactive surveillance is a type of active surveillance in which health system electronic data or other complementary data are systematically collected in as close to real time as possible and regularly monitored automatically resulting in spatial and/or temporal anomaly detection.[1]

Predictive modeling is a name given to a collection of mathematical techniques having in common the goal of finding a mathematical relationship between a target, response, or "dependent" variable and various predictor or "independent" variables with the goal in mind of measuring future values of those predictors and inserting them into the mathematical relationships to predict future values of the target variable.[33]

Proactive surveillance is a type of active surveillance using routinely collected real-time data as a predictive tool to model potential health system outcomes and enhance system preparedness and response.[1]

Pharmacosurveillance is a term used to refer to the monitoring of drug safety, for example, by means of spontaneous adverse-effect reporting systems, case–control and cohort studies.[34]

Canadian Primary Care Sentinel Surveillance Network is a primary care research initiative, which is the first pan-Canadian multidisease electronic medical record surveillance system. They collect health information from electronic medical records in the offices of participating primary care providers.[35]

Google Flu Trends is a web service operated by Google that provides near real-time estimates of flu activity for a number of countries and regions around the world based on aggregated search queries.

Some of these estimates have been validated through comparison with official historic influenza data from the relevant country or region.[36]

CHAPTER 6

Work Process Analysis Framework is a methodological framework for evaluating and improving public health practice performance by identifying existing and missing processes and determining causal effects.[1]

Logic model is a logic model frame used to separate surveillance components into individual program and evaluation elements, including inputs, outputs, intermediate outcomes, and long-term outcomes. The logic model is also a yardstick for ideal implementation of the surveillance system and depicts the standard system components identified by authoritative sources (e.g., World Health Organization, CDC).[1]

Performance indicators are items of information collected at regular intervals to track the performance of a system.[37]

Work process tree is a diagram that incorporates work processes identified through the established guidance and evaluation data collected from system stakeholders. Work process trees are composed of sequential tasks needed to complete a given surveillance activity and inform graphical representations that illustrate gaps in the surveillance system. This tool also provides the basis for inputs that can be used for an ingredient-style costing approach.[1]

CHAPTER 7

Surveillance systems evaluation performs comprehensive measurements of relevant attributes (over time or in a single effort) in order to verify whether the system is still "fit for purpose" and recommend improvements.[38]

Trigger is a term for an event that is the cause of a particular action, process, or situation.[39]

Data quality monitoring is the monitoring of the "quality" of data collected, which includes accuracy and validity, reliability, confidentiality and security, legibility, currency and timeliness, accessibility, meaning or usefulness, and completeness.[40]

The European Surveillance System is a flexible metadata-driven system for collection, validation, cleaning, analysis, and dissemination of data. Its key aims are data analysis and production of outputs for public health action. All EU member states (28) and EEA countries (3) report their available data on communicable diseases (52) to the system.[41]

European Centre of Disease Prevention and Control (ECDC) is a European Union agency, founded in 2005, which aims to strengthen Europe's defenses against infectious diseases.[42]

CHAPTER 8

Socioeconomic determinants of health are the complex, integrated, and overlapping social structures and economic systems that are responsible for most health inequities. These social structures and economic systems include the social environment, physical environment, health services, and structural and societal factors. Social determinants of health are shaped by the distribution of money, power, and resources throughout local communities, nations, and the world.[43]

Return on investment is a financial ration that measures the benefit or gain generated relative to the amount of money invested.[44]

Cost analyses is the act of breaking down a cost summary into its constituents and studying and reporting on each factor.[45]

Global public good are goods and services that are "nonrival" and "nonexcludable". In other words, no one can be excluded from their benefits and their consumption by one person does not diminish consumption by another. Public goods become global (sometimes called international public goods) in nature when the benefits flow to more than one country and no country can effectively be denied access to those benefits.[46]

Results based financing (RBF) is any program that rewards the delivery of one or more outputs or outcomes by one or more incentives, financial or otherwise.[47]

Cost–Benefit analysis is the comparison of costs and achieved benefits, where both costs and benefits are expressed in monetary terms. The usual rule in cost–benefit analysis is for the benefit–cost ratio (B/C) to exceed unit or for $(B - C) > 0$.[48]

Cost-effectiveness analysis is a form of economic evaluation where costs are expressed in money terms but consequences are expressed in physical units. It is used to compare different ways of achieving the same objective.[48]

CHAPTER 9

Workforce is a term for all the people working or available to work in a country, in a industry, or on a project.[49]

Competency is a term for the measurable or observable knowledge, skills, abilities, and behaviors critical to successful job performance.[50]

Public health is an organized effort by society, primarily through its public institutions, to improve, promote, protect, and restore the health of the population through collective action. It includes services such as health situation analysis, health surveillance, health promotion, prevention, infectious disease control, environmental protection and sanitation, disaster and health emergency preparedness and response, and occupational health, among others.[51]

Workforce capacity is a term for the ability of a country or an organization to ensure sufficient staffing levels to accomplish its work processes and successfully deliver its products or services to the targeted group or population.[52]

Field Epidemiology and Laboratory Training Program is a program that focuses on assisting countries to build sustainable capacity for detecting and responding to health threats and to develop expertise so that disease outbreaks can be detected locally and prevented from spreading. The CDC works with regional partners and ministries of health to develop such programs, which are modeled after the CDC's Epidemic Intelligence Service.[53]

Epidemic Intelligence Service (EIS) is a US 2-year postgraduate training program of service and on-the-job learning for health professionals interested in the practice of applied epidemiology. EIS officers are on the public health frontlines, conducting epidemiologic investigations, research, and public health surveillance both nationally and internationally.[54]

Epidemiologists are public health professionals who investigate patterns and causes of disease and injury in humans. They seek to reduce the risk and occurrence of negative health outcomes through research, community education, and health policy.[55]

Field epidemiologists are public health epidemiologists who, when a problem is unexpected, must travel to and work in the field to solve the problem, and the extent of the investigation is likely to be limited because of the imperative for timely intervention.[56]

Council of State and Territorial Epidemiologists (CSTE) is an organization of member states and territories representing public health epidemiologists. CSTE works to establish more effective relationships among state and other health agencies. It also provides technical advice and assistance to partner organizations and to federal public health agencies such as the Centers for Disease Control and Prevention (CDC).[57]

CHAPTER 10

Standards are the established, accepted, and evidence-based technical specifications or bases for comparison.[58]

Governance are the structures, rules, and processes used by society to shape and apply power to identify and achieve objectives.[59]

Public health emergency of international concern is an extraordinary event which is determined to constitute a public health risk to other states through international spread of diseases and to potentially require a coordinated international response.[60]

World Health Assembly (WHA) is the decision-making body of WHO. It is attended by delegations from all WHO member states and focuses on a specific health agenda prepared by the Executive Board. The main functions of the WHA are to determine the policies of the organization, appoint the director general, supervise financial policies, and review and approve the proposed program budget. The Health Assembly is held annually in Geneva, Switzerland.[61]

World Organization for Animal Health (OIE) is an intergovernmental organization responsible for improving animal health worldwide. The World Trade Organization (WTO) recognizes it as a reference organization and in 2013 had a total of 178 member countries.[62]

Food and Agriculture Organization (FAO) is an intergovernmental organization, which is made up of 194 member nations, two associate members and one member organization, the European Union. It focuses on achieving five strategic objectives: help eliminate hunger, food insecurity and malnutrition; make agriculture, forestry and fisheries more productive and sustainable; reduce rural poverty; enable inclusive and efficient agricultural and food systems; and increase the resilience of livelihoods to disasters.[63]

IHR Focal Points is the national center, designated by each State Party, which shall be accessible at all times for communications with the WHO IHR Contact Points.[60]

Asia Pacific Strategy for Emerging Diseases (APSED) is a common strategic framework for countries and areas of the Asia Pacific region to strengthen their capacity to manage and respond to emerging disease threats. Building on the achievements of the original APSED (2005), the updated APSED (2010) is intended to further support progress toward meeting the obligations under the International Health Regulations (IHR, 2005) and consolidate gains already made in establishing collective regional public health security.[64]

Global Outbreak Alert and Response Network (GOARN) is a technical collaboration of existing institutions and networks that pool human and technical resources for the rapid identification, confirmation, and response to outbreaks of international importance. The network provides an operational framework to link this expertise and skill to keep the international community constantly alert to the threat of outbreaks and ready to respond.[65]

International Network of Food Safety Authorities (INFOSAN) is a joint initiative between WHO and the Food and Agriculture Organization (FAO) of the United Nations. This global network includes 181 member states. Each has a designated INFOSAN Emergency Contact Point for communication between national food safety authorities and the INFOSAN Secretariat regarding urgent events. The network aims are to (1) promote the rapid exchange of information during food safety-related events, (2) share information about important food safety-related issues of global interest, (3) promote partnership and collaboration between countries, and (4) help countries strengthen their capacity to manage food safety risks.[66]

Global Early Warning System (GLEWS) is a joint system that builds on the added value of combining and coordinating the alert and disease intelligence mechanisms of OIE, FAO, and WHO for the international community and stakeholders to assist in prediction, prevention and control of animal disease threats, including zoonosis, through sharing of information, epidemiological analysis, and joint risk assessment.[67]

Terrestrial Animal Health Code is a code that sets out standards for the improvement of animal health and welfare and veterinary public health worldwide, including through standards for safe international trade in terrestrial animals (mammals, birds, and bees) and their products. The health measures in the Terrestrial Code are used by the veterinary authorities of importing and exporting countries to provide for early detection, reporting and control agents that are pathogenic to animals or humans, and to prevent their transfer via international trade in animals and animal products, while avoiding unjustified sanitary barriers to trade.[68]

International Health Regulations (2005) is an updated binding instrument of international law that entered into force in June 2007, which aims to "to prevent, protect against, control and provide a public health response to the international spread of disease in ways that are commensurate with and restricted to public health risks, and which avoid unnecessary interference with international traffic and trade."[60]

CHAPTER 11

Global public health security is the need to reduce the vulnerability of people around the world to emerging and re-emerging risks to health, particularly those that cross international borders.[69]

Emerging infectious diseases are broadly defined as infections that have newly appeared in a population or have existed but are rapidly increasing in incidence or geographic range. EIDs can encompass: (1) a recognized infection spreading to new areas or populations; (2) the discovery that a known disease is caused by infection; (3) a previously unrecognized infection appearing in areas where the habitat is changing (e.g., deforestation); (4) a new infection resulting from change(s) in existing microorganisms (e.g., mutation); and (5) a recognized infection, re-emerging in a form resistant to treatment, or as a result of a breakdown in public health prevention measures.[70]

Biological weapons are harmful biological agents used as a weapon to cause death or disease usually on a large scale.[71]

ProMED-mail (PMM), a listserv established in 1994 as a mechanism to identify emerging disease outbreaks. PMM receives reports of public health events in humans, animals, and plants from its subscribers who report information from many different sources including personal observation, written or electronic reports, the news media, and various open websites.[72]

HealthMap is an electronic computer-based mechanism that collects online information about outbreaks from real-time surveillance reports of ProMED-mail, and from many other open electronic sources as well.[73]

Global Public Health Intelligence Network (GPHIN), developed in 1999, is a secure, nonpublic web application that collects information about public health events of potential international significance.[74]

CHAPTER 12

Statist is a public health perspective concerned primarily with the security and stability of the state.[75]

Globalist is the public health governance perspective concerned primarily with the well-being of individuals and communities.[75]

Human security is the concern with human life and dignity. Human security focuses on two aspects: safety from chronic threats, such as hunger, disease, and repression, and protection from sudden and hurtful disruptions in the patterns of daily life.[76]

Viral sovereignty is a sovereign state's ownership rights over pathogens found within its borders.[77]

Universal Declaration of Human Rights is a milestone document in the history of human rights in which the declaration was proclaimed by the United Nations General Assembly in Paris on December 10, 1948, General Assembly resolution 217 A (III) as a common standard of achievements for all peoples and all nations. It sets out, for the first time, fundamental human rights to be universally protected.[78]

Smart public health governance the combination of hard and soft governance strategies in public health.[1]

CHAPTER 13

Cooperation is the action or process of working together to the same end.[79]

Multicountry disease surveillance networks are public health surveillance networks that involve coordination and/or collaboration across multiple countries in the prevention, detection, and response to specific diseases.[1]

Pandemic Influenza Preparedness (PIP) Framework is a framework that brings together WHO member states, industry, other stakeholders, and WHO to implement a global approach to pandemic influenza preparedness and response. Its key goals include (1) to improve and strengthen the sharing of influenza viruses with human pandemic potential and (2) to increase the access of developing countries to vaccines and other pandemic-related supplies. It became effective on May 24, 2011.[80]

CHAPTER 14

Interspecies transmission is the movement of a pathogen between species.[1]

Field sampling the collection of human, animal, and ecologic samples and data at predetermined times.[1]

Diagnostic testing is any type of laboratory test that is performed to aid in the diagnosis or detection of disease.[1]

Information management is the entry of data and management of information from one or more sources and the distribution of that information to one or more audiences.[1]

Mekong Basin Diseases Surveillance (MBDS) network is a cross-border collaboration including Cambodia, China, Myanmar, Lao PDR, Thailand, and Vietnam that has been attempting to combat and control outbreaks of disease through collaborative regional surveillance, reporting, joint outbreak investigation, and capacity building since 2001.[81]

Emerging Pandemic Threats Program was created in 2009 by the US Agency for International Development (USAID) to improve detection, identification, and response for emerging zoonosis. The program consists of four overall projects: PREDICT, RESPOND, IDENTIFY, and PREVENT, and also includes the Center for Disease Control (CDC), all working in concert to build local, regional, and national One Health capacity for disease detection, diagnosis, risk reduction, and response.[82]

OIE/FAO Network of Expertise on Animal Influenza (OFFLU) is the OIE-FAO global network of expertise on animal influenza that works to reduce the negative impacts of animal influenza viruses by promoting effective collaboration between animal health and human health experts.[83]

FoodNet (formerly known as C-EnterNet) is a program developed to improve Canada's food safety surveillance. It is composed of three food safety surveillance sites that collects detailed information about food-borne illness in Canadians and traces those illnesses back to their sources whether in food, water, or animals.[84]

Canadian Integrated Program for Antimicrobial Resistance Surveillance (CIPARS) monitors trends in antimicrobial use and antimicrobial resistance in selected bacterial organisms from human, animal, and food sources across Canada.[85]

Canary Database A database developed by Yale University (Occupational and Environmental Medicine, School of Medicine) that selects, curates, and indexes thousands of scientific studies from MEDLINE, CAB Abstracts, and Agricola to collate the evidence for animals as "early warning" sentinels of human health hazards.[86]

CHAPTER 15

Biosurveillance is the process of gathering, integrating, interpreting, and communicating essential information related to all-hazards threats or disease activity affecting human, animal, or plant health to achieve early detection and warning, contribute to overall situational awareness of the health aspects of an incident, and to enable better decision-making at all levels.[87]

Emerging pathogens are the causative agent(s) of an infectious disease whose incidence is increasing following its appearance in a new host population or whose incidence is increasing in an existing population as a result of long-term changes in its underlying epidemiology.[88]

Information and Communication Technology (ICT) is the technology of the production, manipulation, storage, and communication of information using computers and microelectronics.[89]

Information sharing is the ability to conduct multijurisdictional, multidisciplinary exchange of health-related information and situational awareness data among federal, state, local, territorial, and tribal levels of government, and the private sector.[90]

Transparency refers to the release of information by institutions, which is relevant to evaluating those institutions and allows citizens and markets to hold institutions accountable for their policies and performance.[91]

Collaboration is the act of working together to achieve a common goal or complete a task.[92]

National Strategy for Biosurveillance is the US Government's approach to strengthening the national biosurveillance enterprise. The approach builds on existing biosurveillance concepts and capabilities in seeking to enable more rapid detection, knowledge, and characterization of human, animal, or plant disease activity to enhance incident situational awareness.[87]

CHAPTER 16

Health care encounter monitoring is electronic monitoring of any care for active duty or beneficiaries (defined as those that have access to benefits, such as retirees and family members) paid for by the Department of Defense (DoD).[1]

Reportable medical events are health conditions that must be monitored and reported according to DoD guidance. This list is influenced by CDC's notifiable events list and includes events identified as representing significant military threats.[93]

Field activities include food and water monitoring, sewage treatment, waste management activities, vector and rodent surveillance and control, disease and battle injury monitoring, determination of occupational and environmental exposures, and monitoring of psychological health status.[1]

Deployment surveillance is a type of surveillance that is required by the US Congress in response to concerns from veterans. Questionnaires are used to identify conditions that may need further clinical support or intervention and also for analytic and trend health surveillance purposes.[94]

Environmental and occupational monitoring is the DoD's effort to document the extent and short-/long-term consequences of military environmental and occupational exposures.[95]

The Global Emerging Infections Surveillance and Response System (GEIS) program is a division of the Armed Forces Health Surveillance Center. The GEIS network and its partners support a wide range of global surveillance efforts through a holistic approach that includes surveillance activities to prevent, detect, and respond to infectious diseases; training and capacity building; research innovation and integration; and coordination, communication, and collaboration among GEIS partners to facilitate responsive information sharing.[1]

DoD Cooperative Biological Engagement Program (CBEP) is a DoD program that works with partner countries to dismantle, destroy, and prevent the sale, theft, diversion, or use of biological weapons and also to enhance the partner country's capability to survey, detect, diagnose, identify, secure, and report pathogens, diseases, or events of security concern.[1]

DoD Chemical Biological Defense Program (CBD) was established by the DoD to provide state-of-the-art defense capabilities to allow military forces of the USA to operate and successfully complete missions in chemical and biological warfare environments.[96]

Reference laboratory is a laboratory that provides authoritative test results. For example, the World Health Organization has a network of reference laboratories.[1]

Force Health Protection are all measures taken by commanders, supervisors, individual Service members, and the MHS to promote, protect, improve, conserve, and restore the mental and physical well-being of Service members across the range of military activities and operations. These measures enable the fielding of a healthy and fit force, prevention of injuries and illness and protection of the force from health hazards, and provision of medical and rehabilitative care to those who become sick or injured anywhere in the world.[1]

CHAPTER 17

Association Any organization of people who share similar interests, professions, or other commonality.[1]

Partnership is an association or two or more persons or entities typically involving close cooperation to achieve common goals.[1]

Nongovernmental organizations (NGO) is any nonprofit, voluntary group of citizens organized on a local, national, or international level that performs service, educational, or humanitarian functions, advocates or monitors policies, and/or encourages informed decision-making.[1]

Capacity building assistance (CBA) refers to activities that provide guidance, support, and technical assistance to people and organizations to strengthen capacity in a designated area (e.g., to deliver public health services).[1]

Technical assistance is a form of aid designed to provide expertise needed to promote surveillance practice. It can include sending experts to teach skills and help solve problems in specialized areas.[1]

Workforce development refers to education and training programs for participants in the workforce to build their competencies—knowledge, skills, and aptitudes—to perform their jobs more effectively.[1]

CHAPTER 18

Clinician A health care practitioner having direct contact with and responsibility for patients (as opposed to one involved with theoretical or laboratory studies).[1]

Electronic laboratory reporting (ELR) is the automated transmission of laboratory-related data from commercial, public health, hospital, and other laboratories to state and local public health departments through an electronic health records (EHR) system or Laboratory Information Management System (LIMS).[11]

Electronic health record (EHR) is a longitudinal electronics health record of patient health information generated by one or more encounters in any care delivery setting. Included in this information are patient demographics, progress notes, problems, medications, vital signs, past medical history, immunizations, laboratory data, and radiology reports.[98]

US Outpatient Influenza-Like Illness Network (ILINET) is a US CDC surveillance system based solely on voluntary reporting by clinical providers.[1]

Pay for performance is a term that in health care refers to giving financial incentives to clinicians for better health outcomes, such as lowering blood pressure or counseling that results in cessation of smoking.[1]

CHAPTER 19

Community engagement is the process of working collaboratively with and through groups of people affiliated by geographic proximity, special interest, or similar situations to address issue affecting the well-being of those people.[99]

Nontraditional partners are partners outside a given sector or field.[1]

CHAPTER 20

Interoperability is the ability of two or more systems or components to exchange information and to use the information that has been exchanged following logical, process, and technical parameters.[100]

Technical interoperability is the ability of two or more information and communication technology applications to accept data from each other and perform a given task in an appropriate and satisfactory manner without the need for extra operator intervention.[101]

Semantic interoperability is the ability to ensure that the precise meaning of exchanged information is unambiguously interpretable by any other system, service, or user.[101]

Process interoperability is the ability to communicate and exchange information accurately, effectively, securely, and consistently between different information technology systems, software applications, and networks in various settings, and exchange data such that clinical or operational purpose, context, and meaning of the information are preserved and unaltered.[102]

Data exchange is the process of sending and receiving data in such a manner that the information content or meaning assigned to the data is not altered during the transmission.[103]

Health information systems (HIS) is a system that provides the underpinnings for decision-making and has four key functions: (1) data generation, (2) compilation, (3) analysis and synthesis, and (4) communication and use. The health information system collects data from health and other relevant sectors, analyses the data and ensures their overall quality, relevance, and timeliness, and converts the data into information for health-related decision-making.[104]

Electronic medical records (EMR) are digital versions of a paper charts that contain all of a patient's medical history from one practice. An EMR is mostly used by providers for diagnosis and treatment.[105]

CHAPTER 21

Causation is the relationship between cause and effect; causality.[106]

Data fusion is a process dealing with the association, correlation, and combination of data and information from single and multiple sources to achieve refined position and identity estimates, and complete and timely assessments of situations and threats as well as their significance.[107]

Big Data is a marketing term for data that are larger in volume, have high movement or delivery characteristics, and can vary in structure and source.[1]

Data streams tend to describe data that are in motion. Surveillance data are now valuable to examine in real time while they are moving between systems.[1]

Data storms describe when data are coming in high velocity from many different directions at once into a surveillance system or analysis.[1]

Data quality is a generalized term for describing data that are usable in a consistent manner. There are multiple characteristics around data quality that stem from understanding structure, format, correlation, transport, and existence of the data involved.[1]

Next-generation sequencing, massively parallel or deep sequencing, are related terms that describe a DNA sequencing technology, which has revolutionized genomic research. Using NGS an entire human genome can be sequenced within a single day.[108]

Data warehouse is an integrated information-storage area that consists of a data repository bringing together multiple databases from various data sources, and a report-generating facility.[104]

Data pools describe when we have aggregated or closely integrated sets of data usually located in the same computing center or servers. The term is most useful when discussing federated integration of data across many data pools to create one data view from many sources.[1]

CHAPTER 22

Ecosystem is a system, or a group of interconnected elements, formed by the interaction of a community of organisms with their environment.[109]

Modularity is where a system is created from subcomponents that can be reused in different configurations or independently replaced to change the characteristics of a technology system without redesigning the complete system.[1]

Meaningful use is the use of certified EHR technology in a meaningful manner (e.g., electronic prescribing); ensuring that the certified EHR technology is connected in a manner that provides for the electronic exchange of health information to improve the quality of care; and that in using certified EHR technology the provider must submit to the Secretary of Health & Human Services (HHS) information about quality of care and other measures.[110]

Healthcare-associated infection (HAI) is a localized or systemic condition resulting from an adverse reaction to the presence of an infectious agent(s) or its toxin(s). There must be no evidence that the infection was present or incubating at the time of admission to the acute care setting.[111]

Sociotechnical ecosystem is another way of describing singularity, where surveillance knowledge is served by the close marriage of social behaviors, human interaction and understanding, and technology information delivery systems.[112]

Integration is the verb compared to Interoperability being a noun when thinking about connecting systems together for a specific purpose usually for data exchange. The action of integration happens at a technical level more than a logical one to bring one or many components of a system together to function as one, communicate together, or create a systems of systems.[1]

eMeasures are standardized performance measures in an electronic format. eMeasures help ensure that measures are consistently defined, implemented, and compatible across clinical IT systems to promote higher quality and more appropriate care delivery.[113]

CHAPTER 23

Data visualization is the graphical display of abstract information for two purposes: sense-making (also called data analysis) and communication. Important stories live in our data and data visualization is a powerful means to discover and understand these stories, and then to present them to others.[114]

Analytics is the systematic computational analysis of data or statistics.[115]

Databases are technology architecture components that specialize in the persistence and manipulation of data in specific technology structures allowing many types of inquiry systems to manipulate the information stored.[1]

Geographic Information System (GIS) is a collection of computer hardware, software, and geographic data for capturing, managing, analyzing, and displaying all forms of geographically referenced information. GIS provides a common analytical framework in which public health authorities can understand problems and formulate a response, improving incident management and health planning.[116]

Spatial analysis is the process of examining the locations, attributes, and relationships of features in spatial data through overlay and other analytical techniques in order to address a question or gain useful knowledge. Spatial analysis extracts or creates new information from spatial data.[117]

Information processing is the science concerned with gathering, manipulating, storing, retrieving, and classifying recorded information.[118]

Open question and answer system describes technology systems that allow humans to interact with information and derive knowledge and understanding in a normal way. The human asks questions and a technology systems should enable that to be as easy as possible to advance the humans understanding.[1]

Dengue trends is a Google application that uses near real-time search query data to create an index of dengue incidence that is a linear proxy for traditional surveillance. Studies have shown that GDT correlates highly with dengue incidence in multiple countries on a large spatial scale.[119]

CHAPTER 24

Simplicity is the amount and variety of data, users, organizations receiving case reports, and integrated systems; level of effort to collect, manage, analyze, and disseminate the data; staff training requirements; as well as time needed for system maintenance that contribute to the ease of operation of a public health surveillance system.[120]

Flexibility is the ability of public health surveillance system to adapt to changes in operation or information requirements quickly, with minimal investment of additional resources.[120]

Data quality refers to the "completeness and validity of the data recorded."

Acceptability is the "willingness of persons and organizations to participate in the surveillance system" that may be ascertained by measuring the participation rate of subjects and agencies, completeness of interview and forms, reporting rates, and timeliness of reports.[120]

Sensitivity is the proportion of cases or events that are targets of surveillance that are detected.[120]

Predictive value positive is the proportion of cases or events detected that are actually the target of the detection system.[120]

Representativeness of a surveillance system is determined by assessing a health-related event as it pertains to a certain demography, considering available sources of data, such as death certificates, laboratory results, and medical records, to judge if the trend of that health-related event in reported cases matches actual events.[120]

Timeliness is the measure of speed between timed intervals between various steps in the surveillance process, such as the interval between the onset of a health-related event and the initial report to the public health agency responsible for follow-up.[120]

Stability of a surveillance system is its ability to operate and provide data without system failure. Measure of stability includes the amount of time and resources needed for system maintenance and operation, including any system outages and lags.[120]

Cost of a surveillance system may refer to direct costs of operation, including the staff, equipment, training, software, etc. involved in operating the surveillance system, and indirect costs related to case-related follow-up, such as treatment or outbreak investigations.[120]

Utility of a surveillance system is based on its ability to detect and characterize health-related events and subsequently inform the development of prevention and control programs, policies, and research.[120]

National Institute of Technology (NIST) is a US federal agency involved in the development and application of technologies, measurements, and standards.[121]

Health Level 7 (HL7) is an organization that develops electronic health data exchange and integration standards and frameworks to facilitate interoperability between surveillance systems.[122]

Youth Risk Behavior Surveillance System (YRBSS) is a surveillance system that monitors six types of risk behaviors linked to the leading causes of mortality and morbidity in youth and adults.[123]

Behavioral Risk Factor Surveillance System (BRFSS) is a CDC telephone survey conducted to collect state-based data on health-related risk behaviors, chronic conditions, and use of preventive health care services.[124]

Pregnancy Risk Assessment Monitoring System (PRAMS) is a surveillance system to monitor maternal attitudes and experiences from before to shortly after pregnancy.[125]

CHAPTER 25

Transmission modeling uses mathematical representations to relate and simulate disease transmission variables for the purpose of analyzing surveillance data and forecasting outcomes of interventions.[1]

Data mining uses computer programs to progressively learn from massive and diverse data about how patterns of single variables or combinations of variables relate to patterns of disease.[1]

Transmission models are used to analyze the dissemination of infections through populations. They differ from risk factor epidemiology models and most data mining models by using systems theory to formulate mechanistic feedbacks between variables and the individuals or populations modeled.[1]

Differential equation (DE) models use deterministic approaches that predict expected mean system behavior for very large populations.[1]

Agent-based (AB) models use individuals instead of continuous population segments; when an infected and a susceptible individual encounter each other, there is some chance that transmission may take place.[1]

Parameters are fixed theoretical relationships in models that govern how the values of variables change over time.[1]

Inference robust assessment (IRA) is a type of assessment that is performed by comparing an inference across different model forms.[126]

Identifiability analysis focuses on what data are needed to make a control decision using a causal system model.[1]

CHAPTER 26

Genotype is to characterize phenotypes (e.g., physical traits) by determining variations in genetic markers of an organism.[1]

Pathogen sequence data is a record of the whole genomic sequence for pathogens studied for identification of genes whose expression triggers disease in host organisms.[1]

Disease transmission modeling is conducted using a mathematical causal system model representing infection transmission.[1]

Genetic sequence data are a nearly complete genomic record of an organism studied for identification of genes and mechanics for gene expression.[1]

Genetic pathogen surveillance is surveillance of genetic markers in pathogens that can facilitate early detection of outbreaks or clusters through investigation of genetic divergence in chains of transmission, and characterize expression of pathogen behaviors and traits such as antimicrobial resistance.[1]

Multilocus sequence testing (MLST) sequences a set of housekeeping genes with slow rates of change to characterize bacterial and parasitic pathogens.[1]

Phylodynamics analyzes how the evolution of pathogens and immune responses to pathogens relate to dynamic patterns of infection within hosts or across populations.[127]

Phylodynamic theory explains how the forces affecting pathogen evolution in individuals and in populations affect the spread of infection over time and the patterns of genetic sequences that result from those forces.[1]

Basic coalescent theory uses a simple Wright–Fisher model of neutral evolution to construct continuous entity models of the processes by which separate lines of evolution converge in the direction from the present to the past.[128]

Coalescent analyses make inferences about broad populations from relatively small numbers of samples since each pair in a sample reflects a unique path back to a most recent common ancestor.[1]

Flow model phylogeography is a second level of systems analysis with genetic data that fit models of pathogen flows between populations without modeling the transmission system processes behind these flows. Most often, phylogeographic models do not detail population pathogen size, incidence, or prevalence in the populations between which flow is modeled. If they do, they use the simple population models of coalescent theory to do so.[129–132]

Analytic phylodynamics is a third level of systems analyses. It fits models of infection transmission systems to genetic sequence data.[1]

Population sequence patterns are patterns of commonality and divergence in genetic sequences between members of a population.[1]

CHAPTER 27

Analytics involve the systematic use of data and related insights developed through applied analytical methods (e.g., statistical, contextual, quantitative, predictive, cognitive, and other [including emerging] models) to drive evidence-based decision-making for planning, management, measurement, and learning.[133]

Predictive analytics allow for forecasting and planning. Predictive analytics can anticipate risk and find relationships in health data not apparent with descriptive analytics alone.[134]

Prescriptive analytics suggest possible interventions. Prescriptive analytics utilize available data, information, and knowledge from several domains including public health, medicine, economics, management, and others to inform decision-making in situations of uncertainty.[135]

Data governance is the specification of decision rights and an accountability framework to encourage desirable behavior in the valuation, creation, storage, use, archival, and deletion of data and information.[136]

Data acquisition practices ensure that data are captured in a usable form and include consistent documentation of metadata.[137]

Data standardization is the adoption of common health vocabularies, formats, representations, and definitions to facilitate the exchange and use of data in interoperable and integrated electronic information systems[138]

Data integration is the merger of data from internal and external data sources into an individual-centric data structure optimized for analysis.[1]

Common Data Models are codified standards to define the format and content of clinical observation data so that all software, devices, and protocols that implement the CDM standard can be utilized.[139]

Biomedical Translational Research Information System (BTRIS) is a resource available to the NIH intramural community that brings together clinical research data from the Clinical Center and other NIH Institutes and Centers. BTRIS provides clinical investigators with access to identifiable data for subjects on their own active protocols, while providing all NIH investigators with access to data (1976–present) without personal identifiers across all protocols.[140]

SNOMED CT is a systematically organized, computer processable clinical health care terminology for electronic health records (EHR) and contains more than 311,000 active concepts with unique meanings and formal logic-based definitions organized into hierarchies.[141]

ICD-10-CM is the standard diagnostic tool for epidemiology, health management, and clinical purposes.[142]

Surveillance, Management, and Real-time Trends (SMaRT) system used by the state of Louisiana is an intelligent approach to data analytics for health outcomes and performance monitoring.[143]

Open Government Directive directs executive departments and agencies to take specific actions to implement the principles of transparency, participation, and collaboration.[144]

Health Data Initiative is a public–private collaboration that encourages innovators to utilize health data to develop applications to raise awareness of health and health system performance and spark community action to improve health.[1]

Electronic Medical Record Support for Public Health (ESP) is a platform that consists of software that loads EMR data extracted from clinicians' proprietary systems, analyzes these data for events of public health interest, and electronically communicates findings to public health agencies.[145]

CHAPTER 28

Predictive surveillance is a type of surveillance that uses state-of-the-art computer models and algorithms to predict the presence or absence of a pathogen in a geographic area.[1]

Static data are data the system captures once to help generate predictions.[1]

Dynamic data are the data the system captures periodically to update predictions.[1]

CHAPTER 29

Health Equity is the attainment of the highest level of health for all people. Achieving health equity requires valuing everyone equally with focused and ongoing societal efforts to address avoidable inequalities, historical and contemporary injustices, and the elimination of health and health care disparities.[146]

Social determinants are the circumstances in which people grow, live, work, and age, and the systems put in place to deal with illness.[43]

Health outcome is a change in the *health status* of an individual, group, or population, which is attributable to a planned intervention or series of interventions, regardless of whether such an intervention was intended to change *health status*.[147]

Millennium Development Goals (MGDs) are eight goals that all 191 UN member states have agreed to try to achieve by the year 2015. The United Nations Millennium Declaration, signed in September 2000 commits world leaders to combat poverty, hunger, disease, illiteracy, environmental degradation, and discrimination against women. The MDGs are derived from this Declaration, and all have specific targets and indicators.[148]

Gender equality is the absence of discrimination—on the basis of a person's sex—in providing opportunities, in allocating resources and benefits, or in access to services.[149]

Health Metrics Network (HMN) was launched in 2005 as a network of global, regional, and country partners dedicated to strengthening national HIS and harmonizing approaches to collect, collate, analyze, and use health data to inform decisions and programming. [104]

CHAPTER 30

Point-of-care diagnostics refers to when patient specimens assayed at or near the patient with the assumption that test results will be available instantly or in a very short time frame to assist caregivers with immediate diagnosis and/or clinical intervention.[150]

Internet of Things is a computing concept that describes a future where everyday physical objects will be connected to the internet and be able to identify themselves to other devices.[151]

System for Early warning based on Emergency Data (SEED) was a collaborative project of the GVK Emergency Management and Research Institute (EMRI), India, and GEOMED Research, Germany, funded by the German Federal Ministry of Education and Research (BMBF) and Indian Council of Medical Research (ICMR) to systematically explore the use of emergency data for syndromic surveillance in India.[152]

CHAPTER 31

Disease eradication is the permanent reduction of new infection to zero, with interventions no longer needed.[1]

Human rights are rights inherent to all human beings, whatever our nationality, place of residence, sex, national or ethnic origin, color, religion, language, or any other status. We are all equally entitled to our human rights without discrimination. These rights are all interrelated, interdependent, and indivisible.[153]

Strengthening Health Delivery Systems (SHDS) in Central and West Africa is funded by the US Agency for International Development (USAID) and works in collaboration with the World Health Organization/AFRO to improve health systems in 20 countries of Central and West Africa.[154]

Vital registration (VR) systems/vital statistics system is defined by the United Nations "as the total process of (a) collecting information by civil registration or enumeration on the frequency or occurrence of specified and defined vital events, as well as relevant characteristics of the events themselves and the person or persons concerned, and (b) compiling, processing, analyzing, evaluating, presenting, and disseminating these data in statistical form."[155]

Expanded Program of Immunizations (EPI) is a WHO program with the goal of universal access to all relevant vaccines for all at risk. The program aims to expand the targeted groups to include older children, adolescents, and adults and work in synergy with other public health programs in order to control disease and achieve better health for all populations, particularly the underserved populations.[156]

REFERENCES

1. Definition provided by the chapter author.
2. U.S. Centers for Disease Control and Prevention. About antimicrobial resistance. Antibiotic/antimicrobial resistance. CDC, <http://www.cdc.gov/drugresistance/about.html/>; 2015.
3. Data management, <http://www.businessdictionary.com/definition/data-management.html/>; 2015.
4. Data Analysis, <http://ori.hhs.gov/education/products/n_illinois_u/data-management/datopic.html/>; 2015.
5. Adams DA, Gallagher KM, Jajosky RA, Kriseman J, Sharp P, Anderson WJ, et al. Summary of Notifiable Diseases - United States, 2011. MMWR Morb Mortal Wkly Rep 2013;60(53):1–117.
6. U.S. Centers for Disease Control and Prevention. Surveillance Strategy. 2014.
7. National Program of Cancer Registries (NPCR). Informatics, <http://www.cdc.gov/cancer/npcr/informatics/>; 2015.
8. Meaningful Use. Electronic Laboratory Reporting (ELR), <http://www.cdc.gov/ehrmeaningfuluse/elr.html/>; 2015.
9. Morbidity and Mortality Weekly Report (MMWR), <http://www.cdc.gov/mmwr/about.html/>; 2015.

10. Health Information Privacy. HITECH Act Enforcement Interim Final Rule, <http://www.hhs.gov/>; 2013. [2015].
11. National Notifiable Disease Surveillance System (NNDSS), <http://wwwn.cdc.gov/nndss/>; 2015.
12. BioSense Program. BioSense, <http://www.cdc.gov/biosense/>; 2015.
13. National Vital Statistics System, <http://www.cdc.gov/nchs/nvss.html/>; 2015.
14. About CDC 24-7. Our History - Our Story, <http://www.cdc.gov/about/history/index.html/>; 2015.
15. World Health Organization. National Passive Surveillance, <http://www.who.int/immunization/monitoring_surveillance/burden/vpd/surveillance_type/passive/en/>; 2014. [2015].
16. World Health Organization. Sentinel Surveillance, <http://www.who.int/immunization/monitoring_surveillance/burden/vpd/surveillance_type/sentinel/en/>; 2014, [2015].
17. One Health I. About the One Health Initiative.
18. World Health Organization. Community-based surveillance and case containment activities, <http://www.who.int/dracunculiasis/eradication/strategy/en/>; 2014. [2015].
19. Henning KJ. What is syndromic surveillance? MMWR Morb Mortal Wkly Rep 2004;53:5–11.
20. World Health Organization/Western Pacific Region. A Guide to Establishing Event-based Surveillance. Geneva: World Health Organization; 2008.
21. Razuri H, Romero C, Tinoco Y, Guezala MC, Ortiz E, Silva M, et al. Population-based active surveillance cohort studies for influenza: lessons from Peru. Bull World Health Organ 2012;90(4):318–20.
22. Hampton LM, Zell ER, Schrag S, Cohen AL. Sentinel versus population-based surveillance of pneumococcal conjugate vaccine effectiveness. Bull World Health Organ 2012;90(8):568–77.
23. Witt CJ, Richards AL, Masuoka PM, Foley DH, Buczak AL, Musila LA, et al. The AFHSC-Division of GEIS Operations Predictive Surveillance Program: a multidisciplinary approach for the early detection and response to disease outbreaks. BMC Public Health 2011;11(Suppl. 2):S10.
24. Ameri AA, Henderick S, Jones B, Mariner J. Introduction to participatory epidemiology and its application to highly pathogenic avian influenza participatory disease surveillance: a manual for participatory disease contributors. Regal Press Kenya Limited: 2009.
25. Jost CC, Mariner JC, Roeder PL, Sawitri E, Macgregor-Skinner GJ. Participatory epidemiology in disease surveillance and research. Rev Sci Tech 2007;26(3):537–49.
26. Garcia-Abreu A, Halperin W, Danel I. Public health surveillance toolkit: a guide for busy task managers. In: Development Communications Division EAV-P, editor; The World Bank; 2002.
27. Dunn J, Pryor J, Saketa S, Delai W, Buadromo E, Kishore K, et al. Laboratory-based Salmonella surveillance in Fiji, 2004–2005. Pac Health Dialog 2005;12(2):53–9.
28. Bauer SM. Psychoneuroimmunology and cancer: an integrated review. J Adv Nurs 1994;19(6):1114–20.
29. van de Ven JP, Smailhodzic D, Boon CJ, Fauser S, Groenewoud JM, Chong NV, et al. Association analysis of genetic and environmental risk factors in the cuticular drusen subtype of age-related macular degeneration. Mol Vis 2012;18:2271–8.
30. Haibe-Kains B, Desmedt C, Loi S, Culhane AC, Bontempi G, Quackenbush J, et al. A three-gene model to robustly identify breast cancer molecular subtypes. J Natl Cancer Inst 2012;104(4):311–25.
31. Buffler PA, Kwan ML, Reynolds P, Urayama KY. Environmental and genetic risk factors for childhood leukemia: appraising the evidence. Cancer Invest 2005;23(1):60–75.
32. Global Health Protection & Security. What Is Integrated Disease Surveillance and Response (IDSR)? <http://www.cdc.gov/globalhealth/healthprotection/ghsb/idsr/what/default.html/>; 2015.
33. Dickey DA. Introduction to Predictive Modeling with Examples. SAS Global Forum 2012;2012:1–14.
34. World Health Organization. Introduction to Drug Utilization Research. Geneva: World Health Organization; 2003.p. 49.
35. Canadian Primary Care Sentinel Surveillance Network. About CPCSSN, <http://cpcssn.ca/about-cpcssn/>; 2015.
36. Google Flu Trends. FAQ, <http://www.google.org/flutrends/about/faq.html/>; 2015.
37. Fitz-Gibbon, Carol Taylor, Eds. Performance Indicators. England: Routledge; 1990.
38. Control ECfDPa. Data quality monitoring and surveillance system evaluation: A handbook of methods and applications. Stockholm: ECDC; 2014.
39. Trigger. Oxford Dictionaries. 2015.
40. World Health Organization. Improving data quality: a guide for developing countries. Philippines: World Health Organization; 2003.
41. The European Surveillance System (TESSy), <http://ecdc.europa.eu/en/activities/surveillance/tessy/Pages/TESSy.aspx/>; 2015.
42. ECDC. About Us, <http://ecdc.europa.eu/en/aboutus/Pages/aboutus.aspx/>; 2015.
43. WHO. Closing the gap in a generation: health equity through action on the social determinants of health. Final Report of the Commission on Social Determinants of Health. Geneva: World Health Organization; 2008.
44. Inc. Return on Investment (ROI), <http://www.inc.com/encyclopedia/return-on-investment-ROI.html/>; 2015.
45. Cost Analysis. Merriam-Webster: Encyclopaedia Britannica; 2015.
46. World Health Organization. Global Public Goods, <http://www.who.int/trade/glossary/story041/en/>; 2010. [2015].
47. Mission, <http://www.rbfhealth.org/mission/>; 2015.
48. World Health Organization. Health Systems Strengthening Glossary, <http://www.who.int/healthsystems/hss_glossary/en/index2.html/>; 2011. [2015].
49. Workforce. American Heritage Dictionary of the English Language. 5th ed. Houghton Mifflin Harcourt; 2011.
50. Washington State Human Resources. Competencies, <http://www.hr.wa.gov/WorkforceDataAndPlanning/WorkforcePlanning/Competencies/Pages/default.aspx/>; 2015.
51. La salud pública en las Americas. nuevos conceptos, análisis del desempeño y bases para la acción. Revista do Instituto de Medicina Tropical de São Paulo. 2003;45:102.
52. Workforce Capacity, <http://www.baldrige21.com/BALDRIGE_GLOSSARY/BN/Workforce_Capacity.html/>; 2007. [2015].
53. U.S. Centers for Disease Control and Prevention. Global Health. Field Epidemiology Training Program, <http://www.cdc.gov/globalhealth/fetp/>; 2015.
54. U.S. Centers for Disease Control and Prevention. Epidemic Intelligence Service, <http://www.cdc.gov/eis/index.html/>; 2015.
55. Statistics USBoL. Epidemiologists, <http://www.bls.gov/ooh/life-physical-and-social-science/epidemiologists.html/>; 2014. [2015].
56. Greg MB, ed. Field epidemiology. 2nd ed. New York: Oxford University Press; 2002.
57. Epidemiologists CoSaT. About CSTE, <http://www.cste.org/?page=About_CSTE/>; 2015.
58. Last JM. A Dictionary of Public Health. Oxford University Press; 2007.
59. Bevir M. Encyclopedia of Governance. Thousand Oaks, CA: SAGE Publications, Inc; 2007.
60. WHO. International Health Regulations (2005). 2nd ed. Geneva: World Health Organization; 2008.
61. WHO. World Health Assembly, <http://www.who.int/mediacentre/events/governance/wha/en/>; 2015.
62. The World Organisation for Animal Health. About Us, <http://www.oie.int/about-us/>; 2015.
63. Food and Agriculture Organization of the United Nations. About FAO, <http://www.fao.org/about/what-we-do/en/>; 2015.
64. Emerging Disease Surveillance and Response. Asia Pacific Strategy for Emerging Diseases (APSED, 2010), <http://www.wpro.who.int/emerging_diseases/APSED2010/en/>; 2015.
65. WHO. Global Outbreak Alert and Response Network (GOARN), <http://www.who.int/ihr/alert_and_response/outbreak-network/en/>; 2015.
66. World Health Organization. International Food Safety Authorities Network (INFOSAN). World Health Organization; 2007.

67. About GLEWS, <http://www.glews.net/about-glews/>; 2015.
68. World Organisation for Animal Health. Terrestrial Animal Health Code, <http://www.oie.int/international-standard-setting/terrestrial-code/>; 2015.
69. Rodier G, Greenspan AL, Hughes JM, Heymann DL. Global public health security. Emerg Infect Dis 2007;13(10):1447–52.
70. Morse SS. Factors in the emergence of infectious diseases. Emerg Infect Dis 1995;1(1):7–15.
71. Biological Weapon. Merriam-Webster, <http://www.merriam-webster.com/>; May 2015.
72. ProMED mail. About ProMED-mail, <http://www.promedmail.org/aboutus/>; 2015.
73. About HealthMap, <http://www.healthmap.org/site/about/>; 2015.
74. Mykhalovskiy E, Weir L. The Global Public Health Intelligence Network and early warning outbreak detection: a Canadian contribution to global public health. Can J Public Health 2006;97(1):42–4.
75. Davies SE. Global Politics of Health. 1st ed. Cambridge, Malden: MA Polity Press; 2010.
76. United Nation Development Programme. Human Development Report. 1994, <http://hdr.undp.org/en/content/human-development-report-1994/>; 1994. [2015].
77. Mullis K. Playing Chicken with Bird Flu: "Viral Sovereignty," the Right to Exploit Natural Genetic Resources, and the Potential Human Rights Ramifications. Am. U. Int'l L. Rev 2009;24(5):943–67.
78. United Nations. Universal Declaration of Human Rights, <http://www.ohchr.org/en/udhr/pages/introduction.aspx/>; 2015.
79. Cooperation. Oxford Dictionaries, <http://www.oxforddictionaries.com/>; May 2015.
80. WHO. Pandemic Influenza Framework, <http://www.who.int/influenza/pip/en/>; 2011.
81. Phommasack B, Jiraphongsa C, Ko Oo M, Bond KC, Phaholyothin N, Suphanchaimat R, et al. Mekong Basin Disease Surveillance (MBDS): a trust-based network. Emerg Health Threats J 2013;6. doi: 10.3402/ehtj.v3406i3400.19944.
82. Bogich TL, Chunara R, Scales D, Chan E, Pinheiro LC, Chmura AA, et al. Preventing pandemics via international development: a systems approach. PLoS Med 2012;9(12):e1001354.
83. OFFLU OIE/FAO. Network of expertise on animal influenza, <http://www.offlu.net/>; 6 June 2014.
84. FoodNet Canada (formerly known as C-EnterNet). Reducing the burden of gastrointestinal disease in Canada, <http://www.phac-aspc.gc.ca/foodnet-canada/overview-apercu-eng.php/>; 2006. [2015].
85. Canadian Integrated Program for Antimicrobial Resistance Surveillance (CIPARS), <http://www.phac-aspc.gc.ca/cipars-picra/index-eng.php/>; 2007. [2015].
86. Canary Database. Animals as Sentinels of Human Environmental Health Hazards, <http://canarydatabase.org/about/description/>; 2015.
87. National Strategy for Biosurveillance. Washington, DC: The White House; 2012.
88. Woolhouse ME. Population biology of emerging and re-emerging pathogens. Trends Microbiol 2002;10(Suppl. 10):S3–7.
89. Information Technology. Dictionary.com, <http://www.dictionary.reference.com/>; 2015.
90. U.S. Centers for Disease Control and Prevention. Public Health Preparedness Capabilities: Capability 6: Information Sharing. U.S. Centers for Disease Control and Prevention, Atlanta, Georgia; 2011.
91. The World Bank. Public Sector Development. Anti-corruption and Transparency, <http://web.worldbank.org/WBSITE/EXTERNAL/COUNTRIES/LACEXT/EXTLACREGTOPPUBSECGOV/0,,contentMDK:20830474~pagePK:34004173~piPK:34003707~theSitePK:832592,00.html>; 2015.
92. Collaboration. Collins English Dictionary, <http://www.collinsdictionary.com/>; May 2015.
93. Armed Forces Reportable Medical Events Guidelines and Case Definitions, <https://www.afhsc.mil/documents/pubs/documents/TriService_CaseDefDocs/ArmedForcesGuidlinesFinal14Mar12.pdf> 2012.
94. Comprehensive Health Surveillance. In: Department of Defense Directive, editor. 2013.
95. DeFraites RF, Richards EE. Assessing potentially hazardous environmental exposures among military populations: 2010 symposium and workshop summary and conclusions. Mil Med 2011;176(Suppl. 7):1–112.
96. 2013 Department of Defense Chemical and Biological Defense Annual Report to Congress. In: Chemical and Biological Defense Program, editor. U.S. Department of Defense, Washington, DC; 2013.
97. Association of State and Territorial Health Officials. History of ASTHO, <http://www.astho.org/About/History/>; 2014.
98. Healthcare Information and Management Systems Society (HIMSS). Electronic Health Records, <http://www.himss.org/library/ehr/>; 2015.
99. Community Engagement. Definitions and Organizing Concepts from the Literature, <http://www.cdc.gov/phppo/pce/part1.html/>; 2015.
100. IEEE Standard Computer Dictionary. A Compilation of IEEE Standard Computer Glossaries. IEEE Xplore; 1991.
101. eHealth Governance Initiative. On Semantic and Technical Interoperability. 2012.
102. Amos P. Interoperability within Health & Social Care Systems. Information Standards Board for Health and Social Care; 2008.
103. OECD Glossary of Statistical Terms. Data Exchange, <http://stats.oecd.org/glossary/detail.asp?ID=1355>; 2015.
104. Health Metrics Network. Framework and standards for country health information systems. 2nd ed. Geneva: WHO; 2008.
105. Benefits of EHRs. What is an Electronic Medical Records (EMR)? <http://www.healthit.gov/providers-professionals/electronic-medical-records-emr/>; 2015.
106. Causation. Oxford Dictionaries, <http://www.oxforddictionaries.com/>; May 2015.
107. White FE. Data Fusion Lexicon. San Diego, CA: Data Fusion Subpanel; 1991.
108. Behjati S, Tarpey PS. What is next generation sequencing? Arch Dis Child Educ Pract Ed 2013;98(6):236–8.
109. Ecosystem. Dictionary.com, <http://www.dictionary.reference.com/>; May 2015.
110. Centers for Disease Control and Prevention. Meaningful Use, <http://www.cdc.gov/ehrmeaningfuluse/introduction.html/>; 2015.
111. Horan TC, Andrus M, Dudeck MA. CDC/NHSN surveillance definition of health care-associated infection and criteria for specific types of infections in the acute care setting. Am J Infect Control 2008;36(5):309–32.
112. Software Engineering Institute. Ultra-Large-Scale Systems: The Software Challenge of the Future. Pittsburgh, PA: Carnegie Mellon; 2006.
113. Submitting eMeasures for NQF Endorsement (eMeasures), <http://www.qualityforum.org/Projects/e-g/eMeasures/Electronic_Quality_Measures.aspx/>; 2015.
114. Few S. Data Visualization for Human Perception. In: Soegaard MaD, Rikke Friis, editors. The Encyclopedia of Human-Computer Interaction. 2nd ed. Aarhus, Denmark: The Interaction Design Foundation; 2014.
115. Analytics. Oxford Dictionaries, <http://www.oxforddictionaries.com/>. [2015].
116. National Association of Country and City Health Officials. Glossary of Public Health Informatics Organizations, Activities, and Terms, <http://www.naccho.org/topics/infrastructure/informatics/glossary.cfm/>; 2015.
117. GIS Dictionary. Spatial Analysis, <http://support.esri.com/en/knowledgebase/GISDictionary/term/spatial analysis/>. [2015].
118. Information Processing. The Free Dictionary, <http://www.thefreedictionary.com/>; May 2015. [Farlex].
119. Gluskin RT, Johansson MA, Santillana M, Brownstein JS. Evaluation of Internet-based dengue query data: Google Dengue Trends. PLoS Negl Trop Dis 2014;8(2):e2713.
120. German RR, Armstrong G, Birkhead GS, Horan JM, Herrera G, Waller MN. Updated guidelines for evaluating public health surveillance systems. MMWR Recomm Rep 2001;50:1–35.
121. NIST General Information, <http://www.nist.gov/public_affairs/general_information.cfm/>; 2015.

122. Health Level Seven International. About HL7, <http://www.hl7.org/about/index.cfm?ref=nav/>; 2015.
123. Adolescent and School Health. Youth Risk Behavior Surveillance System (YRBSS), <http://www.cdc.gov/healthyyouth/data/yrbs/index.html/>; 2015.
124. Behavioral Risk Factor Surveillance System. BRFSS Frequently Asked Questions (FAQs), <http://www.cdc.gov/brfss/about/brfss_faq.html/>; 2015.
125. PRAMS Pregnancy Risk Assessment Monitoring System. What is PRAMS? <http://www.cdc.gov/prams/>; 2015.
126. Koopman JS. Infection transmission science and models. Jpn J Infect Dis 2005;58(6):S3–8.
127. Pybus OG, Rambaut A. Evolutionary analysis of the dynamics of viral infectious disease. Nat Rev Genet 2009;10(8):540–50.
128. Wakeley J. Coalescent Theory: An Introduction. Greenwood Village, Colorado: Roberts and Company Publishers; 2008.
129. Lemey P, Rambaut A, Drummond AJ, Suchard MA. Bayesian phylogeography finds its roots. PLoS Comput Biol 2009;5(9):e1000520.
130. Lemey P, Rambaut A, Welch JJ, Suchard MA. Phylogeography takes a relaxed random walk in continuous space and time. Mol Biol Evol 2010;27(8):1877–85.
131. Lemey P, Suchard M, Rambaut A. Reconstructing the initial global spread of a human influenza pandemic: A Bayesian spatial-temporal model for the global spread of H1N1pdm. PLoS Curr 2009;1:RRN1031.
132. Bielejec F, Rambaut A, Suchard MA, Lemey P. SPREAD: spatial phylogenetic reconstruction of evolutionary dynamics. Bioinformatics 2011;27(20):2910–2.
133. Cortada J, Gordon D, Lenihan B. The Value of Analytics in Healthcare: From Insights to Outcomes. Somers, NY: IBM Global Services; 2012.
134. Raghupathi W, Raghupathi V. An Overview of Health Analytics. J Health Med Informat 2013;4(132).
135. Crafts M. Application of Integrated Health Analytics in a Regulatory Environment. National Predictive Modelling Summit; 2012.
136. Sun H. Enterprise Information Management: Best Practices in Data Governance. Redwood Shores, CA: Oracle Corporation; 2011.
137. Rhoads J, Ferrara L. Transforming Healthcare Through Better Use of Data. Falls Church, VA: Global Institute for Emerging Healthcare Practices; 2012.
138. Health Information Technology Standards. Data Standards, <http://www.phdsc.org/standards/health-information/D_Standards.asp/>; 2015.
139. Common Data Model. Observational Medical Outcomes Partnership, <http://omop.org/CDM/>; 2015.
140. Welcome to BTRIS, <http://www.ncbi.nlm.nih.gov/pubmed/>; 2015.
141. SNOMED CT, <http://www.ihtsdo.org/snomed-ct/>; 2015.
142. WHO. International Classification of Diseases (ICD), <http://www.who.int/classifications/icd/en/>; 2014. [accessed May 30, 2015].
143. 2012 Public Health Annual Report. A Year of Innovation in Public Health Information and Technology. 2012.
144. Open Government, <http://www.data.gov/open-gov/>; 2014.
145. Klompas M, McVetta J, Lazarus R, Eggleston E, Haney G, Kruskal BA, et al. Integrating clinical practice and public health surveillance using electronic medical record systems. Am J Prev Med 2012;42(6 Suppl. 2):S154–62.
146. HHS. Health Equity & Disparities, <http://www.minorityhealth.hhs.gov/npa/templates/browse.aspx?lvl=1&lvlid=34/>; 2015.
147. Health Promotion Glossary. Geneva: World Health Organization; 1998.
148. WHO. Millennium Development Goals (MDGs), <http://www.who.int/topics/millennium_development_goals/en/>; 2014. [2015].
149. WHO. Gender, equity, and human rights, <http://www.who.int/gender-equity-rights/en/>; 2015.
150. Ehrmeyer SS, Laessig RH. Point-of-care testing, medical error, and patient safety: a 2007 assessment. Clin Chem Lab Med 2007;45(6):766–73.
151. Internet of Things (IoT), <http://www.techopedia.com/definition/28247/internet-of-things-iot/>; 2010. [2015].
152. Institute GEMaR, mbH GRF. System for Early warning based on Emergency Data (SEED), <http://www.geomed-research.eu/GVK EMRI-Geomed_Leaflet.pdf/>; May 2015.
153. What are Human Rights? <http://www.ohchr.org/en/issues/pages/whatarehumanrights.aspx/>; 2015.
154. Brownlee A, French DM, Neuhauser L. Project for Strengthening Health Delivery Systems (SHDS) in Central and West Africa: applied research program. Public Health Rev 1984;12(3–4):297–300.
155. World Health Organisation. Civil registration and vital statistics (CRVS) systems, <http://www.emro.who.int/civil-registration-statistics/about/what-are-civil-registration-and-vital-statistics-crvs-systems.html/>; 2015.
156. WHO. The Expanded Programme on Immunization, <http://www.who.int/immunization/programmes_systems/supply_chain/benefits_of_immunization/en/>; 2013. [2015].

INDEX

E

F

G

N

O

P

R

S

T